MANUAL OF CLINICAL PROBLEMS IN PEDIATRICS
WITH ANNOTATED KEY REFERENCES

MANUAL OF CLINICAL PROBLEMS IN PEDIATRICS
WITH ANNOTATED KEY REFERENCES

SECOND EDITION

EDITED BY

KENNETH B. ROBERTS, M.D.

The Johns Hopkins University School of Medicine; University of Maryland School of Medicine; Sinai Hospital of Baltimore, Baltimore

LITTLE, BROWN AND COMPANY   BOSTON/TORONTO

In memory of John T. Hayford, Jr., M.D., and Susanne Hogue Deas, M.S.W., and with prayers of health for Ellen, Sharyn, and Dennis: May those who use the information in this book apply it wisely and gently.

CONTENTS

Contributing Authors   xiii

Preface to the Second Edition   xv

Preface to the First Edition   xvii

I. EMERGENCIES

1. Cardiopulmonary Arrest and Resuscitation   3
Kenneth B. Roberts

2. Bacteremia and Septicemia   6
Kenneth B. Roberts

3. Meningitis   9
Kenneth B. Roberts

4. Upper Airway Obstruction   13
Kenneth B. Roberts

5. Respiratory Failure and Status Asthmaticus   16
Dennis C. Stokes

6. Congestive Heart Failure   19
Robert D. White and Jean S. Kan

7. Diabetic Ketoacidosis   21
John T. Hayford, Jr.,* and Margaret E. Mohrmann

8. Acute Abdomen   24
Kenneth B. Roberts

9. Acute Renal Failure   27
Richard A. Cohn

10. Reye Syndrome   29
Kenneth B. Roberts

11. Increased Intracranial Pressure   31
William R. Leahy, Jr.

12. Status Epilepticus   34
William R. Leahy, Jr.

13. Head Trauma   36
William R. Leahy, Jr.

14. Accidents   39
Evan Charney

15. Fever and Antipyretics   42
Kenneth B. Roberts

16. Lead Poisoning   45
John T. Hayford, Jr.,* and Evan Charney

17. Child Abuse   48
Robert D. White

18. Death, Dying, and Mourning   51
Kenneth B. Roberts

*Deceased

19. Sudden Infant Death Syndrome   55
Robert D. White

II. GROWTH, DEVELOPMENT, AND BEHAVIOR

20. Physical Growth   61
Margaret E. Mohrmann and John T. Hayford, Jr.*

21. Infant Nutrition   65
Robert D. White

22. Failure to Thrive   69
Margaret E. Mohrmann

23. Obesity   71
Margaret E. Mohrmann

24. Development and Retardation   74
Kenneth B. Roberts and Eileen P. G. Vining

25. Attention Deficit Disorder   78
Kenneth B. Roberts

26. Sleep   82
Kenneth B. Roberts

27. Bowel Training and Constipation   85
Evan Charney

28. Bladder Control and Enuresis   88
Kenneth B. Roberts

29. Recurrent Pain Syndromes: Abdominal Pain, Headache, and Chest Pain   92
Evan Charney

30. Sexual Development   97
Margaret E. Mohrmann and John T. Hayford, Jr.*

III. THE NEONATE

31. Assessment of the Newborn   105
Robert D. White

32. Respiratory Distress Syndrome   107
Robert D. White

33. Chronic Pulmonary Disease   110
Robert D. White

34. Cyanotic Heart Disease   112
Robert D. White and Jean S. Kan

35. Heart Failure in the Neonate   116
Robert D. White and Jean S. Kan

36. Transient Metabolic Disturbances   118
Robert D. White

37. Neonatal Seizures   121
Robert D. White

*Deceased

38. **Hyperbilirubinemia**   124
Robert D. White

39. **Erythroblastosis**   128
Robert D. White

40. **Nutrition in the Ill Neonate**   130
Robert D. White

41. **Necrotizing Enterocolitis**   134
Robert D. White

42. **Surgical Emergencies**   136
Robert D. White

43. **Congenital Infections**   141
Robert D. White

44. **Neonatal Sepsis**   146
Robert D. White

45. **Bleeding**   150
Robert D. White

46. **Congenital Anomalies**   153
Robert D. White

IV. CARDIOVASCULAR DISORDERS

47. **Dysrhythmias**   159
Robert D. White and Jean S. Kan

48. **Myopericarditis**   163
Margaret E. Mohrmann

49. **Bacterial Endocarditis**   167
Kenneth B. Roberts

50. **Ventricular Septal Defect**   170
Robert D. White and Jean S. Kan

51. **Tetralogy of Fallot**   172
Robert D. White and Jean S. Kan

52. **Transposition of the Great Arteries**   175
Robert D. White and Jean S. Kan

53. **Patent Ductus Arteriosus**   177
Robert D. White and Jean S. Kan

54. **Rheumatic Fever**   179
Kenneth B. Roberts

55. **Hypertension**   182
Margaret E. Mohrmann

V. RESPIRATORY DISORDERS

56. **Upper Respiratory Infection**   189
Kenneth B. Roberts

57. **Otitis Media**   192
Kenneth B. Roberts

58. Bronchiolitis 195
Kenneth B. Roberts
59. Pneumonia 198
Kenneth B. Roberts
60. Asthma 201
Kenneth B. Roberts
61. Cystic Fibrosis 205
Dennis C. Stokes

VI. GASTROINTESTINAL DISORDERS

62. Biliary Atresia and Neonatal Hepatitis 213
Robert D. White
63. Hepatitis 215
Kenneth B. Roberts
64. Chronic Diarrhea and Malabsorption 218
Margaret E. Mohrmann
65. Ulcerative Colitis 224
Kenneth B. Roberts
66. Crohn Disease 227
Kenneth B. Roberts

VII. RENAL, FLUID, AND ELECTROLYTE DISORDERS

67. Hypernatremic Dehydration 233
Kenneth B. Roberts
68. Hematuria and Proteinuria 235
Margaret E. Mohrmann
69. Acute Poststreptococcal Glomerulonephritis 239
Kenneth B. Roberts
70. Hemolytic-Uremic Syndrome 241
Kenneth B. Roberts
71. Nephrotic Syndrome 244
Richard A. Cohn
72. Urinary Tract Infection 248
Richard A. Cohn
73. Chronic Renal Failure 252
Richard A. Cohn

VIII. ENDOCRINE, METABOLIC, AND GENETIC DISORDERS

74. Congenital Adrenal Hyperplasia 259
John T. Hayford, Jr.,* and Margaret E. Mohrmann
75. Thyroid Disorders 262
John T. Hayford, Jr.,* and Margaret E. Mohrmann

*Deceased

76. Hypoglycemia 266
John T. Hayford, Jr.,* and Margaret E. Mohrmann

77. Diabetes Mellitus 269
John T. Hayford, Jr.,* and Margaret E. Mohrmann

78. Metabolic Errors 273
Robert D. White

79. Malformation Syndromes 277
Robert D. White

IX. NEUROMUSCULAR DISORDERS

80. Seizure Disorders 285
William R. Leahy, Jr., and Kenneth B. Roberts

81. Spinal Dysraphism 288
William R. Leahy, Jr.

82. Hydrocephalus 291
William R. Leahy, Jr.

83. Cerebral Palsy 294
Eileen P. G. Vining

X. RHEUMATIC DISORDERS

84. Juvenile Rheumatoid Arthritis 301
Margaret E. Mohrmann

85. Systemic Lupus Erythematosus 305
Margaret E. Mohrmann

86. Other Rheumatic Disorders 309
Margaret E. Mohrmann

XI. HEMATOLOGIC DISORDERS

87. Iron Deficiency 315
Dennis C. Stokes and Evan Charney

88. Sickle Cell Disease 319
Kenneth B. Roberts

89. Hemophilia 323
Kenneth B. Roberts

90. Idiopathic Thrombocytopenic Purpura 325
Kenneth B. Roberts

91. Henoch-Schönlein Syndrome 328
Kenneth B. Roberts

XII. NEOPLASTIC DISORDERS

92. Leukemia 335
Kenneth B. Roberts

*Deceased

93. Wilms Tumor 338
Margaret E. Mohrmann

94. Neuroblastoma 341
Margaret E. Mohrmann

95. Hodgkin Disease 345
Margaret E. Mohrmann

96. Non-Hodgkin Lymphoma 348
Margaret E. Mohrmann

97. Brain Tumors 351
Margaret E. Mohrmann

98. Malignant Bone Tumors 354
Margaret E. Mohrmann

XIII. IMMUNITY AND INFECTIOUS DISEASES

99. Immune Deficiency 359
Kenneth B. Roberts

100. Immunizations and Vaccine-Preventable Diseases 362
Kenneth B. Roberts

101. Infections of Bones and Joints 369
Kenneth B. Roberts

102. Infectious Mononucleosis 372
Kenneth B. Roberts

103. Tuberculosis 375
Kenneth B. Roberts

104. Rocky Mountain Spotted Fever 378
Kenneth B. Roberts

105. Streptococcal Infections 380
Kenneth B. Roberts

106. Enteric Infections 383
Kenneth B. Roberts

107. Gonorrhea 387
Kenneth B. Roberts

Index 391

CONTRIBUTING AUTHORS

Evan Charney, M.D.
The Johns Hopkins University School of Medicine; University of Maryland School of Medicine; Sinai Hospital of Baltimore, Baltimore

Richard A. Cohn, M.D.
Northwestern University Medical School; Children's Memorial Hospital, Chicago, Illinois

John T. Hayford, Jr., M.D.*
University of Iowa College of Medicine; University of Iowa Hospitals and Clinics, Iowa City

Jean S. Kan, M.D.
The Johns Hopkins University School of Medicine; The Johns Hopkins Hospital, Baltimore, Maryland

William R. Leahy, Jr., M.D.
The Johns Hopkins University School of Medicine, Baltimore; Neurological Medicine, P.A., Hyattsville, Maryland

Margaret E. Mohrmann, M.D.
Medical University of South Carolina College of Medicine; Medical University Hospital, Charleston

Kenneth B. Roberts, M.D.
The Johns Hopkins University School of Medicine; University of Maryland School of Medicine; Sinai Hospital of Baltimore, Baltimore

Dennis C. Stokes, M.D.
University of Tennessee Center for the Health Sciences; Saint Jude Children's Research Hospital, Memphis

Eileen P. G. Vining, M.D.
The Johns Hopkins University School of Medicine; The Johns Hopkins Hospital, Baltimore, Maryland

Robert D. White, M.D.
Indiana University School of Medicine; Memorial Hospital, South Bend

PREFACE TO THE SECOND EDITION

A recent alumnus of a northeastern U. S. medical school expressed praise for the first edition of the *Manual* as follows: The elevators at his school's teaching hospital are so notoriously slow that the students and house officers developed an "elevator library," the idea being to use the waiting and transit time profitably. The *Manual of Clinical Problems in Pediatrics* was not only "elected" to this library but was held in high esteem, since it made possible the acquisition of a clinical orientation to a disorder between beginning the trek to the emergency department and the time of arrival.

The compliment is accepted with pride—but with reservation as well. The format of the first edition was what we intended (basic for the students, references for the house officers), but the focus was skewed. It appeared we were interested only in children with disorders affecting various organ systems and not in all children and the aspects of growth, development, and behavior that make pediatrics vital. In the second edition, we have reoriented several chapters and added others, creating a part on growth, development, and behavior to help establish some balance. And the thread can be detected throughout the rest of the *Manual* as well.

In the second edition, as in the first, we have combined the points of view of generalist and specialist in each chapter. We greatly appreciate the input of various consultants, who reviewed text and provided valuable comment on accuracy and currency: Drs. Jacob Felix, Barbara Howard, Alan Lake, Allen Schwartz, Edward Sills, and Jerry Winkelstein. In addition, Drs. Evan Charney, Richard Cohn, Margaret Mohrmann, and Patti Vining graciously reviewed chapters by their fellow contributors. And each contributor accepted the editor's pencil with admirable grace. Thank you all.

Contrary to our expectations (and, I daresay, those of our families and colleagues), revising the *Manual* took a great deal of time and focused attention. We are indebted to those around us and to Little, Brown and Company for patient support through the project. Again, our gratitude and praise to Laraine Fisher, who word-processed our taped and stapled scraps into a second edition with efficiency, accuracy, and skill, correcting our errors without sacrificing speed or our egos. And, when it came down to the wire, Shelley Schaffer came to the rescue; she was still typing long after even the house staff had gone to sleep (and that *is* above and beyond the call, isn't it!). For her help, for her cheer, and for her support: a most sincere thank you. (I hope her next all-nighter brings her more fun.)

K. B. R.

PREFACE TO THE FIRST EDITION

We are constantly asked by junior medical students, "What book should I get for Pediatrics?" Often, what we recommend is an encyclopedia; what they need is a dictionary. Our house officers, after their first taste of sleep deprivation, rapidly abandon the massive texts in favor of a manual in one pocket, a handbook in the other, and a request for key articles to photocopy (and, perchance, to read). This volume attempts to meet the needs of both groups.

One hundred clinical problems in pediatrics are considered in this manual. For each, there is a brief text designed to present an overview and an orientation rather than an exhaustive review. In addition, more than 2,000 references have been selected to augment the text and are categorized and annotated to guide the reader; special consideration has been given to articles in the most widely available journals and to reviews (editorial or comprehensive) with useful bibliographies. Specifics concerning treatment are not detailed in the text; the reader should consult the referenced articles or the companion *Manual of Pediatric Therapeutics* in this Little, Brown and Company series.

To assure accuracy, currency, and perspective, each section was either written by a pediatrician with special knowledge in the given area and reviewed by a generalist or vice versa. The editor is particularly grateful to the contributors for their responsiveness to the exhortation to "keep the text basic, suggest advanced readings in the reference section," and for their generous cooperation in making suggested changes. Drs. Evan Charney and Margaret Mohrmann helped in the task of editing; I am greatly in their debt for their masterly assistance. Other pediatricians who reviewed and provided valuable comment on portions of the manuscript are Drs. Arnold Capute, Jacob Felix, Jerome Paulson, Richard Talamo, David Valle, and Jerry Winkelstein.

Drs. Verdain Barnes, John Littlefield, and Robert Drachman helped initiate and encourage this project. Ms. Kathleen O'Brien (of Little, Brown and Company), Mrs. Ellen Roberts, and Dr. Evan Charney deserve special thanks for their confidence and patient support through the many months of preparation of this volume. Credit for completion of the book belongs to Laraine Fisher: we submitted rough copy to her, and she somehow made it into a book. If the quality of the contents comes close to her degree of secretarial skill, we will be proud indeed.

K. B. R.

I. EMERGENCIES

1. CARDIOPULMONARY ARREST AND RESUSCITATION
Kenneth B. Roberts

Cardiopulmonary arrest deserves its premier position in this manual, being the most important and certainly the most dramatic emergency in children. Underlying causes include respiratory disorders, trauma, sudden infant death syndrome, congenital heart disease, sepsis, metabolic disturbances, anesthesia and other drugs, drowning, neuromuscular diseases, and others. Although cessation of cardiac activity may appear clinically to be a sudden, catastrophic event, there are often signs of impending arrest. Respiratory distress deserves particular attention, since most cardiac arrests in children are preceded by respiratory insufficiency. In addition, glucose and electrolyte abnormalities, which may have serious consequences, are often preventable or recognizable before becoming clinically apparent. Children at risk for hypoxia, hypoglycemia, and hyperkalemia require appropriate monitoring and observation.

It is axiomatic that the earlier effective resuscitation is instituted, the better the prognosis. If the patient has not been hypoxic prior to cardiopulmonary arrest, there is considered to be a period of about 4 minutes before discernible brain damage occurs; since hypoxia is usual in children prior to cardiac arrest, there may be even less of a "grace period" in this age group. A rough estimate of when arrest occurred is obtained by examination of the pupils, which start to dilate 45 seconds after effective circulation ceases and are usually completely dilated by 1 minute and 45 seconds.

The mnemonic A, B, C gives the initial steps in resuscitation: Airway, Breathe, Circulate. Patency of the airway should be ensured by lifting the mandible and manually clearing the pharynx, if necessary. Suction and intubation may be advantageous, but resuscitation must not be delayed because equipment is not immediately available. As soon as a clear airway is established, breathing for the patient must begin. Inattention to this principle has been noted as the most apparent error in resuscitation and the one to which failure to survive is most often attributed. Again, although equipment, such as a self-filling bag with oxygen, is desirable, promptness of ventilation is paramount; mouth-to-mouth or mouth-to-tube breathing can deliver adequate oxygen (exhaled air is 16–17% oxygen).

The mainstay of artificial circulation is so-called closed-chest cardiac massage; one seeks not to massage but to compress the thorax. This is usually preceded in adults by a precordial "thump" because of its value in the treatment of ventricular dysrhythmia. The maneuver is not routine in children, however, because ventricular dysrhythmias are uncommon in children, and the "thump" is ineffective in anoxic asystole (the most common cause of arrest in children) and hypovolemic shock.

The precise technique of chest compression depends on the size of the patient. The procedure is performed in newborns and infants by encircling the chest with both hands and then exerting pressure with the thumbs over the precordium and midsternum. The technique used in older children is similar to that used in adults, except that the base of the palm should rest higher on the sternum to avoid lacerating the liver. The process is most efficiently accomplished with the patient on a hard surface, since if it is to be effective, the chest must be "squeezed" and intrathoracic pressure increased. In adults, proper technique can produce a peak systolic pressure greater than 100 mm Hg, but since the diastolic pressure approaches 0, mean pressure seldom exceeds 40 mm Hg. This produces a carotid blood flow of one-fourth to one-third of normal; it is clear that with inadequate compression, this will be even lower, and integrity of the central nervous system will be compromised. It is therefore imperative to monitor the adequacy of chest compression by palpation of the carotid or femoral pulse.

These ABCs, which should begin as soon as cardiopulmonary arrest is diagnosed, share three important features: (1) none requires equipment; (2) all must be instituted promptly; and (3) all can be done by a single person. During this phase of resuscitation, a return of reactivity of the pupils is a sign of adequate cardiorespiratory support.

The next step in the resuscitation process involves pharmacologic agents, the most useful of which is epinephrine. This drug increases myocardial contractility, elevates perfusion pressure, lowers defibrillation threshold, and restores myocardial conduction in some cases of electromechanical dissociation. In the absence of effective circulation, the epinephrine should be injected into a major central vein or directly into the heart

3

rather than into a peripheral vein; instillation through an endotracheal tube appears to be effective and is rapidly replacing intracardiac injections in many centers. Sodium bicarbonate is frequently administered; it was once recommended routinely to combat the acidosis of cardiopulmonary arrest, but concerns have been expressed about the futility and hazards of such therapy. Acidosis in the central nervous system may worsen after bicarbonate administration, and the patient is exposed to the added risk of hyperosmolarity. Ventilation with effective cardiac massage is usually sufficient to control acidosis; bicarbonate therapy cannot be substituted for adequate, vigorous cardiopulmonary resuscitation. If resuscitation has not been successful with the maneuvers that have been described, accurate ECG diagnosis is required. Asystole is more common in children than fibrillation, but if fibrillation is demonstrated, specific therapy (Xylocaine or electrical defibrillation) is available. Sinus bradycardia or atrioventricular block with bradycardia may respond to atropine; widened QRS complexes or tall, peaked T waves suggestive of hyperkalemia warrant a trial of a calcium salt, which will enhance ventricular conduction and increase myocardial contractility. Isoproterenol or dopamine may be required for ongoing circulatory support.

The most important single prognostic indicator is the duration and degree of anoxia the patient has sustained. Signs of neurologic impairment that are present immediately following resuscitation are often striking but may be transient; their persistence for more than 1 hour is a more ominous indicator of significant neurologic damage. The outcome is most favorable when cardiopulmonary arrest is recognized promptly and effective resuscitative measures are instituted immediately.

Reviews
1. Anthony, C., Crawford, E., and Morgan, B. Management of cardiac and respiratory arrest in children. *Clin. Pediatr.* (Phila.) 8:647, 1969.
   Still the best review dealing with children.
2. Standards and guidelines for cardiopulmonary resuscitation and emergency cardiac care. *J.A.M.A.* 244:453, 1980.
   Excellent, thorough (56-page) review of all aspects, including special consideration of infants and children (p. 472).
3. Orlowski, J. Cardiopulmonary resuscitation in children. *Pediatr. Clin. North Am.* 27:495, 1980.
   Step-by-step management, with explicit comparisons to resuscitation of adults.

Specific Causes of Arrest
4. Salem, M., et al. Cardiac arrest related to anesthesia. *J.A.M.A.* 233:238, 1975.
   A review of 73 cases; 33 percent mortality.
   Also see specific chapters (e.g., Respiratory Failure and Status Asthmaticus).

Specific Aspects of Resuscitation
5. Thaler, M., and Stobie, G. An improved technic of external cardiac compression in infants and young children. *N. Engl. J. Med.* 269:606, 1963.
   Encircle chest and apply pressure to midsternum to avoid laceration of liver. (Technique in newborns: J. Pediatr. 86:781, 1975.)
6. Taylor, G., et al. Importance of prolonged compression during cardiopulmonary resuscitation in man. *N. Engl. J. Med.* 296:1515, 1977.
   Prolonged compression is more effective than rapid rate.
7. Pennington, J., Taylor, J., and Lown, B. Chest thump for reverting ventricular tachycardia. *N. Engl. J. Med.* 283:1192, 1970.
   Article and accompanying editorial by same authors (p. 1223) state rationale and results.
8. Chameides, L., et al. Guidelines for defibrillation in infants and children. *Circulation* 56:502A, 1977.
   Excellent, brief overview by American Heart Association committee.
9. Gutgesell, H., et al. Energy dose for ventricular defibrillation of children. *Pediatrics* 58:898, 1976.
   Start with 2 watt-seconds/kg and double if necessary.
10. Nugent, S., Laravuso, R., and Rogers, M. Pharmacology and use of muscle relaxants in infants and children. *J. Pediatr.* 94:481, 1979.
    Read this before having to intubate.

11. Greenberg, M., Roberts, J., and Baskin, S. Use of endotracheally administered epinephrine in a pediatric patient. *Am. J. Dis. Child.* 135:767, 1981.
    A case report; other drugs given E-T with apparent success include naloxone (Ann. Emerg. Med. 9:289, 1980), diazepam (Ann. Emerg. Med. 11:242, 1982), and atropine (Ann. Emerg. Med. 11:546, 1982).
12. Driscoll, D., Gillette, P., and McNamara, D. The use of dopamine in children. *J. Pediatr.* 92:309, 1978.
    When additional cardiovascular support is needed.(Evaluation of dobutamine: J. Pediatr. 100:977, 1982; extensive, two-part review of shock in children: J. Pediatr. 101:163, 319, 1982.)
13. Rogers, M. New developments in cardiopulmonary resuscitation. *Pediatrics* 71:655, 1983.
    Attention directed to the relationship between chest compression, cardiac output, intracranial pressure, and intracranial perfusion. (For more on recent understanding of the mechanisms of brain injury during arrest and implications for treatment, see J.A.M.A. 251: 1586, 1984.)
14. Lowenstein, S., et al. Cardiopulmonary resuscitation by medical and surgical house officers. *Lancet* 2:679, 1981.
    In simulated cardiopulmonary arrests, no house officer of the 45 tested received a passing score in basic life support. (Benefits of a designated pediatric resuscitation team: J. Pediatr. 84:152, 1974.)

Acidosis and Bicarbonate Therapy
15. Chazan, J., Stenson, R., and Kurland, G. The acidosis of cardiac arrest. *N. Engl. J. Med.* 278:360, 1968.
    The respiratory component is more severe than the metabolic component.
16. Berenyi, K., Wolk, M., and Killis, T. Cerebrospinal fluid acidosis complicating therapy of experimental cardiopulmonary arrest. *Circulation* 52:319, 1975.
    Bicarbonate does not diffuse across the blood-brain barrier as readily as does carbon dioxide.
17. Bishop, R., and Weisfeldt, M. Sodium bicarbonate administration during cardiac arrest. *J.A.M.A.* 235:506, 1976.
    Ventilation per se, without bicarbonate, is adequate. (Bicarbonate without ventilation is not: J. Pediatr. 80:671, 1972; also, bicarbonate use can cause hyperosmolarity: Am. J. Med. 56:162, 1974.) Recent review: Ann. Emerg. Med. 13:781, 1984.

Outcome
18. Cole, S., and Corday, E. Four-minute limit for cardiac resuscitation. *J.A.M.A.* 161:1454, 1956.
    The classic, establishing the limit if "complete cerebral recovery" is to be achieved.
19. Fillmore, S., Shapiro, M., and Killip, T. Serial blood gas studies during cardiopulmonary resuscitation. *Ann. Intern. Med.* 72:465, 1970.
    Emphasizes the need for prompt, effective ventilation.
20. Willoughby, J., and Leach, B. Relation of neurological findings after cardiac arrest to outcome. *Br. Med. J.* 3:437, 1974.
    The prognostic value of the findings of a neurologic examination 1 hour after arrest.
21. Weinberger, H., van der Wonde, R., and Maier, H. Prognosis of cortical blindness following cardiac arrest in children. *J.A.M.A.* 179:126, 1962.
    The prognosis is not as bad as it might appear acutely.
22. Torphy, D., Minter, M., and Thompson, B. Cardiorespiratory arrest and resuscitation of children. *Am. J. Dis. Child.* 138: 1099, 1984.
    Challenges the notion that children are more resistant than adults to the ill effects of cardiopulmonary arrest. (See companion editorial, p. 1097.)
23. Freeman, J., and Rogers, M. On death, dying, and decisions. *Pediatrics* 66:637, 1980.
    Useful thoughts to consider when resuscitation efforts are "partially successful." (More on brain death: N. Engl. J. Med. 299:338,393, 1978; Ann. Intern. Med. 94:389, 1981; and Am. J. Dis. Child. 137:545, 1983. On "Do not resuscitate" orders: Ann. Intern. Med. 96:660, 1982. On the persistent vegetative state: Am. J. Dis. Child. 138:128, 1984.)

2. BACTEREMIA AND SEPTICEMIA
Kenneth B. Roberts

In order for bacteria to infect the bloodstream, they must first bypass the defenses of the skin and mucous membranes and then escape phagocytosis in the extravascular tissues; they travel via the lymphatics to regional lymph nodes and, if not contained by the nodes, gain access to the venous circulation. The liver and spleen play a major role in "filtering" bacteria from the blood; the spleen is predominant if there is no preexisting circulating antibody to the organism. This filtering process can be overwhelmed by a large inoculum of bacteria; residual organisms are phagocytized by white blood cells in the circulation, at alveolar capillary sites in the lungs, and in the tissues. The following factors therefore predispose the host to bacteremia: (1) loss of integrity of the external defenses (e.g., major burns, gastrointestinal ulceration, intravenous catheter); (2) inadequate phagocytic or immune function (e.g., immunosuppressive drugs, neutropenia, immune deficiency disorders); (3) impaired reticuloendothelial function (e.g., splenectomy, sickle cell disease); and (4) an overwhelming inoculum (e.g., perforated intestine). Bacteremia is a dynamic process, a balance between multiplication, invasion, and clearance of organisms; in most patients, host defenses predominate, and bacteremia is a transient phenomenon.

Bacteremia and septicemia are not synonymous. Bacteremia refers only to the presence of organisms in the blood; septicemia adds the connotation of severe illness. The distinction has been highlighted by recent studies reporting that over 3 percent of febrile infants have bacteremia while not appearing sufficiently ill to warrant hospitalization. (Rates as high as 13 percent are documented in "nonseptic-appearing" infants, with fever, leukocytosis, and no apparent focus of bacterial infection.) The causative organism in the majority of these infants is *Streptococcus pneumoniae; Haemophilus influenzae* is the next most common. Since both of these pyogenic bacteria cause meningitis in infants and children (see Chapter 3), their presence in the blood is of great concern; there is no way at present to determine whether or not septicemia or meningitis will develop in a given child with bacteremia.

The clinical signs of septicemia are nonspecific and difficult to define. Generally, the child has high fever and is quite ill; the words *toxic* and *septic* are often used to describe the child's appearance. The white blood cell count is usually elevated (or markedly decreased), and there may be vacuoles or "toxic granulations" in the polymorphonuclear leukocytes. In neonates and very young infants, the signs of septicemia may be considerably more subtle (see Neonatal Sepsis, Chapter 44).

When septicemia is suspected, treatment must be instituted immediately, prior to bacteriologic confirmation. The age and condition of the patient provide reasonable guides to the pathogens most likely to be responsible for clinical disease. In newborns, group B streptococci and gram-negative bacilli are the most frequent bacteria, followed by staphylococci. In immunosuppressed hosts, gram-negative bacilli predominate, particularly *Pseudomonas, Escherichia coli,* and *Klebsiella* strains; *Staphylococcus aureus* is also common. In children with inadequate splenic function (congenital or operative absence of the spleen, or "functional asplenia," as in children with sickle cell disease), the pneumococcus is the usual cause of sepsis; the incidence of *H. influenzae* septicemia in these children is also increased. Certain bacteria are associated with specific foci of infection, as discussed in the sections Pneumonia (Chap. 59), Meningitis (Chap. 3), Infections of the Bones and Joints (Chap. 101), Urinary Tract Infection (Chap. 72), and Bacterial Endocarditis (Chap. 49). Certain skin lesions suggest infection with specific organisms: petechiae/purpura (*Neisseria meningitidis,* the meningococcus), pustules (*Staphylococcus aureus*), small lesions with necrotic centers (*Neisseria gonorrhoeae,* the gonococcus), ecthyma gangrenosum (*Pseudomonas*), and Rose spots (*Salmonella typhosa*).

A gram-stained specimen of pus from any source, or an aspirate from a skin lesion, or a smear of the "buffy coat" of blood may demonstrate the organism. Newer techniques—such as latex agglutination, countercurrent immunoelectrophoresis (CIE), and the limulus test for endotoxin—may help but in general have been less rewarding when applied to blood than when applied to other body fluids (cerebrospinal or pleural fluid). When possible, multiple blood cultures should be obtained prior to treatment.

In practice, it is often necessary to administer more than one antibiotic until the bacterium is identified and sensitivity testing is accomplished. Penicillin is the drug of choice for sepsis due to the pneumococcus or meningococcus, a penicillinase-resistant penicillin (e.g., nafcillin, methicillin, oxacillin) for the staphylococcus, chloramphenicol for *H. influenzae,* and an aminoglycoside (e.g., gentamicin, tobramycin) for the commonly isolated gram-negative bacilli, excluding *Salmonella. Pseudomonas* infection, particularly if the host is immunosuppressed, is best treated with the synergistic combination of an aminoglycoside and a penicillin with anti-*Pseudomonas* activity (e.g., ticarcillin, carbenicillin).

The most serious complication of bloodstream infection is the syndrome of septic shock, characterized by the hypoperfusion of vital organs. Metabolic acidosis and tissue starvation may be profound, resulting from an inadequate blood supply and mitochondrial injury. Endothelial cells are damaged, leading to edema and acting as a nidus for thrombus formation; platelets adhere to the damaged cells, fibrin is deposited, and a cycle is established that can lead to disseminated intravascular coagulation (DIC). In addition, both pathways of complement are activated, and there is potent stimulation for both vasodilatation and constriction, producing the characteristic findings of hypotension and poor peripheral circulation. Poor perfusion and DIC, in some cases complicated by adrenal hemorrhage, may result in the clinical state of purpura fulminans, with 40 to 80 percent mortality. The meningococcus is the most frequent cause of septic shock in normal hosts, but an identical syndrome may be caused by gram-negative bacilli (including, rarely, *H. influenzae* and—particularly in patients with deficient splenic function— by the pneumococcus.

If shock complicates the course of septicemia, consideration is given to the administration of corticosteroids or heparin or both, along with antibiotics. Enthusiasm for corticosteroids stems from the observation that patients who die with a fulminant course of purpura and shock may have adrenal hemorrhage at autopsy (Waterhouse-Friderichsen syndrome). Adrenal insufficiency does not usually occur in "uncomplicated" septicemia, however, so the administration of corticosteroids is usually limited to patients in shock. Heparin therapy appears to improve the bleeding due to DIC in some patients, but it does not affect the high mortality.

Supportive therapy includes the infusion of intravenous fluids and, if necessary, pressors, such as isoproterenol or dopamine. Attention to respiratory care is crucial, since respiratory failure is a major mode of death.

The high morbidity and mortality associated with septicemia and its complications are improved—but by no means eliminated—by early recognition and aggressive therapy. Approaches to prevention include chemoprophylaxis and immunization. Rifampin chemoprophylaxis, for example, is generally prescribed for close contacts of patients with meningococcal disease and is recommended for some contacts of patients with invasive *H. influenzae* disease; the ability of chemoprophylaxis to prevent septicemia on a large scale is obviously limited. Bacterial vaccines effective against *H. influenzae,* meningococci (groups A and C), and multiple types of pneumococci are all promising, but the vaccines developed to date are not effective in infants less than 2 years of age.

Mechanisms
1. MacCabe, W., Treadwell, T., and De Maria, A. Pathophysiology of bacteremia. *Am. J. Med.* 75(1B):7, 1983.
   Part of the proceedings of a symposium on clinical and microbiologic advances in infectious diseases; other articles in the supplement address clinical microbiology of bacteremia (p. 2), host factors in bacteremia (p. 19), and improved methods of detection and isolation (pp. 26, 31), and more.
2. Hyslop, N., and McCluskey, R. Case records of the Massachusetts General Hospital 36-1975. *N. Engl. J. Med.* 293:547, 1975.
   Mechanisms considered in a young adult with fatal sepsis 10 years after splenectomy.

Diagnosis
3. Washington, J. Blood cultures: Principles and techniques. *Mayo Clin. Proc.* 50:91, 1975.
   Practical aspects of collection, processing, and interpretation.
4. Reik, H., and Rubin, S. Evaluation of the buffy-coat smear for rapid detection of bacteremia. *J.A.M.A.* 245:357, 1981.

Of blood samples "positive" by culture, nearly 12 percent were "positive" by buffy coat smear; a positive smear portends a grave prognosis. (Organisms may even be seen in peripheral blood smear: Am. J. Med. 55:851, 1973.)

Bacteremia

5. Winchester, P., Todd, J., and Roe, M. Bacteremia in hospitalized children. *Am. J. Dis. Child.* 131:753, 1977.
   Nearly two-thirds of "positive" blood cultures contained "contaminants;" data describing the remaining one-third are well presented.
6. Everett, E., and Hirschmann, J. Transient bacteremia and endocarditis prophylaxis: A review. *Medicine* (Baltimore) 56:61, 1977.
   Quantifies the risk of bacteremia following procedures.
7. Teele, D., et al. Meningitis after lumbar puncture in children with bacteremia. *N. Engl. J. Med.* 305:1079, 1981.
   A continuing dilemma considered.

"Walk-in" Clinic Bacteremia Studies

8. Teele, D., Marshall, R., and Klein, J. Unsuspected bacteremia in young children: A common and important problem. *Pediatr. Clin. North Am.* 26:773, 1979.
   Summarizes this group's several studies; start here.
9. McCarthy, P., et al. History and observation variables in assessing febrile children. *Pediatrics* 65:1090, 1980.
   Degree of illness judged by playfulness, alertness, and consolability; much of the information comes from watching the child's eyes: Pediatrics 67:687, 1981. (Value of assessing the child's functional status: J. Pediatr. 99:231, 1981.)
10. Carroll, W., et al. Treatment of occult bacteremia: A prospective randomized clinical trial. *Pediatrics* 72:608, 1983.
    Support for the use of "expectant antibiotic therapy" for children with certain risk factors for bacteremia.
11. Caspe, W., Chamudes, O., and Louie, B. The evaluation and treatment of the febrile infant. *Pediatr. Infect. Dis.* 2:131, 1983.
    Focus is on the first 2 months of life; largest series to date. (Perspective editorial: Am. J. Dis. Child. 137:1143, 1983.)

Pneumococcus

12. Klein, J. The epidemiology of pneumococcal disease in infants and children. *Rev. Infect. Dis.* 3:246, 1981.
    Part of a 200-page symposium on the pneumococcus.
13. Cole, F., Saryan, J., and Smith, A. The risk of additional systemic bacterial illness in infants with systemic *Streptococcus pneumoniae* disease. *J. Pediatr.* 99:91, 1981.
    In a retrospective review, 11 percent of infants with pneumococcal sepsis had an additional systemic bacterial illness.
14. Granoff, D. Pneumococcal vaccine in children. *Clin. Pediatr.* (Phila.) 19:96, 1980.
    The good news, the bad news, and "tentative recommendations." (The new "expanded" pneumococcal vaccine: Med. Lett. Drugs Ther. 25:91, 1983.)
    Also see reference 8.

Haemophilus influenzae

15. Dajani, A., Asmar, B., and Thirumoorthi, M. Systemic *Haemophilus influenzae* disease: An overview. *J. Pediatr.* 94:355, 1979.
    Particular attention is paid to the various sites of involvement.
16. Marks, M. Antibiotic therapy of serious *Haemophilus* infections—a continuing problem. *J. Pediatr.* 98:910, 1981.
    A brief editorial lamenting the failure of cefamandole to dependably "cover" the cerebrospinal fluid; looks ahead to moxalactam (as in Pediatrics 71:187, 1983).
    Also see reference 8.

Meningococcus

17. Peltola, H. Meningococcal disease: Still with us. *Rev. Infect. Dis.* 5:71, 1983.
    An extensive review (20 pages, 166 references).

18. Dashefsky, B., Teele, D., and Klein, J. Unsuspected meningococcemia. *J. Pediatr.* 102:69, 1983.
    Less common than occult bacteremia caused by S. pneumoniae *or* H. influenzae; *appears to be less benign, too.*
19. Edwards, M., and Baker, C. Complications and sequelae of meningococcal infections in children. *J. Pediatr.* 99:540, 1981.
    Focus on suppurative, allergic, and neurologic complications.
20. Toews, W., and Bass, J. Skin manifestations of meningococcal infection. *Am. J. Dis. Child.* 127:173, 1974.
    *No skin lesions in 14 percent; 75 percent with generalized maculopapular rash or petechiae; 11 percent with purpura. Meningitis was most frequent in the first group, death in the third group. (*Haemophilus influenzae *can produce similar skin lesions:* Pediatrics *72:469, 1983.)*
21. Stiehm, E., and Damrosch, D. Factors in the prognosis of meningococcal infection. *J. Pediatr.* 68:457, 1966.
    Five prognostic signs, with grave prognosis if three or more are present.

Salmonella
22. Hyams, J., et al. *Salmonella* bacteremia in the first year of life. *J. Pediatr.* 96:57, 1980.
    The risk of Salmonella *bacteremia is highest in the first year of life (*J. Infect. Dis. *143:743, 1981); metastatic foci may be more common in first few months of life (*Am. J. Dis. Child. *135:1096, 1981.)*

Septic Shock
23. Perkin, R., and Levin, D. Shock in the pediatric patient. *J. Pediatr.* 101:163, 1982.
    A two-part review of pathophysiology, monitoring, and therapy. (For a short review of the hemodynamics and pathogenesis of septic shock, see J.A.M.A. *250:3324, 1983.)*
24. Yabek, S. Management of septic shock. *Pediatr. Rev.* 2:83, 1980.
    Modern management. (Also see Pediatr. Clin. North Am. *30:365, 1983.)*
25. Sheagren, J. Septic shock and corticosteroids. *N. Engl. J. Med.* 305:456, 1981.
    Editorial review of controversy. (Help reverse shock but not reduce mortality. N. Engl. J. Med. *311:1137, 1984; Naloxone, anyone?* J. Infect. Dis. *142:229, 1980.)*
26. Corrigan, J. Heparin therapy in bacterial septicemia. *J. Pediatr.* 91:695, 1977.
    Heparin may help control bleeding from DIC but it does not reduce mortality.
27. Knaus, W. Changing the cause of death. *J.A.M.A.* 249:1059, 1983.
    An editorial accompanying the article "Failure of intensive care unit support to influence mortality from pneumococcal bacteremia" (page 249); discusses what an ICU can do and what it cannot do. (The focus is on adults but the perspective in the editorial makes valuable reading nevertheless.)

Antibiotics
28. Speck, W., and Blumer, J. (eds.). Symposium on anti-infective therapy I. *Pediatr. Clin. North Am.* 30(1), 1983.
    A collection of 16 articles on the various commonly used (and not so commonly used) agents.

3. MENINGITIS
Kenneth B. Roberts

During infancy and childhood (but beyond the neonatal period), the greatest risk for meningitis is between 6 and 12 months of age; 90 percent of cases occur between 1 month and 5 years of age. Three organisms cause 90 percent of these cases; *Haemophilus influenzae* type b; *Neisseria meningitidis;* and *Streptococcus pneumoniae.* Of these, *H.*

influenzae is by far the most common, responsible for 2 to 6 times as many cases as the meningococcus or the pneumococcus. The risk of *H. influenzae* meningitis prior to school age is between 1 in 300 and 1 in 1600 and is higher in infants and children of low socioeconomic status. Pneumococcal meningitis is 5 to 6 times more common in blacks than in Caucasians, and children with sickle cell disease are at particular risk (36 times the risk for black children without sickle cell disease, 314 times the risk for whites); the rate in children with sickle cell disease under age 6 approaches 1 percent per year.

The signs and symptoms of meningitis are variable and depend on the age of the patient. In infants, whose cranial sutures are still open, fever, vomiting, irritability, lethargy, convulsions, and bulging of the fontanelle may be present; during the first 2 years of life in particular, the findings are often subtle or nonspecific. In older children, focal neurologic signs, such as a sixth nerve palsy, may be more prominent, and signs of meningeal irritation, such as nuchal rigidity, Kernig's sign, or Brudzinski's sign, are usually present.

Examination of the cerebrospinal fluid (CSF) is mandatory if there is clinical suspicion of meningitis. In most cases of bacterial meningitis, there is an increased number of white cells in the CSF, usually well over 100 per cu mm, with a predominance of polymorphonuclear leukocytes. The glucose level in the CSF is reduced (hypoglycorrhachia), usually to below 40 mg/dl and less than half the concentration of the serum glucose; the protein level in the CSF is elevated. Organisms are visible in gram-stained specimens in the majority of cases. *H. influenzae* is a gram-negative, pleomorphic organism; meningococci are bean-shaped, gram-negative diplococci that usually orient with the concave surfaces apposed; pneumococci are lancet-shaped, gram-positive cocci that may also appear in pairs but with end-to-end orientation. Bacterial products may be identified by rapid techniques: capsular polysaccharide by latex agglutination or countercurrent immunoelectrophoresis (CIE), endotoxin by the limulus lysate test. It is vital to recognize that none of the features described above is a sine qua non for the diagnosis of bacterial meningitis: any can be "normal" in a given patient, and, on very rare occasions, meningitis is present in the absence of any of these changes. The definitive diagnosis is established bacteriologically.

Meningitis may be caused by agents other than pyogenic bacteria, including viruses (aseptic meningitis), *Mycobacterium tuberculosis,* fungi, and neoplasms. These situations are generally associated with fewer, mostly mononuclear, cells in the CSF. Early in the course of viral meningitis, polymorphonuclear leukocytes may predominate; a specimen of CSF obtained 6 to 8 hours after the initial evaluation usually demonstrates the characteristic "shift" to mononuclear cells. The protein and glucose concentrations are usually normal, but meningitides caused by tuberculosis, mumps, and some enteroviruses are notable exceptions.

Treatment of bacterial meningitis must be instituted without delay, prior to bacteriologic confirmation. Chloramphenicol and ampicillin are administered parenterally in large doses until identification of the organism and antibiotic-susceptibility testing are complete and permit selection of a single drug. Supportive care is crucial and is aimed toward prevention and treatment of complications, the most important of which initially is increased intracranial pressure (see Increased Intracranial Pressure, Chap. 11). Focal neurologic signs occur in approximately 10 to 15 percent of the patients; sixth nerve palsies usually resolve in the first day or two of hospitalization, but gross focal neurologic signs are associated with sequelae still detectable after discharge from the hospital. Seizures occur in about one-fourth of children, two-thirds of whom have their seizures before treatment is instituted. Seizures beyond the third hospital day portend an unfavorable prognosis. Antidiuretic hormone secretion causes hyponatremia, commonly noted at the time of admission; severe water intoxication with seizures can usually be prevented by restricting the intake of fluids and electrolytes. Intracranial inflammation may cause cavernous sinus thrombosis, subdural effusions, or hydrocephalus. Other complications and sequelae include ataxia, deafness, and mental retardation. When the results of psychologic testing of school-age survivors of meningitis are included in assessing the sequelae of infection, less than one-half the children appear normal when compared with their siblings.

Mortality in bacterial meningitis remains 5 to 10 percent despite prompt administration of antibiotics in appropriate doses and vigorous supportive therapy. Bacterial polysaccharide vaccines are being developed for the prevention of meningitis. Those currently available are of limited usefulness because of their low immunogenicity in infants under the age of 2, the group at greatest risk.

Reviews

1. Bell, W., and McCormick, W. *Neurologic Infections in Children* (2nd ed.). Philadelphia: Saunders, 1981.
   A general discussion of bacterial meningitis, with chapters on the meningitides caused by specific organisms.
2. Feigin, R., and Dodge, P. Bacterial meningitis: Newer concepts of pathophysiology and neurologic sequelae. *Pediatr. Clin. North Am.* 23:541, 1976.
   Many practical aspects, well covered; Feigin also has an excellent, thorough general review in R. Feigin, and J. Cherry (eds.), Textbook of Pediatric Infectious Disease. Philadelphia: Saunders, 1981.

Epidemiology

3. Fraser, D., et al. Risk factors in bacterial meningitis: Charleston County, South Carolina. *J. Infect. Dis.* 127:271, 1973.
   Infants from poor families had a higher incidence of H. influenzae meningitis than infants from more wealthy families. Infants under 4 years of age with sickle cell disease had a rate of pneumococcal meningitis of nearly 1 percent per year.
4. Parke, J., et al. The attack rate, age incidence, racial distribution, and case fatality rate of Hemophilus influenzae type b meningitis in Mecklenburg County, North Carolina. *J. Pediatr.* 81:765, 1972.
   There was 1 case per 1600 children under 6 years of age. The attack rate for black infants was 4 times that for white children.

Diagnosis

5. Petito, F., and Plum, F. The lumbar puncture. *N. Engl. J. Med.* 290: 225, 1974.
   A brief editorial reviewing the practical aspects of the procedure.
6. Gururaj, V., et al. To tap or not to tap. . .*Clin. Pediatr.* (Phila.) 12:488, 1973.
   A chart review of 709 children who underwent lumbar puncture and an attempt to find the formula for predicting a "positive" tap; none was found. The signs and symptoms in bacterial meningitis, viral meningitis, and no meningitis are displayed and contrasted. (What else causes a stiff neck? See Clin. Pediatr. [Phila.] 21:559, 1982.)
7. Onorato, I., Wormser, G., and Nicholas, P. "Normal" CSF in bacterial meningitis. *Case reports and a review of the literature; "normal" CSF (cell count, protein and glucose values, and gram-stained smear) neither excludes early bacterial meningitis nor precludes its development. ("Correcting" WBC count for RBCs not valid: Am. J. Clin. Pathol. 82:95, 1984; Arch. Neurol. 41:1084, 1984.)*
8. Donald, P., Malan, C., and van der Walt, A. Simultaneous determination of cerebrospinal fluid glucose and blood glucose concentrations in the diagnosis of bacterial meningitis. *J. Pediatr.* 103:413, 1983.
   The values in patients with bacterial meningitis (119) are compared with those in patients with aseptic meningitis (97) or no meningitis (133); data are well displayed. "Realistic lower limits of 'normal'" proposed: CSF-blood glucose ratio of 40 percent or an absolute CSF glucose concentration of 40 mg/dl. (Differential diagnosis of low CSF sugar: Pediatrics 58:67, 1976; mechanisms for low CSF sugar in meningitis: Pediatrics 44:1, 1969.)
9. Provine, H., and Gardner, P. The gram-stained smear and its interpretation. *Hosp. Pract.* 9(10):85, 1974.
   A review of the procedure, with color illustrations of what to expect. (Also see P. Gardner and H. Provine, Manual of Acute Bacterial Infections: Early Diagnosis and Treatment (2nd ed.). Boston: Little, Brown, 1984.)
10. Lewin, E. Partially treated meningitis. *Am. J. Dis. Child.* 128:145, 1974.
    An editorial review; concludes that it is rare for oral antibiotic treatment prior to diagnosis to alter all CSF parameters; briefly reviews adjunct laboratory tests. (Update on rapid diagnostic techniques: Pediatr. Infect. Dis. 1:366, 1982.)

Treatment

11. Kaplan, S., and Feigin, R. Treatment of meningitis in children. *Pediatr. Clin. North Am.* 30:259, 1983.
    A treatment plan is proposed, including aspects of supportive care.
12. McCracken, G. Management of bacterial meningitis in infants and children: Current status and future prospects. *Am. J. Med.* 76(5A):215, 1984.
    A review of newer antibiotics and modalities of treatment.
13. Fulginiti, V. Treatment of meningitis in a very young infant. *Am. J. Dis. Child.* 137:1043, 1983.
    A one-page editorial review of problems in selecting initial therapy for the treatment of meningitis in infants 0 to 8 weeks of age; recommendations offered.
14. Durack, D., and Spanos, A. End-of-treatment spinal tap in bacterial meningitis: Is it worthwhile? *J.A.M.A.* 248:75, 1982.
    Not worthwhile in review of 165 cases. (Similar conclusion: Pediatrics 67:188, 1981.)

Complications

15. Feigin, R., and Kaplan, S. Inappropriate secretion of antidiuretic hormone in children with bacterial meningitis. *Am. J. Clin. Nutr.* 30:1482, 1977.
    Common (58%) and associated with neurologic sequelae.
16. Benson, P., et al. The prognosis of subdural effusions complicating pyogenic meningitis. *J. Pediatr.* 57:670, 1960.
    As common in pneumococcal as in H. influenzae *meningitis; tapping was associated with cessation of seizures in 60 percent and with relief of irritability, but did not seem to help fever, lethargy, coma, or signs of recurrent or persistent meningeal infection.*
17. Bodino, J., et al. Computed tomography in purulent meningitis. *Am. J. Dis. Child.* 136:495, 1982.
    When to look and what you see. (Also see J. Pediatr. 96:820, 1980.)
18. Rutman, D., and Wald, E. Fever, in *Haemophilus influenzae* type b meningitis. *Clin. Pediatr.* (Phila.) 20:192, 1981.
    Distinguishes secondary fever from prolonged fever; only the latter associated with higher rate of neurologic complications.

Sequelae

19. Sell, S. Long term sequelae of bacterial meningitis in children. *Pediatr. Infect. Dis.* 2:90, 1983.
    A review, with discussion of each sequela individually. (New data regarding hearing loss: N. Engl. J. Med. 311:869, 1984.)

Prevention

20. Nelson, J. How preventable is bacterial meningitis? *N. Engl. J. Med.* 307:1265, 1982.
    An editorial review of communicability and prevention. ("Guidelines for dealing with the guidelines" regarding Haemophilus: J. Pediatr. 105:761, 1984.)

Aseptic Meningitis

21. Feigin, R., and Shackelford, P. Value of repeat lumbar puncture in the differential diagnosis of meningitis. *N. Engl. J. Med.* 289:571, 1973.
    A repeat lumbar puncture in 6 to 8 hours confirmed the impression of aseptic meningitis in 87 percent.
22. Singer, J., et al. Management of central nervous system infections during an epidemic of enteroviral aseptic meningitis. *J. Pediatr.* 96:559, 1980.
    More than 450 patients in a 3-month period; findings presented. (Also see reference 6.)
23. Sells, C., Carpenter, R., and Ray, C. Sequelae of central-nervous-system enterovirus infections. *N. Engl. J. Med.* 293:1, 1975.
    A frequently quoted article suggesting that aseptic meningitis is not as benign as commonly thought when contracted in the first year of life; interpretation questioned, p. 609. (Also see Pediatrics 67:811, 1981.)

4. UPPER AIRWAY OBSTRUCTION
Kenneth B. Roberts

Because of its size and structure, the upper airway in infants and children produces clinically apparent signs (such as stridor) with even a mild degree of obstruction. Resistance to air flow is proportional to the radius of the airway to the fourth power (r^4) if flow is laminar, to the fifth power (r^5) if flow is turbulent. Thus, a small amount of narrowing of an already small airway can greatly compromise flow. Moreover, the submucosa is "loose," which is conducive to the accumulation of edema fluid, but the confines of the airway are rigid and cartilaginous; any accumulation, then, encroaches on the lumen of the airway. A final factor contributing to the vulnerability of the infant to upper airway obstruction is the short distance between the pharynx and the trachea; compromise that in an adult can be localized to a relatively short portion of the upper airway may appear more generalized in the very small infant.

Many ways of organizing a differential diagnosis of the 30 to 40 causes of upper airway obstruction have been proposed: by age of the patient; by relationship of the lesion to the airway (intrinsic-extrinsic); by the level of the lesion (supraglottic-glottic-subglottic); or by the pathophysiologic process producing upper airway obstruction (e.g., infectious, neoplastic). In practice, however, the clinician uses all these simultaneously to arrive at the most likely diagnosis, recognizing that all but a few causes are uncommon.

Laryngomalacia and *congenital stridor* are terms used for an entity that usually is manifest in the first few months of life. Characteristically, the infant appears to be normal except for stridor, which is particularly audible when the infant is supine or excited. With additional airway compromise, such as during episodes of upper respiratory tract infection, the stridor may be accentuated, and the infant may require medical attention. Direct laryngoscopy reveals the epiglottis, arytenoid cartilage, and aryepiglottic folds to be "floppy" and drawn into the larynx during inspiratory effort. The condition commonly becomes more severe during the first year of life but then gradually improves, with complete clinical recovery.

The most common cause of upper airway obstruction in infants is *viral croup*. The majority of cases occur between October and April in infants 3 months to 3 years of age; boys outnumber girls 2 to 1. The signs and symptoms of upper airway obstruction appear after several days of upper respiratory tract infection. The child has stridor and the characteristic barking, croupy cough; retractions and dyspnea, with increased efforts during inspiration, are present. Anxiety usually exacerbates the infant's difficulties, and there may be progression to fatigue, restlessness, and air hunger. The respiratory rate is a good estimate of the arterial oxygen tension: as the respiratory rate increases from 20 to 45, arterial PO_2 decreases linearly from 90 to 60 mm Hg. The respiratory rate does not reflect the PCO_2, which is usually normal despite the hypoxia; an explanation for the disproportionate hypoxia is that the marked inspiratory effort with upper airway obstruction creates sufficient intrathoracic negative pressure to cause pulmonary edema.

Tracheostomy or intubation has been performed in up to 13 percent of hospitalized patients with croup in some older reports; mortality has been as high as 2.7 percent. Various agents, including corticosteroids, have been administered in an effort to reduce mortality and the need for tracheostomy, but no controlled study has provided convincing evidence that these goals are accomplished by corticosteroid therapy. Racemic epinephrine does not affect the duration of hospitalization, but it does provide rapid transient relief; repeated courses, frequently administered, have been used to forestall—and in some cases obviate—the need for tracheostomy. Antibiotics are not warranted in the usual uncomplicated case of croup; parainfluenza virus is the usual etiologic agent. Humidity, given by vaporizer or inhalation of steam at home or by "croup tent" in the hospital, is the time-honored mainstay of therapy. The duration of the illness is from 1 to 14 days; 13 percent of patients have a recurrence.

Spasmodic croup is an entity of unknown pathogenesis; many presume it to be allergic. Episodes are brief, begin in the evening, occur without a prodromal upper respiratory infection (URI), and tend to be recurrent.

A more serious form of infection-produced upper airway obstruction is *epiglottitis*. Two-thirds of patients are between ages 3 and 7; males again predominate 2 to 1. The course of the illness in children with epiglottitis is notoriously brief—a matter of hours from the onset of symptoms to total airway obstruction. There is no prodrome; sore throat and fever develop, and within hours the child assumes a characteristic posture, with protrusion of the jaw, drooling, refusal to swallow, muffled phonation, and an anxious appearance. On presentation, one-half the patients are agitated, and one-half are limp. The degree of severe prostration out of proportion to the duration of symptoms is characteristic and should suggest the clinical diagnosis of epiglottitis.

Attempts to visualize the epiglottis by forcible depression of the tongue may precipitate total airway obstruction and are therefore contraindicated. When the diagnosis is in question, a lateral x-ray film of the neck is a reliable means of detecting swelling of the epiglottis without the risk associated with direct visualization. Mortality can be reduced from 24 to 2 percent by the provision of an airway; nasotracheal intubation or tracheostomy should be performed "semielectively" for each patient with epiglottitis as soon as possible. Unlike croup, which often lasts for several days, epiglottitis is a brief illness when successfully treated, and the mechanical airway need be provided only for a short time (less than a day or two for most patients). Epiglottitis is caused by *Haemophilus influenzae* type b; at present, chloramphenicol is the antibiotic of choice. Racemic epinephrine and corticosteroids are of no value in this disease.

Since infants and toddlers commonly explore their world by taste as well as by touch, ingested and aspirated foreign bodies are a problem in this age group. The anatomic site of the foreign body is the gastrointestinal tract twice as often as the respiratory tract. The common areas of obstruction are the esophagus at the level of the cricopharyngeal muscle, the aortic arch, and the gastric inlet; less common sites are the pylorus and the distal duodenum proximal to the ligament of Treitz. In the respiratory tract, foreign bodies tend to lodge in the bronchi more commonly than in the trachea or the larynx. Foreign bodies in the respiratory tract are removed at bronchoscopy.

General

1. Hollinger, P., and Johnston, K. Factors responsible for laryngeal obstruction in infants. *J.A.M.A.* 143:1229, 1950.
   Facts and figures.
2. Green, M. *Pediatric Diagnosis* (3rd ed.). Philadelphia: Saunders, 1980. P. 489.
   A short general discussion of stridor and an extensive differential diagnosis.
3. Davis, H., et al. Acute upper airway obstruction: Croup and epiglottitis. *Pediatr. Clin. North Am.* 28:859, 1981.
   Includes the general approach to acute upper airway obstruction and differential diagnosis in addition to discussion of croup and epiglottitis. (Other Pediatr. Clin. North Am. *reviews: 26:931, 1979, and 26:565, 1979.)*

Croup

4. Denny, F., et al. Croup: An 11-year study in a pediatric practice. *Pediatrics* 71:871, 1983.
   Parainfluenza virus continues to be the main cause, although other agents get into the act.
5. Newth, C., et al. The respiratory status of children with croup. *J. Pediatr.* 81:1068, 1972.
   The respiratory rate is a good indicator of PaO_2. The decrease in PaO_2 is disproportionate to the degree of hypercapnea, suggesting the presence of pulmonary edema. (Suggestion confirmed: Pediatrics *59:695, 1977.)*
6. Taussig, L., et al. Treatment of laryngotracheobronchitis (croup). *Am. J. Dis. Child.* 129:790, 1975.
   Racemic epinephrine is of acute, short-lived benefit, but it does not shorten the duration of the disease. (Confirmed: Am. J. Dis. Child. *132:484, 1978. Nebulization is as good as IPPB:* J. Pediatr. *101:1028, 1982.)*
7. Tunnessen, W., and Feinstein, A. The steroid-croup controversy: An analytic review of methodologic problems. *J. Pediatr.* 96:751, 1980.
   Nine studies analyzed for quality of design. (Steroids effective in spasmodic croup but not in infectious: Am. J. Dis. Child. *137:941, 1983.)*
8. Loughlin, G., and Taussig, L. Pulmonary function in children with a history of laryngotracheobronchitis. *J. Pediatr.* 94:365, 1979.

Children with croup in the past had higher rate of bronchial reactivity irrespective of allergy or baseline function. (Similar findings: Am. Rev. Resp. Dis. *122:95, 1980.)*

Epiglottitis

9. Rapkin, R. The diagnosis of epiglottitis: Simplicity and reliability of radiographs of the neck in the differential diagnosis of the croup syndrome. *J. Pediatr.* 80:96, 1972.
   Pediatricians can reliably assess epiglottis by x-ray study.
10. Myers, M. More on treatment of epiglottitis. *J. Pediatr.* 83:168, 1973.
    A summary of 17 reported series (with references), demonstrating a reduction in mortality associated with provision of an airway (2% versus 24%).
11. Rapkin, R. Nasotracheal intubation in epiglottitis. *Pediatrics* 56:110, 1975.
    One of many papers expressing a preference for routine nasotracheal intubation (by a previous advocate of tracheostomy).
12. Adair, J., and Ring, W. Management of epiglottitis in children. *Anesth. Analg.* 54:622, 1975.
    No place for racemic epinephrine. The epiglottis returns to normal quickly on therapy, within 12 to 14 hours, permitting early extubation or decannulation.
13. Rothstein, P., and Lister, G. Epiglottitis: Duration of intubation and fever. *Anesth. Analg.* 62:785, 1983.
    Mean duration of intubation was 36 hours but with marked variation between patients; authors recommend direct observation of epiglottis before extubation.

Foreign Bodies

14. Baker, S., and Fisher, R. Childhood asphyxiation by choking or suffocation. *J.A.M.A.* 244: 1343, 1980.
    A review of deaths in Maryland, 1970–1978, by age and object; recommendations offered. (For a review of childhood asphyxiation by food objects, see J.A.M.A. *251:2231, 1984.)*
15. Greensher, J., and Mofenson, H. Emergency treatment of the choking child. *Pediatrics* 70:110, 1982.
    One of three articles addressing the controversy between the Heimlich maneuver (pp. 113, 120) and back blows—chest thrust (p. 110). Also see the subsequent commentaries by Day: Pediatrics *71:300, 976, 1983.*
16. Kosloske, A. Tracheobronchial foreign bodies in children: Back to the bronchoscope and a balloon. *Pediatrics* 66:321, 1980.
    Forget inhalation and postural drainage. (Author's experience with 41 children: Am. J. Dis. Child. *136:924, 1982; series of 200 cases:* Am. J. Dis. Child. *134:68, 1980.)*

Other

17. Quinn-Bogard, A., and Potsic, W. Stridor in the first year of life. *Clin. Pediatr.* (Phila.) 16:913, 1977.
    A review of 63 infants, approximately one-half of whom had either congenital subglottic stenosis, laryngomalacia, or unilateral vocal cord paralysis; 16 less common conditions were seen in the other 33 patients. (For a review of congenital anomalies of the larynx, with color photographs, see Am. J. Dis. Child. *138:35, 1984.)*
18. Smith, G., and Cooper, D. Laryngomalacia and inspiratory obstruction in later childhood. *Arch. Dis. Child.* 56:345, 1981.
    Pulmonary function test abnormalities persist long after stridor is no longer audible.
19. Marshak, G., and Grundfast, K. Subglottic stenosis. *Pediatr. Clin. North Am.* 28:941, 1981.
    Considers both congenital and acquired stenosis.
20. Jones R., Santos, J., and Overall, J. Bacterial tracheitis. *J.A.M.A.* 242:721, 1979.
    Characteristically, preschool children with high fever, toxicity, and purulent tracheal secretions; usually caused by S. aureus. *(Also see* Clin. Pediatr. *[Phila.] 22:407, 1983; also called membranous laryngotracheobronchitis:* Pediatrics *70:705, 1982.)*
21. McCook, T., and Felman, A. Retropharyngeal masses in infants and young children. *Am. J. Dis. Child.* 133:41, 1979.
    Six case reports, with x rays, and discussion of differential diagnosis.
22. Gross, S., and Nieburg, P. Ludwig angina in childhood. *Am. J. Dis. Child.* 131:291, 1977.

Reminder about an uncommon entity. (In young adults: J.A.M.A. *243:1171, 1980.)*

23. Mandel, E., and Reynolds, C. Sleep disorders associated with upper airway obstruction in children. *Pediatr. Clin. North Am.* 28:897, 1981.
    Discusses etiology and pathophysiology, clinical and laboratory findings, diagnosis and treatment.

5. RESPIRATORY FAILURE AND STATUS ASTHMATICUS
Dennis C. Stokes

Acute respiratory failure in infants and children is the most common medical emergency faced by those caring for children. Although respiratory failure is usually defined operationally as synonymous with need for mechanical ventilatory assistance (based on a $PCO_2 > 65$ mm Hg), it should be recognized that any degree of hypoxia or hypercapnea signifies that numerous compensatory mechanisms have failed. The most common underlying causes of respiratory failure in the first 2 years of life are pneumonia, upper airway obstruction, and status asthmaticus; the most frequent in older children are status asthmaticus, heart disease, and accidents (e.g., drowning, smoke inhalation). Although the ensuing discussion focuses on status asthmaticus, the same general considerations apply in any disorder that may progress to respiratory failure: required are an understanding of the pathophysiology of the process, adequate assessment of the clinical status of the patient, and institution of rational supportive treatment.

Status asthmaticus is a clinical state in which a patient's asthma has become refractory to outpatient management, determined most often by lack of response to epinephrine. Status asthmaticus is rarely an acute event; more often, it has its beginnings in the previous days or weeks, with the patient's (or his physician's) inattention to symptoms or misuse of medications. Failure to recognize status asthmaticus leads to continued futile attempts at outpatient management. The duration of symptoms in asthma influences the severity and ease of reversing the physiologic abnormalities; thus, delay in hospitalization and appropriate therapy can lead to disastrous results, including death.

The factors that must be evaluated in the acute asthmatic patient include the promptness of response to the usual outpatient pharmacologic agents, recent history of symptoms, past history of severe asthma, and presence of complicating factors such as fatigue, steroid dependence, infection, and anxiety.

The pathophysiology of acute severe asthma involves widespread obstruction of predominately larger airways by bronchiolar smooth-muscle spasm, mucosal edema, and mucous secretions; of these, extensive mucous plugging is the most frequently found in autopsy series. This progressive mucous plugging probably accounts for the relationship between the duration of symptoms and diminished responsiveness to therapy. Uneven distribution of ventilation produced by uneven airway obstruction leads to ventilation-perfusion mismatching and hypoxemia; the PO_2 falls early, well before the arterial PCO_2 starts to rise. Increased alveolar ventilation—the result of hypoxemia, stimulation of intrapulmonary stretch receptors, and anxiety—produces a reduced PCO_2. It is only when either (1) respiratory efforts are inadequate, due to fatigue or oversedation, or (2) the progressive increase in physiologic "dead space" (areas not participating in gas exchange but still ventilated) cannot be overcome by increased overall ventilation, that arterial PCO_2 begins to rise to normal or—more ominously—above normal. The initial fall and later rise of PCO_2 is important to recognize, since a "normal" PCO_2 may represent the critical period of a worsening course. A mixed metabolic and respiratory acidosis then occurs, with further tissue hypoxia, aggravated by the increased metabolic demands of breathing (due both to the increased rate and the increased work of breathing at high lung volumes).

Physical signs of impending respiratory failure may be misleading if one presumes that decreases in retractions and wheezing indicate improvement; they may in fact indicate maximal hyperexpansion with little air exchange and may demand emergency measures. Sternocleidomastoid retractions are a reliable indicator of the severity of obstruction; also signs of severe disease are cyanosis despite the administration of oxygen, changes in consciousness (hypoxic agitation or hypercapneic somnolence), and the presence of pulsus paradoxus. Measurement of arterial oxygen and carbon dioxide tensions and pH is essential and provides quantitative data both for initial evaluation and for monitoring response to therapy.

Respiratory failure is usually an avoidable complication of status asthmaticus if pharmacologic treatment to reverse airway obstruction is early and vigorous. Currently, management includes supplemental oxygen (bronchodilator therapy may initially produce a fall in PO_2), continuous intravenous theophylline, and adrenergic agents. Newer, more selective beta-2 adrenergic agents, such as salbutamol or metaproterenol, are often used instead of epinephrine. Delivery of these bronchodilators by the aerosol route is particularly effective. The role of corticosteroids in the management of acute asthma remains controversial, since steroids do not result in greater improvements in lung function than sympathomimetic agents.

Infection is a frequent precipitating factor in status asthmaticus, although fever and atelectasis commonly occur without other evidence of infection. The hazards of empirical antibiotic therapy must be weighed against the evidence that infection is a frequent contributing factor in deaths due to asthma.

Dehydration as a result of poor intake or vomiting, coupled with hyperventilation, is common with severe asthma and should be corrected rapidly to prevent worsening or acidosis. Attempts to overhydrate in order to "liquefy" inspissated mucous plugs are futile, however, and, because of the large negative pleural pressures in acute asthma, may result in pulmonary edema. Adequate humidification of inspired oxygen and vigorous pulmonary toilet are the preferred methods of mobilizing secretions; physiotherapy has no effect in reversing bronchospasm, however.

Nebulizers are widely used to deliver pharmacologic agents directly to the airways. Intermittent positive pressure breathing (IPPB) has been used in the past but is now recognized as hazardous, since the lungs are maximally distended, and positive airway pressure may produce pneumothorax or pneumomediastinum and is associated with increased mortality.

Respiratory acidosis developing during acute asthma is an ominous sign. There is evidence that acidosis limits the effectiveness of bronchodilator therapy. Although the administration of bicarbonate appears attractive, the potential risks in the absence of effective ventilation are well documented: the bicarbonate is converted to carbon dioxide that cannot be "blown off," so that the blood PCO_2 may rise even higher; the blood-brain barrier is freely diffusible to carbon dioxide (but not bicarbonate), resulting in worsening of central nervous system acidosis. If ventilation is improved, by mechanical ventilation or improvement in pulmonary function, a "rebound" metabolic alkalosis may result as PCO_2 falls.

For the child in whom the arterial PCO_2 is above 65 mm Hg or whose course suggests increasing fatigue or persistent severe hypoxemia, endotracheal intubation and assisted ventilation are necessary. Continuous intravenous infusion of isoproterenol has been used successfully in some children with a rising PCO_2 to forestall or obviate the need for mechanical ventilation. Continuous ECG monitoring during this therapy is mandatory because of the risk of cardiac dysrhythmias. Controlled ventilation with a volume-limited respirator, low inspiratory flow rates, and neuromuscular paralysis is usually effective for the patients who require mechanical support; assisted (patient-initiated) ventilation is less useful in children, since they frequently fail to coordinate with the ventilator. High peak pressures may be required in severe airway obstruction, and there is a high risk of "barotrauma"-related complications, including subcutaneous emphysema (23%), pneumothorax (7%), and tension pneumothorax and cardiac tamponade (3%).

With presently available therapy, death from status asthmaticus should be a rare event. When it occurs, it is usually associated with infection, oversedation, drug toxicity, or inadequate doses of drugs. Although death is rare, morbidity, both physical and emotional, is not, emphasizing the need for preventive management.

Reviews

1. Downes, J., et al. Acute respiratory failure in infants and children. *Pediatr. Clin. North Am.* 19:423, 1972.
   A successful general approach to the therapy of respiratory failure from various causes (97 references).

2. Seibert, E., and Weiss, E. Status Asthmaticus. In E. Weiss and M. Segal (eds.), *Bronchial Asthma: Mechanisms and Therapeutics* (2nd ed.) Boston: Little, Brown, 1985.
   An excellent source for in-depth reviews.
3. Heiser, M., and Downes, J. Acute Respiratory Failure in Infants and Children Due to Lower Respiratory Tract Obstructive Disorders. In W. Shoemaker, et al. (eds.), *Textbook of Critical Care.* Philadelphia: Saunders, 1984.
   The text also contains sections on other major causes of respiratory failure (e.g., infections, drowning).
4. Newth, C. Recognition and management of respiratory failure. *Pediatr. Clin. North Am.* 26:617, 1979.
   Includes 60 references. (Also see Pediatr. Rev. 3:247, 1982.)

Assessment
5. McFadden, E., Kisen, R., and deGroot, W. Acute bronchial asthma: Relations between clinical and physiologic manifestations.*N. Engl. J. Med.* 288:221, 1973.
   In adults, sternocleidomastoid muscle retraction was consistently correlated with severe impairment of pulmonary function, while dyspnea and wheezing were not; holds true for children, too (Pediatrics *58:537, 1976).*
6. Rebuck, A., and Pengelly, L. Development of pulsus paradoxus in the presence of airway obstruction. *N. Engl. J. Med.* 288:66, 1973.
   Found in patients breathing at very high lung volumes, with high intraalveolar pressures limiting right ventricular filling.
7. Downes, J., et al. Arterial blood gases and acid-base disorders in infants and children with status asthmaticus. *Pediatrics* 42:238, 1968.
   The sequence of blood gas changes.
8. Ownby, D., et al. Attempting to predict hospital admission in acute asthma. *Am. J. Dis. Child.* 138:1062, 1984.
   Initial peak flow and duration of symptoms appear to be predictive when applied to a group of patients but not for admission of individual patients.

Therapy
9. Loughnan, P., et al. Pharmacokinetic analysis of the disposition of intravenous theophylline in young children. *J. Pediatr.* 88:874, 1976.
   How to achieve and maintain therapeutic levels of theophylline intravenously. (A frequent problem is the need to administer aminophylline to children who have recently received oral theophylline: J. Pediatr. 97:301, 1980; serum levels should be obtained and sympathomimetics used alone until a safe dosage can be determined: J. Pediatr. 98:678, 1981.)
10. Pierson, W., Bierman, C., and Kelley, V. A double-blind trial of corticosteroid therapy in status asthmaticus. *Pediatrics* 54:282, 1972.
    Improvement in hypoxemia, but not in FEV_1 compared with controls. (Also see J. Pediatr. 96:596, 1980.)
11. Chang, N., and Levison, H. The effect of a nebulized bronchodilator administered with or without intermittent positive pressure breathing on ventilatory function in children with cystic fibrosis and asthma. *Am. Rev. Respir. Dis.* 106:867, 1972.
    Isoproterenol administered by IPPB was no more effective than administration by a powered nebulizer. (For a general review of aerosolized bronchodilators useful in acute asthma, see Am. Rev. Resp. Dis. 122:89, 1980.)
12. Wood, D., et al. Intravenous isoproterenol in the management of respiratory failure in childhood status asthmaticus. *J. Allergy Clin. Immunol.* 50:75, 1972.
    Effective (also see Am. J. Dis. Child. 130:39, 1976), but poses the risk of cardiac dysrhythmias and myocardial ischemia (J. Pediatr. 92:776, 1978).

Complications
13. Bierman, C. Pneumomediastinum and pneumothorax complicating asthma in children. *Am. J. Dis. Child.* 114:42, 1967.
    May occur spontaneously or as complication of ventilator management. ("Controlled hypoventilation" to minimize barotrauma: Am. Rev. Respir. Dis. 129:385, 1984.)

14. Stalcup, A., and Mellins, R. Mechanical forces producing pulmonary edema in acute asthma. *N. Engl. J. Med.* 297:592, 1977.
    Marked negative pleural pressures favor accumulation of interstitial fluid.

Outcome

15. Buranakul, G., et al. Causes of death during acute asthma in children. *Am. J. Dis. Child.* 128:343, 1974.
    Infection, oversedation, drug toxicity, and inadequate therapy.

6. CONGESTIVE HEART FAILURE
Robert D. White and Jean S. Kan

Congestive heart failure (CHF) that has its onset in childhood after the newborn period may be caused by congenital cardiac abnormalities (e.g., aortic stenosis, pulmonic stenosis, coarctation of the aorta), by acquired heart disease (e.g., rhythm abnormalities, myocarditis, cardiomyopathy, rheumatic heart disease, mitral valve prolapse, hypertension), or by noncardiac disorders (e.g., anemia, metabolic disease, drug toxicity). The mechanism of CHF in these disorders relates to: (1) an increased work load of the heart (pressure overload, as in aortic stenosis, or volume overload, as in AV valve regurgitation), (2) altered myocardial function (e.g., from myocarditis, myocardial ischemia), or (3) a combination of both factors.

In the pediatric age group, tachypnea and cardiomegaly are the most consistent signs of CHF; it is rare for heart failure to be present without them. Tachycardia, exercise intolerance (manifested in infants as rapid fatigue during feedings), diaphoresis, hepatomegaly, and a diastolic gallop are also present in a majority of patients; no one of these signs is specific for CHF, but as a symptom complex they are quite distinctive. Edema and rales are frequently present in children, but are uncommon in infants; isolated ("pure") right or left ventricular failure may also be found in children, but infants usually have signs of biventricular failure.

The signs and symptoms of CHF reflect the body's compensatory attempts to improve myocardial function or decrease the work load of the heart. Cardiomegaly is the result of ventricular dilatation. Tachypnea and rales reflect pulmonary venous congestion due to elevated left ventricular end-diastolic pressure (which increases myocardial contractility through the Frank-Starling mechanism); similarly, peripheral edema and hepatomegaly reflect elevated right ventricular end-diastolic pressure. Diastolic filling of the ventricle under these conditions produces an S3 or S4 (less specifically called a "gallop" rhythm), due to reduced ventricular compliance. Tachycardia, diaphoresis, and peripheral vascular vasoconstriction are the result of increased sympathetic tone, which improves cardiac function through inotropic and chronotropic stimulation of the myocardium. Exercise intolerance and salt and water retention are produced in part by reduction of blood flow to the muscles and kidneys, respectively, when cardiac output is decreased.

The history, physical examination, and laboratory evaluation of a patient with CHF are directed toward diagnosis of the underlying disorder and assessment of the severity of heart failure. Laboratory evaluation should include serum electrolytes and tests to exclude anemia and kidney disease; the measurement of blood gases is also indicated in patients with moderate or severe distress. The chest radiograph and ECG are helpful in estimating cardiac chamber enlargement, pulmonary vascular congestion, and disorders of cardiac rhythm; the latter can be further defined by 24-hour Holter monitoring and stress ECG, if necessary. The two-dimensional echocardiogram defines cardiac structure and assesses myocardial function and chamber size. Cardiac catheterization is indicated to define structural abnormalities prior to surgical correction or to evaluate the physiologic effects of myocardial stimulation with inotropic agents or vasodilators.

Definitive treatment of CHR is control or resolution of the underlying disorder. In children with cardiac disorders, this may entail correction of the anatomic lesion, placement of a pacemaker for control of bradydysrhythmias, or cardiac transplantation. If definitive therapy is not immediately feasible, palliative treatment may improve cardiac function and decrease metabolic requirements of the body. Dobutamine is a potent cardiac stimulant that may be administered intravenously in the acute phase of myocardial support in an intensive care setting. Digoxin, a cardiac glycoside, is a positive inotropic agent that may be indicated for long-term therapy of disorders that impair myocardial contractility directly or through chronic overload of the heart. Hypokalemia and myocardial ischemia increase the toxicity of digitalis glycosides. Digoxin toxicity is uncommon in children but should be considered in the presence of bradydysrhythmias (sinus bradycardia, heart block, supraventricular ectopic beats) or persistent nausea and vomiting; ventricular dysrhythmias are rare in children with digoxin toxicity. Afterload reduction decreases the work load of the heart and should be considered in severe cases of myocardial dysfunction. Acutely, intravenous therapy with nitroprusside may be considered in an intensive care setting. Long-term oral therapy (e.g., with prazosin, hydralazine, or captopril) may result in symptomatic improvement.

Metabolic demands on the heart may be reduced by activity restriction and oxygen administration. Salt restriction and diuretic therapy may improve symptoms of systemic and pulmonary venous congestion but should be used with caution, since diuretics may significantly decrease the preload of the heart and thereby impair cardiac output through the Frank-Starling mechanism.

The prognosis for a patient with CHF depends primarily on the type and severity of the underlying disorder. Some disorders are relentlessly progressive (e.g., hypoplastic left heart syndrome, cor pulmonale), but in most patients a degree of symptomatic improvement can be achieved with medical management. Subsequently, spontaneous improvement or resolution is common in certain disorders (ventricular septal defect, patent ductus arteriosus, myocarditis), and correction of many others is possible through surgery (e.g., structural heart disease) or medical intervention (as in anemia and kidney disease).

Reviews

1. Braunwald, E. Heart failure: Pathophysiology and treatment. *Am. Heart J.* 102:486, 1981.
   Distillation of a lifetime of thought and research. (For a review by this author of current issues for research, see Am. J. Cardiol. 51: 603, 1983.)
2. Artman, M., Parrish, M., and Graham, T. Congestive heart failure in childhood and adolescence: Recognition and management. *Am. Heart J.* 105:471, 1983.
   Includes discussion of postoperative management. (Also see Pediatr. Rev.1:321, 1980.)
3. Keith, J., Rowe, R., and Vlad, P. *Heart Disease in Infancy and Childhood* (3rd ed.). New York: Macmillan, 1978.
   Most thorough discussion of nonanatomic causes of heart failure.

Biochemical and Hemodynamic Alterations

4. Katz, A. Congestive heart failure: Role of altered myocardial cellular control. *N. Engl. J. Med.* 293:1184, 1975.
   Is heart failure a protective mechanism for the overworked heart?
5. Cannon, P. The kidney in heart failure. *N. Engl. J. Med.* 296:26, 1977.
   Details renovascular, hormonal, and neural alterations.
6. Rook G., et al. Folic acid deficiency in infants and children with heart disease. *Br. Heart J.* 35:87, 1973.
   Folate and iron deficiency anemias are common.

Medical Management

7. Smith, T., and Haber, E. Digitalis. *N. Engl. J. Med.* 289:945, 1010, 1063, 1125, 1973.
   Thorough! Contains 336 references. (For a current update by the author, see Hosp. Pract. 19(3):67, 1984.)
8. Friedman, W., and George, B. New concepts and drugs in the treatment of congestive heart failure. *Pediatr. Clin. North Am.* 31:1197, 1984.
   Discussion of therapy to influence preload, contractility, and afterload, with age-related considerations.

9. Singh, S. Clinical pharmacology of digitalis glycosides: A developmental viewpoint. *Pediatr. Ann.* 5(9):81, 1976.
   The unique pharmacology of digitalis in children is emphasized.
10. Cohn, J. Indications for digitalis therapy: A new look. *J.A.M.A.* 229:1911, 1974.
    Digitalis is not always indicated in patients with heart failure. (Also see J. Pediatr. 92:867, 1978, and 106:66, 1985.)
11. Vanderhoof, J., et al. Continuous enteral feedings: An important adjunct to the management of complex congenital heart disease. *Am. J. Dis. Child.* 136:825, 1982.
    Weight gain doubled using this technique.
12. Maron, B., et al. Hypertrophic cardiomyopathy in infants: Clinical features and natural history. *Circulation* 65:7, 1982.
    Asymmetric septal hypertrophy was present in 80 percent.

Transplant Surgery
13. Reitz, B. Heart-lung transplantation: A review. *Heart Transplantation* 1:291, 1981.
    Minimum age requirements continue to decline.

7. DIABETIC KETOACIDOSIS
John T. Hayford, Jr., and Margaret E. Mohrmann

Diabetic ketoacidosis (DKA) is a life-threatening complication of diabetes mellitus (see Chap. 77), characterized by inadequate insulin activity, hyperglycemia, dehydration, metabolic acidosis, and ketosis. Hyperglycemia is the consequence of both decreased glucose utilization and augmented hepatic gluconeogenesis. In the absence of insulin, glucose is an obligate extracellular molecule; as the serum concentration of glucose rises, water is drawn from the intracellular compartment to maintain extracellular isotonicity, and intracellular dehydration results. The osmotic diuresis that accompanies the hyperglycemia leads to depletion of extracellular water as well. Inadequate insulin activity also permits accelerated lipolysis and oxidation of the free fatty acids to β-hydroxybutyric and acetoacetic acids, which induce a metabolic acidosis. (Acetone is also formed and gives a fruity odor to the patient's breath, but it does not contribute to the acidosis.) Variable degrees of lactic acidosis are also usually present. Insulin lack is the primary abnormality, but concentrations of glucagon, cortisol, growth hormone, and epinephrine are increased, and each hormone's anti-insulin activity contributes to the physiologic derangements.

Diabetic ketoacidosis is not difficult to recognize in a child with known diabetes who is dehydrated, hyperventilating, and obtunded. Diagnostic confusion is more likely in the child whose diabetes has not yet been recognized. Even in the ketosis-prone child with diabetes, however, the physician must consider alternative explanations for the clinical findings, such as Reye syndrome, toxic ingestion (especially salicylate or alcohol), and central nervous system infection or trauma. Persistent vomiting may suggest gastroenteritis or, with abdominal pain, acute appendicitis. The diagnosis of diabetes (if not already established) is suggested by a history of polyuria, polydipsia, polyphagia with weight loss, and lack of evidence for alternative diagnoses. Diabetic ketoacidosis is confirmed by the presence of hyperglycemia, acidosis, ketonuria, and ketonemia.

The initial evaluation includes assessment of circulatory status (pulse, blood pressure, peripheral perfusion) and degree of clinical dehydration. A careful search for a site of infection is made, since infection is often the event that triggers DKA. Electrolyte concentrations, blood gas tensions, and blood pH are determined to define the severity of acidosis and the degree of compensation, and to provide a baseline potassium concentration. (If hyperlipemia is present, the concentration of electrolytes will be artifactually lowered.)

The acute management of DKA is directed at correction of dehydration, acidosis, and hyperglycemia. Multiple treatment protocols have been proposed, but two principles must be applied in all cases: (1) Dehydration and acidosis are the metabolic derangements that will cause death imminently unless simple treatment is given promptly, and fluid therapy must not be delayed pending the administration of insulin or determination of electyrolyte concentrations. (2) All treatment protocols are merely guidelines for therapy and require modification according to the patient's response; careful monitoring of clinical and laboratory changes is essential for the successful management of DKA.

Sufficient fluid must be administered intravenously to replace the deficit (usually 5–7% of body weight in adolescents, more in younger children) and supply maintenance requirements, with attention to continued increased urinary losses due to the continued osmotic diuresis. An initial bolus of isotonic fluid is given rapidly to expand the vascular compartment and improve the poor peripheral circulation. Rehydration of the child with DKA (or other cause of hypertonic dehydration) must be carried out with caution to avoid potentially fatal cerebral edema. Because of large intracellular fluid losses, the child with DKA is almost invariably potassium-depleted at the time of diagnosis, although the serum potassium concentration is usually normal or elevated. Administration of insulin and correction of acidosis may result in severe hypokalemia, reflected by flat or inverted T waves on the ECG and requiring prompt intravenous potassium therapy. Early potassium supplementation, begun when the child first voids, usually prevents the fall to dangerously low concentrations.

Specific therapy for the acidosis of DKA remains controversial. Frequently, dramatic improvement results simply from initial expansion of extracellular fluid volume and reestablishment of adequate peripheral perfusion. An elevation in blood pH following bicarbonate administration may be attended by worsening acidosis in the central nervous system, since CO_2 diffuses across the blood-brain barrier but HCO_3 does not. Furthermore, the organic acids in DKA, in contrast to metabolic acidosis from other causes, are metabolized to bicarbonate. Thus, administration of "additional" bicarbonate may result in a late alkalosis. Bicarbonate may have a place in the treatment of DKA, but only in the more severe degrees of acidosis (pH less than 7.10–7.15), which may be associated with myocardial depression. If bicarbonate is given, the dosage is calculated to bring the pH only to the range of 7.2; slow infusion is preferable to bolus injection.

The administration of insulin is an essential but frequently abused aspect of therapy in DKA, especially when insufficient consideration is given to fluid and electrolyte management. Insulin therapy protocols are of two types: traditional high-dose and more recent low-dose regimens. The former are based on clinical observations of low mortality in patients receiving 1.0–1.5 units/kg subcutaneously. Low-dose protocols are designed to provide predictable, constant physiologic concentrations of circulating insulin. The concerns about a state of "insulin resistance" associated with acidosis, increasing patient age, or previous insulin requirements have been demonstrated by the success of these protocols to be unjustified. Continuous intravenous infusion allows close titration of the insulin dose to metabolic needs and results in a predictable rate of fall in blood glucose (approximately 80–100 mg/dl/hour). Moreover, the problems of erratic absorption from subcutaneous sites during dehydration and later "release" of insulin are obviated. Excessive insulin along with massive infusions of glucose-free fluid may precipitously drive glucose, potassium, and water intracellularly, leading to the three early complications of therapy: hypoglycemia, hypokalemia, and cerebral edema. All three are rare with careful management. Cerebral edema is particularly noteworthy because it may be irreversible; its pathogenesis is not always totally explicable.

Reviews
1. Sperling, M. Diabetic ketoacidosis. *Pediatr. Clin. North Am.* 31:591, 1984.
   An excellent, comprehensive, up-to-date review.
2. Schade, D., and Eaton, R. Diabetic ketoacidosis: Pathogenesis, prevention and therapy. *Clin. Endocrinol. Metab.* 12:321, 1983.
   A lucid review with appropriate emphasis on prevention.
3. Foster, D., and McGarry, J. The metabolic derangements and treatment of diabetic ketoacidosis. *N. Engl. J. Med.* 309:159, 1983.
   An elegant, concise explication of the abnormalities of glucose metabolism and ketogenesis. (Also see Ann. Intern. Med. 88:681,1978.)
4. Schwartz, R. Diabetic ketoacidosis and coma. *Pediatrics* 47:902, 1971.
   A comprehensive review of pathophysiology and clinical problems; treatment based on high-dose insulin protocol.

Evaluation

5. Campbell, I., et al. Abdominal pain in diabetic metabolic decompensation: Clinical significance. *J.A.M.A.* 233:166, 1975.
   Be suspicious of a cause other than DKA if HCO_3 is greater than 10 mEq/liter.
6. Stephens, J., Sulway, M., and Watkins, P. Relationship of blood acetoacetate and B-hydroxybutyrate in diabetes. *Diabetes* 20:485, 1971.
   Ratio of the two changes with therapy; since only acetoacetate is measured by usual methods, improvement may not be apparent by a test for "ketones" (but will be reflected in pH, HCO_3, and clinical response).

Electrolytes

7. Katz, M. Hyperglycemia-induced hyponatremia: Calculation of expected serum sodium depression. *N. Engl. J. Med.* 289:843, 1973.
   The serum sodium concentration decreases 1.6 mEq/liter for each 100 mg/dl increase in serum glucose.
8. Soler, N., et al. Electrocardiogram as a guide to potassium replacement in diabetic ketoacidosis. *Diabetes* 23:610, 1974.
   Useful.
9. Fisher, J., and Kitabchi, A. A randomized study of phosphate therapy in the treatment of diabetic ketoacidosis. *J. Clin. Endocrinol. Metab.* 57:177, 1983.
   The only significant difference between treated and untreated groups was lower ionized calcium levels in those receiving phosphate; a study reported in Am. J. Dis. Child. *137:241, 1983, showed no benefit from phosphate supplementation. (For a review of the clinical and biochemical effects of phosphate depletion, see* Hosp. Pract. *12(3):121, 1977.)*

Acidosis

10. Adrogue, H., et al. Plasma acid-base patterns in diabetic ketoacidosis. *N. Engl. J. Med.* 307:1603, 1982.
    A study and discussion of the nature of the acidosis, especially in reference to whether it is a "pure" anion gap acidosis.
11. Lever, E., and Jaspan, J. Sodium bicarbonate therapy in severe diabetic ketoacidosis. *Am. J. Med.* 75:263, 1983.
    A comparison study showing no advantage to the use of bicarbonate; the two classic articles on possible neurologic complications of alkali therapy are in N. Engl. J. Med. *277:605, 1967, and 284:283, 1971.*
12. Kaye, R. Diabetic ketoacidosis: The bicarbonate controversy. *J. Pediatr.* 87:156, 1975.
    An editorial review of the physiology of problems with and indications for bicarbonate administration in DKA.

Insulin

13. Lightner, E., Kappy, M., and Revsin, B. Low-dose intravenous insulin infusion in patients with diabetic ketoacidosis: Biochemical effects in children. *Pediatrics* 60:681, 1977.
    A simple and successful protocol. (Also see J. Pediatr. *87:846, 1975, for a slightly different method.)*
14. Edwards, G., et al. Effectiveness of low-dose continuous intravenous insulin in diabetic ketoacidosis. *J. Pediatr.* 91:701, 1977.
    A comparison of low-dose intravenous and high-dose intermittent subcutaneous administration; the former is "at least as effective," with less hypokalemia. (For other series supporting the use of a low-dose regimen, see J. Pediatr. *89:560, 1976, and Am. J. Dis. Child. 133:523, 1979.)*
15. Tamborlane, W., and Genel, M. Discordant correction of hyperglycemia and ketoacidosis with low-dose insulin infusion. *Pediatrics* 61:125, 1978.
    With low-dose insulin infusion, blood glucose concentration is lowered faster than ketones are cleared.
16. Weber, M., and Abbassi, V. Continuous intravenous insulin therapy in severe diabetic ketoacidosis: Variations in dosage requirements. *J. Pediatr.* 91:755, 1977.
    Not every child responds to the "usual" protocol; modifications may be needed.

Cerebral Edema

17. Arieff, A., and Kleeman, C. Studies on mechanisms of cerebral edema in diabetic comas: Effects of hyperglycemia and rapid lowering of plasma glucose in normal rabbits. *J. Clin. Invest.* 52:571, 1973.
    One mechanism by which cerebral edema may be produced; the clinical implications are clear.
18. Rosenbloom, A., et al. Cerebral edema complicating diabetic ketoacidosis in childhood. *J. Pediatr.* 96:357, 1980.
    Case reports plus literature review and speculative discussion of etiology; further discussion in a letter and reply in J. Pediatr. *98:674, 1981.*

8. ACUTE ABDOMEN
Kenneth B. Roberts

Abdominal pain is a common, usually self-limited problem in children, but it is dangerous to presume that abdominal pain represents a benign illness, since in the child whose pain signals the need for operative intervention, delay in diagnosis may be catastrophic. It is imperative that certain important diagnoses be entertained whenever abdominal pain is the complaint. In the newborn the acute abdomen may reflect obstruction or perforation: specific entities include necrotizing enterocolitis, malrotation, volvulus, congenital bands, atresias, meconium ileus, and aganglionic megacolon. Septicemia is also an important consideration in this age group. Between the ages of 1 month and 2 years, intussusception and incarcerated inguinal hernias must be considered. The infant with intussusception has colicky pain, draws up his legs as the intense pain comes, and then rests quietly between episodes. Characteristically, a sausage-shaped mass is palpable in the right upper quadrant, representing a portion of ileum trapped within the colon. Mucosal fragments and blood are passed per rectum, giving the stool the appearance of currant jelly. Not all intussusceptions are "classic," however, and recent reports have reemphasized "painless" intussusception. A barium enema examination is not only diagnostic but may be therapeutic as well, since raising the bag of barium 36 inches above the child often provides sufficient hydrostatic pressure to reduce the intussusception; greater heights may result in perforation and therefore are not used. Even in patients requiring laparotomy to reduce the intussusception, it is unusual to find pathologic "lead point" areas, such as a Meckel diverticulum, and the cause usually remains unclear.

After the age of 2 years, appendicitis is the principal diagnostic consideration in the acute abdomen. Appendicitis can and does occur during infancy, but is so uncommon that the correct diagnosis is usually not suspected until the appendix has perforated and the infant has become quite ill. In the somewhat older child, as in the adult, pain begins periumbilically and then migrates to the right lower quadrant. Vomiting is common only as a secondary sign, as in infants with intussusception; the occurrence of pain *prior* to the onset of vomiting is an important diagnostic feature. The presence of fever and neutrophilic leukocytosis is not a sine qua non for the diagnosis, since they are often not present in early disease; rather, they are correlated with late gangrenous changes or actual perforation of the appendix.

The initial step in the pathogenesis of appendicitis is considered to be obstruction of free communication between the appendix and the cecum. Venous congestion produces edema, which perpetuates the congestion, leading to ischemic necrosis and ultimately to perforation, with spillage of intestinal contents into the peritoneum. When engorgement alone is present, periumbilical pain is produced; later, as the peritoneum is irritated, the pain is referred to the right lower quadrant, and cutaneous hyperesthesia and rebound tenderness may be demonstrated. The location of the appendix will determine the presence or absence of other signs, such as pain on stretching the iliopsoas muscle, or urinary findings as a result of contact between the inflamed appendix and the right ureter.

Diagnostic clues on x-ray examination include the absence of gas in the right lower quadrant, scoliosis, presence of a "sentinel loop," and signs of ileus, perforation, or peritonitis. In addition, because of the importance of obstruction in the pathophysiology of appendicitis, much attention has been directed to fecoliths. It seems clear that in patients with established fecoliths in the appendix, the risk of the development of appendicitis, often with perforation, is increased, leading some authors to urge strongly that elective appendectomy be performed in any patient with a radiographically demonstrable "appendicolith."

Because the morbidity with appendicitis increases when gangrene or perforation occurs, early diagnosis and operative intervention have been stressed, and a removal rate of normal appendixes up to 20 percent has not been considered excessive. In the past decade, a period of in-hospital observation for patients whose clinical diagnosis is uncertain has been shown to permit a reduction in the rate of "negative" appendectomies without an increase in the rate of perforation.

Even when the diagnosis of appendicitis is clear, the time taken to prepare the acutely ill, dehydrated, febrile child for surgery is well worthwhile. If gangrene or perforation of the appendix is suspected clinically, the preoperative administration of antibiotics is a logical adjunct to fluid therapy. Postoperatively, peritoneal drains are not beneficial and appear to prolong the duration of fever. Early in the course, gram-negative sepsis is an uncommon but life-threatening complication; wound infection, though much less serious, is frequent following perforation or gangrene of the appendix, occurring in approximately 18 percent of patients. Intraabdominal abscesses are later complications in 2 to 6 percent of these patients, the result of persistent combined aerobic and anaerobic infection. Antibiotics alone may be insufficient to treat this complication, and reexploration is commonly required.

The clinical picture of appendicitis may be mimicked exactly in children by the disorder designated *acute mesenteric lymphadenitis*. The pain in this condition is often severe, but the child typically does not appear as ill as one with appendicitis. Close observation and repeated examinations usually permit differentiation of the two conditions, although laparotomy may be required. The visualized lymph nodes are acutely inflamed, often described as "succulent." Bacteria, such as streptococci and members of the *Yersinia* group, and viruses have been implicated.

Other serious causes of severe abdominal pain in childhood are myriad and include basilar pneumonia, pyelonephritis, pericarditis, herpes zoster, rheumatic fever, sickle cell anemia, Henoch-Schönlein syndrome, food poisoning, and metabolic disorders, such as hyperlipidemia, hypoglycemia, porphyria, and diabetic ketoacidosis. Torsion of the testis or ovary and pelvic inflammatory disease must be considered in the pubertal child. A detailed history and careful physical examination are the main tools in establishing at least a tentative diagnosis and identifying the child who requires immediate surgical attention.

General

1. Silen, W. *Cope's Early Diagnosis of the Acute Abdomen.* New York: Oxford University Press, 1979.
   A revision of Dr. Cope's classic.
2. Green, M. *Pediatric Diagnosis* (3rd ed.). Philadelphia: Saunders, 1980.
   The chapter on abdominal pain briefly considers more than 80 causes of acute abdominal pain (p. 325).

Appendicitis

3. Holgersen, L., and Stanley-Brown, E. Acute appendicitis with perforation. *Am. J. Dis. Child.* 122:288, 1971.
   A study of 100 cases. Earlier diagnosis and intervention are required! (Parent versus physician factors in delay of diagnosis: Pediatrics 63:37, 1979.)
4. White, J., Santillana, M., and Haller, J. Intensive in-hospital observation: A safe way to decrease unnecessary appendectomy. *Am. Surg.* 41:739, 1975.
   The "negative" appendectomy rate declined from 15 to 2 percent without an increase in perforation rate. (Early surgery rather than observation urged to decrease perforation rate: Pediatrics 70:414, 1982.)
5. Neuhauser, E. Acute appendicitis: The x-ray examination. *Postgrad. Med.* 45:64, 1969.
   Appendicoliths illustrated. (Barium enema proposed and illustrated: J. Pediatr. 92:451, 1978.)

6. Shaul, W. Clues to the early diagnosis of neonatal appendicitis. *J. Pediatr.* 98:473, 1981.
   Cutaneous, radiographic and urinary "clues" described.
7. Bartlett, R., Eraklis, A., and Wilkinson, R. Appendicitis in infancy. *Surg. Gynecol. Obstet.* 130:99, 1970.
   Uncommon and difficult under age 2 years. (Radiographic clues in this age group: Am. J. Dis. Child. *118:687, 1969.)*
8. Williamson, W., Bush, R., and Williams, L. Retrocecal appendicitis. *Am. J. Surg.* 141:507, 1981.
   Of nearly 500 patients with appendicitis, 21.8 percent had a retrocecal appendix; this group had relatively straightforward clinical presentations. The 2.5 percent who had a retroperitoneal, *retrocecal appendix had a more atypical presentation.*
9. Stone, H., et al. Perforated appendicitis in children. *Surgery* 69:673, 1971.
   Aspects of diagnosis are considered; preoperative administration of antibiotics is urged.
10. Stone, H. Bacterial flora of appendicitis in children. *J. Pediatr. Surg.* 11:37, 1976.
    Correlates clinical and bacteriologic findings; data are well presented with clear tables. (Same author on significance of anaerobes: Ann. Surg. *181:705, 1975.)*
11. Bartlett, J., et al. Therapeutic efficacy of 29 antimicrobial regimens in experimental intraabdominal sepsis. *Rev. Infect. Dis.* 3:535, 1981.
    Antibiotics active against coliforms prevent early sepsis; those active against Bacteroides fragilis *prevent late abscesses.*

Intussusception

12. Gierup, J., Jorulf, H., and Livaditis, A. Management of intussusception in infants and children: A survey based on 288 consecutive cases. *Pediatrics* 50:535, 1972.
    Stresses the limitations of the classic presentation in diagnosis. (Another large series: J. Pediatr. Surg. *6:16, 1971.)*
13. Rachmel. A., et al. Apathy as an early manifestation of intussusception. *Am. J. Dis. Child.* 137:701, 1983.
    Once thought to be a late sign, it appears the "knocked-out" appearance may be present early, too.
14. Rosenkrantz, J., et al. Intussusception in the 1970's: Indications for operation. *J. Pediatr.* 12:367, 1977.
    Barium enema was successful in more than 50 percent of attempts; peritonitis and obstruction are indications to bypass the x-ray department and proceed to the operating room.

Other Causes

15. Knight, P., and Vassy, L. Specific diseases mimicking appendicitis in childhood. *Arch. Surg.* 116:744, 1981.
    What the children who do not have appendicitis at laparotomy do have. (Also see Am. J. Surg. *144:335, 1982.)*
16. Blattner, R. Acute mesenteric lymphadenitis. *J. Pediatr.* 74:479, 1969.
    A short comment.
17. Nord, K., Rossi, T., and Lebenthal, E. Peptic ulcer in children. *Am. J. Gastroenterol.* 75:153, 1981.
    Gastric ulcers were more common than duodenal (17 : 11 ratio); cimetidine was no better than antacids.
18. Jordan, S., and Ament, M. Pancreatitis in children and adolescents. *J. Pediatr.* 91:211, 1977.
    Another uncommon cause to consider.
19. Shafer, M., Irwin, C., and Sweet, R. Acute salpingitis in the adolescent female. *J. Pediatr.* 100:339, 1982.
    Etiology, diagnosis, and treatment (11 pages, 83 references). For a discussion of both acute and chronic causes of abdominal pain in adolescent girls, see Pediatr. Rev *4:281, 1983.*
20. Williamson, R. Death in the scrotum: Testicular torsion. *N. Engl. J. Med.* 296:338, 1977.

*A one-page editorial review of the incidence, pathogenesis, course, and management.
(Nuclear scan may be helpful in diagnosis: Am. J. Dis. Child. 136:831, 1982.)
Also see specific chapters.*

9. ACUTE RENAL FAILURE
Richard A. Cohn

Acute renal failure (ARF) represents an abrupt decrease in renal function with consequent inability to maintain normal electrolyte, urea, creatinine, water, and acid-base balance. The hallmarks are oliguria (< 200 ml/sq m/day), acidosis, hyperkalemia, and azotemia. Causes may be classified as follows: *prerenal,* e.g., renal hypoperfusion due to hypovolemia, hypotension, or heart failure; *postrenal,* e.g., obstructive uropathy, stones, or tumors; or *renal,* i.e., parenchymal disorders of the kidney. The renal disorders are: (1) acute tubular necrosis (ATN), representing significant ischemic injury; (2) nephrotoxic injuries from drugs (indomethacin, gold, cis-platinum), chemical poisons (e.g., ethylene glycol, carbon tetrachloride, mercury), antibiotics (e.g., cephalosporins, aminoglycosides, penicillins), or endogenous metabolites (e.g., hypercalcemia, hyperuricemia, and myoglobinuria); and (3) a variety of disorders, such as the hemolytic-uremic syndrome, rapidly progressive glomerulonephritis, acute interstitial nephritis, and vasculitis.

The initial diagnostic consideration is to exclude prerenal and postrenal causes of ARF, since they are often reversible; if untreated, prerenal failure can develop into ATN. In addition, patients with stable chronic renal failure may have an acute deterioration in renal function due to dehydration, urinary tract infection, hypertension, obstruction, electrolyte imbalance, or acidosis, which, if successfully treated, may obviate the need for dialysis.

Laboratory studies can aid in separating prerenal causes from primary renal tubular dysfunction. In the former, the kidney responds "normally" to hypoperfusion by conserving salt and water, with resulting oliguria, high urine osmolality, and normal findings on urinalysis; the urine–plasma creatinine ratio is greater than 30, and the urinary sodium concentration is less than 20 mEq/liter. The fractional excretion of sodium (FE_{Na}) is less than 1 percent. In ATN, salt and water conservation is impaired, with ensuing isosthenuria, a urine-plasma creatinine ratio less than 20, a urinary sodium concentration greater than 30 mEq per liter and the FE_{Na} more than 2 percent; casts and protein and cellular elements are often seen in the urine. Occasionally, patients with ATN are not oliguric, although their degree of renal functional impairment may be as great as those with oliguria.

Three factors may participate in the pathophysiology of ATN; the relative contribution of each is controversial: (1) Mechanical intratubular obstruction to urine flow may occur from toxic injuries, myoglobinuria, urate nephropathy, and so on, causing low urinary flow and increased resorption of filtered solutes and water. (2) Alternatively, significant hypoxic injury to tubular epithelial cells may result in augmented resorption of filtrate from tubular lumens directly into peritubular capillaries (the "passive backflow" theory). (3) Damage to tubular cells with increased salt delivery to the macula densa of the distal tubule stimulates local renin-angiotensin release, leading to glomerular arteriolar constriction and a diminished glomerular filtration rate.

Diagnosis of cause of ARF and treatment usually are approached in a stepwise fashion. First, remediable causes of ARF are corrected: hypotension, dehydration, sepsis, heart failure, and other causes of renal hypoperfusion as suggested by the history and physical findings must be appropriately managed. Then, if obstruction within the urinary tract appears likely, it must be excluded; ultrasonography, cystourethrography, and retrograde pyelography of one kidney, particularly in the presence of anuria or intermittent polyuria, may be required.

Established ARF often requires 14 to 21 days to resolve, and during this period therapy is directed toward reestablishing homeostasis. Fluids are replaced in proportion to insensible losses plus urine output. Minimal sodium—and often no potassium—replacement is necessary. Phosphate-binding antacids and alkali therapy may be required to correct hyperphosphatemia and acidosis. Nutritional considerations include protein of high biologic quality (essential amino acids) and sufficient caloric intake to minimize catabolism. Dosages of drugs excreted by the kidney must be modified in proportion to the severity of ARF. Infectious complications, a leading cause of death in ARF, are minimized by removing unnecessary indwelling tubes (especially urinary catheters); prophylactic antibiotics are to be avoided. Finally, dialysis is indicated when fluid, electrolyte, and uremic problems become unmanageable with conventional medical therapy (see Chap. 73, Chronic Renal Failure).

Prophylaxis with mannitol and furosemide in high-risk patients (e.g., prior to open heart surgery) may prevent the development of ARF. Similarly, these drugs have averted full-blown renal failure when given to patients with impending ARF, but only after restoration of effective circulating volume. When unsuccessful in reversing ARF, mannitol and furosemide may convert the course from oliguric to nonoliguric, facilitating clinical management of the patient.

Recovery is heralded by the onset of diuresis and may result in extreme polyuria, necessitating careful electrolyte, fluid, and drug therapy as renal function improves. Most children regain normal renal function, but some, particularly those with glomerular and vascular disorders, may have hypertension or a reduction in renal function or urinary concentrating ability as a permanent sequela.

Pathophysiology

1. Levinsky, M. G. Pathophysiology of acute renal failure. *N. Engl. J. Med.* 296:1453, 1977.
   A concise review of mechanisms (5 pages, 76 references).
2. Thurau, K., and Boylan, J. W. Acute renal success: The unexpected logic of oliguria in acute renal failure. *Am. J. Med.* 61:308, 1976.
   Evidence that the renin-angiotensin system is a major regulating factor in ARF is presented.

Clinical Concepts in Acute Renal Failure

3. Arbeit, L., and Weinstein, W. Acute tubular necrosis-pathophysiology and management. *Med. Clin. North Am.* 65:147, 1981.
   A 16-page review.
4. Counahan, R., et al. Presentation, management, complications and outcome of acute renal failure in childhood: Five years' experience. *Br. Med. J.* 1:599, 1977.
   A comprehensive review of 72 episodes of ARF.
5. Harrington, J. T., and Cohen, J. J. Acute oliguria. *N. Engl. J. Med.* 292:89, 1975.
   A short review of causes and management.
6. Anderson, R. J., et al. Nonoliguric acute renal failure. *N. Engl. J. Med.* 296:1134, 1977.
   A comparison of oliguric and nonoliguric ARF.

Special Clinical Settings

7. Chesney, R. W., et al. ARF: An important complication of cardiac surgery in infants. *J. Pediatr.* 87:381, 1975.
   Acute renal failure developed in almost 10 percent of infants undergoing a cardiac operation.
8. Lynch, R. E., Kjellstrand, C. M., and Coccia, P. F. Renal and metabolic complications of childhood non-Hodgkin's lymphoma. *Semin. Oncol.* 4:325, 1977.
   A review of ARF associated with childhood malignancy: causes, treatment, and prevention.
9. Jain, R. Acute renal failure in the neonate. *Pediatr. Clin. North Am.* 24:605, 1977.
   A review of causes, mechanisms, and treatment of ARF in early life (12 pages, 86 references).

Prognosis

10. Hodson, E., Kjellstrand, C., and Mauer, S. Acute renal failure in infants and children: Outcome of 53 patients requiring hemodialysis treatment. *J. Pediatr.* 93:756, 1978.
    Prognosis related to cause of ARF.

Differential Diagnosis
11. Oken, D. On the differential diagnosis of acute renal failure. *Am. J. Med.* 71:916, 1981.
12. Espinel, C., and Gregory, A. Differential diagnosis of acute renal failure. *Clin. Nephrol.* 13:73, 1980.
   Two papers comparing tests that aid in diagnosis.

10. REYE SYNDROME
Kenneth B. Roberts

In 1963, Reye proposed a new disease entity of encephalopathy with fatty degeneration of viscera based on his findings in 21 children. Since that time, thousands of cases have been identified, and Reye syndrome has received wide attention.

The clinical features are stereotyped. There is a prodrome, usually a mild respiratory illness, followed 3 to 7 days later by vomiting, which may be severe and include hematemesis. Shortly thereafter, signs of encephalopathy are noted, with generalized withdrawal in mild cases and agitation progressing to delirium and decerebrate posturing in more severe cases. The cerebrospinal fluid is normal, but there are marked abnormalities of liver function, including elevation of serum SGOT, SGPT, and blood ammonia concentrations, and prolongation of prothrombin time (without evidence of disseminated intravascular coagulation); notably, the serum bilirubin concentration is normal. There is usually a respiratory alkalosis at the time of diagnosis (caused by hyperventilation), partly compensated by metabolic acidosis; acidosis may predominate in the very young or very ill.

Differential diagnosis is usually not difficult; the normal cerebrospinal fluid and bilirubin render encephalitis and fulminant hepatitis unlikely. The pattern of serum amino acid concentrations is helpful in distinguishing Reye syndrome from entities with similar clinical findings. The ultimate support for the diagnosis is the histologic appearance of the liver. Small fat droplets are contained in each cell, with insignificant inflammation and no individual cell necrosis. The brain similarly reveals the lack of inflammation, but edema and anoxic neuronal degeneration are evident. At the ultrastructural level, the basic abnormality appears to be a disturbance in the mitochondria.

The cause of Reye syndrome is unknown. The available epidemiologic clues are a marked predilection for Caucasians and for children, winter occurrence, self-limited course, the nature of the metabolic abnormalities, and the observation that asymptomatic contacts of cases have elevations of serum transaminase concentrations. Since cases cluster following outbreaks of influenza and chickenpox, it has been proposed that Reye syndrome represents a postinfectious reaction. Environmental factors, such as toxins, and host factors, such as subclinical defect in ammonia metabolism, may also play a role. There is an association between salicylate therapy during the prodromal illness and the development of Reye syndrome, but it is not clear whether this is simple association or cause-and-effect. Current recommendations advise against the administration of salicylate during bouts of chickenpox and influenza.

The period of liver and central nervous system swelling lasts 3 to 6 days after the onset of the vomiting. The liver is palpably enlarged in only half the patients and may not be felt at first, only to develop its soft, smooth, round-edged enlargement on the second or third day. The laboratory abnormalities, like the clinical ones, return to normal within the week. Different authors have proposed various staging systems for classifying the degree of central nervous system swelling. The most complete is Lovejoy's five-stage system, coupling with a five-grade electroencephalographic system the clinical progression from lethargy (stage 1) to disorientation (stage 2), coma (stage 3), rigidity (stage 4), and arrest (stage 5). There has not been general acceptance of any one classification scheme.

Many modalities have been proposed for the treatment of Reye syndrome, including peritoneal dialysis, exchange transfusion, and alphaketoacid infusion, but it is not clear that any is better than vigorous supportive therapy. The chemical abnormalities, including the elevated blood ammonia concentration, return to normal in the first few days, with or without specific therapy. Management includes the supportive therapy appropriate for a patient in hepatic failure. Cerebral edema, the major cause of death, occurs before papilledema becomes evident; direct monitoring of intracranial pressure and early aggressive treatment of pressure elevations seem to be major recent advances in therapy. Gross bleeding is generally not a problem in patients with Reye syndrome, despite the deficiency in clotting factors produced by the liver. Hypoglycemia is a common feature in affected infants and is treated with intravenous glucose. The early vomiting does not require treatment, since it is self-limited. Fever and seizures may be difficult to control, particularly late in the course.

The prognosis for survival seems to correlate with the degree of central nervous system involvement and the peak serum ammonia concentration. Sequelae, more common in infants than in adolescents, include motor and memory deficits and mental retardation.

The Public Health Service currently considers Reye syndrome the most common virus-associated disease of the central nervous system in the United States. Polio and measles, formerly the most common, have been controlled by vaccination efforts. No means of preventing Reye syndrome is currently available.

The Classic

1. Reye, R., Morgan, G., and Baral, J. Encephalopathy and fatty degeneration of the viscera: A disease entity in childhood. *Lancet* 2:749, 1963.
   A study of 21 patients.

Reviews

2. Dodge, P., et al. Diagnosis and treatment of Reye's syndrome. *J.A.M.A.* 246:2441, 1981.
   The consensus of a panel of experts convened by the N.I.H.; responses to 15 questions summarized.
3. Trauner, D. Reye's syndrome. *Curr. Probl. Pediatr.* 12(7), 1982.
   Extensive (26-page), readable review. (Even more extensive: Adv. Pediatr. 22:175, 1976; 54 pages, 184 references.)
4. Volk, D. Reye's syndrome: An update for the practicing physician. *Clin. Pediatr.* (Phila.) 20:505, 1981.
   Comes complete with a protocol for staging and management.
5. La Montagne, J. Summary of a workshop on disease mechanisms and prospects for prevention of Reye's syndrome. *J. Infect. Dis.* 148:943, 1983.
   A review of the epidemiology and metabolic aspects, concluding that further delineation of risk factors is top priority.

Epidemiology/Diagnosis

6. Sullivan-Bolyai, J., and Corey, L. Epidemiology of Reye syndrome. *Epidemiol. Rev.* 3:1, 1981.
   This extensive review (26 pages, 163 references) goes beyond age, sex, race, and socioeconomic status to consider etiology and areas in which "the epidemiologic method" may help. (National surveillance summary: Pediatrics 70:895, 1982.)
7. Lichtenstein, P., et al. Grade I Reye's syndrome: A frequent cause of vomiting and liver dysfunction after varicella and upper-respiratory-tract infection. *N. Engl. J. Med.* 309:133, 1983.
   Of 19 children with elevated liver enzyme concentrations but "a paucity of neurologic findings" after chickenpox or URI, 14 had liver biopsy evidence of Reye syndrome.
8. Corey, L., et al. Diagnostic criteria for influenza B-associated Reye's syndrome: Clinical vs. pathologic criteria. *Pediatrics* 60:702, 1977.
   Under appropriate epidemiologic circumstances, biopsy confirmation of the diagnosis is not necessary (in sporadic cases, biopsies may be required: J. Pediatr. 87:869, 1975).
9. Romshe, C., et al. Amino acid pattern in Reye syndrome: Comparison with clinically similar entities. *J. Pediatr.* 98:788, 1981.
   Noninvasive (unlike liver biopsy) and helpful in differential diagnosis.
10. Schwartz, A. The coagulation defect in Reye's syndrome. *J. Pediatr.* 78:326, 1971.
    Liver factors (I, II, V, VII, IX, X) are abnormal; factor VIII and platelets are normal; no fibrin split products are present.

Etiology/Pathogenesis

11. DeLong, G., and Glick, T. Encephalopathy of Reye's syndrome: A review of pathogenetic hypothesis. *Pediatrics* 69:53, 1982.
    Assesses role of hyperammonemia, fatty and organic acidemia, generalized derangement of mitochondrial structure and function, and lactic acidosis, indicting ammonia; therapeutic implications discussed.
12. Fulginiti, V., et al. Aspirin and Reye syndrome. *Pediatrics* 69:810, 1982.
    The American Academy of Pediatrics Committee on Infectious Diseases finds high likelihood that aspirin contributes to causation of Reye syndrome; rebuttal in same issue (p. 822) questions interpretation of data. (More on the "scientific uncertainties": J.A.M.A. 249:1311, 1983; to the pathologist, fatal salicylate intoxication and Reye syndrome are indistinguishable: Lancet 1:326, 1983.)

Staging/Survival/Sequelae

13. Huttenlocher, P. Reye's syndrome: Relation of outcome to therapy. *J. Pediatr.* 80:845, 1972.
    A popular, four-stage system based on clinical findings.
14. Lovejoy, F., et al. Clinical staging in Reye syndrome. *Am. J. Dis. Child.* 128:36, 1974.
    A five-stage system, including electroencephalographic as well as clinical findings.
15. Fitzgerald, J., et al. The prognostic significance of peak ammonia levels in Reye syndrome. *Pediatrics* 70:997, 1982.
    Mortality was 0 percent if ammonia was less than 5 times normal compared to 41 percent if ammonia level was higher; patients who needed more aggressive therapy could be distinguished from those not needing such intervention, usually within 4 hours of admission. (Also see N. Engl. J. Med. 311:1539, 1984.)
16. Boutros, A., et al. Reye syndrome: A predictably curable disease. *Pediatr. Clin. North Am.* 27:539, 1980.
    A new classification based on intracranial pressure is proposed; aggressive management of ICP is discussed.
17. Brunner, R., et al. Neuropsychologic consequences of Reye syndrome. *J. Pediatr.* 95:706, 1979.
    Outcome correlates with extent of clinical disease.
18. Shaywitz, S., et al. Long-term consequences of Reye syndrome: A sibling-matched, controlled study of neurologic, cognitive, academic, and psychiatric function. *J. Pediatr.* 100:41, 1982.
    Sequelae were more frequent in younger patients.

Treatment

19. Shaywitz, B., Rothstein, P., and Venes, J. Monitoring and management of increased intracranial pressure in Reye syndrome: Results in 29 children. *Pediatrics* 66:198, 1980.
    Apparent benefit of ICP monitoring, controlled respiration, mannitol, and barbiturates is presented. (Pentobarbital coma and hypothermia: J. Pediatr. 100:663, 1982.)
20. Wiegand, C., et al. The management of life-threatening hyperammonia: A comparison of several therapeutic modalities. *J. Pediatr.* 96:142, 1980.
    Hemodialysis is superior to exchange transfusion or peritoneal dialysis.
21. DeVivo, D., Keating, J., and Haymond, M. Reye syndrome: Results of intensive supportive care. *J. Pediatr.* 87:875, 1975.
    Emphasizes the importance of general supportive care (see also Pediatrics 60:708, 1977).

11. INCREASED INTRACRANIAL PRESSURE

William R. Leahy, Jr.

Intracranial pressure is a balance between the volume of the intracranial contents and the space available. Raised pressure may be regarded as a result of a space-occupying mass or excessive blood, cerebrospinal fluid (CSF), or brain volume in the rigid calvarium. Processes responsible include tumor, abscess, hematoma, obstruction to CSF flow (hydrocephalus), or brain swelling (vascular engorgement within the brain or parenchymal swelling).

The two entities most commonly responsible for increasing intracranial pressure in the newborn are brain swelling secondary to perinatal hypoxia or trauma, and congenital hydrocephalus. In older infants and children, the likely causes are the following: meningitis; trauma or complications of trauma, such as epidural and subdural hematoma; brain tumor (usually infratentorial in location); and "toxic" or metabolic encephalopathy (e.g., Reye syndrome, lead poisoning). Pseudotumor cerebri is an additional consideration in older children and adolescents.

The signs and symptoms vary somewhat with the age of the patient. This is largely because the cranium is able to expand until approximately age 10. Once the sutures fuse, however, intracranial contents must shift to accommodate increased volume of any one of the various compartments.

The cardinal manifestations of raised pressure in adults and older children are the following: generalized, early morning headache; insidious vomiting, projectile in type and often unassociated with nausea; extraocular muscle dysfunctions, such as unilateral or bilateral abducens palsy; papilledema; and motor disturbances. In infants, however, the signs are more subtle, such as irritability, restlessness, lethargy, or stupor; papilledema is rare, and motor signs are variable and may include hypotonia or hypertonia, focal paresis, or opisthotonus. A principal finding of elevated intracranial pressure in infants is rapid enlargement of the head and a bulging fontanelle. The characteristic "Cushing triad" of bradycardia, hypertension, and irregular respiration may or may not be present.

Prompt diagnostic procedures must be undertaken when raised intracranial pressure is suspected. Plain skull x-ray films may demonstrate splayed sutures in the young child, erosion or enlargement of the sella turcica in the older child. An electroencephalogram may help in localizing mass lesions, such as tumors, hematomas, or abscesses.

Further tests, such as brain scan and the more invasive studies—arteriography, pneumoencephalography, or ventriculography—may be necessary in selected cases to delineate the location of the disturbance. Computerized axial tomography (CAT scan) offers a safe examination that is most rewarding in the investigation of raised pressure; since the size and shape of the ventricular system are well visualized, a mass lesion with attendant edema that distorts the ventricles is easily appreciated, and the difference between hydrocephalus and generalized edema is seen clearly.

Measurements of serum electrolytes, glucose, calcium, and blood ammonia, liver function tests, and a search for toxic substances may be indicated in selected patients.

The lumbar puncture is potentially a dangerous procedure when signs of raised intracranial pressure are present. If a mass lesion is considered likely, the lumbar puncture is contraindicated because of the potential for tentorial or tonsillar herniation. However, in infants or children suspected of having meningitis, encephalitis, or subarachnoid hemorrhage, the lumbar puncture is essential for diagnostic and therapeutic information. The clinician must therefore weigh the risks against the benefits of the procedure.

Initial therapy is directed at stabilization of vital functions. This requires the correction of life-threatening situations such as hypoxia and shock. Frequent, careful observations of vital signs are essential, and serial neurologic examinations must be done. In an attempt to minimize focal or generalized edema, intravenous fluids are restricted.

Various medications have been used to decrease cerebral swelling; rational selection of an agent is based on whether the underlying process is vasogenic or cytotoxic. Vasogenic edema is associated with focal pathologic conditions, such as trauma, tumors, abscesses, or vascular accidents, and is most often discrete; dexamethasone is usually considered the drug of choice. Cytotoxic processes, such as hypoxia, hypernatremia, and Reye syndrome, cause diffuse cerebral swelling; osmotically active agents such as 20% mannitol, glycerol, or 30% urea are used and produce cellular dehydration of normal as well as abnormal central nervous system tissue. Osmotic agents may also be beneficial in the preoperative period when excision of mass lesions is contemplated. The diuretics acetazolamide and furosemide are sometimes used, particularly in posttraumatic (operative and nonoperative) cerebral edema. Hyperventilation leads to a decrease in cerebral blood flow and thereby to a decrease in pressure; the therapeutic use of this modality requires intubation and controlled mechanical ventilation. Hypothermia and "barbiturate coma" may be used to decrease cerebral metabolism during a period of cerebral edema presumed to be self-limited.

Several systems to monitor intracranial pressure directly have been introduced during the past decade. Some measure the pressure in the subdural or epidural space; others, by means of an indwelling intraventricular catheter, both measure and permit the therapeutic release of CSF. Such systems should prove invaluable in defining the best method for medical management of raised pressure in a given clinical situation.

The prognosis in raised intracranial pressure is dependent on several factors, such as the nature of the underlying cause, the duration of elevation, and complications such as herniation. An aggressive approach in diagnostic evaluation and therapeutic intervention is essential.

Reviews

1. Hahn, J. Cerebral edema and neurointensive care. *Pediatr. Clin. North Am.* 27:587, 1980.
   Definition and brief discussion of pathophysiology, aspects of monitoring and therapy; excellent review.
2. Bruce, D., et al. Cerebrospinal fluid pressure monitoring in children: Physiology, pathology and clinical usefulness. *Adv. Pediatr.* 24:233, 1977.
   A comprehensive review of the physiology and anatomy of increased intracranial pressure, including the techniques for monitoring and measuring intracranial pressure, therapy, and clinical indications. (For a shorter, more recent review by this author, see Pediatr. Rev. *4:217, 1983.)*
3. Bell, W., and McCormick, W. *Increased Intracranial Pressure in Children.* (2nd ed.). Philadelphia: Saunders, 1978.
   A classic in-depth review.

Specific Entities

4. Brown, J., and Habel, A. Toxic encephalopathy and acute brain swelling in children. *Dev. Med. Child Neurol.* 17:659, 1975.
   A review of causes, pathology, clinical aspects, and management.
5. Weisberg, L., and Chutorian, A. Pseudotumor cerebri of childhood. *Am. J. Dis. Child.* 131:1243, 1977.
   A study of 38 children reviewing different modes of therapy: 16 spontaneously improved or improved with repeat lumbar puncture; 16 received steroid therapy, and 12 of these 16 were better in a shorter period of time.
6. Ahlskog, J., and O'Neill, B. Pseudotumor cerebri. *Ann. Intern. Med.* 97:249, 1982.
   An extensive review discussing characterization, outcome, and management of patients with pseudotumor cerebri (83 references). Only 4 to 12 percent had severe persistent visual loss.

Experimental Studies

7. Klatzo, I. Neuropathological aspects of brain edema. *J. Neuropathol. Exp. Neurol.* 26:1, 1967.
   One of the initial and classic works in brain edema.

Diagnostic Study

8. Kistler, J., et al. Computerized axial tomography: Clinico-pathological correlations. *Neurology* (Minneap.) 25:201, 1975.
   A review of 10 patients, illustrating the benefit of CAT.

Medical Management

9. Venes, J. Intracranial pressure monitoring in perspective. *Child's Brain* 7:236, 1980.
   An update on methods of monitoring, the use of steroids, and barbiturate therapy. Although the incidence of complications in monitoring is low and monitoring has proven useful in management, a beneficial effect on outcome has not clearly been demonstrated.
10. Marshall, L., et al. The outcome with aggressive therapy in severe head injuries. Part I: The significance of intracranial pressure monitoring. *J. Neurosurg.* 50:120, 1979.

Analysis of 100 patients with severe head injury treated in a uniform manner with aggressive medical and surgical management.

11. Gudeman, S., et al. Failure of high-dose steroid therapy to influence intracranial pressure in patients with severe head injury. *J. Neurosurg.* 51:301, 1979.
    High-dose steroid (40 mg q6h of methylprednisolone) given during therapy for elevated intracranial pressure had no beneficial effects on ICP or periventricular elasticity; side effects of gastric hemorrhage and hyperglycemia with glucosuria led to untoward effects, however.

12. Mickell, J. Intracranial pressure: Monitoring and normalization therapy in children. *Pediatrics* 59:606, 1977.
    A study of 42 children with increased intracranial pressure from various causes; the effects of ventricular drainage, hyperventilation, glycerol, therapeutic hypothermia, and barbiturates are noted.

13. Long, D., Hartmann, J., and French, L. The response of human cerebral edema to glucosteroid administration. *Neurology* (Minneap.) 16:521, 1977.
    A clinical and electromicroscopic study.

14. Shenkin, H., et al. Clinical methods of reducing intracranial pressure. *N. Engl. J. Med.* 282:1465, 1970.
    The role of cerebral circulation and methods of controlling it are discussed, including hyperventilation.

12. STATUS EPILEPTICUS
William R. Leahy, Jr.

Status epilepticus is a state of persistent or recurrent seizures without intervals of consciousness. Mortality is estimated at 3 to 20 percent, and morbidity is substantial, establishing status epilepticus as a true medical emergency.

In children receiving anticonvulsant therapy, noncompliance or changes in the medication regimen and intercurrent infections seem to constitute the most frequent precipitating causes of status epilepticus. In patients without previous seizures, status epilepticus may be associated with a multitude of acute disorders, including anoxia, systemic or central nervous system infections, cranial trauma, neoplasm, or severe metabolic disturbance with encephalopathy.

The pathophysiology of status epilepticus is unclear. Severe physiologic disturbances, each a consequence of the repeated seizures, contribute to the hazards of this state and may themselves precipitate seizure activity; these disturbances include hypoxia, hyperpyrexia, acidosis, hypotension, and hypoglycemia. Added to these systemic alterations are cellular changes, such as edema of cerebral cells. These factors collectively may explain the self-sustaining nature of the repeated, persistent, and often refractory seizures. Vomiting and aspiration constitute a further compromising, sometimes fatal complication.

Prompt attention must be directed toward: (1) the institution of general supportive measures, (2) the cessation of seizure activities, and (3) a thorough investigation of the causes precipitating the prolonged seizure state.

General supportive measures include ensuring a patent airway, protecting the body against injury, and establishing an intravenous route for the administration of appropriate drugs and hydration. Vital signs must be carefully monitored and the patient observed for signs of respiratory failure or worsening neurologic status.

The rapid termination of convulsions requires the intravenous administration of anticonvulsants. Diazepam is considered by many the drug of choice. It acts rapidly, but the effect is poorly sustained. The drug should be given slowly to avoid the serious complications of apnea, bradycardia, or hypotension. Phenobarbital has a slower onset of action but is effective for a much longer period than diazepam and may be continued as a maintenance anticonvulsant after the acute episode. Phenobarbital, in the doses usually administered to control status epilepticus, will decrease the level of consciousness and may depress respirations, particularly when used in conjunction with diazepam. Phenytoin has been used for status epilepticus. Depression of respirations and a decrease in the level of consciousness are not problems encountered with the usual doses; the drug is a myocardial depressant, however, and cardiac monitoring should be performed during intravenous administration. Other drugs have also been used successfully, including valproic acid, administered per rectum or through a nasogastric tube, and paraldehyde, given per rectum, intramuscularly, or by intravenous infusion.

Investigation of the cause of status epilepticus requires a thorough evaluation of the history and prompt laboratory studies. In patients receiving anticonvulsant medication chronically, blood levels of these drugs should be measured. Determination of electrolytes, glucose, calcium, and urea nitrogen should also be made to diagnose treatable conditions. Lumbar puncture is necessary in the child suspected of having meningitis or encephalitis. More extensive studes, such as brain scan, computerized axial tomography, and arteriography, should be limited to patients suspected of having mass lesions.

Recent experimental work indicates that sustained seizure activity per se may have damaging effects on neurons, and it appears that the longer the duration of seizures, the more difficult control becomes. Thus, recognition of the severity of the problem must be prompt and the approach to therapy rapid and aggressive.

Reviews

1. Rothner, A., and Erenberg, G. Status epilepticus. *Pediatr. Clin. North Am.* 27:593, 1980.
   A broad discussion of the types of status epilepticus and therapy.
2. Oppenheimer, E., and Rosman, N. Seizures in childhood: An approach to emergency management. *Pediatr. Clin. North Am.* 26:837, 1979.
   A comprehensive review and practical approach to status epilepticus, recurrent seizures, and nonepileptic disorders with recommendations for evaluation and therapy.
3. Delgado-Escueta, A., et al. Management of status epilepticus. *N. Engl. J. Med.* 306:1337, 1982.
   A brief review with specific recommendations.
4. Barbosa, E., and Freeman, J. Status epilepticus. *Pediatr. Rev.* 4:185, 1982.
   A readable review. (For a review of management of status epilepticus in the same journal, see Pediatr. Rev. 1:219, 1980.)

Experimental Studies

5. Duffy, T., et al. Cerebral energy metabolism during experimental status epilepticus. *J. Neurochem.* 24:925, 1975.
   Evidence that seizures lead to focal alteration in neuronal energy potentials is presented.
6. Meldrum, B., and Horton, R. Physiology of status epilepticus in primates. *Arch. Neurol.* 28:1, 1973.
7. Meldrum, B., et al. Systemic factors in epileptic brain damage. *Arch. Neurol.* 29:82, 1973.
   These two studies indicate that even when all physiologic parameters are controlled, seizures per se have a deleterious effect on the central nervous system, and that after approximately 25 minutes of activity, the seizures may become self-perpetuating.

Drugs for Therapy

8. Cloyd, J., et al. Status epilepticus: The role of intravenous phenytoin. *J.A.M.A.* 244:1479, 1980.
   Excellent review of a drug for preventing recurrence of seizures during status.
9. Wilder, B., et al. Efficacy of intravenous phenytoin in the treatment of status epilepticus: Kinetics of central nervous system penetration. *Ann. Neurol.* 1:511, 1977.
   Penetration into brain tissue and the cerebrospinal fluid is rapid; status epilepticus was treated effectively in 9 of 10 patients without adverse effect on sensorium or cardiorespiratory centers.
10. Wallis, W., et al. Intravenous dilantin in the treatment of acute repetitive seizures. *Neurology* (Minneap.) 18:513, 1968.
    Success and failure were related to the cause of status epilepticus.

11. Bailey, D., and Fenichel, G. The treatment of prolonged seizure activity with intravenous diazepam. *J. Pediatr.* 73:923, 1968.
   Effective in nearly 90 percent, but two patients stopped breathing!
12. Bostrom, B. Paraldehyde toxicity during treatment of status epilepticus. *Am. J. Dis. Child.* 136:414, 1982.
   Hopefully, you won't need this.
   Also see Seizure Disorders, Chapter 80.

13. HEAD TRAUMA
William R. Leahy, Jr.

Accidents constitute the leading cause of death during childhood. A high percentage of these deaths result from craniocerebral trauma and its various complications. Trauma may also produce serious effects on the developing nervous system, with residual impairment, both physical and mental.

Clinical manifestations depend on the extent and location of cerebral injury. The most frequent syndromes are minor trauma with preservation of consciousness, concussion, contusion, and fractures. Less common, but more devastating, are subdural and epidural hematomas.

Minor head trauma without a history of loss of consciousness and without focal neurologic signs is common and may be followed by vomiting, pallor, irritability, or lethargy.

Concussion is the next most common injury to the nervous system. It is defined as a transient and rapidly reversible state of neuronal dysfunction associated with loss of consciousness that occurs immediately on injury to the head. Amnesia for the event and for a variable period prior to the event is a common phenomenon.

Contusion is focal bruising or tearing of cerebral tissue accompanied by parenchymatous hemorrhage and edema in the area of injury. The most frequently affected sites are the ventral surfaces of the frontal lobe and the inferolateral aspects of the temporal lobes. Such injury is often associated with focal disturbances in strength or sensation, or, if more extensive, with increased intracranial pressure.

Most linear fractures of the skull are of no therapeutic import per se; they are, however, an indicator of the intensity of the trauma and, on the basis of location and extent, of the possible complications to be anticipated. Fractures extending across the course of the middle meningeal artery, across the sagittal sinus, violating the orbit or paranasal sinuses, or involving the rim of the foramen magnum may be associated with a neurologic deficit. Basilar fractures may be associated with leakage of cerebrospinal fluid into the auditory or nasal passages and therefore provide ready access of organisms from the skin or respiratory tract to the subarachnoid space. The vast majority of basilar fractures are not visualized radiographically, but the presentation of bleeding from the nasopharynx, hemotympanum, or postauricular ecchymosis should prompt consideration of the diagnosis.

Depressed skull fractures require prompt medical attention and surgical intervention.

A less common sequela of blunt trauma is the subdural hematoma, i.e., a collection of blood between the dura and the cerebral mantle. Such hematomas may present either in the acute period or in a more chronic phase. The signs and symptoms of cerebral compression from acute hematoma evolve within hours or days after injury. The presentation may be that of altered level of consciousness, symptoms and signs of intracranial hypertension, or a focal deficit. The management of acute subdural hematoma is surgical evacuation; therapy of the more slowly developing chronic subdural hematoma remains controversial.

A rare but often fatal consequence of cranial trauma is the epidural hematoma. The source of bleeding may be arterial or venous. The sequence of events may be varied after injury, but characteristically the child has a brief period of unconsciousness at the time of injury and then returns to normal (a lucid interval), only to suffer a progressive decline a number of hours later, with alteration in the level of consciousness, onset of focal neurologic signs, and, often, drastic changes in vital signs. Prompt surgical therapy is necessary.

A thorough history of the traumatic episode and the initial examination usually permit the physician to classify the type of injury. Often, however, questions remain regarding the severity of the trauma and thus the extent of the diagnostic evaluation that is necessary. The majority of children with mild head trauma can safely be observed at home by competent parents. Children who may require observation, evaluation, or treatment in the hospital include the following: those with altered consciousness at the time of initial examination or unconsciousness for a period of time; with a depressed skull fracture; with an unclear or suspicious history of the circumstances of injury, raising the possibility of child abuse; with a focal or diffuse neurologic disturbance.

Children hospitalized with head trauma require close observation, with attention to the level of consciousness and vital signs. Serial neurologic examinations may detect evolution of a pattern of general worsening of the neurologic status; particularly noteworthy is the development of lateralizing signs or change in pupillary size or function.

Most available diagnostic studies are of limited value in children with head trauma. Roentgenography, electroencephalography, computerized axial tomography, and angiography should be reserved for confirmation of suspected complications of craniocerebral trauma. Computerized tomography is the safest and most efficacious method of defining intracranial pathology and should be performed if clinical status worsens.

Seizures in the first week after injury occur in about 5 percent of patients hospitalized for head trauma; the incidence in children under 5 is almost twice that. Seizures are more common during the first week; they are often limited to focal motor attacks, are less likely to recur, and have a more benign prognosis than those occurring at a later stage.

The capacity for recovery depends on several factors, particularly age, coma duration, and the site of maximal involvement. Common disabilities noted during the recovery phase are retrograde amnesia, behavioral changes (such as increase in aggressiveness), sleep disturbance, and some decrease in intellectual ability. Overall, functional recovery following head injury in children, even after drastic neurologic dysfunction, is in general remarkably good.

Reviews

1. Rosman, N., et al. Acute head trauma in infancy and childhood. *Pediatr. Clin. North Am.* 26:707, 1979.
   An excellent, comprehensive review of anatomy, management, and syndromes associated with head injuries with an especially good table on medical management of acute intracranial pressure.
2. Raphaely, R., et al. Management of severe pediatric head trauma. *Pediatr. Clin. North Am.* 28:715, 1980.
   A good, brief review with emphasis on medical therapy of increased intracranial pressure, barbiturate coma, and attendant withdrawal syndrome; the outcome and recovery of 120 children are reviewed.
3. Singer, H., and Freeman, J. Head trauma for the pediatrician. *Pediatrics* 62:819, 1978.
   A brief overview of basic information.
4. Jennett, B. Head injuries in children. *Dev. Med. Child Neurol.* 14:137, 1972.
   A review of management of uncomplicated head injury with specific attention to posttraumatic epilepsy.
5. Bruce, D., and Schut, L. The value of CAT scanning following pediatric head injury. *Clin. Pediatr.* (Phila.) 19:719, 1980.
   Clinical review of the criteria for CT scanning.

Skull Fractures

6. Einhorn, A., and Mizrahi, E. Basilar skull fractures in children. *Am. J. Dis. Child.* 132:1121, 1978.
   To treat or not to treat with antibiotics: CNS infections did not occur in children not treated with antibiotics.

7. Bell, R., and Loop, J. The utility and futility of radiographic skull examination for trauma. *N. Engl. J. Med.* 284:236, 1971.
   Clinical examination rather than routine x-ray films is stressed. (Also see Pediatrics 69:139, 1982.)

8. Rothman, L., et al. The spectrum of growing skull fracture in children. *Pediatrics* 57:26, 1976.
   Four illustrative cases are discussed. (Also see Am. J. Dis. Child. 129:1197, 1975.)

Complications of Head Trauma

9. Bruce, D., et al. Diffuse cerebral swelling following head injuries in children: The syndrome of "malignant brain edema." *J. Neurosurg.* 54:170, 1981.
   Serial CT scans have provided a description of this devastating clinical entity of rapid deterioration in injured children who are initially conscious. The pathophysiology is suspected to be vasodilatation and initial hyperemia leading to ischemia and death.

10. Grossman, R. Treatment of patients with intracranial hematomas. *N. Engl. J. Med.* 304:1540, 1981.
    Editorial review, accompanying article on traumatic acute subdural hematoma, subtitled "Major mortality reduction in comatose patients treated within four hours," p. 1511.

11. Gutierrez, F., et al. Delayed onset of acute post-traumatic subdural effusion. *Am. J. Dis. Child.* 128:327, 1974.
    The cases of six children with problems after skull fracture.

12. Milley, J., et al. Neurogenic pulmonary edema in childhood. *J. Pediatr.* 94:706, 1979.
    A review of the pathophysiology and therapy of an unusual but serious clinical event related to severe head trauma.

Treatment

13. Cooper, P., et al. Dexamethasone and severe head injury: A prospective double-blind study. *J. Neurosurg.* 51:307, 1979.
    Dexamethasone had no significant effect on morbidity and mortality.
    Also see Increased Intracranial Pressure, Chapter 11.

Prognosis

14. Bruce, D., et al. Outcome following severe head injuries in children. *J. Neurosurg.* 48:679, 1978.
    The outcome of 53 children was compared with statistics from other clinical centers. One-third of the children were noted to develop diffuse late brain swelling.

15. Brink, J., et al. Physical recovery after severe closed head trauma in children and adolescents. *J. Pediatr.* 97:721, 1980.
    A 1-year review of morbidity and mortality in 344 head injured children: 73 percent were improved, 10 percent were dependent in self-care, 9 percent were totally dependent, and 8 percent never regained consciousness; those in coma less than 3 months did considerably better. (Also see Pediatrics 71:756, 1983.)

16. Levin, H., et al. Long-term neuropsychological outcome of closed head injury. *J. Neurosurg.* 50:412, 1979.
    An adult-oriented review of 27 patients identified specific disabilities despite good overall recovery; noted were problems with memory, language, and personality/social adjustments.

17. Clifton, G., et al. Neurologic course and correlated computerized tomography findings after severe closed head injury. *J. Neurosurg.* 52:611, 1980.
    In a study of 124 patients with closed head injuries, the peak times of death were within 48 hours and after 7 days. Rapid deterioration was most often related to delayed intracranial hematomas, which could be visualized on CT scanning.

18. Jennett, B. Trauma as a cause of epilepsy in childhood. *Dev. Med. Child. Neurol.* 15:56, 1973.
    "Early" and "late" seizures have different prognostic significance.

14. ACCIDENTS
Evan Charney

Accidents are the leading cause of death in childhood after the neonatal period, accounting for more fatalities than all other causes combined. The fact that there are several hundred nonfatal accidents for every fatal one suggests something of the enormity of this health problem in human and economic terms. The fatalistic view that accidents are "an act of God" and not inherently controllable is similar to the way infectious diseases were thought of a century ago; and, as with infectious disease, improved information should lead to increased understanding and better control. Although it is unrealistic to expect that all accidental deaths can be prevented, a reduction in the annual death rate by 25 percent in childhood would save as many children as die from childhood leukemia and other malignancies combined.

Motor vehicle deaths account for the single largest number of accidental fatalities—one-half of accidental deaths between 5 and 14 years of age and two-thirds of accidental deaths from 15 to 24 years of age. The rate of automobile-related fatalities increases sharply throughout childhood, particularly in adolescence. (In fact, the overall accidental death rate in this century has not decreased at all for 15- to 24-year-olds, largely due to automobile deaths, while it has decreased by one-half in all other age groups.)

Drowning is the second most common cause of accidental death throughout childhood. The number of fatal drownings has decreased slightly over the past three decades—about 4,000 per year, a figure that represents significant improvement in swimming safety, since many more people today use swimming pools and have access to lake and ocean bathing than in the past.

Burns are the next most frequent cause of accidental death, killing 1,500 children annually. These deaths, primarily the result of house fires, are most common between 1 and 4 years of age. The fatalities are due to smoke inhalation and respiratory failure, hypovolemic shock and renal failure (from fluid loss through the burned skin), and overwhelming infection, contributed to by impaired immunocompetence in the severely burned patient. Serious but nonfatal burns affect 150,000 children annually; these are particularly tragic injuries, which often require long periods of hospitalization, repeated surgery, and extensive rehabilitation, with major psychologic sequelae for the child and family.

Poisonings are the fourth most common cause of accidental death in childhood. There are at least 200 nonfatal cases for every poisoning fatality, and although the management of poisonings (particularly in toddlers) occupies a significant amount of patient, family, and physician time, the fatality rate for poisonings is only one-tenth that for motor vehicle deaths and one-third that for drowning. Moreover, recovery from poisoning is usually complete, unlike the residual morbidity often complicating a burn injury. Although many more toddlers than older children are accidentally poisoned, 577 of the 695 fatal poisonings in 1978 were adolescent suicides, which have tripled in frequency over the past two decades.

The variation by sex in injury and case fatality rates is striking; boys have twice the accident death rate of girls (4 times the rate between 15 and 24 years of age, largely due to motor vehicle deaths). This sex ratio holds true for death from drowning, firearms, and toxic ingestions, but the rates are approximately equal for burn fatalities.

A number of studies have helped define common antecedents in the behavior of adults and children involved in accidents: families in which a child has sustained a serious accident have a higher proportion of acute and chronic illness, and the mother, in particular, is often preoccupied or absent from the home; boys who have accidents are more likely to be described as risk takers or as having recently undergone stress. These studies have increased our understanding of the psychology of accidents, but have been difficult to translate into specific preventive action.

A conceptual approach to the problem that has gained considerable support in the past decade considers strategies for "injury control" rather than (or in addition to) "accident prevention." Accidents may or may not be preventable; injury control focuses on specific countermeasures to prevent or reduce the frequency and severity of injuries and their sequelae. For example, a crash-activated air bag in an automobile will not prevent the accident but will significantly reduce injury. Another important concept considers an "active-passive" dimension—how much volitional involvement is required of a person to avoid an accident. In general, countermeasures that reduce or remove the hazard and those that do not require individual cooperation to be effective have been the most successful. For example, in Great Britain, a law that required safety grilles in front of fireplaces markedly reduced the number of burns sustained by children. In the United States, limiting the number of children's aspirin tablets in a single bottle and, somewhat later, the introduction of a safety cap did more to decrease deaths from salicylate poisoning than did the earlier establishment of a network of poison information centers. Perhaps the most dramatic example of the effectiveness of a single preventive act was the decline in motor vehicle deaths by 20 percent in a single year—from 55,000 to 46,000 in 1974—following the lowering of the speed limit to 55 miles/hour.

Efforts to alter the behavior of children and adults to prevent accidents have not been productive, especially when conducted at a general community level. Health information (just providing facts) is less successful than health education, which aims to alter the subject's behavior in a specific fashion. For example, an intensive year-long, community-wide education program on accident prevention conducted in Rockland County, New York, did not reduce the number of accidental injuries reported to hospitals and physicians; in a separate study, television viewers exposed to carefully designed and repeatedly shown advertisements to buckle up their seat belts failed to do so. More focused educational efforts—e.g., an individual pediatrician advising patients that proper infant seat restraints be installed in the family car and used—have been somewhat more successful. Attempts to mandate seat belt use by law have been gaining in popularity in the United States, and nearly all states now have mandatory child safety seat laws, with some evidence of significant increase in use, particularly by infants. However, even in states with such laws, the majority of adults and older children are not safely restrained as passengers in automobiles.

In summary, control strategies that emphasize changes in the environment that are not dependent on repeated individual cooperation for efficacy are likely to be the most successful ones (e.g., for automobile accidents, the installation of crash-activated air bags; for burns, the permanent installation of home smoke detectors.) Carefully directed educational efforts are important as well (e.g., most drownings occur in nonswimmers, and teaching a child to swim may "immunize" him against that risk).

The role of physicians in the management of accidental injury is an important one. Once a serious injury has occurred, physicians are involved as clinicians. In the strategy of accident prevention, they must be teachers for their own patients and, in the public arena, advocates for reforms that will protect all children from such injuries.

General

1. National Safety Council. *Accident Facts.* Chicago: National Safety Council, 1982.
   Compendium of statistics on accidents in the United States published every few years; valuable data on the nature of and trends in accidental injury. (Also see Baker, S., O'Neill, B., and Karpf, R. The Injury Fact Book Lexington: Heath, 1984.)
2. Westfelt, J. Environmental factors in childhood accidents: A prospective study in Goteborg, Sweden. *Acta Paediatr. Scand. (Suppl.)* 291, 1982.
   One in seven children sustained an accident in a 1-year period. For comparable U.S. data, see Am. J. Public Health 74:1340, 1984.
3. Berger, L. Childhood injuries: Recognition and prevention. *Curr. Prob. Pediatr.* 12(1), 1981.
   A broad review, ranging from definition, concepts, and general approaches to specific types of injuries and countermeasures. (Also see Adv. Pediatr. 29:471, 1982, for a well-written overview of trends and an assessment of countermeasures, with discussion of the pediatrician's role as educator and public advocate.)
4. Haddon, W. Advances in the epidemiology of injuries as a basis for public policy. *Publ. Health Reports* 95:411, 1980.
   Reviews his theory: countermeasures for injury control should focus on reducing the transfer of energy.
5. Ross Roundtable on Critical Approaches to Common Problems. *Preventing Childhood Injuries.* Columbus, Ohio: Ross Laboratories, 1982.

Series of presentations by experts in the field. Practical approaches using the injury control concept.

Motor Vehicle Accidents

6. Scherz, R. Fatal motor vehicle accidents of child passengers from birth through 4 years of age in Washington State. *Pediatrics* 68:572, 1981.
   In 39,500 accidents over a decade, only 14 percent of children were restrained; fatality rate in this group was 93 percent lower than in nonrestrained children.
7. Centers for Disease Control. State action to prevent motor vehicle deaths and injuries among children and adolescents. *M.M.W.R.* 31:488, 1982.
   Laws not only increase use of car safety seats (Am. J. Public Health 71:163, 1981) and seat belts (Am. J. Dis. Child. 137:582, 1983), but reduce deaths (55%) and injuries (30%). Also see J.A.M.A. 252:2571, 1984.
8. Reisinger, K., et al. Effect of pediatrician's counseling on infant restraint use. *Pediatrics* 67:201, 1981.
   Strong positive effect demonstrated over controls when message was repeated over first 2 months of life; differences diminished thereafter as both groups attained 50 percent use.
9. Karwacki, J., and Baker, S. Children in motor vehicles: Never too young to die. *J.A.M.A.* 242:2849, 1979.
   Fatal injury rate highest for those less than 1 year of age.
10. Agran, P., and Dunkle, D. Motor vehicle occupant injuries to children in crash and non-crash events. *Pediatrics* 70:993, 1982.
    Of 548 nonfatal injuries, 15 percent occurred in "noncrash events" (sudden stops, swerves). Seat restraint use would have attenuated or eliminated injury.
11. Centers for Disease Control. Alcohol related highway fatalities among young drivers. *M.M.W.R.* 31:641, 1982.
    Young people 16 to 24 years old accounted for 48 percent of all highway fatalities but were only 17 percent of U.S. population. Alcohol was a factor in 38 percent. (Summarized in Clin. Pediatr. [Phila.] 22:449, 1983.)
12. Robertson, L., et al. A controlled study of the effect of television messages on safety belt use. *Am. J. Public Health* 64:1071, 1974.
    The results of general health education, even when well done, are disappointing. An important study of what doesn't work.
13. Robertson, L., and Zador, P. Driver education and fatal crash involvement of teenaged drivers. *Am. J. Public Health* 689:959, 1978.
    Identifies an apparent paradox: Because driver education leads to more 16- and 17-year-old licensed drivers, it results in more fatal accidents; moreover, 18 and 19 year olds with or without prior driver education have similar fatal accident rates. Ergo, eliminating high school driver education should reduce fatalities. See p. 954 (same issue) for rebuttal and Am. J. Public Health 70:599, 1980, for substantiation.

Drowning

14. Giammona, S. Drowning: Pathophysiology and management. *Curr. Probl. Pediatr.* 1(7), 1971.
    A good review (with extensive references) on management.
15. Modell, J. *The Pathophysiology and Treatment of Drowning and Near Drowning.* Springfield, Ill.: Thomas, 1971.
    The pathophysiology of drowning is discussed.
16. Modell, J. Biology of drowning. *Annu. Rev. Med.* 29:1, 1978.
    Brief but useful overview of pathophysiologic changes by an expert in the field.
17. Conn, A., Edmonds, J., and Barker, G. Cerebral resuscitation in near drowning. *Pediatr. Clin. North Am.* 26:691, 1979.
    Analyzes factors affecting cerebral recovery and outlines vigorous approach to management.
18. Dietz, P., and Baker, S. Drowning: Epidemiology and prevention. *Am. J. Public Health* 64:303, 1974.
    An interesting analysis of 117 drowning deaths in Maryland.

19. Frates, R. Analysis of predictive factors in the assessment of warm-water near-drowning in children. *Am. J. Dis. Child.* 135:1006, 1981.

    Of 42 children submerged in warm water, all who arrived in the emergency room in coma with fixed and dilated pupils died or had major neurologic sequelae. (Also see the companion editorial for a succinct review of the data on prognostic factors, p. 998.)

20. Laughlin, J., and Eigen, H. Pulmonary function abnormalities in survivors of near drowning. *J. Pediatr.* 100:26, 1982.

    Residual lung injury noted in 9 of 10 cases studied 6 months to 8.5 years later.

21. Pearn, J. Secondary drowning in children. *Br. Med. J.* 281:1103, 1980.

    Of 94 children, 5 had deterioration of pulmonary function hours after initially successful resuscitation.

Burns

22. Trunkey, D., and Parks, S. Burns in children. *Curr. Probl. Pediatr.* 6(3), 1976.

    A good overview of the problem, with practical guidelines; 48 pages, 84 references.

23. Moncrief, J. Burns. *N. Engl. J. Med.* 288:444, 1973.

    A pathophysiologic approach to burn management is presented; 88 references.

24. Denling, R. Fluid resuscitation after major burns. *J.A.M.A.* 250:1438, 1983.

    Outlines rationale for and current guidelines in fluid management.

25. Katcher, M. Scald burns from hot tap water. *J.A.M.A.* 246:1219, 1981.

    Reviews risk factors. Reducing hot water heater temperature would prevent almost all cases.

Poisoning

26. Gilman, A.G., Goodman, L., and Gilman, A. *The Pharmacological Basis of Therapeutics* (6th ed.). New York: Macmillan, 1980.

    A basic and continually useful text.

27. Gosselin, R., et al. *Clinical Toxicology of Commercial Products* (5th ed.). Baltimore: Williams & Wilkins, 1984.

    Another basic guide to the management of specific poisonings; identifies ingredients in commercial products.

28. Scherz, R. (ed.). The management of accidental childhood poisoning. *Pediatrics* 54:323, 1974.

    A collection of seven articles on various topics, from the unknown poison (p. 336) to specific agents. (Also see the American Academy of Pediatrics, Handbook of Common Poisonings in Children. HEW publication No. (FDA) 76–7004, 1976.)

29. Clarke, A., and Walton, W. Effect of safety packaging in aspirin ingestion by children. *Pediatrics* 63:687, 1979.

    Reported ingestions decreased 43 to 56 percent, deaths declined 21 to 24 percent; the authors consider the relative contributions of safety packaging and other factors.

Other

30. Dershewitz, R., and Williamson, J. Prevention of childhood household injuries: A controlled clinical trial. *Am. J. Public Health* 67:1148, 1978.

    An education program in the physician's office aimed at parents with young children failed to reduce household hazards.

31. Baker, S., and Fisher, R. Childhood asphyxiation by choking or suffocation. *J.A.M.A.* 244:1343, 1980.

    A review of deaths in Maryland, 1970–1978, by age and object; recommendations offered. (For a review of childhood asphyxiation by food objects, see J.A.M.A. 251:2231, 1984; also see Upper Airway Obstruction, Chapter 4.)

15. FEVER AND ANTIPYRETICS
Kenneth B. Roberts

Perhaps the most common and the most distressing sign of childhood illness to both parents and pediatricians is fever. Although the cause is usually viral, self-limiting, and benign, fever is considered synonymous with disease and thus often elicits considerable concern. The physician's responsibility is to establish a correct diagnosis and initiate treatment if indicated, meanwhile ensuring that the child is comfortable. A more long-term goal is parental education about the use of thermometers and the meaning of fever.

It is generally accepted that 37.0°C (98.6°F) is "the normal" body temperature, but it should be clear that body temperature is like other biologic phenomena in that not every member of the population has exactly the same temperature. It should be noted specifically that infants, on the average, have a higher basal temperature than do older children or adults; 50 percent of 18-month-olds have daily temperatures in excess of 37.8°C (100.0°F) without associated illness. Only after age 2 does the downward trend begin, reaching a "normal" 37.0°C during adolescence. Oral temperatures are generally 0.5 to 0.6°C lower than rectal temperatures, and a probe inserted 14 cm into the rectum will record a temperature as much as 1.3°C higher than that measured by the usual clinical thermometer placed only 2 to 6 cm inside the rectum.

Fever of any magnitude in neonates may be the only sign of sepsis; in infants 7 to 24 months of age, there appears to be a higher incidence of bacteremia if the temperature is above 39.5°C. In older children, fever may persist for days or weeks and still be of obscure cause; the designation *fever of unknown origin (FUO)* should be applied only when fever has persisted for more than 3 weeks. (Some authors are content with 2 weeks as in adults, but in children, many viral infections will persist past 14 days.) Infections (such as tuberculosis), cancer (especially leukemia), and collagen-vascular disorders (especially juvenile rheumatoid arthritis) must be thought of in the differential diagnosis of fever of unknown origin, but the majority of children will prove to have a more common illness, although perhaps with an unusual presentation. Despite the increasing availability of sophisticated tests, including nuclear scans, the history and physical examination remain the most discriminating tools in formulating a diagnosis.

Although fever may portend serious illness, it is rarely harmful per se. It causes an increase in the basal metabolic rate of approximately 12 percent per degree centigrade elevation above 37.8°C, and the associated insensible loss of water may lead to dehydration if there is no compensatory increase in fluid intake. The pulse rate increases approximately 20 to 25 beats /minute/°C of fever, which may be deleterious to a myocardium already strained because of cardiac disease or anemia. Seizures are a common concern, but current feeling generally is that "febrile seizures" may be associated more with a rapid rise in temperature than with the absolute height attained, although it is unusual for convulsions to occur if the maximal temperature is 39°C (102°F) or less. Febrile seizures are often associated with the initial fever spike in an illness and uncommonly occur twice in the same illness, so it is unclear how much antipyretics contribute in the prevention of convulsions.

Many authors have argued teleologically and on the basis of in vitro experiments that fever might be beneficial in the presence of infectious agents. In some specific bacterial diseases, notably neurosyphilis, fever therapy has been clinically effective, and multiplication of some viruses is limited by elevation of the temperature from 37 to 40°C (98.6–104°F). Yet it seems that presently available data are insufficient to establish an advantage of fever to the infected host.

The most compelling reason to reduce fever under the usual conditions in childhood is patient discomfort. Certain antipyretic measures, such a sponging with ice water, may not only be ineffective because of shivering and increased thermogenesis but may also produce more discomfort than the untreated fever and are therefore to be discouraged. The two pharmacologic agents most frequently used to reduce fever are acetylsalicylic acid (aspirin) and acetaminophen. Both are presumed to act by interfering with prostaglandin synthesis and, in equivalent doses, have equivalent effects; the toxicities associated with these agents are markedly different, however.

Salicylate in large amounts uncouples oxidative phosphorylation, producing a metabolic acidosis. It also acts directly on the respiratory center, causing a hyperpnea that can result in respiratory alkalosis, particularly in adults and older children. In severe salicylate intoxication, the acidosis usually supervenes and may be profound, increasing toxicity in the central nervous system. Alkalinization protects against central nervous system toxicity, increases the amount of salicylate that can be eliminated in the urine, and is thus a major goal in the management of salicylate intoxication. Two pharmacologic principles should be kept in mind in the assessment and management of a child who has ingested a large dose of salicylate. First, absorption through the gastrointestinal tract is not instantaneous. Thus, the peak level is not reached immediately after ingestion, but comes after a delay; this is considered in the Done nomogram, which depicts the relationship of salicylate concentration in the serum to the severity of clinical intoxication, by its omission of any values prior to 6 hours after ingestion. A second pharmacologic feature, peculiar to aspirin and other compounds such as phenytoin, is the change in pharmacokinetics that occurs at high serum levels, with prolongation of half-time suggesting a saturation phenomenon. Prior to the widespread use of child safety caps, aspirin was the most common harmful ingestion in children; while in most series it is no longer first, it is still close to it.

Acetaminophen became popular in the 1960s as a "harmless" alternative to aspirin, free from the bothersome side effects noted with salicylate (notably, gastric irritation and platelet dysfunction), and less likely to cause serious poisoning. It is clear that acetaminophen is not harmless, however: large overdoses can be fatal. Deaths result from fulminant liver damage, the signs and symptoms of which are characteristically delayed 2 to 3 days. Of the various regimens proposed to treat acetaminophen overdose, *N*-acetylcysteine has been the most widely accepted.

General

1. Cone, T. Diagnosis and treatment: Children with fevers. *Pediatrics* 43:290, 1969.
   A general overview, including not only where to insert the thermometer but also how far and for how long.
2. Bayley, N., and Stolz, H. Maturational changes in rectal temperatures of 61 infants from 1 to 36 months. *Child Dev.* 8:195, 1937.
   Is 37°C (98.6°F) the normal temperature of all infants? Pull this oldie out of your library's archives!
3. Tandberg, D., and Sklar, D. Effect of tachypnea on the estimation of body temperature by an oral thermometer. *N. Engl. J. Med.* 308:945, 1983.
   The oral temperature is lowered by tachypnea even when the patient is not obviously mouth breathing.
4. Kluger, M. Fever. *Pediatrics* 66:720, 1980.
   Brief review of pathophysiology and role in disease. (Also see reference 8; for a longer exposition of same topic, see Ann. Intern. Med. 91:261, 1979; Am. J. Med. 72:799, 1982 [20 pages, 253 references]; J. Infect. Dis. 149:339, 1984.)
5. Banco, L., and Veltri, D. Ability of mothers to subjectively assess the presence of fever in their children. *Am. J. Dis. Child.* 138:976, 1984.
   At least as good as "temperature strips," studies of which are referenced.
6. Schmitt, B. Fever phobia. *Am. J. Dis. Child.* 134:176, 1980.
   Misconceptions of parents about fevers, many learned from health care providers.

Antipyresis: General

7. Done, A. Treatment of fever in 1982: A review. *Am. J. Med.* 74(6a):27, 1983.
   The pros and cons of treatment.
8. Stern, R. Pathophysiologic basis for symptomatic treatment of fever. *Pediatrics* 59:92, 1977.
   Matching mechanisms and treatments.
9. Steele, R., et al. Evaluation of sponging and of oral antipyretic therapy to reduce fever. *J. Pediatr.* 77:824, 1970.
   Sponging and an antipyretic are more effective than either alone, but sponging is a source of increased discomfort.

Antipyretics

10. Rumack, B. (ed.). Aspirin and acetaminophen: A comparative view for the pediatric patient, with particular regard to toxicity, both in therapeutic dose and overdose. *Pediatrics* 62:866, 1978.
    A collection of 13 articles, detailing pharmacokinetics, comparative effect, toxicity, pathophysiology and management of overdose, and more; the place to begin.
11. Done, A., Yaffe, S., and Clayton, J. Aspirin dosage for infants and children. *J. Pediatr.* 95:617, 1979.
    Reviews pharmacokinetics and proposes a new aspirin dosage schedule.

12. Lasagna, L., and McMahon, F. (eds.). New perspectives on aspirin therapy. *Am. J. Med.* 74(6a), 1983.

    A collection of articles (16) on the various uses of aspirin.

13. Fulginiti, V., et al. Aspirin and Reye syndrome. *Pediatrics* 69:810, 1982.

    The American Academy of Pediatrics Committee on Infectious Diseases finds high likelihood that aspirin contributes to causation of Reye syndrome; rebuttal in same issue (p. 822) questions interpretation of data. (More on the "scientific uncertainties": J.A.M.A. 249:1311, 1983.)

14. Gaudreault, P., Temple, A., and Lovejoy, F. The relative severity of acute versus chronic salicylate poisoning in children: A clinical comparison. *Pediatrics* 70:566, 1982.

    "Chronic" poisoning was more severe; note that chronic meant repeated doses over a period exceeding 12 hours.

15. Clarke, A., and Walton, W. Effect of safety packaging in aspirin ingestion by children. *Pediatrics* 63:687, 1979.

    Reported ingestions decreased 43 to 56 percent, deaths declined 21 to 24 percent; the authors consider the relative contributions of safety packaging and other factors.

16. Prescott, L., et al. Intravenous N-acetylcysteine: The treatment of choice for paracetamol poisoning. *Br. Med. J.* 4:1097, 1979.

    The authors' experience in 100 cases of acetaminophen (paracetamol) overdose.

Fever of Unknown Origin

17. Feigin, R., and Shearer, W. Fever of unknown origin in children. *Curr. Probl. Pediatr.* 6(10), 1976.

    More than the title promises: review of fever, treatment, and fever of unknown origin (65 pages, 279 references).

18. Kleiman, M. The complaint persistent fever: Recognition and management of pseudo fever of unknown origin. *Pediatr. Clin. North Am.* 29:201, 1982.

    A valuable adjunct to reference 17, detailing management of the child purported to have FUO but who in fact does not.

19. Long, S. Approach to the febrile patient with no obvious focus of infection. *Pediatr. Rev.* 5:305, 1984.

    A good entree to the problem of acute unexplained febrile illness. (Also see Bacteremia and Septicemia, Chapter 2, and other specific sections.)

16. LEAD POISONING

John T. Hayford, Jr., and Evan Charney

Lead, an element with no known therapeutic use, has long been recognized as a toxic substance. In the past, the problem of concern has been overt encephalopathy, but recent data suggest that lead may cause more subtle neurologic deficits as well, even at levels formerly thought "safe." More sensitive and specific diagnostic evaluations continue to be developed to detect the presence of an increased body burden of lead and to monitor the effects on physiologic processes.

The average blood lead level in the United States population appears to have decreased in the past decade, presumably related to the reduced lead content of gasoline. However, as many as 4 percent of children between 6 months and 5 years of age (the group at highest risk) still have blood lead levels greater than 30 μg/dl, the value now considered potentially hazardous. Elevated levels are more commonly found at all ages among urban, low income, and black persons. For example, 18.6 percent of central city black children less than 5 years of age have blood lead concentrations greater than 30 μg/dl.

There are multiple sources of lead in the environment: lead in food, water, and air account for a "basal intake," entering the body directly by ingestion or inhalation, or indirectly by hand contamination and repetitive mouthing typical of young children. In general, the total amount of lead absorbed from these combined sources is less than 200 μg/day, and blood lead levels will then remain under 20 μg/dl. Where environmental dust and dirt contamination with lead are increased—notably in deteriorated urban settings—blood lead elevations between 30 and 60 μg/dl are more common. In such an environment, a minority of young children may have overtly toxic blood levels ($>$ 70 μg/dl) due to pica (the habitual ingestion of nonfood objects) for lead-contaminated paint chips or dirt. Nutritional status influences the amount of ingested lead that is absorbed from the gastrointestinal tract: deficiencies of iron, protein, calcium, and vitamin D can increase absorption fivefold.

Inorganic lead enters and leaves the body chiefly through the gastrointestinal tract; 10 percent is absorbed (up to 40% in children) and distributed into three body pools. Bone is the largest reservoir, with 90 percent of body lead incorporated in hydroxyapatite crystals, but without effect on the skeletal architecture. The bone marrow and soft tissues are a second body pool, with more active turnover than that in bone. Clinically, the most important pool is the rapidly exchangeable lead in red blood cells and parenchymal organs. The central nervous system is freely permeable to soluble lead, and animal studies indicate no threshold to lead accumulation in the central nervous system; these studies also demonstrate that central nervous system lead is relatively difficult to mobilize.

The impairment in erythropoiesis caused by lead does not result in a profound anemia but does provide an opportunity to assess metabolic injury. Lead interferes with sulfhydryl-containing enzymes and thereby disrupts the synthesis of the heme porphyrin structure from aminolevulenic acid. Many tests have been proposed to measure accumulated metabolites as quantitative reflections of the disruption of hemoglobulin synthesis, the most popular currently being the determination of free erythrocyte protoporphyrin (EP). Although elevation of free erythrocyte protoporphyrin occurs in other conditions of ineffective erythropoiesis, such as iron deficiency, sickle cell disease, and thalassemia major, a blood value greater than 10 times normal is virtually diagnostic of lead-induced metabolic injury. Since EP determination is inexpensive and can be performed reliably on capillary blood samples, it is currently the screening method of choice. Children whose whole blood EP levels are greater than 50 μg/dl should then have a determination of blood lead concentration.

The clinical manifestations of early lead intoxication are subtle and relatively nonspecific. Anorexia, vomiting, intermittent abdominal pain, and constipation are common gastrointestinal complaints. Central nervous system toxicity is reflected by lethargy, irritability, ataxia, and clumsiness; more severe expressions include stupor, refractory convulsions, and increased intracranial pressure. Anemia with basophilic stippling is a late sign associated with more severe toxicity. Similarly, Fanconi syndrome of urinary abnormalities reflects severe and usually chronic intoxication. Dense metaphyseal lines seen on x-ray films of the proximal fibula, scapula, distal ulna, and iliac crests may be evident as well but must be distinguished from growth lines.

The neurologic sequelae of severe lead intoxication have been recognized for many years, with up to 40 percent of affected children having residual neurologic deficits, such as mental retardation, a "cerebral palsy," or a seizure disorder. The risks of such sequelae have been related to the severity of the intoxication, and children presenting with ataxia, seizures, or encephalitis are at highest risk. Recent epidemiologic data in conjunction with more refined assessments of lead burden suggest that lead may be a cause of subtle psychoneurologic deficits in children, even when peak blood lead levels have been below 60 μg/dl. There appears to be an association between modest lead level elevation in the first years of life and hyperactivity, abnormal behavior, irritability, and abnormal fine motor, adaptive, and language function manifest in the early school years. If there is a toxic effect associated with low-level ingestion among a large group of exposed children, it is possible that a particular subset of these children are especially affected; perhaps they are selected by the intensity or the duration of exposure at key points in their development.

Therapy for lead intoxication involves both environmental and medical management. An investigation of the child's environment to determine and eliminate the source(s) of lead is mandatory. It often requires aggressive efforts by the physician, social worker, and public health agencies to remove the child from the source(s) of lead and ensure environmental "detoxification." Current methods of home hazard abatement involve removing all peeling or deteriorated lead-containing interior and exterior surfaces of the child's home and careful cleanup of residual lead-contaminated dust. Hazard abatement strategies are currently undergoing reassessment as the minimum "safe" blood level for children has been progressively lowered.

Medical management is based on administration of chelating agents to bind soft-tissue lead stores and accelerate their excretion. Calcium EDTA and dimercaprol (British anti-lewisite, BAL) are the mainstays of current therapy, with the dosage and administration schedule depending on the clinical and biochemical findings. BAL is used in cases of severe lead intoxication to decrease the likelihood of precipitating acute lead encephalopathy during the initial mobilization of the lead burden. Both drugs must be given parenterally and are potentially toxic. Penicillamine, an investigational drug for heavy metal mobilization, is administered orally but is less effective than BAL or EDTA and so is not suitable treatment for acute or severe lead intoxication. It is probably effective in long-term chelation therapy, however.

The following four recommendations are adapted from guidelines of the Centers for Disease Control and the Surgeon General of the United States for screening and treatment:

1. All children who live in or visit old, dilapidated buildings should have screening (by erythrocyte protoporphyrin with confirmation of high levels by venous blood lead level determination) beginning at 1 year of age and repeated, depending on degree of risk, through age 6 years.
2. Any child with continued whole blood lead levels between 30 and 49 μg/dl should be considered to have moderate lead poisoning, should have current sources of exposure to lead investigated and corrected, and should be followed closely to ensure that higher blood lead levels or clinical symptoms do not develop.
3. All children with blood lead levels 50 to 69 μg/dl should have diagnostic tests for metabolic and clinical evidence of lead poisoning and be treated immediately if such evidence is present. Under careful supervision, chelation therapy may be indicated even if the child is asymptomatic.
4. All children with blood lead levels greater than 70 μg/dl should be hospitalized immediately and treated with chelating agents.

Reviews

1. Angle, C., and McIntire, M. Children: The barometer of environmental lead. *Adv. Pediatr.* 29:3, 1982.
   An excellent review of sources of lead in the environment with interesting historical references. The title of the article is perceptive: If environmental contamination exists children will be the first affected.
2. Chisolm, J., and O'Hara, D. *Lead Absorption in Children.* Baltimore: Urban & Schwarzenberg, 1982.
   Report of a conference with 21 chapters covering metabolism and toxicity; pertinent environmental, behavioral, and social factors; and practical strategies for case management.
3. Nriagu, J. Saturnine gout among Roman aristocrats: Did lead poisoning contribute to the fall of the Empire? *N. Engl. J. Med.* 308:660, 1983.
   Contaminated wine may have done in the Caesars and the Roman Empire. An excellent reference for those lulls in cocktail party conversation.

Prevalence and Sources

4. Mahaffey, K., et al. National estimates of blood lead levels: United States, 1976–1980. *N. Engl. J. Med.* 397:573, 1982.
   The best data currently available suggest that 4 percent of children less than 5 years of age are affected. Mean blood lead levels in the United States appear to be decreasing over this time period.
5. Annest, J., et al. Chronological trend in blood lead level between 1976 and 1980. *N. Engl. J. Med.* 308:1373, 1983.
   The 37 percent reduction in levels noted can be explained by reduced lead content of gasoline.
6. Charney, E., Sayre, J., and Coulter, M. Increased lead absorption in inner city children: Where does the lead come from? *Pediatrics* 65:226, 1980.
   Multiple mechanisms (inhalation of airborne lead, pica for paint or dirt, hands

contaminated with house dust) all contribute in preschool inner city children. (Home lead dust control lowers blood lead levels of affected children: N. Engl. J. Med. *309:1089, 1983.)*

7. Roels, H., et al. Exposure to lead by the oral and pulmonary routes of children living in the vicinity of a primary lead smelter. *Environ. Research* 22:81, 1980.
   An important study, documenting that hand contamination and inhalation of airborne lead both account for blood lead elevation in school age children.

8. Baker, E., et al. Lead poisoning in children of lead workers: Home contamination with industrial dust. *N. Engl. J. Med.* 296:260, 1977.
   "Fouling one's own nest" is the term Chisolm uses for this mechanism of childhood lead poisoning.

9. Ziegler, E., et al. Absorption and retention of lead by infants. *Pediatr. Res.* 12:29, 1978.
   Infants less than 2 years of age absorbed 42 percent of ingested lead; in previous studies adults absorbed only 10 percent.

Central Nervous System Effects

10. Goldstein, G., Asbury, A., and Diamond, I. Pathogenesis of lead encephalopathy. *Arch. Neurol.* 31:382, 1974.
    Uses an animal model for the vascular toxicity of lead and a study of CNS transport.

11. Rutter, M. Raised lead levels and impaired cognitive/behavioral functioning: A review of the evidence. *Dev. Med. Child Neurol. [Suppl.]* 22:1, 1980.
    A thorough and balanced assessment: critical review of over 200 studies (as of 1979) that consider at what point the hazard begins. (Updated in Rutter, M., and Jones, R. Lead vs. Health Chichester: Wiley, 1983.)

12. Needleman, H., et al. Deficits in psychologic and classroom performance of children with elevated dentine lead levels. *N. Engl. J. Med.* 300:689, 1979.
    Major study suggesting that (presumably) low level exposure in early childhood impairs later psychologic test and school performance. Both supported (Dev. Med. Child Neurol. 23:567, 1981, J. Pediatr. 102:523, 1983) and refuted (Pediatrics 67:911, 1981) by subsequent studies.

Toxicity Assays

13. Chisolm, J., Barrett, M., and Harrison, H. Indicators of internal dose of lead in relation to derangement in heme synthesis. *Johns Hopkins Med. J.* 137:6, 1975.
    An analysis of the interrelationships and sensitivities of various tests for evaluating the body lead burden and its significance.

14. Chisolm, J., Barrett, M., and Mellits, E. Dose effect and dose response relationships for lead in children. *J. Pediatr.* 87:1152 [Suppl.], 1975.
    A review of toxicity and body lead burden.

Treatment

15. Piomelli, S., et al. Management of childhood lead poisoning. *J. Pediatr.* 105:523, 1984.
    Expert consensus on specifics of chelation therapy and environmental intervention.

16. Preventing lead poisoning in young children: A statement by the Center for Disease Control. *J. Pediatr.* 93:709, 1978.
    Definitions of levels of toxicity and recommended environmental and clinical therapy.

17. CHILD ABUSE
Robert D. White

Recognition and management of child abuse by the pediatrician demands a full measure of clinical acumen, skill, and diplomacy. The results of a battering may be immediately apparent or so subtle as to be overlooked for years. Therapy is difficult, and success depends on patient and sympathetic treatment of the entire family to interrupt a cycle of aggression usually initiated decades before the birth of the patient. This disease, to a greater extent than most, exemplifies the roles of the pediatrician as child advocate and family counselor.

The incidence of child abuse probably exceeds 50,000 cases per year in the United States. One-fourth of fractures and 10 to 15 percent of trauma in children under 3 years of age are "nonaccidental." Death by battering occurs in 2000 children yearly, while 3 times that number suffer permanent brain damage.

The cause of child abuse defies simple classification. It seems clear that most abused children are "exceptional," but this description includes not only demanding, hand-icapped, or chronically ill infants, but highly intelligent and active children as well. Many aberrant personality traits can be found retrospectively in abusive parents, but most are sufficiently common in the general population to make accurate identification of a battering parent extremely difficult prior to one or more episodes of abuse. Many abusive parents were themselves beaten in childhood; thus, aggression toward their own children is often less an expression of hatred than a learned response to anger or adversity.

The diagnosis of child abuse requires a high index of suspicion by the examining physician. In only a few cases does a malevolent, hostile parent bring to the physician a child with the classic signs of subdural hematoma and multiple fractures in various stages of healing; far more often, the battered child is one of several patients in a crowded emergency room or office with a minor bruise, burn, or laceration, accompanied by attentive parents. Abuse should be considered in a child under 3 years of age with any form of trauma (except from an automobile accident), especially when the history of the trauma is vague or discrepant, or when there has been a delay in seeking medical attention. Child abuse or neglect should also be considered in the differential diagnosis of "failure to thrive." In addition, evidence of battering may take many unusual forms, such as retinal hemorrhage, duodenal hematoma, drug overdosage (usually with sedatives), and sexual abuse.

Evidence of previous trauma should be searched for during general examination of the child, and the previous medical record should be thoroughly reviewed for a pattern of repeated trauma. Many cases of child abuse are missed because only cursory attention is given to these portions of the medical evaluation during treatment for traumatic injuries. In some situations, a series of radiographs of the skull, extremities, and ribs is indicated to demonstrate old fractures, metaphyseal abnormalities, or subperiosteal hemorrhages that would otherwise be missed. Discussion with parents of the circumstances surrounding an unusual or suspicious injury must be thorough but should be devoid of any hint of accusation.

When abuse is evident or highly suspicious, steps must be taken to protect the child from the dangerous environment; the child should be hospitalized, even if the actual injury is minor. Removal of the child from the home allows a cooling-off period for the parents, as well as time to evaluate the family environment in adequate depth. The physician should carefully document the injuries suffered (photographs are very helpful), the history given by the parents, and the medical therapy rendered. Notification of state authorities is mandatory but should be done without accusation. As pointed out earlier, the stereotypical malevolent parent is rarely seen; most parents who batter their children are also capable of loving them and caring for them well when intervention by medical and social personnel is offered with understanding and sympathy.

Therapy is directed toward rehabilitation of the family unit whenever possible. Psychologic evaluation of the parents delineates the emotional framework and the stresses that promote battering; the parents' understanding of their own behavior may be a major therapeutic step. When the parents are able to enjoy their child and have a secure resource to turn to when stress mounts, it may be safe to return the child to the home. Continued liaison, as with a trained home visitor, is advisable to provide the parents with competent, ongoing support and to serve as an "early warning device" to detect the potential recurrence of abuse. This approach appears capable of reducing the risk of subsequent battering to less than 5 percent, but such programs are not available in many areas. Parents' groups have formed in some communities to help fill this void. The failure to provide ongoing support has serious consequences; when an abused child returns to the home without therapeutic intervention, the risk of further abuse is approximately 50 percent with death resulting in up to 10 percent of children.

Reviews
 1. Kempe, C., Child abuse: The pediatrician's role in child advocacy and preventive pediatrics. *Am. J. Dis. Child.* 132:255, 1978.
    The shared experience of a lifetime.
 2. Taylor, L., and Newberger, E. Child abuse in the international year of the child. *N. Engl. J. Med.* 301:1205, 1979.
    An international perspective, encouraging efforts on many fronts.
 3. Rauser, A. (ed.). Symposium on child abuse. *Pediatrics* 57:771, 1973.
    A practical discussion. Also reviewed in Pediatr. Ann. *13(10), 1984.*
 4. Non-accidental injury in children. *Br. Med. J.* 4:656, 1973.
    A brief framework for diagnosis and management is presented.
 5. George, J. Spare the rod: A survey of the battered-child syndrome. *Forensic Sci.* 2:129, 1973.
    An interesting section on legal implications.
 6. Newberger, E., and Hyde, J., Jr. Child abuse: Principles and implications of current pediatric practice. *Pediatr. Clin. North Am.* 22:695, 1975.
    The sociologic aspects of abuse are considered in depth.
 7. Bittner, S., and Newberger, E. Pediatric understanding of child abuse and neglect. *Pediatr. Rev.* 2:197, 1981.
    Very good section on the psychopathology, stresses, and situations that trigger abuse.

Series
 8. Lauer, B., Ten Broeck, E., and Grossman, M. Battered child syndrome: Review of 130 patients with controls. *Pediatrics* 54:67, 1974.
    Emotional and physical neglect are much more pervasive than battering.
 9. Smith, S., and Hanson, R. 134 battered children: A medical and psychological study. *Br. Med. J.* 3:666, 1974.
    The danger to siblings of abused children should not be overlooked.

Specific Aspects of Abuse
10. Caffey, J. The whiplash shaken infant syndrome: Manual shaking by the extremities with whiplash-induced intracranial and intraocular bleedings, linked with residual permanent brain damage and mental retardation. *Pediatrics* 54:396, 1974.
    The title tells it all; cogent argument for funduscopic examination of every ill or injured infant.
11. Kempe, C. Uncommon manifestations of the battered child syndrome. *Am. J. Dis. Child.* 129:1265, 1975.
    A brief listing of some of the more bizarre forms of abuse.
12. Powell, G., Brasel, J., and Blizzard, R. Emotional deprivation and growth retardation simulating idiopathic hypopituitarism: I. Clinical evaluation of the syndrome. *N. Engl. J. Med.* 276:1271, 1967.
    Neglect as an often subtle but important form of abuse.
13. Money, J. The syndrome of abuse dwarfism (psychosocial dwarfism or reversible hyposomatotropism). *Am. J. Dis. Child.* 131:508, 1977.
    A macabre case report serves as the focal point for an insightful discussion of this type of abuse. (Also see Clin. Pediatr. *[Phila.] 21:587, 1982.)*
14. Ayoub, C. and Pfiefer, D. Burns as a manifestation of child abuse and neglect. *Am. J. Dis. Child.* 133:910, 1979.
    Accidental burns secondary to extreme neglect were as common as nonaccidental burns.
15. Pascoe, J., et al. Patterns of skin injury in non-accidental and accidental injury. *Pediatrics* 64:245, 1979.
    Bruises over the trunk were significantly more common in abused children. (Also see Am. J. Dis. Child. *133:906, 1979.)*

Specific Aspects of Abuse: Sexual Abuse
16. Kempe, C. Sexual abuse: Another hidden pediatric problem. *Pediatrics* 62:382, 1978.
    An explosion of information has occurred on this once hidden problem. (Also see Pediatr. Rev. *4:93, 1982; J.A.M.A. 242: 1761, 1979; Am. J. Dis. Child. 136:129, 142, 1982, and 134:255, 1980; and N. Engl. J. Med. 302:319, 348, 1980.)*

17. Orr, D., and Prietto, S. Emergency management of sexually abused children: The role of the pediatric resident. *Am. J. Dis. Child.* 133:628, 1979.
Worthwhile reading for any primary care physician.

Specific Aspects of Abuse: Long-Term Follow-Up
18. Martin, H., et al. The development of abused children. *Adv. Pediatr.* 21:25, 1974.
Neurologic abnormalities were found in more than 50 percent. (Also see Pediatrics *59:273, 1977.)*
19. Green, A. Self-destructive behavior in battered children. *Am. J. Psychiatry* 135:579, 1978.
Learned behavior.
20. Green, F. Child abuse and neglect: A priority problem for the private physician. *Pediatr. Clin. North Am.* 22:329, 1975.
A brief and concise outline management.
21. Fontana, V., and Robison, E. A multidisciplinary approach to the treatment of child abuse. *Pediatrics* 57:760, 1976.
"Intensive care" of the family unit.
22. Leake, A., and Smith, D. Preparing for an testifying in a child abuse hearing. *Clin. Pediatr.* (Phila.) 16:1057, 1977.
Good preparation helps the physician and the child. (Also see Am. J. Dis. Child. *134:503, 1980.)*
23. Rosenfeld, A., and Newberger, E. Compassion vs control: Conceptual and practical pitfalls in the broadened definition of child abuse. *J.A.M.A.* 237:2086, 1977.
Trying to find the appropriate balance between understanding abusive parents' needs and rights, and yet preventing further harm to the child. (Also see Pediatrics *65:180, 358, 1980; and* Am. J. Dis. Child. *133:691, 1979.)*

Prevention
24. Klein, M., and Stern, L. Low birth weight and the battered child syndrome. *Am. J. Dis. Child.* 122:15, 1971.
Suggests that abuse of premature infants after discharge may be largely an iatrogenic problem.
25. Helping mothers to love their babies. *Br. Med. J.* 2:595, 1977.
Perhaps current hospital care, even of full-term infants, fosters later abuse and neglect.
26. Kempe, C. Approaches to preventing child abuse: The health visitors concept. *Am. J. Dis. Child.* 130:941, 1976.
An eloquent appeal for a reordering of medical and social priorities.
27. Lealman, G., et al. Prediction and prevention of child abuse: An empty hope? *Lancet* 1:1423, 1983.
At-risk families were identified and counseled, but the rate of abuse was not reduced.

18. DEATH, DYING, AND MOURNING
Kenneth B. Roberts

During the past decade, the popular writings of Dr. Elisabeth Kübler-Ross stimulated much interest in death and dying. Dr. Ross identified several important principles, chief among which is our inability (at any age) to conceive of our own death, a psychologic limitation reinforced by our death-denying society. She proposed that a terminally ill patient knows the seriousness of his condition whether or not he is told and would like his physician to acknowledge the gravity of the disease—but not to remove hope. Above all, she stressed, the fear of abandonment, of being alone, is worse than the fear of death.

Dr. Ross also described five psychologic "stages" through which dying patients progress: denial, anger, bargaining, depression, and acceptance. It is important to recognize that these stages typify the reaction not only to death but also to any perceived major loss. Thus, the parents of a newborn with Down syndrome and the older child who learns of intended parental separation are likely to progress through the same five stages in some form.

Management of a sick child—whether or not his illness is fatal—includes providing reassurance that pain will be controlled, that a capable adult will provide care, and that the child will not be abandoned. It often requires a conscious effort by medical personnel to maintain communication with a seriously ill child; the inability to effect a cure is frustrating and disheartening, and may be personally (professionally) threatening. The child may ask questions that make adults uncomfortable; as with other emotionally charged subjects, it is important to ascertain the child's level of understanding before answering. Just as one needs to know the child's frame of reference to answer appropriately "Where do babies come from?" one should similarly determine the fantasies of the questioner before responding to "Is Jimmy going to die?" or "Am *I* going to die?" Often, the physician or parent will discover that the child's concern is not death per se, but mutilation, pain, or being left alone, and reassurance about such matters can be both honest and effective.

What children (and adults) understand about death and the coping behaviors they employ are age-related. In very young children, separation and death are more or less equivalent: both result in the absence of a loved one on whom the child depends. By age 3 to 5, boys and girls are aware of sex differences and may become concerned about mutilation of their bodies; death is considered a dramatic event that happens to strangers. The preschool child also has a sense of magical omnipotence, which can be the source of much guilt, because he believes that all occurrences stem from his own wishes or deeds; e.g., the death of a newborn brother or sister may be interpreted as "his fault" because he wished to remain an only child. In early school years, the few facts that the child gleans are woven together with rich, often terrifying fantasies. Until age 10, the child usually considers death a reversible process; that is, the dead person is able to return to life at will. The adolescent is capable of recognizing that death is both irreversible and universal; it has been demonstrated that he may be able to comprehend the implications of fatal illness and make decisions about the termination of his life. The teenager struggling for independence views fatal illness as an unjust intrusion into a personal world in which he perceives himself to be all-powerful; death is a "punishment." The young adult typically responds to death with feelings of rage. The reaction of the middle-aged adult is characterized by intellectual acceptance but emotional denial, in contrast to that of a person of more advanced age, in whom personal assessment leads more naturally to an acceptance of death, although often with a lack of understanding of the appropriate age-related behavior of younger persons.

The popular phrase "death and dying" overlooks consideration of the important areas of mourning and grief. The goal of "grief work" is "emancipation from the bondage to the deceased," involving readjustment to life without the loved one and reinvestment of the self in new relationships. The anguish is revealed in a variety of somatic signs, including sighing respirations, digestive symptoms, feelings of being "choked up," and complaints of exhaustion, coupled with patterns of constant but nonproductive activity. Less well-recognized features, which may cause a mourner to fear he is "losing his mind with grief," are perceptions that the deceased is still present ("I can still hear the baby crying sometimes"), overwhelming guilt, and hostile reactions to friends who attempt to give comfort. The process of grieving is a slow one. Each season brings its own memories, and special holidays and anniversaries may be difficult for years. All too commonly, parents do not resolve their grief; instead, they may create a "replacement child."

It is important to recognize that individuals grieve differently; some are overtly emotional, others more stoic. Gender stereotypes may create expectations. Communication between parents can become strained and the sense of isolation deepened. Children usually do not express their sense of loss by overt "grieving" as adults do but may become more demanding of attention; parents may have difficulty accepting such behavior, seeing it as uncaring and self-centered. The physician sensitive to these issues can provide a valuable service to the family by acknowledging different styles and by fostering communication.

Chronic illness provides an opportunity for preparation for death; progression through the five stages usually begins at the time of diagnosis. Although "anticipatory grief" is of benefit to the parents, shortening their period of mourning following the child's death, premature separation may make the child's final days more frightening and more lonely. Moreover, if the child survives a potentially fatal episode, his parents may have difficulty accepting him as still living ("Lazarus syndrome"), or they may perceive him as particularly fragile and become excessively protective of him ("vulnerable child syndrome"). The physician's responsibility is to ensure both the physical and the emotional comfort of the child and to provide guidance for the grieving parents.

Most infants and children who die do not have chronic diseases, however; rather, they are the victims of accidents or sudden infant death syndrome. Acceptance of the unexpected death is particularly difficult, since there has been no anticipatory grief, no opportunity for the parents to work through the five stages gradually. Incapacitation may be prolonged, and the follow-up visit is of special importance. The physician's role is to help parents face their loss and to guide them through the many difficult months of grief work.

The physician should meet with the family of a deceased child 2 to 3 months after the death to answer lingering questions (and review autopsy results), to assess the members' level of functioning, and to assist in the mourning process. His role is to listen, to support, to sanction mourning behavior, and to give assurance that surprising and disturbing feelings are signs not of insanity but of grief.

Reviews

1. Kübler-Ross, E., Wessler, S., and Avioli, L. On death and dying. *J.A.M.A.* 221:174, 1972.
   A resumé of the 1969 book with same title, discussing why we have so much trouble facing death, and proposing five stages of dying: denial, anger, bargaining, depression, and acceptance.
2. Sahler, O., and Friedman, S. The dying child. *Pediatr. Rev.* 3:159, 1981.
   A readable review that touches many relevant issues from child's concepts to management.

Child's Concept of Death

3. Easson, W. Care of the young patient who is dying. *J.A.M.A.* 205:203, 1968.
   Describes the stages in children and physician (adult): the best descriptions are of the preschool years, adolescence, and beyond.
4. Green, M. Care of the dying child. *Pediatrics* 40:492, 1967.
   Emphasizes that a child asking about his own death wonders "Am I safe?" "Will I be alone?" "Will you make me feel all right?"
5. Yudkin, S. Children and death. *Lancet* 1:37, 1967.
   A good description of the terrifying mix of fact and fantasy in 3- to 7-year-old children and an expression of concern for the child whose fears are reasonable.
6. Spinetta, J., Rigler, D., and Karon, M. Anxiety in the dying child. *Pediatrics* 52:841, 1973.
   The focus is on children 6 to 10 years old; data are presented to show that hospitalized children with leukemia are more anxious than matched controls with chronic but nonfatal illness (as outpatients, too: Pediatrics *56:1034, 1975).*
7. Childers, P., and Wimmers, M. The concept of death in early childhood. *Child Dev.* 42:1299, 1971.
   Discussions with 75 children age 4 to 10 revealed an increasing trend toward acceptance of death as universal (100% by age 9), but fewer than one-third at age 4 to 9 and fewer than two-thirds at age 10 believed that death is irreversible (irrevocable).
8. Schowalter, J., Ferholt, J., and Mann, N. The adolescent patient's decision to die. *Pediatrics* 51:97, 1973.
   It may well be a mature one.

Approach to Fatal Disease

9. Vernick, J., and Karon, M. Who's afraid of death on a leukemic ward? *Am. J. Dis. Child.* 109:393, 1965.
   Includes a discussion of the staff's feelings. The authors advocate telling the child the diagnosis and present an example of "how to." (For additional brief, helpful notes about handling the individual child, see Pediatrics *40:518, 1967.)*

10. Waller, D., et al. Coping with poor prognosis in the pediatric intensive care unit. *Am. J. Dis. Child.* 133:1121, 1979.
    Dealing with parental denial; also see editorial p. 1119. (Denial may have a positive function: J. Pediatr. *99:401, 1981.)*
11. Howell, D. A child dies. *J. Pediatr. Surg.* 1:2, 1966.
    A sensitive presentation of the author's approach: anticipate the child's needs and questions and address them ("the best defense is a good defense").
12. Wessel, M. The primary physician and the death of a child in a specialized hospital setting. *Pediatrics* 71:443, 1983.
    The role of the primary care provider in a tertiary setting.
    Also see Leukemia, Chapter 92.

Grief, Mourning, and Parents
13. Lindemann, E. Symptomatology and management of acute grief. *Am. J. Psychiatry* 101:141, 1944.
    Five (perhaps six) pathognomonic features of grief and a definition of "grief work" (mourning) are presented. (Poignant illustrations of the principles, elicited from group sessions with parents after their child's death: J. Pediatr. *88:140, 1976.)*
14. Cassel, E. The nature of suffering and the goals of medicine. *N. Engl. J. Med.* 306:639, 1982.
    Distinguishes pain from suffering; required reading.
15. Schulman, J., and Rehm, J. Assisting the bereaved. *J. Pediatr.* 102:992, 1983.
    Many practical suggestions. (What to do visit by visit: Clin. Pediatr. [Phila.] *20:466, 1981.)*
16. Mandell, F., McAnulty, E., and Reece, R. Observations of paternal response to sudden unanticipated infant death. *Pediatrics* 65:221, 1980.
    A pattern often different than the maternal response.
17. Friedman, S. Psychological aspects of sudden unexpected death in infants and children. *Pediatr. Clin. North Am.* 21:103, 1974.
    Differences between anticipated loss and unexpected loss are discussed, followed by superb commentary by Bergman (p. 115).
18. Speck, W., and Kennell, J. Management of perinatal death. *Pediatr. Rev.* 2:59, 1980.
    Review, ranging from stillbirth (also see J. Pediatr. *93:869, 1978) to follow-up meetings (utilized if offered:* Pediatrics *64:665, 1979; content:* Pediatrics *62:166, 1978.) Also see* Pediatrics *62:96,100, 1978, for comments for physicians and for parents.*

Siblings, Replacements, Overprotection
19. Weston, D., and Irwin, R. Preschool child's response to death of infant sibling. *Am. J. Dis. Child.* 106:564, 1963.
    Discussion of the child's concerns, interaction with grieving parents, and change in roles. (Also see Pediatrics *72:652, 1983.)*
20. Schowalter, J. How do children and funerals mix? *J. Pediatr.* 89:139, 1976.
    The child's wishes are often the best guide. (Same author, same topic: Pediatr. Rev. *1:337, 1980.)*
21. Poznanski, E. The "replacement child": A saga of unresolved parental grief. *J. Pediatr.* 81:1190, 1972.
    A case history to remind us of this entity as representing ineffective coping.
22. Green, M., and Solnit, A. Pediatric management of the dying child: III. Reactions to the threatened loss of a child: A vulnerable child syndrome. *Pediatrics* 34:58, 1964.
    Overprotection of the child with a fatal illness or of a surviving sibling is discussed.

Generalizability
23. Butler, A. There's something wrong with Michael: A pediatrician-mother's perspective. *Pediatrics* 71:446, 1983.
    Articulate and sensitive description of feelings and dynamics.

24. Miller, L. Toward a greater understanding of the parents of the mentally retarded. *J. Pediatr.* 73:699, 1968.

    Parents react to the diagnosis of mental retardation with "grief"; so do parents told of the need to transfer a neonate to a regional center: N. Engl. J. Med. *294:975, 1976.*

25. Kappelman, M., and Black, J. Children of divorce: The pediatrician's responsibility. *Pediatr. Ann.* 9:342, 1980.

    Age/stage-specific responses. (Also see Pediatr. Rev. *1:211, 1980;* N. Engl. J. Med. *305:557, 1981; for a discussion of the effects of parental death, see* Pediatrics *72:645, 1983.)*

Physicians

26. Schowalter, J. Death and the pediatric house officer. *J. Pediatr.* 76:706, 1970.

    A description of 10 house officers through the "period of impact," the "period of battle," and the "period of defeat."

27. Sahler, O., McAnarney, E., and Friedman, S. Factors influencing pediatric interns' relationships with dying children and their parents. *Pediatrics* 67:207, 1981.

    The child's age, neurologic status, and duration of illness.

28. Wiener, J. Attitudes of pediatricians toward the care of fatally ill children. *J. Pediatr.* 76:700, 1970.

    Varies with the age of the physician (see reference 3).

---

19. SUDDEN INFANT DEATH SYNDROME
Robert D. White

For centuries, infections were the leading cause of death in infancy. Now, with the development and extensive use of antibiotics and vaccines, other causes of infant mortality are increasingly apparent. Foremost among these is the sudden infant death syndrome (SIDS), which at present is the leading cause of postneonatal infant mortality, with an incidence of approximately two cases per 100,000 live births, or 7000 cases per year, in the United States. These deaths are, by definition, sudden, unexpected, and unexplained, even after a careful autopsy. Although the cause of this disease or group of diseases remains obscure, the recent surge of medical interest in SIDS has identified several promising avenues of research into identification of infants at risk and prevention of mortality.

Sudden infant death syndrome has several notable epidemiologic characteristics. Almost 90 percent of cases are in infants 1 to 6 months of age. Virtually all deaths occur while the infant is asleep, and although signs of vigorous activity are occasionally present, there is no warning cry. Infants nearly always appear to have been in good health, although in half, an upper respiratory infection has been present in the week prior to death. Viruses can be isolated from the nasopharynx and stool of infants with SIDS more often than from control infants, but there is no evidence of sepsis due to either viral or bacterial agents. The syndrome is most common during the winter months, in lower socioeconomic groups, in prematurely born infants, and in males.

The pathologic findings of SIDS are provocative. Intrathoracic petechiae are present in about 90 percent of the infants, often associated with pulmonary congestion, edema, and microscopic areas of mild inflammation. Some investigators have found thickening of the pulmonary arterial musculature, prolonged retention of brown fat and extramedullary hematopoeisis, and changes in the carotid bodies, all suggestive of chronic hypoxemia. On the other hand, the thymus and adrenals show no evidence of chronic stress, and the bladder and rectum are usually empty, indicating an acute agonal event.

Theories of causation for SIDS abound. Most of these have been suggested on the basis of observations made in a small number of patients and subsequently refuted by data from larger series. Several appear compatible with most of the observed epidemiologic and pathologic findings, however, and remain plausible. One theory proposes that death is due to respiratory insufficiency, possibly secondary to acute upper airway obstruction by laryngospasm or muscular relaxation of the oropharynx; this is consistent with the sudden, silent death during sleep and the striking localization of petechiae, presumably secondary to strongly negative intrathoracic pressures developed during agonal gasps. An alternative hypothesis proposes neurogenic imbalance, either in brainstem control of respiration or in the autonomic nervous system; this theory is attractive because it provides an explanation for the observed excess of premature infants and infants with neurologic abnormalities, and because it implies a chronic disorder, consistent with the changes found in the pulmonary vasculature, carotid body, and brown fat. A third possibility is that SIDS is the result of a fatal cardiac arrhythmia, which is also consistent with a sudden, silent death. It is difficult to prove or disprove any of these hypotheses, because of the sudden, unexpected nature of SIDS; one, all, or none could be correct, in whole or part.

The pediatrician's role in SIDS is important, and extends well beyond the care of the infant (see Death, Dying, and Mourning, Chap. 18). The events preceding death should be recorded thoroughly and compassionately. The parents should be informed of the provisional diagnosis, emphasizing that SIDS is a definite, although poorly understood, clinical entity; that an autopsy should be performed to confirm the diagnosis; and that blaming themselves for the child's death is unwarranted. Extended counseling for the parents is vital. The counselor should understand the patterns of parental grief and must be comfortable with his own feelings about death. Invaluable support is also available from parents' groups that have been organized in most major cities.

Occasionally, an infant is successfully resuscitated from a SIDS-like incident. These so-called near-misses present a serious dilemma in management. Infectious and metabolic disorders should be ruled out as possible causes of the acute episode. Seizures, arrhythmias, gastroesophageal reflux, and prolonged sleep apnea are often impossible to exclude with certainty, but should be investigated nevertheless. Fatal episodes occur subsequently in approximately 10 to 25 percent of infants with a previous near-miss; prevention of SIDS, even in this high-risk group, is not yet possible. The decision to send an infant home, with or without an apnea or heart rate monitor, or to observe him in the hospital for a prolonged period must be made with the knowledge that each choice carries obvious risks but no certain benefit. The parents' capabilities and their informed choice help determine the course of management.

Reviews

1. Valdes-Dapena, M. Sudden infant death syndrome: A review of the medical literature 1974–1979. *Pediatrics* 66:597, 1980.
   Concentrates on recent research into causation.
   Also see N. Engl. J. Med. *306:959, 1022, 1982, and* Pediatr. Clin. North Am. *29:1241, 1982.*

2. Brady, J. Sudden infant syndrome: The physician's dilemma. *Adv. Pediatr.* 30:635, 1983.
   Also see N. Engl. J. Med. *306:959, 1982, and* Pediatr. Clin. North Am. *29:1241, 1982.*

Theories of Causation

3. Tonkin, S. Sudden infant death syndrome: Hypothesis of causation. *Pediatrics* 55:650, 1975.
   Does the unique anatomy and physiology of the infant oropharynx predispose to airway obstruction during rapid eye movement sleep?

4. Steinschneider, A. Nasopharyngitis and prolonged sleep apnea. *Pediatrics* 56:967, 1975.
   Do upper respiratory tract infections cause sleep apnea and SIDS?

5. Shannon, D., Kelly, D., and O'Connell, K. Abnormal regulation of ventilation in infants at risk for sudden-infant-death syndrome. *N. Engl. J. Med.* 297:747, 1977.
   In 11 near-miss cases the infant hypoventilated during quiet sleep, and 3 of these infants later died of SIDS.

6. Naeye, R. Sudden infant death. *Sci. Am.* 242(April): 56, 1980.
   Summarizes author's earlier studies suggesting that subtle abnormalities in oxygenation, growth, and temperament precede death in apparently healthy babies. (For a contrasting view, see Pediatrics *73:646, 1984.)*

7. Jeffery, H., Rahilly, P., and Read, D. Multiple causes of asphyxia in infants at high risk for sudden infant death. *Arch. Dis. Child.* 58:92, 1983.

Further evidence that asphyxia may be a common link between several predisposing factors and sudden death.

8. Root, A., and Lee, W. Sudden infant death syndrome and triiodothyronine: Clarification of a relationship. *J. Pediatr.* 102:251, 1983.
   Another footnote in the long search for the cause of a marker for SIDS.
9. Peterson, D. Evolution of the epidemiology of sudden infant death syndrome. *Epidemiol. Rev.* 1:97, 1980.
   A most difficult jigsaw puzzle.
10. Guntheroth, W. The QT interval and sudden infant death syndrome. *Circulation* 66:502, 1982.
    Outlines the methodologic problems with establishing this association.
11. Denborough, M., Galloway, G., and Hopkinson, K. Malignant hyperpyrexia and sudden infant death. *Lancet* 2:1068, 1982.
    New, attractive theories continue to sprout.
12. Arnon, S., et al. Intestinal infection and toxin production by *Clostridium botulinum* as one cause of sudden infant death syndrome. *Lancet* 1:1273, 1978.
    The veil falls from one cause (albeit uncommon) of SIDS.
13. Peterson, D., Chinn, N., and Fisher, L. The sudden infant death syndrome: Repetitions in families. *J. Pediatr.* 97:265, 1980.
    Lightning does strike twice. (Also see N. Engl. J. Med. 302:517, 1980.)

Infantile Apnea

14. Guilleminault, C., et al. Abnormal polygraphic findings in near-miss sudden infant death. *Lancet* 1:1326, 1976.
    These infants had respiratory obstruction and apnea and asystole. (Also see Pediatrics 64:882, 1979, and N. Engl. J. Med. 309:107, 1983.)
15. Keeton, B., et al. Cardiac conduction disorders in six infants with "near-miss" sudden infant deaths. *Br. Med. J.* 2:600, 1977.
    Includes 1 infant with an upper respiratory tract infection and apnea and an arrhythmia.
16. Herbst, J., Book, L., and Bray, P. Gastroesophageal reflux in the "near-miss" sudden infant death syndrome. *J. Pediatr.* 92:73, 1978.
    Gastric reflux (often without vomiting) may produce severe apnea in early infancy.
17. Friedman, S., et al. Statement on terminology from the National SIDS Foundation. *J. Pediatr.* 99:664, 1981.
    Renaming the "near-miss" syndrome.
18. McBride, J. Infantile apnea. *Pediatr. Rev.* 5:275, 1984.
    Also see N. Engl. J. Med. 309:107, 1983, and Am. J. Dis. Child. 136:1012, 1982.
19. Southall, D. Home monitoring and its role in the sudden infant death syndrome. *Pediatrics* 72:133, 1983.
    For additional thoughts on the role of monitors, see Pediatrics 61:511, 663, 665, 1978.
20. Black, L., Hersher, L., and Steinschneider, A. Impact of the apnea monitor on family life. *Pediatrics* 62:681, 1978.
    An assessment of the "psychic cost." (Also see Pediatrics 66:37, 1980, and 74:323, 1984.)

Management

21. Krein, N. Sudden infant death syndrome: Acute loss and grief reactions. *Clin. Pediatr.* (Phila.) 18:414, 1979.
    An excellent guide for counseling parents, regardless of the cause of death. (Also see Pediatrics 62:160, 1978; Arch. Dis. Child. 58:467, 1983; and Pediatr. Clin. North Am. 21:103, 1974—the advice is timeless.)
22. Mandell, F., McAnulty, E., and Reece, R. Observations of paternal response to sudden unanticipated infant death. *Pediatrics* 65:221, 1980.
    Beneath the stoic exterior, fathers undergo extensive grief—often missed or misunderstood by wives, doctors, and friends.
23. Mandell, F., and Wolfe, L. Sudden infant death syndrome and subsequent pregnancy. *Pediatrics* 56:774, 1975.
    Infertility secondary to psychologic factors is common.

II. GROWTH, DEVELOPMENT, AND BEHAVIOR

20. PHYSICAL GROWTH

Margaret E. Mohrmann and John T. Hayford, Jr.

The growth of a child occurs in four phases—fetal, infant, juvenile, and adolescent—that are distinguished by differences in controlling influences, characteristic growth velocity, and factors commonly responsible for abnormal growth.

The size of an infant at birth, which correlates poorly with his ultimate adult height, is affected primarily by maternal size and secondarily by other intrauterine factors, such as maternal nutrition and use of tobacco and alcohol, placental adequacy, and intrauterine infection. Children who suffer a growth-retarding insult during the early fetal period of active cell division do not show "catch-up" growth in the postnatal period; growth potential is irrevocably lost. On the other hand, if growth is slowed in the third trimester, a time of cell enlargement rather than division and differentiation, later compensatory growth frequently occurs and growth potential may be realized.

During the first 12 to 24 months after birth, the time of greatest postnatal growth velocity, the infant "seeks his own curve." That is, by the age of 2 years, the child's stature reflects his own genetic endowment rather than his mother's size and health. Growth during the remainder of childhood occurs at a rate of 5 to 7 cm/year, along the percentile band achieved by 24 months. Adolescence is characterized by an abrupt, short-lived increase in growth velocity (the "growth spurt"), mediated by gonadal hormones and resulting in an adult height that may to some degree be predictable by the parental heights.

Differential rates of growth of various body parts result in marked changes in body proportions during childhood; the school-aged child is not only bigger than the infant but also quite different in appearance. Head growth, for example, a passive phenomenon reflecting growth of the brain, is rapid in early infancy but is largely completed in the first years of life. As the rest of the body continues growing, the head comprises a decreasing fraction of total body size and weight. Also, the limbs grow faster than the trunk throughout childhood; the upper to lower segment ratio decreases from 1.7 at birth to 1.0 at 10 years of age. This disparity in growth velocity between the limbs and the trunk may be most visible during the pubertal growth spurt; the rapid growth of the limbs often produces a gangling appearance, and the child has to wait for trunk growth to catch up in order to "grow into his arms and legs."

Another factor contributing to the changing appearance with age is the relationship of height velocity to weight velocity. During the final trimester of gestation, weight velocity exceeds height velocity, so a full-term newborn looks fat compared to a prematurely born infant. During early childhood, the relationship is reversed, and height velocity exceeds weight velocity. This may be a source of great concern to parents who see their "fat, healthy" baby becoming "skinny," despite reassurance from the physician that their child's height and weight are both progressing normally on the growth curve. Just before puberty, the pattern changes again: weight velocity exceeds height velocity, and children tend to look chubby. During the adolescent growth spurt, height velocity greatly exceeds weight velocity, explaining the "loss of baby fat" at this age.

Full expression in postnatal life of an individual's genetically determined growth potential depends on the normal integration of numerous factors; thus, failure to reach that potential may be due to one of a myriad of possible causes. In infancy, growth failure is generally considered as the syndrome of "failure to thrive" (see Chap. 22).

Growth failure, or short stature, in childhood and adolescence is defined by a height that is less than the third percentile for age. Evaluation must include a detailed history, including parental heights, and a meticulous physical examination. A growth curve, if available, gives invaluable information about the onset of growth deceleration and the presence or absence of a normal growth velocity (at least 5 cm/year). Skeletal maturation is assessed by measurement of body proportions (arm span, upper to lower segment ratio) and by radiographic estimation of bone age. Selection of other laboratory tests is directed by the history and physical examination.

The most common cause of short stature is a genetically limited growth potential: *familial short stature*. This diagnosis implies the absence both of inherited pathologic conditions and of any other growth-retarding abnormality in organ function. Children with familial short stature may be either small or normal in size at birth, but by 2 years of age they are below the third percentile in height and remain there while they grow at an adequate rate to an ultimate height that is consistent with parental heights. Bone age is within the limits of normal for chronologic age, and puberty occurs at the normal time.

Constitutional delay of growth and adolescence is the next most common cause of retarded growth. As in familial short stature, there is no pathologic disorder; these two normal variants together comprise 90 percent of children evaluated for short stature. The child with constitutional delay has a normal birth weight and length and a gradual growth deceleration to a point at or below the third percentile by 2 to 3 years of age, followed by consistent growth at a rate only slightly more than 5 cm/year. Documentation of an adequate growth rate is necessary to rule out an acquired deficiency of pituitary hormones. Bone age is consistent with height age rather than with chronologic age. Sexual development is delayed, with puberty occurring at a time appropriate for the bone age. A normal, though delayed, growth spurt occurs, resulting in an adult height compatible with parental heights. Constitutional growth delay appears to occur more often in males than in females; these children usually present in the early teenage years, a time when many children are beginning puberty and the physical discrepancies of delayed maturation become most evident.

Reassurance that normal sexual development will occur and that a normal adult height will be attained is the only therapy needed in the majority of cases; regular follow-up is essential for psychologic support of the patient and family and for confirmation of the diagnosis. Stimulation of somatic growth and sexual development with anabolic steroids (androgens) may occasionally be indicated in a child with disabling psychosocial problems stemming from delayed growth.

Primordial dwarfism is found in a heterogeneous group of disorders, including placental insufficiency and many dysmorphic syndromes, with or without chromosomal abnormalities. The characteristic features of primordial dwarfism are intrauterine growth retardation with low birth weight, low growth velocity, and short adult stature. Affected children appear to have a decreased growth potential that is independent of familial influences; this may be due to a defect in the responsiveness of somatic tissues to growth-promoting factors or to an irreparable interruption of cell multiplication early in fetal life. Bone age and sexual maturation are usually consistent with chronologic age. Although large doses of human growth hormone may produce some growth in certain children with primordial dwarfism, medical intervention is generally of no value.

Gonadal dysgenesis (XO karyotype, Turner syndrome, see p. 98) is characterized by short stature, the cause of which is uncertain. In some series it is the most common diagnosis in females referred to pediatric endocrinology clinics for evaluation of short stature. The often subtle nature of Turner syndrome in childhood requires that a chromosome analysis be done in every female with nonfamilial short stature.

Chronic systemic disorders frequently result in abnormal somatic growth. Pulmonary, cardiovascular, and central nervous system diseases are usually easily identified as causes of retarded growth, but gastrointestinal and renal diseases are often less obvious causes. Inflammatory bowel disease may present with short stature as the predominant complaint; bowel symptoms may be absent, atypical, or mild but less distressing than the growth failure. Renal tubular acidosis and renal parenchymal destruction secondary to urinary tract obstruction and infection are subtle, frequently overlooked causes of growth failure; screening evaluation of renal function should be done in all patients with nonfamilial short stature. The bone age is usually somewhat retarded in chronic systemic disease; abnormalities in the growth curve reflect the age at onset and severity of the disease. Control or correction of the primary disease can frequently restore normal growth.

Skeletal abnormalities, either heritable (e.g., chondrodysplasia) or acquired (e.g., rickets), are usually obvious causes of short stature. Specific diagnoses are confirmed primarily by x-ray studies.

Although *endocrine disorders* usually result in abnormal growth, they are uncommon causes of growth failure because they are uncommon diseases in childhood. Hypothyroidism in childhood causes marked growth retardation, the severity of which varies with both the degree of thyroid hypofunction and the age at onset; bone age and skeletal proportions are retarded more than height. The child with short stature due to isolated growth hormone (GH) deficiency or hypopituitarism has normal proportions, immature facies, and a characteristic abdominal apron of fat; bone age is consistent with, or somewhat more advanced than, height age. Although GH deficiency is usually idiopathic or familial, a tumor of the sellar or suprasellar region causing pituitary failure must be excluded. A profoundly disordered psychosocial environment has been clearly implicated as a cause of growth failure ("deprivation dwarfism"), characterized by very low levels of circulating pituitary hormones; removal of the child from the abnormal environment results in dramatic catch-up growth and a rapid return of hormone levels to normal.

Hormone excess is an even less common cause of short stature than hormone deficiency. Endogenous or exogenous glucocorticoid excess must be considered, although Cushing syndrome due to an adrenal or pituitary tumor is rare in children. Prematurely increased sex steroids (primarily androgens) from adrenals or gonads cause not only precocious sexual development but also rapid growth, followed by early cessation of growth due to premature epiphyseal fusion, and consequent short adult stature.

Unusually tall stature, which is perceived as a problem primarily when it occurs in females, is almost always a consequence of genetic endowment. It may rarely be a manifestation of a marfanoid syndrome or the result of an excess of growth hormone ("pituitary gigantism").

Despite the fact that abnormal stature, per se, is not a disease and is most often not due to a disease, it may be considered a significant affliction by both the child and his or her family. The physician, patient, and parents must carefully weigh the possible benefit of growth stimulation (for example, by anabolic steroids in a boy with constitutional delay of growth) or growth suppression (for example, by high-dose estrogen therapy in a girl with a projected adult height over 6 ft), the possible risks of such therapy, and the potential psychologic consequences of the abnormal stature.

Normal Growth

1. Smith, D. *Growth and Its Disorders*. Philadelphia: Saunders, 1977.
   Excellent basic chapter on the stages of normal growth, followed by detailed discussions of the causes of abnormal growth; includes many helpful tables of standards not only for height but also for upper-lower segment ratios, growth velocity, and height prediction based on midparental height.
2. Widdowson, E., and McCance, R. A review: New thoughts on growth. *Pediatr. Res.* 9:154, 1975.
   Time of onset, duration, and severity of a growth-retarding insult determine future capability of regaining normal stature.
3. Smith, D., et al. Shifting linear growth during infancy: Illustration of genetic factors in growth from fetal life through infancy. *J. Pediatr.* 89:225, 1976.
   Describes the growth patterns of infants "seeking their own curve."
4. Underwood, L., and Van Wyck, J. Hormones in Normal and Aberrant Growth. In R. Williams (ed.), *Textbook of Endocrinology* (6th ed.). Philadelphia: Saunders, 1981.
   An excellent review of how hormones modulate somatic growth.
5. Phillips, L., and Vassilopoulou-Sellin, R. Somatomedins. *N. Engl. J. Med.* 302:371, 438, 1980.
   A detailed and extensively referenced review of the GH-induced effectors of cellular growth. (Also see Adv. Pediatr. 28:293, 1981; for a review of these and other "growth factors," see Am. J. Dis. Child. 133:419, 1979; for a discussion of somatostatins, inhibitors of GH release, see N. Engl. J. Med. 309:1495, 1556, 1983.)

Abnormal Growth: Reviews

6. Frasier, S. Short stature in children. *Pediatr. Rev.* 3:171, 1981.
   Comprehensive, well-organized review of etiologies and evaluation; much of this information, plus a brief discussion of tall stature, can be found in Pediatr. Clin. North Am. 26:1, 1979.
7. Bacon, G., et al. *A Practical Approach to Pediatric Endocrinology* (2nd ed.). Chicago: Year Book, 1982.
   The chapter on abnormal growth is a very well-referenced review.
8. Rimoin, D., and Horton, W. Short stature. *J. Pediatr.* 92:523, 697, 1978.
   A thoughtful two-part review of the causes and the evaluation of short stature.
9. Dorst, J., et al. The radiologic assessment of short stature–dwarfism. *Radiol. Clin. North Am.* 10:393, 1972.
   Sorting out the causes of dwarfism by radiologic examination.

Constitutional Delay

10. Horner, J., Thorsson, A., and Hintz, R. Growth deceleration patterns in children with constitutional short stature: An aid to diagnosis. *Pediatrics* 62:529, 1978.
    Deceleration occurs in infancy, with normal growth velocity thereafter; thus, an otherwise healthy child who is "crossing percentile lines" during the first 2 years of life does not necessarily require evaluation for growth failure.
11. Gordon, M., et al. Psychosocial aspects of constitutional short stature: Social competence, behavior problems, self-esteem, and family functioning. *J. Pediatr.* 101:477, 1982.
    Children with constitutional delay of growth had lower self-esteem and more behavior problems than children of normal stature.

Primordial Dwarfism

12. Beck., G., and van den Berg, B. The relationship of the rate of intrauterine growth of low birth weight infants to later growth. *J. Pediatr.* 86:504, 1975.
    The small-for-dates infant has the greatest likelihood of persistent growth retardation.
13. Fitzhardinge, P., and Stevens, E. The small-for-date infant: 1. Later growth patterns. *Pediatrics* 49:671, 1972.
    The rate of growth in the first 6 months is a better predictor of later childhood growth than is birth weight.

Systemic Disease

14. Mehrizi, A., and Drash, A. Growth disturbance in congenital heart disease. *J. Pediatr.* 61:418, 1962.
    A retrospective review of infants with cardiac lesions and growth failure.
15. Rosenthal, S., et al. Growth failure and inflammatory bowel disease: Approach to treatment of a complicated adolescent problem. *Pediatrics* 72:481, 1983.
    A comprehensive picture of the pathogenesis (primarily undernutrition) and treatment possibilities (control of disease and dietary supplementation); the effects of therapy on growth have also been described in Pediatrics *55:459, 1975, and 59:717, 1977.*
16. Nash, M., et al. Renal tubular acidosis in infants and children. *J. Pediatr.* 80:738, 1972.
    A diagnosis to be considered in evaluating a child because of growth failure.

Endocrine Dysfunction

17. Root, A., Bongiovanni, A., and Eberlein, W. Diagnosis and management of growth retardation with special reference to the problem of hypopituitarism. *J. Pediatr.* 78:737, 1971.
    A good review, with emphasis on endocrinologic causes.
18. Van Wyck, J., and Underwood, L. Growth hormone, somatomedins, and growth failure. *Hosp. Pract.* 13(8):57, 1978.
    Thorough discussion of theory and practice.
19. Frasier, S. A review of growth hormone simulation tests in children. *Pediatrics* 53:929, 1974.
    Still-current overview. (For an assessment of the exercise test, see Pediatrics *62:526, 1978; for a comparison study showing the smallest number of false-positive results with the combination of levodopa and propranolol as stimulators, see* Am. J. Dis. Child. *133:931, 1979.)*
20. Powell, G., Brasel, J., and Blizzard, R. Emotional deprivation and growth retardation simulating idiopathic hypopituitarism. *N. Engl. J. Med.* 276:1271, 1279, 1967.
    A study of 13 patients, all with a distinctive history, endocrinologic picture, and clinical course.
21. Elders, M. Glucocorticoid therapy in children: Effect on somatomedin secretion. *Am. J. Dis. Child.* 129:1393, 1975.
    A possible explanation for glucocorticoid-induced growth failure.

Tall Stature

22. Reiter, E. The "too tall" child. *Pediatr. Rev.* 5:119, 1983.
    A review of available means of predicting adult height and the efficacy of estrogen

therapy in suppressing growth. (Also see Pediatrics *62:1189, 1196, 1202, and 1210, 1978.)*

Therapy

23. Ad Hoc Committee on Growth Hormone Usage, The Lawson Wilkins Pediatric Endocrine Society, and Committee on Drugs, American Academy of Pediatrics. Growth hormone treatment of children with short stature. *Pediatrics* 72:891, 1983.
    Clarification of the experimental nature of GH use in any but proven GH-deficient children; this is an important counterbalance to the risk of overenthusiastic interpretation of the studies mentioned in reference 24.

24. Frazer, T., et al. Growth hormone-dependent growth failure. *J. Pediatr.* 101:12, 1982.
    This study (and others: Pediatrics *71:576, 1983, and J.* Pediatr. *99:868, 1981) describes a small number of short children with normal GH levels and low serum somatomedin concentrations who respond to injections of GH with accelerated growth and an increase in somatomedin levels. (These two effects cannot be correlated:* Pediatrics *71:324, 1983). (For reports of GH therapy in "short normal" children, see N. Engl. J. Med. 305:123, 1981, and 309:1016, 1983; for a study of its use in patients with intrauterine growth retardation, see J.* Pediatr. *84:635, 1974.)*

25. Committee on Drugs, American Academy of Pediatrics. Counseling synthetic steroids in short stature without organic disease. *Pediatrics* 53:285, 1974.
    Emphasizes psychologic counseling; gives indications for steroids.

26. Rosenfeld, R., Northcraft, G., and Hintz, R. A prospective, randomized study of testosterone treatment of constitutional delay of growth and development in male adolescents. *Pediatrics* 69:681, 1982.
    Patients treated with testosterone grew at a more rapid rate than those not treated, without a greater acceleration of skeletal maturation. There is no evidence in this or similar studies (J. Pediatr. *82:38, 1973; 86:783, 1975; 94:657, 1979; and* Pediatrics *58:412, 1976) that androgens increase or, when used cautiously, decrease ultimate adult height.*

21. INFANT NUTRITION
Robert D. White

The goal of infant nutrition is maintenance of normal growth, development, and health during the important first year of life. Failure to meet this goal can have far-reaching consequences; nutritional excess in infancy may predispose to obesity later in life, while severe undernutrition has been associated with permanent neurologic damage.

The newborn requires 110 to 120 calories/kg/day to meet the energy needs of basal metabolism, activity, and growth; by the end of the first year, the requirement decreases to 80 to 100 cal/kg/day. Calories are supplied by protein and carbohydrate (4 cal/gm each) and fat (9 cal/gm). *Protein* is essential for synthesis of body tissue. Although protein sources differ in their amino acid composition, digestibility, and utilization, it is estimated that the requirement for protein in the neonatal period is about 2.2 gm/kg/day, decreasing to 1.2 gm/kg/day by the end of the first year. Protein intake in excess of 4 gm/kg/day cannot be fully utilized or stored and may produce harmful accumulation of metabolic by-products. *Fat*, also a "building block" for body tissues and hormones, is an important source of immediate and reserve energy and usually comprises 40 to 50 percent of the dietary calories. A small amount of dietary fat must be supplied as linoleic acid; the remainder may be provided as a combination of saturated and unsaturated fats. *Carbohydrate* is a source of immediate energy, but may also be utilized in the synthesis of fat and protein. Only a minimal amount of carbohydrate is actually necessary in the diet, but human milk and most infant formulas derive 40 to 50 percent of their calories from carbohydrate. Lactose, a disaccharide composed of glucose and galactose, is the predominant carbohydrate of both human and cow milk.

At least 12 *minerals* are essential to humans. Most are supplied in appropriate amounts by standard feeding regimens, but iron requires special attention. Iron-deficiency anemia is common in infants fed nonfortified cow milk-based formulas and may be avoided by the use of fortified formulas, supplemental iron, or human milk; although human milk contains no more iron than cow milk, its iron is much better absorbed. *Vitamins* are important as essential cofactors for many metabolic processes; overzealous administration may be detrimental, however. Both human and unfortified cow milk contain negligible amounts of vitamin D, and fortification or supplementation of this vitamin is therefore necessary to prevent rickets. Other vitamins are provided in appropriate amounts by human milk, but cow milk formulas must be fortified with vitamins A and C. *Water* requirements are usually estimated as 100 to 125 ml/100 cal metabolized and are satisfied by the normal feeding regimens for healthy infants.

Human breast milk is uniquely suited to meet the nutritional requirements that have been listed; with the exception of vitamin D, it is a complete food source for most infants until approximately 6 months of age. Its nutrients are present in a more digestible and less antigenic form than are those of cow milk. Human milk also promotes a bowel flora in which *Lactobacillus* rather than *Escherichia coli* predominates, and it contains immunoglobulins, macrophages, and lysozymes that protect against bacterial infection in the infant. The act of breast feeding itself can create a bond between mother and infant that is particularly satisfying.

Currently, breast feeding is initiated in more than 50 percent of newborns, a figure that has risen steadily over the past decade. Since breast feeding is more common now than a generation ago, experienced grandmothers or relatives may not be available to the nursing mother to help her establish and sustain successful nursing; support from knowledgeable health professionals or others is therefore particularly helpful. Strategies that increase the likelihood of successful breast feeding include initiating nursing immediately post partum, providing rooming-in to allow flexible and frequent nursing, refraining from using formula (and, some believe, water) supplementation, and allowing ad-lib rather than strictly scheduled nursing in the first weeks of life.

Commercial formulas derived from cow milk are the usual alternative to breast feeding; most formulas in current use have been "humanized" to approximate human milk in protein, lactose, and mineral composition, and they are "fortified" with vitamins A, C, and D and iron.

The introduction of solid foods into an infant's diet is a decision based more on folklore than on scientific data. Infants do not need solid food before 4 to 6 months of age, but there is also little evidence that earlier introduction is detrimental. (Feeding solid foods before 3 months of age may be somewhat more time-consuming, however, because of the infant's immature tongue and swallowing reflexes.) Feeding-associated problems are common in the first year of life, and infants with gastroenteritis, colic, and constipation occupy a considerable portion of a pediatrician's office time. These problems tend to be self-limited, rarely produce morbidity, and are said to be less common in breast-fed infants. Management varies from one physician to another but often involves dietary manipulation. In gastroenteritis, for example, because damage to the intestinal mucosa produces transient deficiencies of the enzymes of the mucosal brush border, therapy usually includes temporary removal of milk from the diet and replacement with a solution of monosaccharide and minerals that can be absorbed without digestion. Regeneration of the brush border is usually complete 2 to 3 days after the diarrhea has stopped, and milk feedings can be restarted at this point; since lactase is the last enzyme to regain normal activity, some physicians suggest a lactose-free formula for several days before reinstituting regular feedings.

Formula changes are often recommended in the management of colic and constipation, although the rationale for these manipulations is not always clear. Frequently, the normal pattern of increasing "fussiness" of an infant in the first weeks of life is misinterpreted by new parents as colic, leading to unnecessary intervention. Some cases of "colic" may represent intolerance to cow-milk (cow-milk allergy or congenital lactose intolerance) but these probably constitute only a small minority of cases. Furthermore, since both conditions can be diagnosed clinically (lactose intolerance by demonstration of reducing substances in the stool; cow milk allergy, discussed in the next paragraph), empirical changes of formula need not be considered routine therapy for colic. Constipation in infants can usually be managed by the addition of carbohydrates (cane syrup is a favorite), fruits (e.g., prunes), or nonabsorbable substances (mineral oil, dioctyl sodium sulfosuccinate [Colace]) to the diet, without a change of formula.

Cow milk allergy, while somewhat less common than the preceding problems, is more serious. Cow milk contains several antigenic proteins that have ready access to the infant's circulation because the intestinal mucosa during the neonatal period is highly permeable. Allergy to one or more of these proteins is characterized serologically by formation of specific IgE, IgG, IgM, and IgA antibodies and clinically by chronic diarrhea, eczema, and nasal stuffiness, usually presenting in the first month of life. Its incidence, as estimated by various authors, ranges from 0.3 percent to more than 5 percent, depending on the criteria used for diagnosis. Additional symptoms may include cough, asthma, vomiting, colic, anorexia, and irritability, as well as more serious manifestations such as angioneurotic edema and anaphylaxis. Cow milk allergy is usually treated by replacement of dairy products with vegetable proteins in the diet during the first year of life. Many children appear to lose their allergy to cow milk after infancy, and dairy products can often be reintroduced, although care must be taken not to miss symptoms such as abdominal pain, headache, and hyperactivity, which may indicate continued allergy.

Reviews

1. Fomon, S. *Infant Nutrition* (2nd ed.). Philadelphia: Saunders, 1974.
   The bible of infant feeding.
2. Neumann, C., and Jelliffe, D. (eds.). Symposium on nutrition in pediatrics. *Pediatr. Clin. North Am.* 24(1), 1977.
   Practical discussions of economy, vegetarian diets, federal programs, and office assessment. For symposium on intestinal and liver diseases, including cow milk allergy and other causes of diarrhea, see Pediatr. Clin. North Am. *22(4), 1975.*
3. Report of the task force on the assessment of the scientific evidence relating to infant feeding practices and infant health. *Pediatrics* 74:579, 1984; Current issues in feeding the normal infant. *Pediatrics* 75:135, 1985.
   Multi-article supplements summarize an increasingly complex science.
4. Barness, L., and Pitkin, R. (eds.). Nutrition. *Clin. Perinatol.* 2(2), 1975.
   Emphasis on maternal nutrition as it affects the fetus and infant.
5. Fomon, S., et al. Recommendations for feeding normal infants. *Pediatrics* 63:52, 1979.
   Biochemical rationale for selection of milk, solid foods, and vitamin and mineral supplements.
6. Lawrence, R. Infant nutrition. *Pediatr. Rev.* 5:133, 1983.
   Good discussion of failure to thrive and other difficulties associated with breast feeding.
7. Lebenthal, E., Lee, R., and Heitlinger, L. Impact of development of the gastrointestinal tract on infant feeding. *J. Pediatr* 102:1, 1983.
   Fascinating description of the intestine's biologic clock.

Breast-feeding

8. Weichert, C. Breast-feeding: First thoughts. *Pediatrics* 56:987, 1975.
   Explores negative attitudes toward breast feeding and concludes that many are related to sexual anxieties.
9. Ketts, D., and Jones, E. Breast-feeding. *Curr. Probl. Pediatr.* 13:7, 1983.
   For additional review articles, see Pediatr. Rev. *1:289, 1980;* Pediatr. Res. *16:266, 1982; and* Pediatrics *62:591, 1978.*
10. Kemberling, S. Supporting breast-feeding. *Pediatrics* 63:60, 1979.
    Along with Am. J. Dis. Child. *135:595, 1981;* Pediatrics *68:141, 1981; and* A Gift of Love, *published by the American Academy of Pediatrics for nursing mothers: a cornucopia of valuable advice.*
11. Auerbach, K., and Avery, J. Relactation: A study of 366 cases. *Pediatrics* 65:236, 1980.
    Three-fourths of respondents to this survey had a favorable experience, but there is undoubtedly a bias of selection.
12. Jelliffe, D., and Jelliffe, E. "Breast is best": Modern meanings. *N. Engl. J. Med.* 297:912, 1977.
    A review of the biochemical, anti-infective, and psychologic benefits.
13. Giacoia, G., Catz, C., and Yaffe, S. Environmental hazards in milk and infant

nutrition. *Clin. Obstet. Gynecol.* 26:458, 1983.
   Or how people manage to contaminate a good thing. (For a more thorough discussion of drug transfer in breast milk, see Pediatr. Rev. *2:279, 1981.)*
14. Committee on Drugs, American Academy of Pediatrics. Breast-feeding and contraception. *Pediatrics* 68:138, 1981.
   Lactational amenorrhea is not perfect protection!
15. Berger, L. When should one discourage breast-feeding. *Pediatrics* 67:300, 1981.
   Breast is usually best; exceptions are discussed in this article.
16. Nichols, B., and Nichols, V. Nutritional physiology in pregnancy and lactation. *Adv. Pediatr.* 30:473, 1983.
   Extensive discussion of each nutrient, vitamin, and mineral important to the pregnant or nursing mother.

Formula Feeding

17. Wharton, B., and Berger, H. Bottle-feeding. *Br. Med. J.* 1:1326, 1976.
   A short discussion of the practical aspects.
18. ESPGAN Committee on Nutrition. Guidelines on infant nutrition: I. Recommendations for the composition of an adapted formula. *Acta Paediatr. Scand.* [*Suppl.*] 262, 1977.
   Available data on the nutritional needs of infants are the basis for a recommended composition of a "humanized" formula.
19. Anderson, S., Chinn, H., and Fisher, K. History and current status of infant formulas. *Am. J. Clin. Nutr.* 35:381, 1982.
   Encyclopedic discussion of the many pitfalls discovered during the development of current artificial formulas.
20. Committee on Nutrition, American Academy of Pediatrics. On the feeding of supplemental foods to infants. *Pediatrics* 65:1178, 1980.
   More a function of the child's development than age.

Vitamin and Mineral Supplementation

21. Makin, H., Seamark, D., and Trafford, D. Vitamin D and its metabolites in human breast milk. *Arch. Dis. Child.* 58:750, 1983.
   Summarizes the current debate regarding the need for supplementation.
22. Saarinen, U. Need for iron supplementation in infants on prolonged breast feeding. *J. Pediatr.* 93:177, 1978.
   Infants fed human milk after 6 months of age should probably receive an iron supplement.
23. Committee on Nutrition, American Academy of Pediatrics. Fluoride supplementation: Revised dosage schedule. *Pediatrics* 63:150, 1979.
   One must know the concentration of fluoride in the water supply and consider the child's age in order to prescribe this supplement appropriately.
24. Committee on Nutrition, American Academy of Pediatrics. Vitamin and mineral supplement needs in normal children in the United States. *Pediatrics* 66:1015, 1980.
   Includes biochemical rationale for recommendations.

Colic

25. Brazelton, T. Crying in infancy. *Pediatrics* 29:579, 1962.
   "Colic"? Or normal crying? (Related to management: Pediatrics *74:998, 1984).*

Cow Milk Allergy and Intolerance

26. Eastham, E., and Walker, W. Effects of cow's milk on the gastrointestinal tract: A persistent dilemma for the pediatrician. *Pediatrics* 60:477, 1977.
   Attempts to clarify the confusion surrounding the causes and diagnosis of cow milk allergy; the authors conclude that there are multiple causes and no generally accepted means of diagnosis.
27. Gerrard, J., et al. Cow's milk allergy: Prevalence and manifestations in an unselected series of newborns. *Acta Paediatr. Scand.* [*Suppl.*] 234, 1973.
   Of infants allergic to cow milk, 20 percent were also allergic to soy formula; 30 percent had lost their allergy by 12 months of age.

28. Committee on Nutrition, American Academy of Pediatrics. The practical significance of lactose intolerance in children. *Pediatrics* 62:240, 1978.
   *Summarizes current knowledge about lactose intolerance, with recommendations for
   management.*
29. Fomon, S., et al. Cow milk feeding in infancy: Gastrointestinal blood loss and iron
nutritional status. *J. Pediatr.* 98:540, 1981.
   *It would appear that many infants are intolerant of unmodified cow milk until 5
   months of age, even in the absence of lactase insufficiency.*

---

22. FAILURE TO THRIVE
Margaret E. Mohrmann

Failure to thrive (FTT) in infancy and childhood is a sign found in many disorders,
including acute and chronic organic diseases, disordered parent-child interaction, and
overt child abuse. It is usually defined as weight below the third percentile for age;
however, since this definition applies to 3 percent of the population, the description of a
child as failing to thrive also implies an inadequate rate of weight gain (crossing centile
lines) or an inappropriately low weight-for-height or both, usually in a child less than 2
years of age.

Many children admitted to the hospital with this sign have an obvious organic disease
or disorder, such as congenital heart disease or cerebral palsy, which can partially or
completely explain their failure to thrive; these children are more likely to seek medical
care because of signs and symptoms related to their underlying disease than because of
FTT, however. Of the children without known or obvious organic disease, the majority
are considered to have psychosocial or nonorganic FTT. (Psychosocial FTT is distinguished from the syndrome of psychosocial, or deprivation, dwarfism by the definition
of the latter as short *stature* associated with severe psychosocial deprivation in a child
more than 3 years old.) In a small percentage, FTT is but one manifestation of neglect
and/or abuse. Another 15 to 20 percent have subtle organic disease.

An assumed need to "rule out" covert organic disease in children who are failing to
thrive has often resulted in the use of expensive, time-consuming batteries of diagnostic
tests. It is now clear that the presence of previously undiagnosed organic disease is
indicated by findings from an adequately detailed history and physical examination.
Screening laboratory tests that are not suggested by such findings add little—if
anything—to diagnostic accuracy and may have a detrimental effect on the child's already compromised nutritional status.

The etiology of nonorganic FTT is impossible to define precisely, but there are several
recognized contributing factors. Common to almost all cases is a disturbed mother-child
relationship, the responsibility for which cannot be attributed solely to the mother in
most cases. This basic "incompatibility" is often unveiled or exacerbated by one or a
number of stressors, such as maternal depression, multiple siblings, poverty, and marital
discord. The child thus emotionally deprived generally also has an inadequate caloric
intake, due to anorexia, rumination (self-stimulated regurgitation), a deficient supply of
calories, or some combination of these factors. The relative importance of caloric *versus*
emotional deprivation in producing failure to thrive is debatable and probably varies
considerably among infants.

In children with obvious organic disease whose FTT is out of proportion to the severity
of their affliction, the physician must consider the additional diagnosis of psychosocial
FTT; chronic illnesses and congenital anomalies in infants often make development of a
normal mother-child relationship difficult, and FTT may be the result.

In most instances, the child with FTT that is presumed to be of nonorganic etiology
should be hospitalized to allow close observation of the infant and parents and to facilitate thorough interviewing of the parents, a process that often requires several con-
versations. Most authorities agree that an initial determination of hemoglobin and
hematocrit and a urinalysis are warranted; further laboratory evaluation should be
governed by findings from the history and physical examination, which should include

careful observation and scoring of the child's affect and responses to social overtures. The infant with clinically severe malnutrition requires a careful assessment of nutritional status (using tests such as serum albumin and transferrin levels).

Successful management of the infant with nonorganic FTT involves attention to both nutritional and psychosocial factors. To replace the nutritional deficit and achieve weight gain requires the provision of many more calories than would be needed by a well-nourished infant of the same weight and often requires more calories than would be needed by a well-nourished child of similar height. The degree of malnutrition is the major factor determining the route of administration of calories (enteral or intravenous), the composition of feedings, and the time required to attain an adequate caloric intake. Care of the infant's psychosocial situation requires an intensive team effort, both during the hospitalization and for a prolonged period thereafter, aimed at restoring the parent-child relationship and the healthy functioning of the family as a whole. Except in situations of severe child abuse or psychopathology in a parent, it is essential that the parents be intimately involved in the planning and implementation of the infant's care. Most children, within a few days to a few weeks of admittance, show a significant weight gain (which helps confirm the diagnosis of nonorganic FTT); it is the physician's responsibility to see that the infant's improvement in hospital not be construed by the parents as further evidence of their incompetence.

The ultimate prognosis for an infant with nonorganic FTT, especially in terms of emotional health, appears to be related to socioeconomic status, the chronicity of environmental stresses, whether the mother is depressed or hostile, and whether she perceives the child as ill or "bad." Although it is usually possible for these children to achieve some degree of catch-up growth, most remain somewhat underweight and many manifest behavioral and learning problems later in childhood.

Reviews

1. Berwick, D. Nonorganic failure-to-thrive. *Pediatr. Rev.* 1:265, 1980.
   Well-written summary of recent literature that emphasizes the role of the parents in etiology and treatment and the need for consistent long-term follow-up.
2. Goldbloom, R. Failure to thrive. *Pediatr. Clin. North Am.* 29:151, 1982.
   An excellent review with emphasis on the need for supernormal caloric intake to ensure adequate catch-up growth.
3. English, P. Failure to thrive without organic reason. *Pediatr. Ann.* 7:775, 1978.
   Good concise review of facts and speculations.
4. Barbero, G., and Shaheen, E. Environmental failure to thrive: A clinical view. *J. Pediatr.* 71:639, 1967.
   Gives criteria defining nonorganic FTT and makes important statements about the pivotal role of the physician-parent relationship in treatment.
5. Mitchell, W., Gorrell, R., and Greenberg, R. Failure-to-thrive: A study in a primary care setting. *Pediatrics* 65:971, 1980.
   In this survey of a rural, poor population, the incidence of FTT was almost 10 percent, all due to nonorganic causes. (This is in contrast to surveys from referral hospitals that report organic disease to be the major cause.)
6. Smith, C., and Berenberg, W. The concept of failure to thrive. *Pediatrics* 46:661, 1970.
   A trenchant commentary, emphasizing the need to use the phrase "failure to thrive" as a description rather than a diagnosis.

Evaluation

7. Cupoli, J., Hallock, J., and Barness, L. Failure to thrive. *Curr. Probl. Pediatr.* 10(11), 1980.
   Includes a detailed discussion of the important points to cover in the history and physical examination.
8. Homer, C., and Ludwig, S. Categorization of the etiology of failure to thrive. *Am. J. Dis. Child.* 135:848, 1981.
   A thorough history and physical examination accurately differentiated among psychosocial, organic, and combined etiologies; of interest is that one-half of children with organic disease had a significant psychosocial component to their FTT.

9. Sills, R. Failure to thrive: The role of clinical and laboratory evaluation. *Am. J. Dis. Child.* 132:967, 1978.

   A brief but important survey of 185 children with FTT; the organic causes present in 18 percent of the patients were all indicated by the history and physical examination; laboratory tests often confirmed the organic diagnosis but never revealed unsuspected disease. (Similar results: Arch. Dis. Child. 57:347, 1982.)

10. Rosenn, D., Loeb, L., and Jura, M. Differentiation of organic from nonorganic failure to thrive syndrome in infancy. *Pediatrics* 66:698, 1980.

    Presents an "approach-withdrawal" scale for assessing 6- to 16-month-old infants; initial results in a small number of children suggest that this means of scoring the child's social interactions is helpful in identifying those with nonorganic FTT.

Psychologic Aspects and Outcome

11. Leonard, M., Rhymes, J., and Solnit, A. Failure to thrive in infants: A family problem. *Am. J. Dis. Child.* 111:600, 1966.

    Important for its detailed investigation and presentation of disordered parenting.

12. Pollitt, E., and Eichler, A. Behavioral disturbances among failure-to-thrive children. *Am. J. Dis. Child.* 130:24, 1976.

    Significant differences were found in attitudes toward food and in daily caloric intake between children with FTT and a control group.

13. Hufton, I., and Oates, R. Nonorganic failure to thrive: A long-term follow-up. *Pediatrics* 59:73, 1977.

    Five- to eight-year follow up of 22 children: nearly half of them had behavioral and school problems.

23. OBESITY
Margaret E. Mohrmann

The pervasive problem of obesity and its management has become a source of much controversy and consternation among physicians. Although pediatricians are not usually faced with significant health problems associated with this form of malnutrition, they do have two unique obligations. First, given the fact that a majority of obese juveniles and adolescents remain obese as adults, physicians who care for children must assume considerable responsibility for early education and prevention. Second, it is essential that pediatricians anticipate, recognize, and thoughtfully manage the psychologic problems of the obese child and his family.

Several studies have attempted to link infantile and juvenile obesity with adult obesity; the results are somewhat conflicting. A synthesis of these studies indicates that 20 to 40 percent of overweight infants are overweight in later childhood (less than 10 percent of nonobese infants become obese juveniles) and that almost 80 percent of overweight adolescents are overweight as adults. Further, studies of obese adults indicate that those who were overweight as children tend to be the most severely obese adults and most resistant to treatment.

Obesity in the adult has long been thought to be a factor in a number of chronic diseases, although the question of causation versus association is generally unsettled. The Framingham cardiovascular study showed a 10-fold increase in the incidence of hypertension in obese adults (with all proper guidelines concerning adequate cuff size being followed). The study also showed a significantly increased incidence of all types of cardiovascular disease in obese men and women, regardless of whether hypertension or hyperlipidemia was also present.

In obese children and adults, one may see numerous metabolic derangements, such as impaired glucose tolerance, insulin resistance, hypertriglyceridemia, hypercholesterolemia, hyperadrenocorticism, and a blunted growth hormone response to exercise and other stimulants. These abnormalities, rather than being the cause of the obesity, may all be explained by the overweight condition itself—many of them being related to the enlarged adipocyte's insensitivity to insulin—and are all reversible with weight loss.

Although many practitioners take the view that "a child is fat if he looks fat," the definitive diagnosis of obesity and the measurement of the degree of obesity are not quite that simple. The use of weight may be adequate in many children, especially when correlated with height, but the problem of separating the contribution of lean body mass from that of body fat can make the measurement of total body weight alone difficult to interpret at times. Skin-fold thickness, measured in the triceps and scapular areas, is a considerably more accurate gauge of adiposity, and there are numerous tables of normal standards available; a drawback to the use of this method is the need for accurate calipers. Indexes, such as Quetelets' (W/H^2) and the ponderal index ($\sqrt[3]{W}/H$), are frequently used in obesity studies but are of limited usefulness for the practicing pediatrician. For practical purposes, a child may be considered overweight if he or she is 10 to 20 percent over the ideal weight (50th percentile for height) and obese if more than 20 percent overweight.

There are several uncommon syndromes characterized by obesity, such as the Prader-Willi syndrome (see p. 281), but by far the predominant cause of obesity in childhood is excessive caloric intake. The debatable point is whether "excessive" is an absolute or relative term. There are proponents of the theory who think obesity is caused solely and simply by overeating or by overfeeding in infancy. Others feel that because of some unknown factor—possibly a genetically determined defect in thermogenesis—a "normal" caloric intake may cause obesity in certain persons. In the presence of a normal height (or somewhat accelerated linear growth, not uncommonly seen in obesity), a search for an endocrinologic cause, such as hypothyroidism or Cushing syndrome, is not indicated.

Many attempts have been made to correlate adipocyte mass with the development and maintenance of obesity. The facts appear to be that adipose cell number normally increases gradually until puberty; after that time, only cell size may increase or decrease with weight gain or loss. Theoretically (factually, in the opinion of some), obesity in childhood causes an excessive number of fat cells to be formed, so that the adult is, in a sense, predestined to be obese.

Although many would argue with the data used to support the theory of excessive adipocyte numbers, there is a statistical correlation between childhood and adult obesity, for whatever reason. The best defense against the development of infantile and juvenile obesity is the education of parents in good nutritional habits and toward abolishing the maxim that "a fat baby is a healthy baby." Encouraging breast feeding and advocating the late introduction of solid foods (after 4 months of age, rather than at 1 or 2 months) are two practical ways to help prevent overfeeding.

Once obesity is established, the treatment is difficult, frustrating, and seldom successful. At present, a combination of moderate caloric restriction, increased physical activity, and some form of behavior modification appears to offer the best possibility for long-term success. It is important to remember that during childhood and early adolescence, before linear growth has ceased, any caloric restriction must be undertaken with great caution; the therapist may have to be satisfied with a stabilization of weight, rather than weight loss, in order to maintain linear growth. In general, anorectic drugs have no place in the treatment of childhood obesity. Gastric and jejunoileal bypass operations have been used in a small number of pediatric patients, mostly adolescents, as a "last-resort" treatment of massive obesity. Although these procedures have often been successful in producing weight loss, one must be aware of the numerous medical and psychologic problems associated with them; surgical treatment should probably not be recommended for a child who is less than 250 to 300 percent overweight or who has not had an adequately intensive trial of dietary restriction.

As noted, medical complications of obesity in childhood are unusual. A rare problem is the pickwickian syndrome of massive obesity, alveolar hypoventilation, and cardiac decompensation. The most significant aspects of childhood obesity are the implications for obesity in adulthood and the adverse psychologic effects on the child, who often suffers ridicule and isolation by peers, has a poor self-image, and may be the focal point for pathologic family interactions.

General

1. Committee on Nutrition, American Academy of Pediatrics. Nutritional aspects of obesity in infancy and childhood. *Pediatrics* 68:880, 1981.
   An excellent place to start for a concise but thorough summary of current opinion.

2. Dietz, W. Childhood obesity: Susceptibility, cause, and management. *J. Pediatr.* 103:676, 1983.
   An excellent survey that emphasizes important details of dietary, psychologic, and family therapy.
3. Weil, W. Obesity in children. *Pediatr. Rev.* 3:180, 1981.
   A well-written, thorough discussion of epidemiology, etiology, and treatment. (For another, longer review, see Curr. Probl. Pediatr. 12(11), 1982.)
4. Montagu, A. Obesity and the evolution of man. *J.A.M.A.* 195:105, 1966.
   An anthropologically oriented essay, with the conclusion that obesity can in no way be considered evolutionarily advantageous.
5. Weil, W. Current controversies in childhood obesity. *J. Pediatr.* 91:175, 1977.
   An appropriately skeptical review of all aspects, emphasizing the paucity of facts; an important counterweight to the rest of the literature.
6. Bruch, H. Obesity in childhood. *Am. J. Dis. Child.* 58:457, 1939.
   A classic, often-quoted study of 102 obese children with meticulous analyses of their growth and developmental characteristics (28 pages).

Epidemiology and Etiology

7. Charney, E., et al. Childhood antecedents of adult obesity. *N. Engl. J. Med.* 295:6, 1976.
   A comparison of adult (third-decade) weight with weight up to 6 months; 36 percent of those whose weight was above the 90th percentile at least once in the first 6 months of life are overweight or obese as adults (366 subjects).
8. Zack, P., et al. A longitudinal study of body fatness in childhood and adolescence. *J. Pediatr.* 95:126, 1979.
   The best predictor of adolescent obesity is childhood obesity.
9. Vuille, J.-C., and Mellbin, T. Obesity in 10 year olds: An epidemiologic study. *Pediatrics* 64:564, 1979.
   A well-designed study of 550 Swedish children; the results support the concept of a multifactorial etiology of obesity (factors assessed were early weight gain, appetite, activity, environment, and heredity) but also show differences between the sexes in the relative predictive value of each factor.
10. Kramer, M. Do breast-feeding and delayed introduction of solid foods protect against subsequent obesity? *J. Pediatr.* 98:883, 1981.
    In this study of adolescents, those who were not breast-fed were more likely to be obese. (As counterpoint, a study reported in Am. J. Clin. Nutr. 32:1997, 1979, found no correlation between feeding practices and infant obesity.)
11. Huse, D., et al. The challenge of obesity in childhood. *Mayo Clin. Proc.* 57:279, 285, 1982.
    An interesting study of school children (aged 9–13 years), including intervention and reassessment after 5 years, which produced an attitudinal staging system that may be useful both as outcome predictor and as treatment guide.
12. Smith, D. Adipose Tissue and Obesity. In *Growth and Its Disorders*. Philadelphia: Saunders, 1977.
    A short, informative chapter with emphasis on etiology, the author thinks that the problem is primarily idiopathic and not related to overeating; tables (on the inside back and front covers of the book) include skin-fold thickness standards.
13. Knittle, J. Obesity in childhood: A problem in adipose tissue cellular development. *J. Pediatr.* 81:1048, 1972.
    A good overview, with emphasis on metabolic phenomena and theories of pathogenesis (10 pages, 77 references).

Complications

14. Mann, G. The influence of obesity on health. *N. Engl. J. Med.* 291:178, 226, 1974.
    A very readable (often wry) discussion of fact versus theory with respect to the relationship of obesity to chronic disease and types of therapy (14 pages, 138 references). (For a discussion of the relationship of body weight to morbidity and mortality, see Ann. Intern. Med. 100:285, 1984.)
15. Salans, L., and Wise, J. Metabolic studies of human obesity. *Med. Clin. North Am.* 54:1533, 1970.

A concise review of metabolic derangements in obesity, emphasizing the insulin resistance of the enlarged adipocyte.

16. Hubert, H., et al. Obesity as an independent risk factor for cardiovascular disease: A 26 year follow-up of participants in the Framingham heart study. *Circulation* 67:968, 1983.
    Not only is obesity a significant risk factor in men, but it is now seen to be preceded in importance only by age and blood pressure as an independent risk factor in women.
17. Sims, E., and Berchtold, P. Obesity and hypertension: Mechanisms and implications for management. *J.A.M.A.* 247:49, 1982.
    Strongly recommends attempts to decrease weight and increase physical activity before use of antihypertensive drugs.
18. Ward, W., and Kelsey, W. The Pickwickian syndrome. *J. Pediatr.* 61:745, 1962.
    A good discussion of clinical manifestations and pathophysiology.
19. Stool, S., et al. The "chubby puffer" syndrome. *Clin. Pediatr.* (Phila.) 16:43, 1977.
    Three case reports of upper airway obstruction exacerbated by massive obesity.

Treatment

20. Barnes, H., and Berger, R. An approach to the obese adolescent. *Med. Clin. North Am.* 59:1507, 1975.
    A good, brief discussion of the problem, with differential diagnosis; emphasis on a practical plan of caloric restriction and modification of eating habits; in Pediatr. Clin. North Am. *24:123, 1977, a detailed therapeutic regimen is presented.*
21. Brownell, K., and Stunkard, A. Behavioral treatment of obesity in children. *Am. J. Dis. Child.* 132:403, 1978.
    Best overview of theory and practice; same authors present evidence of importance of nature of parental involvement in treatment in Pediatrics *71:515, 1983.*
22. Rayner, P., and Court, J. The effect of dietary restriction and anorectic drugs on linear growth velocity in childhood obesity. *Postgrad. Med. J.* 51[Suppl. 1]:120, 1975.
    Growth velocity in the group put on a diet and given fenfluramine decreased relative to that in the group on a diet alone and to that in normal subjects.
23. Pugliese, M., et al. Fear of obesity: A cause of short stature and delayed puberty. *N. Engl. J. Med.* 309:513, 1983.
    A reminder of what excessive dieting can do to children.
24. Joffe, S. A review: Surgery for morbid obesity. *J. Surg. Res.* 33:74, 1982.
    For specific information about the results of bypass procedures in children and adolescents, see J. Pediatr. Surg. *9:341, 1974, and 10:51, 1975.*

24. DEVELOPMENT AND RETARDATION
Kenneth B. Roberts and Eileen P. G. Vining

"Growing up" involves three major dynamic processes: growth (see Chap. 20), sexual maturation (see Chap. 30), and development. Development refers to the progressive acquisition of skills and abilities in various spheres of functioning: motor (both gross and fine); social-adaptive; communication; and cognitive. Development does not proceed in each sphere at the same rate, but certain principles are common to all: (1) Development is progressive; the rate may vary from rapid to imperceptible, but the direction is constant. Temporary setbacks may be noted, so-called regressive behavior, but a continued loss of previously attained milestones is abnormal and requires attention. (2) Development is orderly and cumulative; one milestone necessarily follows another in a regular, predictable fashion. For example, motor development proceeds according to neurologic maturation, from head to foot (cephalocaudad progression). Language begins with cooing, then babbling, then words, "jargoning" (the inflection of speech without recognizable speech), sentences, and so forth. Cognitive development also advances in identifiable stages: sensorimotor, preconceptual, intuitive, concrete operations, and formal operations. (3) Development is affected by many factors, including genetic potential, neurologic maturation, overall physical condition, and environmental and emotional orces. The interplay of factors is complex, and each child's uniqueness is preserved despite the apparent stereotyped nature of development; indeed, few children are "average" in all spheres at all times.

Pediatricians need to be able to assess a child's level of functioning in all of the various spheres to portray accurately the child's true capacity, strengths, and weaknesses. Parents, school systems, and government programs look to the pediatrician for guidance; as resources are developed to aid children with developmental problems, there is increased pressure—and reason—to identify children with "handicaps." Knowledge of normal developmental tasks and behavior patterns not only is necessary for assessment but also permits guidance to be consistent with reasonable expectations.

Assessment begins with the history, to determine the presence of recognized "risk factors" (e.g., neonatal asphyxia, sensory or motor handicaps) and construct a timetable of milestones attained. Parental ability to chronicle development is often quite good, although understandably better for recent events than for more distant ones; pediatricians should nevertheless seek to document present abilities by direct examination. The physical examination also includes identification of all major and minor abnormalities to detect the presence of a known syndrome (see Malformation Syndromes, Chap. 79). Tests such as the Denver Developmental Screening Test (DDST) make office screening feasible; more formal testing, using the Cattell or Bayley Scales for infants and the Wechsler Scales for older children, may be required if a problem is suggested by the history, the examination, or the screening tests.

The pattern of delays or abnormalities gives clues to possible causes and thereby directs the further evaluation. Impaired gross motor development, when it is an isolated finding, suggests cerebral palsy (see Chap. 83) or, less commonly, skeletal or neuromuscular disease. Fine motor development requires intact vision as well as extrapyramidal function. Abnormalities of social-adaptive development, often expressed in infancy as failure to thrive (see Chap. 22) and in older children as depression and/or "behavior problems," alert the pediatrician to explore the child's home and family situation. Isolated delay in language demands assessment of the child's hearing. Children may be of normal intelligence and have an attention deficit or specific learning disability (see Chap 25). The greatest developmental concern is more globally impaired cognitive function: mental retardation.

Mental retardation is defined by the American Academy of Mental Deficiency (AAMD) as "significantly subaverage general intellectual functioning (two standard deviations below the normal) existing concurrently with deficits in adaptive behavior, and manifested during the developmental period." "Two standard deviations below the normal" would identify approximately 2.5 percent of the population as "retarded," but recent studies, utilizing the AAMD definition and carefully considering adaptive functioning, suggest an incidence of approximately 1 percent in children under 18 years of age. The majority of retarded persons have an IQ between 50 and 70; there is a high likelihood of retardation in other members of their family and a disproportionate representation of the lower socioeconomic groups. The more severely retarded (IQ below 50) comprise only about 0.3 percent of the population and, except for children with specific syndromes, do not show an increased intrafamilial occurrence and are evenly distributed among socioeconomic groups.

Four grades of retardation severity are distinguished: mild (IQ:55–69), moderate (IQ: 40–54), severe (IQ:25–39), and profound (IQ: < 25). The lower the IQ or the developmental quotient (DQ: [the age level of function/the chronologic age] × 100), the earlier development can be recognized with confidence as being outside the range of normal. Thus, children with mild retardation are often not identified until kindergarten or first grade, while those with moderate retardation are recognized in preschool settings, and those with more severe handicaps are distinguished before age 3.

Children with mild mental retardation (previously called "educably retarded") are usually normal physically and in motor development, but they show a limited ability to generalize concepts well. Appropriate goals for these children include literacy and the ability to read instructional manuals. It is vital that they receive vocational guidance, since they can lead a significantly independent existence; as adults, roughly two-thirds are employed, and 80 percent are married.

Moderately ("trainably") retarded children, with appropriate education, can be taught to read "survival words" (such as STOP), write their name, and learn sufficient arithmetic to be able to conduct their own basic shopping as adults. They usually can handle routine daily functions but often have a tendency to excessive motor activity and perseveration. They require some supervision to negotiate living in a complex society.

The severely retarded often can become independent in terms of self-care, feeding, and toileting, but they require a great deal of supervision. Profoundly retarded children may respond to very structured situations and behavioral management, but many require nursing or custodial care.

Approximately 85 percent of retarded children have at least 1 additional handicap, the recognition of which is important for maximal habilitation. One-half have ambulation problems and upper limb difficulties, one-half have speech problems, and one-half have emotional problems. Problems in toilet training are common and are of longer duration, in accordance with developmental age rather than chronologic age. Visual and hearing deficits and seizures are more frequent than in children of normal intelligence. In addition, 40 percent have chronic organic conditions, such as dental disease, obesity, anemia, heart disease, and diabetes.

An important part of management is the counseling of the family. The physician needs to feel secure in the diagnosis and the likely prognosis and must be able to tailor communication to the family's stage of emotional adjustment. (See Death, Dying, and Mourning, Chap. 18, for related discussion.) Siblings should also be counseled, to help them avoid problems with guilt, resentment, shame, fear that they themselves might also be "defective," and, finally, concern about their long-term responsibilities to their retarded sibling.

Organizations such as the National Association for Retarded Citizens have an important role in the welfare of the retarded. They increase awareness and understanding, develop programs, exert pressure on governmental agencies, and provide a means for parents to work with other parents.

The future for mentally retarded persons depends on their level of competence but also on society's philosophy and goals. The 1971 United Nations Declaration on the Rights of Mentally Retarded Persons states that the mentally retarded person has "to the maximum degree of feasibility, the same rights as other human beings." These include medical care, education, economic security, a decent standard of living, and a chance to live in as normal surroundings as possible; legal decisions have guaranteed all children the right to an appropriate education. Considerable emphasis has been placed on deinstitutionalization and normalization; retarded citizens are remaining with or being returned to their families, to live in the community. This program requires the cooperation of the pediatrician, both in providing medical services and in planning.

Reviews

1. Illingworth, R. *The Development of the Infant and Young Child: Normal and Abnormal.* Edinburgh: Churchill-Livingstone, 1975.
   Basic yet complete. Good descriptions and photos; well-indexed.
2. Knobloch, H., and Pasamanick, B. (eds.). *Gesell and Amatruda's Developmental Diagnosis.* Hagerstown, Md.: Harper & Row, 1974.
   The basic Gesell items, weighted toward the first year of life.
3. Horowitz, F. Child development for the pediatrician. *Pediatr. Clin. North Am.* 29:359, 1982.
   A review of normal development, assessment, and intervention.

General Developmental Assessment

4. Capute, A., and Biehl, R. Functional developmental evaluation: Prerequisite to habilitation. *Pediatr. Clin. North Am.* 20:3, 1973.
   Reviews developmental screening and milestones; presents a parent questionnaire. (Part of a symposium on the habilitation of the handicapped child.)
5. Thorpe, H., and Werner, E. Developmental screening of preschool children: A critical review of inventories used in health and educational programs. *Pediatrics* 53:362, 1974.
   Reviews the DDST, Head Start, and other tests.
6. Frankenburg, W., et al. The newly abbreviated and revised Denver Developmental Screening Test. *J. Pediatr.* 99:995, 1981.

A screening test for a screening test! Using 12 items from the DDST permits identification of all those who require the entire test.

7. Frankenburg, W., et al. The Denver Prescreening Developmental Questionnaire (PDQ). *Pediatrics* 57:744, 1976.

A 5-minute questionnaire derived from DDST items; permitted a 69 percent decrease in the number of full DDST examinations required. Another parent questionnaire: Pediatrics 63:872, 1979.

8. Shonkoff, J., et al. Primary care approaches to developmental disabilities. *Pediatrics* 64:506, 1979.

The majority of pediatricians interviewed did not use screening tests but relied exclusively on clinical judgment and general observations to assess development. (Also see J. Pediatr. 93:524, 1978.) Assessing development in such an informal manner is feasible (Pediatrics 65:614, 1980)—mothers can do it (Am. J. Dis. Child, 136:101, 1982)—but it is fraught with clinical pitfalls, such as being misled by cuteness or normal motor development (Clin. Pediatr. [Phila.] 21:308, 1982).

Assessment: Specific Aspects

9. Capute, A., and Accardo, P. Linguistic and auditory milestones during the first two years of life: A language inventory for the practitioner. *Clin. Pediatr.* (Phila.) 17:847, 1978.

A 32-item evaluation instrument is described. (For another early language milestone scale, see Pediatrics 70:677, 1982.) Delay in speaking should not be ignored; causes and management: Clin. Pediatr. (Phila.) 14:403, 1975. (For reviews of language disorders and hearing-impairment, see Pediatr. Rev. 6:85, 151, 1984.)

10. Hreidarsson, S., Shapiro, B., and Capute, A. Age of walking in the cognitively impaired. *Clin. Pediatr.* (Phila.) 22:248, 1983.

Cognitive level is not the sole criterion for this motor skill.

11. Scheiner, A., and Moomaw, M. Care of the visually handicapped child. *Pediatr. Rev.* 4:74, 1982.

A review of milestones, screening and early identification, developmental aspects of blindness, intervention, education, and the role of the primary care physician. (Also see Pediatr. Rev. 6:173, 1984.)

12. Rosenberger, P. The pediatrician and psychometric testing. *Pediatric. Rev.* 2:301, 1981.

Not only what but when.

Normal Cognitive Development

13. Flavell, J. *Cognitive Development.* Englewood Cliffs, N.J.: Prentice-Hall, 1977.

Piaget's stages of cognitive development made clear.

14. Baroody, A., and Ginsburg, H. Preschoolers' informal mathematical skills. *Am. J. Dis. Child.* 136:195, 1982.

An editorial review of the development of skills such as counting.

15. Bibace, R., and Walsh, M. Development of children's concept of illness. *Pediatrics* 66:912, 1980.

Fits nicely the stages of cognitive development proposed by Piaget. (Also see Pediatrics 67:841, 1981, and, specifically for adolescents' conceptions, Pediatrics 68:834, 1981. The concept of "where babies come from" follows a similar developmental course: responses of children at various ages are presented in Child. Dev. 46:77, 1975. You'll enjoy this one!)

Mental Retardation

16. Grossman, H. (ed.). Symposium on mental retardation. *Pediatr. Clin. North Am.* 15(4), 1968.

Dated in some aspects, but it has good chapters on issues such as physician's role, parental expectations, behavior modification, and education.

Mental Retardation: Etiology and Evaluation

17. Opitz, J. Mental retardation: Biologic aspects of concern to pediatricians. *Pediatr. Rev.* 2:41, 1980.

Emphasis is on etiology and "the workup."

18. Smith, D., and Simons, F. Rational diagnostic evaluation of the child with mental deficiency. *Am. J. Dis. Child.* 129:1285, 1975.
    Classification by cause and by timing of insult (prenatal, perinatal, postnatal unknown) permits an appropriate diagnostic evaluation. (Role of CT scan: J. Pediatr 98:63, 1981.)

19. Townes, P. Fragile-X syndrome: A jigsaw puzzle with picture emerging. *Am. J. Dis Child.* 136:389, 1982.
    An editorial review of what may possibly be the second most common diagnosable cause of mental retardation. (Down syndrome is more common.)

Mental Retardation: Supportive Management

20. Myers, B. The informing interview. *Am. J. Dis. Child.* 137:572, 1983.
    Management begins with "breaking the news"; the author discusses the variou ingredients that interact in the interview.

21. Butler, A. There's something wrong with Michael: A pediatrician-mother's perspective. *Pediatrics* 71:446, 1983.
    An articulate and sensitive description of feelings and dynamics.

22. Miller, L. Toward a greater understanding of the parents of the mentally retarded *J. Pediatr.* 73:699, 1968.
    A superb description of parental reaction and adjustment, with excellent suggestion for counseling.

Mental Retardation/Developmental Delay: Treatment

23. American Academy of Pediatrics. The Doman-Delacato treatment of neurologically handicapped children. *Pediatrics* 70:810, 1982.
    A review of the process, the claims, and the available data; the AAP concludes tha patterning "offers no special merit" and "in some cases there may be harm in its use."

24. Marquis, P. Cognitive stimulation. *Am. J. Dis. Child.* 130:410, 1976.
    A review of educational surveys, animal research, and controlled interventio programs, concluding that programs aimed at preventing "educationa incapacitation" should focus on "optimizing the developmental milieu of the child prior to age 4. (For the "current status" of infant stimulation or enrichment programs the first of four consecutive articles on related issues, see Pediatrics 67:32, 1981.)

25. McCall, R. A hard look at stimulating and predicting development: The cases o bonding and screening. *Pediatr. Rev.* 3:205, 1982.
    The author is skeptical. (Also see editorial on p. 203.)

26. Wright, G. The pediatrician's role in public law 94-142. *Pediatr. Rev.* 4:191, 1982.
    Definitions, issues, and problems. (Focus on education of retarded children. Am. J Dis. Child. 127, 237, 1974.) Also see Attention Deficit Disorder, Chap. 25.

25. ATTENTION DEFICIT DISORDER
Kenneth B. Roberts

Attention deficit disorder (ADD) is the current designation of a syndrome of childhoo formerly referred to by terms such as "minimal brain dysfunction (MBD)," "hyperkineti syndrome," etc. The new nomenclature identifies that inattention, rather than hyper activity, is the central feature of the syndrome; this is of benefit since not all childre with ADD are hyperactive, and those who are tend to become less hyperactive (but no necessarily less inattentive) with time. The syndrome is common, affecting 5 t 10 percent of schoolchildren, and is not limited to any particular social class. In all ag groups, boys are affected 4 to 10 times more commonly than girls.

"Inattention" is defined as three or more of the following: (1) often fails to finish thing he or she starts, (2) often does not seem to listen, (3) easily distracted, (4) difficulty concentrating on schoolwork or other tasks requiring sustained attention, and (5 difficulty sticking to a play activity.

"Impulsivity," another constant feature of ADD, is defined as three or more of the following: (1) often acts before thinking, (2) excessive shifting from one activity to an other, (3) has difficulty organizing work (not due to cognitive impairment), (4) needs a lo of supervision, (5) frequent calling out in class, and (6) difficulty waiting for turn in games or group situations.

The source of this nomenclature, the third edition of the American Psychiatric Association Diagnostic and Statistical Manual of Mental Disorders (known as DSM-III) has three requirements for a diagnosis of ADD in addition to the presence of inattention and impulsivity: (1) onset before age 7 years; (2) duration of at least 6 months; and (3) absence of schizophrenia, affective disorder, or severe or profound mental retardation. Categories are established for "Attention Deficit Disorder with Hyperactivity," "Attention Deficit Disorder Without Hyperactivity," and "Attention Deficit Disorder, Residual Type."

Many children with ADD are clearly hyperactive. (For "hyperactivity," DSM-III requires two or more of the following: (1) runs about or climbs on things excessively, (2) has difficulty sitting still or fidgets excessively, (3) has difficulty staying seated, (4) moves about excessively during sleep, and (5) is always "on the go" or acts as if "driven by a motor".) Commonly, the history is that the child was "colicky" as an infant, with difficulty in falling asleep or general irritability. The hyperactive preschool child may be described as "clumsy," "into everything," and "difficult to discipline." Temper tantrums and a short attention span are characteristic of the affected kindergarten-age child. During adolescence, there is often improvement in the motor symptoms. The history is of particular importance, since the usual physical examination may be misleading: a personal interview with the physician may fail to elicit hyperactive behavior that is readily apparent in a group setting, such as the classroom.

Many children with ADD, although of normal or near-normal intelligence, have learning disabilities. Associated with learning disorders are perceptual deficits, such as difficulty with right-left discrimination, spatial orientation, and hand-eye coordination. Deficits in symbols and language development are common.

Children with ADD may have hyperactivity or learning disabilities; many have both. The differential diagnosis includes such disparate conditions as normal (exuberant) behavior, mental retardation, severe emotional disturbance, vision or hearing deficit, hyperthyroidism, other metabolic disorders (e.g., lead intoxication, hypoglycemia), or neurologic disorders (such as chorea). An accurate diagnosis is of obvious importance, since the treatment for each of these conditions is different.

The goal of the medical history is to try to distinguish the various disorders and to assess the degree of disability. A family history may be positive for ADD, and the information about a previous occurrence may be most helpful in counseling. Attention is often directed toward gestational and perinatal events, though the relevance for any given child with ADD is unclear, contrary to the situation in cerebral palsy. The developmental history is of great importance and should include a description of characteristic behavior at various ages and identify achievements and educational attainments; the social and environmental history focuses on such factors as patterns of discipline, reactions to the child's behavior, and maintenance of friendships.

The physical examination is of value largely to rule out other causes of hyperactivity or learning disability. Although much has been made of inability to perform rapid alternating movements (dysdiadochokinesis), decreased coordination for age, increased mirror movements, and so on, there appears to be a growing disenchantment with these "soft signs" as indicators of "disease," and many clinicians favor spending the examination time determining what the child thinks of himself and his relationship to other people rather than grading performance on the finger-nose test and other such tests. The electroencephalogram does not appear to help in either diagnosis or treatment unless the child has a clinical indication of an abnormality, such as seizures; this rationale extends to other tests, such as echoencephalograms, radioisotope brain scans, karyotyping, and skull roentgenograms.

Psychometric testing is of great importance and should include a determination not only of IQ but also of perceptual ability and reading performance. The status of hearing, speech, and vision should be investigated if there is any question about these abilities. The data-gathering process is incomplete until information has been solicited from the school, which, as previously noted, may be able to provide a more valuable assessment of the child's behavior than the physician during a one-on-one interview.

In planning a course of treatment, it is prudent to consider hyperactivity and learning disability separately. Two classes of chemotherapeutic agents have been used to assist in controlling hyperactive behavior: stimulants, such as methylphenidate (Ritalin) or amphetamines, and tranquilizers. The former reduce purposeless activity and allow better performance, while the latter reduce activity but may impede learning. Many children "respond" to a placebo, but the stimulant drugs have been shown to be more effective. Response to methylphenidate or amphetamines occurs in 60 to 80 percent of the patients and is often dramatic, with observable improvement within a day or two; the effect of these drugs lasts only a matter of hours, however. The following are the three most notable side effects: (1) anorexia initially, coupled with other growth inhibiting effects, resulting in a diminished velocity of height and weight gain; (2) insomnia, which may be minimized by withholding medication after 3 to 4 P.M.; and (3) dysphoria in some children. Primarily because of the natural tendency for hyperactivity to diminish with age and because of concern about decreased growth rate, some authors have advocated limiting medication to school days only; this permits catch-up growth during the summer and allows determination of the age at which the child no longer requires medication. Other authorities emphasize that most learning and social interaction takes place outside the classroom and therefore stress the importance of continuing medication on weekends and vacations.

The response to pharmacologic agents may be limited or augmented by emotional and environmental factors. Counseling of the family to permit venting of frustration, hostility, and guilt feelings is an important part of the management. Assistance is often needed to help the family and child organize daily activities and establish a routine of one-step assignments for the child that can be mastered with repetition. The physician often provides a great service just by lending a sympathetic ear, recognizing the problems posed by a hyperactive child with short attention span, and alleviating guilt by insisting that the mother schedule time for herself. Many programs utilizing various methods and claiming to help the child have become popular; the physician may be asked about dietary manipulations (especially the Feingold diet), patterning therapy, optometric exercises, and other treatments. Converts to the programs are persuasive, but data to support the claims are lacking.

No pharmacologic agents are available that will ensure learning; drugs may make it more feasible for the student to concentrate, but it should be emphasized that control of hyperactivity per se may be insufficient to satisfy the needs of the child with a coexisting learning disorder. Many school systems simply do not have the resources to deal with children with learning disabilities, and those that have such resources suffer from a lack of good data specifying how best to treat each child. Despite the practical limitations, educators agree on certain principles: the need for repetition, the need to build on the child's strengths, the need for more individual attention than can be provided in the ordinary classroom, and the need to keep distracting stimuli to a minimum.

In considering prognosis—as with diagnosis—it is best to separate hyperactivity and learning disability. By adolescence, many of the symptoms of hyperactivity recede, but the child is left with signs and symptoms that are interpreted by some as the "scars" of previous failures and lack of self-control. There is an increased incidence of social disability, including delinquency; this tends to abate by early adulthood. Most studies have demonstrated that the attention and learning disorders persist. Children with higher IQs appear to do better as a group, but even here, it is clear that an early and continued goal of management must be modification of the pattern of persistent and repeated failure. "Cure" seems unattainable; rather, successful adaptation is the desired outcome.

Developmental Disabilities

1. Shaywitz, S., Grossman, H., and Shaywitz, B. Symposium on learning disorders. *Pediatr. Clin. North Am.* 31(2), 1984.
   A collection of 12 articles on ADD, learning disorders, school failure, and more (513 pages).
2. Levine, M. The high prevalence–low severity developmental disorders of schoolchildren. *Adv. Pediatr.* 29:529, 1982.
   An extensive (25-page) review of the problems in defining, diagnosing, and managing the spectrum of disabilities.
3. Levine, M., Busch, B., and Aufseeser, C. The dimension of inattention among children with school problems. *Pediatrics* 73:87, 1982.

Children with primarily attention deficits compared with children with learning problems: significant degree of overlap found.

Attention Deficit Disorder

4. Shaywitz, S., and Shaywitz, B. Evaluation and treatment of children with attention deficit disorders. *Pediatr. Rev.* 6:99, 1984.
   A readable review.
5. Levine, M., and Melmed, R. The unhappy wanderers: Children with attention deficits. *Pediatr. Clin. North Am.* 29:105, 1982.
   A longer review of the concept, the clinical spectrum, and management.
6. Shaywitz, S., Cohen, D., and Shaywitz, B. The biochemical basis of minimal brain dysfunction. *J. Pediatr.* 92:179, 1978.
   A review of the evidence that ADD is caused by a metabolic abnormality of bioactive amines and is under genetic influence.

Evaluation

7. Peters, J., Romine, J., and Dykman, R. A special neurological examination of children with learning disabilities. *Dev. Med. Child Neurol.* 17:63, 1975.
   The "soft signs." (Serious doubt about value of signs raised: Pediatrics *59:584, 1977.)*
8. Rosenberger, P. The pediatrician and psychometric testing. *Pediatr. Rev.* 2:301, 1981.
   When to test, what tests to use, and how to use the results.
9. Connors, C. A teacher rating scale for use in drug studies with children. *Am. J. Psychiatry* 126:884, 1969.
   A simplified way of getting useful data from the teacher. (Don't forget to ask the child: Am. J. Dis. Child. *137:369, 1983.)*

Treatment

10. Shaywitz, S., et al. Psychopharmacology of attention deficit disorder: Pharmacokinetic, neuroendocrine, and behavioral measures following acute and chronic treatment with methylphenidate. *Pediatrics* 69:688, 1982.
    There is a relationship between plasma concentration and clinical response and evidence of a central mechanism. (For more on the physiologic basis of hyperkinesis treated with methylphenidate, see Pediatrics *62:343, 1978.)*
11. Wolraich, M. Stimulant drug therapy in hyperactive children: Research and clinical implications. *Pediatrics* 60:512, 1977.
    Review of available studies on basis of scientific merit.
12. Schowalter, J. Paying attention to attention deficit disorder. *Pediatrics* 64:546, 1979.
    An editorial comment accompanying two studies of the effects of Ritalin, emphasizing different effects at different doses, role of the observer (teacher versus parent), and age-related nature of symptoms.
13. Roche, A., et al. The effects of stimulant medication on the growth of hyperkinetic children. *Pediatrics* 63:847, 1979.
    A review of the literature documents short-term effects but good prognosis for ultimate height and weight.
14. Eisenberg, L. Hyperkinesis revisited. *Pediatrics* 61:319, 1978.
    Editorial discussion of two companion articles (pp. 211, 217) that describe behavior therapy in place of stimulants and point out the overdiagnosis of MBD in the classroom. (Use of stimulants in schoolchildren increased two- to three-fold in the past decade: Clin. Pediatr. [Phila.] *22:500, 1983.)*
15. National Institutes of Health Consensus Developmental Conference. Defined diets and child hyperactivity. *J.A.M.A.* 248:290, 1982.
    A thoughtful review of the evidence plus recommendations for future research. (Also see reference 20.)

Prognosis

16. Hechtman, L., and Weiss, G. Long-term outcome of hyperactive children. *Am. J. Orthopsychiatry* 53:532, 1983.
    A literature review (43 references) concluding that "antisocial behavior," noted in short-term outcome studies usually resolves by adulthood; what persist are low

educational achievement, impulsivity, restlessness, and lower self-esteem and poor social skills than a group of controls.

Learning Disabilities

17. Wender, E. Learning disabilities in children. *Pediatr. Rev.* 3:91, 1981.
    Includes both attention deficit disorder and specific learning disabilities; clearly written with good tables. (Other reviews of learning disabilities: Pediatr. Clin. North Am. *29:121, 1982;* J. Pediatr. *102:487, 1983.)*
18. Kinsbourne, M. School problems. *Pediatrics* 52:697, 1973.
    A chatty, readable orientation.
19. Levine, M. Reading failure and the learning-dyslabeled child. *Pediatrics* 63:817, 1979.
    Nonreaders are a heterogeneous group. (Follow-up studies suggest that 20 to 25 percent of children with mild disabilities early come up to grade level but those with severe disability tend not to improve: J. Am. Acad. Child Psychiatry *21:376, 1982.)*
20. Silver, L. Acceptable and controversial approaches to treating the child with learning disabilities. *Pediatrics* 55:406, 1975.
    A review of special education, medication, psychotherapy, "neurophysiologic retraining" (patterning, optometry, sensory integrative therapy), orthomolecular medicine (megavitamins, hypoglycemia, allergy), alpha-wave conditioning, and food additives. (Brought up to date by Golden: Am. J. Dis. Child. *134:487, 1980.)*
21. Gindin, R. Spelling performance of medical students. *Bull. N.Y. Acad. Med.* 50:1120, 1974.
    A humbling note, dear reader.

School and School Failure

22. Oberklaid, F., and Levine, M. Precursors of school failure. *Pediatr. Rev.* 2:5, 1980.
    A brief review of forces tending to sink the child, the strengths to help keep him afloat, and how the doctor can assess and intervene.
23. Sahler, O. The teenager with failing grades. *Pediatr. Rev.* 4:293, 1983.
    An overview of skills required in school at various ages and a differential diagnosis of school failure; also, a comment on the "art of diagnosis and referral." (Children with low productivity, "developmental output failure," discussed: Pediatrics *67:18, 1981.)*
24. Rutter, M. School influences on children's behavior and development. *Pediatrics* 65:208, 1980.
    For the potential beneficial effects of a pediatrician on the school's behavior and development, see Pediatr. Clin. North Am. *28:643, 1981, or* Pediatr. Rev. *4:82, 1982.*

26. SLEEP
Kenneth B. Roberts

Thirty years ago, rapid eye movements (REMs) were reported to occur during the sleep of infants. Since that time, REM sleep has been confirmed as distinct from quiet, non-REM (NREM) sleep and has been associated with dreaming. NREM sleep has been subclassified into four stages on the basis of the electroencephalogram (EEG). A great deal has been learned about the physiology of sleep, but, with few exceptions, these advances in understanding have not translated directly to aid the clinician; rather, the most valuable tools remain knowledge of normal age- and stage-related patterns and the application of simple behavioral techniques.

Newborns generally sleep approximately 17 out of 24 hours, with even distribution during day- and nighttime hours. The total amount of time spent sleeping per 24 hours does not change much during the first 3 months of life, but the percentage during the nighttime hours increases. By 3 months of age, approximately 70 percent of infants have "settled," that is, they regularly sleep through the night (midnight to 5 A.M.); 83 percent of 6 month olds sleep through the night, and, by 9 months to 1 year, the figure is 90 percent.

Toward the end of the first year, half of the infants who have been sleeping through the night develop "night waking." Video recordings have demonstrated that the majority of infants at this age awaken during the night—but most fall back to sleep quietly. External stimulation or low-sensory threshhold temperament may cause certain infants to waken sufficiently to elicit parental response and create the clinical situation identified as "night waking." A pattern of waking leading to parental attention can be quickly established as a regular nightly event; fortunately for parents, the pattern can usually be extinguished in a few nights to a week of limited attention and acceptance of crying.

As separation becomes a major issue in infancy, bedtime becomes a time of potential conflict. The child may view bedtime as a serious separation; the parent may see it as a respite! At this age, bedtime refusal is common, and bedtime rituals are often initiated, serving as soothing reassurance of affection and a quiet period to facilitate sleep. Objects such as blankets or favorite toys may reduce the separation anxiety associated with bedtime and the physical absence of the parent.

Preschool children commonly express fears relating to bedtime: fear of the dark, of insects, of animals. It is therefore understandable that parents may confuse "night terrors" (pavor nocturnus) with nightmares; these two entities are quite different, however. Children with night terrors characteristically cry out in their sleep and are inconsolable for 10 to 15 minutes; they are glassy-eyed and have no recollection of the event in the morning. Night terrors do not occur in REM sleep, are not content-laden, and are events without adequate psychologic or physiologic explanation. By contrast, nightmares generally occur in somewhat older children and have content ("bad dreams"). Counseling about night terrors includes reassurance that the child is not "working through" a hidden trauma, that the parents are not the cause, that the behavior is not intentional, and that the child will "outgrow" the behavior. Waking the child (often not an easy task!) terminates the episode; in severe cases, diazepam (Valium) can be given to the child at bedtime.

Sleepwalking, sleep talking, and enuresis are all most common during the school-age years. They are more frequent in boys than in girls, the presence of one increases the likelihood of another, and they are all related to the time in the sleep cycle between deep sleep and REM sleep (leading some authors to refer to them as disorders of arousal rather than of sleep). In general, the older the child is at the onset, the more likely there is to be a psychologic cause and the less likely there is to be a spontaneous resolution. Sleepwalking can be dangerous, and the child requires a safe, nighttime environment. (Enuresis is discussed in Chap. 28.)

During adolescence, sleep patterns and the nature of complaints change. The most frequently voiced sleep-related concern of parents is that their teenager seems excessively tired, with spontaneous awakening on schooldays an unusual event and "sleeping 'til noon" on nonschool days commonplace. To many parents, this behavior indicates ill health, perhaps an underlying chronic disease, malignancy, or involvement with drugs. The pattern is frequent enough, however, to be considered an age-related norm. The cause of the altered pattern is not precisely clear. Chronic sleep deprivation may well play a role: teenagers sleep less per night than preteens. The increasing psychologic stress and metabolic requirements related to physical and endocrinologic changes may also be important.

Although parents may be concerned about excessive sleepiness, teenagers themselves, when asked, commonly acknowledge at least occasional difficulty in falling or remaining asleep. The patterns they identify are similar to those experienced by adults, particularly under stress.

The more serious sleep-related disorders, such as narcolepsy, are uncommon. Narcolepsy is characterized by excessive sleepiness, which usually occurs 3 to 4 hours after waking, and by cataplexy, episodes of inability to make voluntary movements although awake. Additional features are disturbed nocturnal sleep and hypnagogic hallucinations; the latter appear to reflect a disorder in the transition from wakefulness to sleep, during which hallucinations, particularly auditory, are quite vivid (as in a dream) and muscle activity is inhibited. True narcolepsy is difficult to treat. Stimulants, such as methylphenidate, have been tried with some success; imipramine has been used for the management of some adjunctive symptoms, such as cataplexy and hypnagogic hallucinations.

Narcolepsy is particularly rare before adolescence. A more likely (although still uncommon) cause of excessive daytime sleepiness in children is the sleep apnea–hypersomnia syndrome. Affected children suffer chronic upper airway obstruction at night, with attendant hypercarbia and hypoxemia. Enuresis and a decline in intellectual functioning may develop. Obstructive tonsils and/or adenoids may be responsible, and otolaryngologic consultation is warranted. In some severe cases, when no anatomic cause for obstruction can be found and removed, tracheostomy has been performed.

Perhaps related to sleep apnea is the sudden infant death syndrome (SIDS; see Chap. 19), which occurs during sleep. One of the many theories proposed to explain SIDS postulates a physiologic disturbance in sleep or in the regulation of respiration during sleep. "Sleep studies" are commonly performed in many centers in an attempt to identify infants at risk for SIDS, and parents of infants considered to be at risk may be advised to monitor their infant during sleep using an apnea alarm or cardiorespiratory monitor.

Reviews

1. Anders, T., Carskadon, M., and Dement, W. Sleep and sleepiness in children and adolescents. *Pediatr. Clin. North Am.* 27:29, 1980.
   Neurophysiology, sleep-wake patterns, and disturbances of sleep.
2. Kales, A., and Kales, J. Sleep disorders: Recent findings in the diagnosis and treatment of disturbed sleep. *N. Engl. J. Med.* 290:487, 1974.
   A still-useful "update" on sleepwalking, night terrors, nightmares, enuresis, narcolepsy, hypersomnia, sleep apnea, insomnia, general medical conditions, and treatment.
3. Anders, T., and Weinstein, P. Sleep and its disorders in infants and children: A review. *Pediatrics* 50:312, 1972.
   An age-related review.
4. Anders, T., and Guilleminault, C. The pathophysiology of sleep disorders in pediatrics. *Adv. Pediatr.* 22:137, 1976.
   A two-part encyclopedic review (37 pages); part I deals with infants, part II with children.

Epidemiology

5. Simonds, J., and Parraga, H. Prevalence of sleep disorders and sleep behaviors in children and adolescents. *J. Am. Acad. Child Psychiatry* 21:383, 1982.
   Prevalence depended on age, sex, socioeconomic status, and medical condition.
6. Price, V., et al. Prevalence and correlates of poor sleep among adolescents. *Am. J. Dis. Child.* 132:583, 1978.
   Of eleventh and twelfth graders, 37.6 percent reported occasional sleep disturbance and 12.6 percent reported chronic and severe sleep disturbance.

Infants

7. Parmalee, A., Wenner, W., and Schulz, H. Infant sleep patterns: From birth to 16 weeks of age. *J. Pediatr.* 65:576, 1964.
   Details on the maturational changes during the first 4 months.
8. Grunwaldt, E., Bates, T., and Guthrie, D. The onset of sleeping through the night in infancy: Relation to introduction of solid food in the diet, birth weight, and position in the family. *Pediatrics* 26:667, 1960.
   The average age was 9.3 weeks; no relationship was found to any of the variables studied.
9. Jones, N., et al. The association between perinatal factors and later night waking. *Dev. Med. Child Neurol.* 20:427, 1978.
   Incriminates "a sub-optimal obstetric history" and exonerates parental behavior.
10. Anders, T. Night-waking in infants during the first year of life. *Pediatrics* 63:860, 1979.
    Through time-lapse videotape recordings, the complexity of "sleeping through the night" and "night-waking" are revealed. Most infants wake up during the night; the issue is what happens then.
11. Carey, W. Night waking and temperament in infancy. *J. Pediatr.* 84:756, 1974.
    Focus on the infant: a correlation is found between night waking and the temperament characteristic of "low sensory threshold." (Also see J. Pediatr. 99:817, 1981, and J. Pediatr. 104:477, 1984.)

Preschoolers

12. Chamberlin, R. Management of preschool behavior problems. *Pediatr. Clin. North Am.* 21:33, 1974.
    Puts sleep-related problems in perspective with other complaints.
13. Beltramini, A., and Hertzig, M. Sleep and bedtime behavior in preschool-aged children. *Pediatrics* 71:153, 1983.
    Age and stage-specific behavior of 1, 2, 3, 4, and 5 year olds described.

Specific Disturbances

14. Kales, A., et al. Somnambulism: Clinical characteristics and personality patterns. *Arch. Gen. Psychiatry* 37:1406, 1980.
    Those who outgrow sleepwalking generally start before age 10 and stop before age 15; adults who sleepwalk generally start later, have a higher frequency of sleepwalking, and sleepwalk earlier in the night. Only the adult group had evident psychopathology.
15. Guilleminault, C., et al. Sleep apnea in eight children. *Pediatrics* 58:23, 1976.
    A syndrome with excessive daytime sleepiness, decrease in school performance, abnormal daytime behavior, recent enuresis, morning headache, abnormal weight, and progressive development of hypertension. Also see J. Pediatr. 100:31, 1982.
16. Mandel, E., and Reynolds, C. Sleep disorders associated with upper airway obstruction in children. *Pediatr. Clin. North Am.* 28:897, 1981.
    A brief review of etiology, pathophysiology, laboratory and clinical findings, diagnosis and treatment.
17. Broughton, R. Sleep disorders: Disorders of arousal? *Science* 159:1070, 1968.
    A summary of the evidence that enuresis, sleep walking, and nightmares occur in "confusional states of arousal" rather than in "dreaming sleep."

Other

18. Finkelstein, J. "Early to bed" or sleep revisited. *Am. J. Dis. Child.* 127:474, 1974.
    An editorial review of the relationship between sleep and hormone release. (For more on circadian rhythms, see N. Engl. J. Med. 309:469, 530, 1983.)
19. Solomon, F., et al. Sleeping pills, insomnia and medical practice. *N. Engl. J. Med.* 300:803, 1979.
    The report of a committee of the Institute of Medicine, National Academy of Science, convened in response to a request by "federal agencies" to review the status of sleeping pills in medical practice.

27. BOWEL TRAINING AND CONSTIPATION
Evan Charney

Bowel training is attained at a median age of between 18 and 24 months in the United States; over 90 percent of children are trained by 30 months, 95 percent by 4 years of age, and 1 or 2 percent have not achieved bowel control by age 5. Firstborns are trained somewhat later than are subsequent children, and boys are several months behind girls in acquiring control. Of those still untrained at age 5 and older, boys outnumber girls by at least 3 to 1.

Toilet training is influenced by social norms as well as physiologic maturation. In western Europe toilet training is instituted early: almost all Swiss children are regularly placed on a potty chair between 6 and 12 months, and bowel control is essentially complete in 60 percent of children by 1 year and 90 percent by 2 years of age. Indeed, in several East African cultures virtually complete bowel and bladder control is reported by 6 months of age, although parents actively participate by anticipating the infant's needs and can trigger defecation-on-command by placing the child in an accustomed position on the mother's outstretched legs.

Opinions about the "correct" time and method of bowel training not only vary throughout the world but have changed in this country over time: in the 1920s and 1930s parents were advised to finish training by 6 to 8 months of age! Over the next decades psychoanalytic theory stressed the potential harm of early and strict bowel training, although that conclusion was largely based on anecdotal and retrospective case data. Current recommendations suggest that training be deferred until the child acquires sufficient developmental skills to be an active participant in the process. The child should be aware of what is required and motivated to cooperate, be able voluntarily to inhibit the defecation reflex, and indicate to the parent a need (or intent) to defecate—skills generally developed by 15 to 18 months of age. When those maturational levels are attained, the child is provided a potty seat; one on the floor enables the child to brace arms and legs so that the levator ani muscles can act most efficiently. The child is urged (not coerced) to sit on the potty once or twice daily for not more than 5 to 10 minutes, and success is heartily praised. With this "child-centered approach" the vast majority of children are trained within a few months. Those regular in temperament and bowel pattern will be trained more rapidly. Family moves, intercurrent illness, and stress can be expected to cause setbacks in the process. Parents who make the training a power struggle or whose children's temperaments are more negative or unpredictable are likely to encounter more difficulty.

Toilet training is not the only issue in bowel function; the frequency and character of stools often are concerns to parents: too few, too many, too hard, too soft. Normal stool frequency and appearance varies in early infancy: after the greenish-black meconium stools of the first 3 or 4 days of life the infant passes a thin transitional stool several times daily for the first week. Thereafter, stools of a breast-fed infant are yellow and semisolid, have little odor, and will vary greatly in number, commonly 8 to 10 per day but occasionally 1 every several days; extremely hard stools are uncommon. Infants fed cow milk formula will have firmer, more brownish, and generally less frequent stools. In both cases stool frequency tends to diminish over the first 3 months of life, from initially 1 per feeding (or more) to 1 every 1 to 3 days. While parents commonly identify this reduced frequency as constipation, problems arise only when stools are hard and dry; the term "constipation" is better reserved for hard rather than infrequent stools. When the stools are hard, anal fissures may develop, and the associated painful anal spasm can initiate a cycle of stool retention and further dessication. A stool softener for several days or, in recurrent cases, use of a bulk cathartic such as Maltsupex may be helpful, and the problem usually resolves. The physician needs to be alert to the child whose bowel pattern (often familial) is one of recurrent episodes of infrequent, dry, hard stools throughout infancy and childhood. Anticipatory counseling should then include intake of a high-fiber diet (bran, graham crackers, fruit, and later, abundant fresh vegetables) and milk intake should be limited. The family can be counseled that exacerbation of the problem is likely to occur during febrile illnesses, when mild dehydration may be reflected in more constipation. In toilet training, the need for a regular and unhurried time on the toilet for these children needs emphasis, so that evacuation is complete. With attention to diet and avoidance of laxatives (except in rare instances), the few percent of children with a tendency to chronic constipation can function well and avoid more serious problems.

A small subgroup of children have very severe chronic constipation. Some may have encopresis, defined as repeated deposition of stool in clothing (or other unorthodox sites) after 4 years of age. Boys outnumber girls with this disorder by 4 or 5 to 1. These chronically constipated children appear to have a constitutional predisposition to infrequent stool passage, possibly related to a disorder of colonic motility; whether this abnormality is a cause or a consequence of chronic stool retention is still unclear. In addition, there are "potentiators" at specific developmental stages in infancy and childhood that may convert this predisposition to a chronic clinical problem: these include inappropriately managed acute constipation and frequent anal fissures, excessive laxative and enema use, and major bowel training conflicts. Fear of using the toilet, prolonged gastroenteritis, parent-child conflicts, family psychopathology, or school stress may result in manifest symptoms in the child's "vulnerable bowel."

In these cases stool retention over time leads to dessication by water absorption in the terminal colon, painful defecation, and further retention. The result is a distention and stretching of the rectum and colon (megacolon) with shortening of the anal canal and disordered function of internal and external sphincters. Seepage of liquid stool around the fecal mass may result in encopresis, at times mistaken for diarrhea. When bowel movements do occur (often only with the aid of enemas), the stool may be enormous in size, reflecting the caliber of the dilated rectum, and can be of sufficient size and volume to block the household plumbing.

Once the problem has evolved to this more serious stage an organized diagnostic and management approach with child and family is required to intervene. First, the family needs to agree to a long-term (6- to 12-month) therapeutic plan, which conveys the extent of commitment required of both physician and family for a successful outcome. A complete history and physical examination should seek out the "potentiators" and rule out organic conditions such as spinal cord anomalies and associated metabolic and developmental conditions (e.g., cerebral palsy, hypothyroidism, chronic urinary tract infection secondary to stasis). Rectal examination to assess anal tone and determine the presence and consistency of stool in the ampulla is indicated, and plain radiographs may be helpful in assessing the extent of stool retention. More extensive laboratory evaluation (barium enema, rectal biopsy, manometrics) should be reserved for the small number of cases not responding to initial management. Although Hirschsprung's disease (aganglionic megacolon) is often considered, it accounts for a small fraction of these cases, almost always characterized by an onset in the neonatal period (delayed passage of meconium) or in early infancy. Second, there should be a complete "clean-out" to clear the colon of retained stool: a several-day process involves laxatives and enemas (several of the references offer specifics), and a follow-up radiograph helps assess its completeness. Third, a long-term program of at least 3 to 6 months' duration, combines regular laxative use (commonly mineral oil), diet instruction, and, most important, regular and undisturbed daily toileting time. Repeat visits are essential to monitor progress, to provide support, and to maximize the child's role in the process as age-appropriate. These visits help sort out the cases requiring more intensive psychotherapy from those in which behavioral and interpersonal conflicts ease as the symptom is controlled. In perhaps two-thirds of these cases laxative use can be markedly reduced or withdrawn after several months. However, relapses can be anticipated, and the chronic nature of the underlying problem needs to be appreciated.

The primary physician has much to offer these families: primary prevention of the problem through identification and guidance in early stages of child development for susceptible children, and long-term intervention and guidance in more severe cases.

Norms in Toilet Training

1. Brazelton, T. A child-centered approach to toilet training. *Pediatrics* 29:121, 1962.
   Landmark study of 1170 children defining norms for an upper middle-class U.S. population; outlines an approach to training still widely recommended.
2. Largo, R., and Stutzle, W. Longitudinal study of bowel and bladder control by day and night in the first six years of life: I. Epidemiology and II. Role of potty training. *Dev. Med. Child Neurol.* 19:598, 607, 1977.
   Data from Switzerland on 413 children. Bowel control can be accelerated by very early training and frequent prompting but advantage is transient. No adverse consequences of early training were identified, however.
3. Bellman, M. Studies on encopresis. *Acta. Paediatr. Scand.* [*Suppl.*] 170, 1966.
   Of 9591 children in Stockholm, 1.5 percent were still not bowel trained by age 7 years.
4. Klackenberg, G. A prospective longitudinal study of children. *Acta Paediatr. Scand.* [*Suppl.*] 224, 1971.
   And yet more from Scandinavia.
5. deVries, M., and deVries, M. Cultural relativity of toilet training readiness: A perspective from East Africa. *Pediatrics* 60:170, 1977.
   With "nurturant conditioning" night and day dryness and bowel control were achieved by 6 months of age!
6. Doleys, D., and Dolce, J. Toilet training and enuresis. *Pediatr. Clin. North Am.* 29:297, 1982.
   Useful review of training techniques with a behavioralist orientation.
7. Azrin, N., and Foxx, R. *Toilet Training in Less Than a Day.* New York: Pocket Books, 1974.
   A no-nonsense behavioralist approach.

Constipation and Encopresis

8. Davidson, M., Kugler, M., and Bauer, C. Diagnosis and management in children with severe and protracted constipation and obstipation. *J. Pediatr.* 62:261, 1963.
   An important early article outlining a regimen for severe case (still widely used): initial complete cleanout and use of large amounts of mineral oil to produce 4 to 6 stools daily. Only those "failing" this phase merit further evaluation for Hirschsprung's disease. Mineral oil is continued for at least 3 months and regular toileting times introduced. Although relapses occurred, the success rate was 90 percent in the 119 cases reported.

9. Levine, M. Children with encopresis: A descriptive analysis. *Pediatrics* 56:412, 1975.
   Valuable description of 102 cases emphasizing heterogeneity of behavioral and developmental characteristics.

10. Levine, M., and Bakow, H. Children with encopresis: A study of treatment outcome. *Pediatrics* 58:845, 1976.
    Considers both physical and psychologic factors in treating a large series of difficult cases. Success correlated with a variety of demographic and clinical variables.

11. Levine, M., Mazonson, P., and Bakow, H. Behavioral symptom substitution in children cured of encopresis. *Am. J. Dis. Child.* 134:663, 1980.
    Fear unfounded that "cure" of encopresis would result in major behavioral deterioration (by removing child's coping symptom): in fact, general improvement in behavior was noted along with relief of incontinence.

12. Levine, M. Encopresis: Its potentiation, evaluation and alleviation. *Pediatr. Clin. North Am.* 29:315, 1982.
    A particularly well-balanced analysis of the problem, with much practical advice on management. Also see Pediatr. Rev. 2:285, 1981.

13. Barr, R., et al. Chronic and occult stool retention: A clinical tool for its evaluation in school-age children. *Clin. Pediatr.* (Phila.) 18:674, 1979.
    Scoring system for presence and extent of stool on plain abdominal radiographs; helpful when constipation is not adequately appreciated by history and physical examination, and in assessing adequacy of clean-out.

14. Olness, K., and Tobin, J. Chronic constipation in children: Can it be managed by diet alone? *Postgrad. Med.* 72:149, 1982.
    Yes, at least in 60 children given raw bran with exclusion of milk products, apples, bananas, rice, and gelatin. Outlines the role of diet in this disorder.

15. Olness, K., McFarland, F., and Piper, J. Biofeedback: A new modality in the management of children with fecal soiling. *J. Pediatr.* 96:505, 1980.
    High success rate in 50 cases, 4 to 15 years of age with imperforate anus or functional constipation; importance of therapist-patient relationship stressed.

16. Newmann, P., DeDominico, L., and Nogrady, M. Constipation and urinary tract infection. *Pediatrics* 52:241, 1973.
    Fecal retention may be associated with urinary stasis and infection.

Manometric Studies

17. Loening-Baucke, V., and Younoszai, M. Abnormal anal sphincter response in chronically constipated children. *J. Pediatr.* 100:213, 1982.
    Abundant manometric data suggest abnormalities in internal sphincter and rectal motility patterns in "functional" constipation. Are these primary or secondary to stretching? Exact role of manometry in management remains to be elucidated. (Also see Arch. Dis. Child. 58:257, 1983; Gastroenterology 77:330, 1979; and Pediatrics 71:774, 1983.)

---

28. BLADDER CONTROL AND ENURESIS
Kenneth B. Roberts

Enuresis is defined as the involuntary passage of urine, but in common usage it is not synonymous with incontinence. Enuresis usually refers to bedwetting, although this would more properly be termed *nocturnal enuresis* and is applied only after the age at which the child is expected to be dry. Primary enuresis is distinguished from secondary enuresis in that a child with the former has never had a sustained period of dry nights (e.g., 3 months), whereas bedwetting in the latter begins after nocturnal dryness has been achieved.

At what age is a child expected to be dry at night? The answer depends on a number of factors, including who is being asked (parents, grandparents, and physicians generally have different expectations), the sex of the child (girls are dry at a younger age than boys), and the child's development in other spheres. Normally, the initial step in the development of urinary continence takes place before 2 years of age, by which age most infants are aware of having voided and can report what has happened. Between 2 and $2\frac{1}{2}$ years, the child develops the ability to sense a full bladder before it is emptied and to initiate voiding from a full bladder. During the next few years, the ability to retain urine voluntarily is mastered, but it is not until $4\frac{1}{2}$ to 6 years that the child can initiate voiding at any degree of bladder fullness or start and stop the urinary stream at will.

Approximately 60 percent of 3-year-old children have mastered the process sufficiently to be dry at night; the incidence of bedwetting at that age, then, is 40 percent. During the next 3 years, the incidence of bedwetting declines to approximately 30 percent at age 4, 20 percent at age 5, and 10 percent at age 6. Of those children who still wet the bed at age 6, approximately 15 percent per year will have a "spontaneous cure," leaving 7 percent of 8 year olds, 3 percent of 12 year olds, and 1 percent of 18 year olds bedwetting more than once a month. Boys outnumber girls at each age by a ratio of 1.5 : 1.

There are many possible causes of enuresis. Each of the following has been implicated: faulty toilet training, developmental (maturational) delay, sleep disorder, inadequate bladder capacity, genitourinary tract abnormality, and systemic disease.

The relationship between toilet training and enuresis is not clear, although considerable discussion over the past several decades has been given both to the optimal timing and the optimal style of conducting the process. The notion of a critical period for learning skills of continence appears to have given way, but many still believe in a "sensitive period." Noncoercive toilet training techniques are felt by supporters to be associated with fewer later difficulties such as enuresis and encopresis (see Chap. 27); conditioning techniques to accomplish training in a short period of time also enjoy great popularity, however. Stress and psychologic pressure(s) appear to play a greater role in secondary enuresis than in primary.

Some children appear to have only a developmental delay in achieving dryness; there is often a family history of a similar situation in a parent.

As noted in Chapter 26, Sleep, enuresis is considered by some to be a disorder of arousal, as are sleepwalking and sleeptalking. That is, enuresis is most likely to occur during the return from deep sleep to light sleep in a somewhat confused state of near-wakefulness. Children with one of the "disorders of arousal" may well have another.

Many children with enuresis have unusually small functional bladder capacities; when asked to retain urine as long as possible, the amount finally voided is less than would be expected. (A rule of thumb is 1 oz/year of age.) Cystometric studies have shown that many of these children with reduced functional capacities have normal bladder capacities when they are anesthetized. Bladder stretching exercises (see p. 90) may help motivated children with this form of enuresis; in such cases, an increase in functional bladder capacity is usually associated with success.

Abnormalities of the genitourinary tract rarely cause bedwetting alone. Enuresis must be distinguished by history from constant dribbling, which may indicate an anomalous insertion of the ureter below the bladder neck (i.e., into the urethra), and from overflow incontinence due to a neurogenic bladder. The onset of enuresis in a previously dry child may signal urinary tract infection, especially in a girl; the enuresis responds to treatment of the infection. Two other medical conditions associated with an increased incidence of enuresis are diabetes insipidus and diabetes mellitus.

The evaluation of a child with enuresis depends heavily on the history. How old is the child, and what developmental and maturational skills have been achieved? Is the enuresis nocturnal, diurnal (daytime), or both? Is this primary or secondary enuresis? What has been the longest dry period to date? Does the child have difficulty voiding, suggesting obstruction of the lower urinary tract? Is there associated bowel or lower limb pathology suggestive of a neurologic disorder? Is there a family history of bedwetting? Is there sufficient social turmoil as to interfere with toilet training? What are the parental attitudes and behaviors regarding the bedwetting: What happens when the child wets the bed? Who is responsible for changing the sheets? What has been tried? And why is help being sought at this particular time?

A complete general physical examination is warranted, with particular emphasis on the neurologic examination and an assessment of the child's behavior. A urine specimen for specific gravity, urinalysis, and culture should be obtained; if lower tract obstruction is suspected, voiding should be observed. Further studies—such as a roentgenogram of the lumbar and sacral spines, an intravenous pyelogram, or a voiding cystourethrogram—need be performed only if history, physical examination, or examination of the urine suggests a lesion.

Treatment begins with reassurance, particularly to the child, that while the enuresis is disturbing and annoying, many children have the same problem and "grow out of it." Further reassurance can be given that, if the child is interested in working on "the problem," the physician can help.

The simplest form of treatment is withholding fluids after dinner and voiding before bedtime; this may be all that is required for some children close to dryness, but it has usually already been tried by families seeking help from the physician. Waking the child before the parents go to bed is also commonly performed and may be helpful in mild cases.

Further intervention depends on the age of the child, associated findings, the level of concern, and family dynamics, including assessment by the physician as to how much cooperation—rather than coercion—will be forthcoming. If the child is younger than age 6, the physician should discuss normal development and maturation of bladder control with the parents and attempt to reach agreement regarding appropriate expectations. For the young school-age child with a small functional bladder capacity, many physicians recommend "bladder stretching exercises." The child is asked to force fluids once each day and to resist the urge to void as long as possible. When the child must void, he practices starting and stopping his stream as he urinates into a measuring cup. The volume is recorded on a calendar; the calendar is also used as a "star chart" to identify dry nights. Rewards are given for appropriate achievements, and the family is encouraged to focus on successes, with praise and reward, rather than on failures.

For school-age children, some clinicians have been successful with hypnosis and imagery, having the child imagine the sensation of bladder fullness, the act of getting out of bed and voiding in the bathroom, and returning to a "nice, dry bed." The child is encouraged to think about this image at bedtime each night.

Of various drugs that have been tried, the most widely used is imipramine (Tofranil), a tricyclic antidepressant. The drug has been demonstrated to be superior to placebo with cure rates between 10 and 50 percent. When used as an antidepressant, imipramine requires weeks for a beneficial effect and is given in divided doses through the day. For treatment of enuresis, however, a single daily dose, given an hour before bedtime, is usually sufficient, and drug effect is recognized within days. The optimal duration of therapy is unknown. Relapses are common once the drug has been discontinued, and some children, initially aided by imipramine, appear to become tolerant to its effects. The manufacturer of the drug has advertised it as "temporary adjunctive therapy in reducing enuresis in children age six years and older," which appears to be an appropriate perspective. The need for monitoring and reporting successes and for assuring social rewards is not lessened by prescribing imipramine; the role of the drug is to facilitate the social process by increasing the chances of success. It should be recognized when prescribing imipramine that overdoses can be quite serious or fatal due to myocardial toxicity.

Conditioning techniques, involving an apparatus such as the "bell and pad" enuresis alarm, are associated with the highest initial cure rates of the various forms of therapy proposed for enuresis (approximately 70%), have a lower relapse rate than imipramine and are safe. The methods involve a form of sensor between the child and the bed that when dampened, sets off an alarm designed to awaken the child.

Whatever treatment plan is prescribed, the physician needs to be aware of the child's self-concept, his abilities, and the pressures on him. Taking these factors into account, the physician, for example, may suggest that the child be responsible for the "extra" laundry caused by wet bed linen; other circumstances may prompt a different suggestion. Since the vast majority of children who wet their beds have a self-limited problem, a major goal is to minimize "emotional scars" by assuaging and redirecting anger, rechanneling frustration, and providing needed support.

Reviews

1. Cohen, M. Enuresis. *Pediatr. Clin. North Am.* 22:545, 1975.
   A readable, 15-page review.
2. Smith, L. Nocturnal enuresis. *Pediatr. Rev.* 2:183, 1980.
   A brief overview.
3. Kolvin, I., MacKeith, R., and Meadows, S. (eds.). Bladder control and enuresis. *Clin. Dev. Med.* 48:49, 1973.
   A collection of 32 chapters (328 pages) on multiple aspects.
4. McLain, L. Childhood enuresis. *Curr. Probl. Pediatr.* 9(8), 1979.
   An extensive review (36 pages, 147 references) of physiology, etiology, "workup," and therapy.

Voiding

5. Kaplan, G., and Brock, W. Voiding dysfunction in children. *Curr. Probl. Pediatr.* 10(8), 1980.
   The anatomy and physiology. (For more on the development of urinary control in children, see J.A.M.A. 172:1256, 1960.)

Epidemiology

6. Oppel, W., Harper, P., and Rider, R. The age of attaining bladder control. *Pediatrics* 42:614, 1968.
   A literature review plus results of a 12-year prospective study of 859 children: notes age of initial dryness, age of final dryness, and the prevalence of dryness. Low birth weight is a risk factor, and the contribution of "relapsers" to the total pool is evident.

Parental Perceptions

7. Haque, M., et al. Parental perceptions of enuresis. *Am. J. Dis. Child.* 135:809, 1981.
   What parents anticipate to be the age of dryness, what they perceive to be the cause of enuresis, and how they manage bedwetting. (Attitudes of parents contrasted with those of physicians: Pediatrics 67:707, 1981.)

Toilet Training

8. Doleys, D., and Dolce, J. Toilet training and enuresis. *Pediatr. Clin. North Am.* 29:297, 1982.
   When and how to toilet train, assessment and treatment of enuresis.
9. Brazelton, T. A child-oriented approach to toilet training. *Pediatrics* 29:121, 1962.
   A gentle approach may produce more dry beds.

Other Issues in Etiology

10. MacKeith, R. Is maturation delay a frequent factor in the origins of primary nocturnal enuresis? *Dev. Med. Child Neurol.* 14:217, 1972.
    The author believes the answer to be no.
11. Broughton, R. Sleep disorders: Disorders of arousal? *Science* 159:1070, 1968.
    Enuresis occurs in a "confusional state or arousal," not in REM sleep. (Also see Sleep, Chap. 26.)
12. Starfield, B. Functional bladder capacity in enuretic and nonenuretic children. *J. Pediatr.* 70:777, 1967.
    The capacity was less in children with enuresis. (Under anesthesia, however, volumes are equal: J. Urol. 105:129, 1971. Increasing the functional bladder capacity is associated with improvement: J. Pediatr. 72:483, 1968.)
13. Seibert, J., et al. Excretory urography for evaluation of enuresis. *Pediatrics* 65:644, 1980.
    The recommendation of the American Academy of Pediatrics Committee on Radiology, the nature and frequency of urinary tract pathology warrants a urine culture—but not radiologic studies—to be a part of "routine" evaluation.

Treatment

14. Schmitt, B. Nocturnal enuresis: An update on treatment. *Pediatr. Clin. North Am.* 29:21, 1982.

Motivational counseling, bladder exercises, alarms, medications, and a perspective on which works best at what age. (Read this.)

15. Glicklich, L. An historical account of enuresis. *Pediatrics* 8:859, 1951.
    A 27-page review of some pretty amazing approaches. (Ah, but what will the future think of us?)

16. Forsythe, W., and Redmond, A. Enuresis and spontaneous cure rate: Study of 1129 enuretics. *Arch. Dis. Child.* 49:259, 1974.
    The rate was 14 to 16 percent per year between 5 and 19 years of age, a figure to be remembered when evaluating various treatment modalities.

17. Marshall, S., Marshall, H., and Lyon, R. Enuresis: An analysis of various therapeutic approaches. *Pediatrics* 52:813, 1973.
    The authors stress involving the child.

18. Dische, S., et al. Childhood nocturnal enuresis: Factors associated with outcome of treatment with an enuresis alarm. *Dev. Med. Child Neurol.* 25:67, 1983.
    "Family difficulties" were the most important predictor of initial success, relapse rate, and long-term success.

19. Imipramine for enuresis. *Med. Lett. Drugs Ther.* 16:22, 1974.
    A brief perspective on Tofranil.

20. Wagner, W., et al. A controlled comparison of two treatments for nocturnal enuresis. *J. Pediatr.* 101:302, 1982.
    Conditioning beat the drug.

21. Olness, K. The use of self-hypnosis in the treatment of childhood nocturnal enuresis. *Clin. Pediatr.* (Phila.) 14:273, 1975.
    Of 40 children taught self-hypnosis, 31 stopped bedwetting, 6 improved, and 3 did not improve; the process is described.

29. RECURRENT PAIN SYNDROMES: ABDOMINAL PAIN, HEADACHE, AND CHEST PAIN

Evan Charney

Recurrent abdominal pain, headache, and chest pain in childhood and adolescence, although distinctly different syndromes, are grouped together here because they share certain features of presentation and management: (1) they occur commonly in childhood, but only a minority of those with symptoms seek medical attention; (2) a minority of those who do seek care have a serious (at times urgent) medical problem that requires prompt identification; (3) in many cases the symptom is associated with an important psychosocial component that must be addressed in order to deal successfully with the problem; and (4) the management involves a very thorough history and physical examination (even if the family is known to the physician), usually a minimum laboratory investigation, and may require a series of scheduled visits over an interval of time before the problem sorts itself out.

Recurrent abdominal pain occurs in 10 to 15 percent of children between 5 and 15 years of age. It is defined as three or more episodes of abdominal pain severe enough to interrupt normal activities and occurring over a period longer than 3 months (Apley). It is chiefly a problem during the school years, with a peak incidence just before puberty in girls and perhaps somewhat earlier in boys.

There are over 100 entities that either can cause or are commonly associated with recurrent abdominal pain and an extensive series of tests would be required to rule them all out. But in a series of 100 hospitalized children only 8 had organic disorders that appeared to have caused their pain: 4 had urologic problems (e.g., recurrent urinary tract infection, hydronephrosis, renal cyst) and 4 had gastrointestinal problems (e.g., duodenal ulcer, Meckel's diverticulum, gallstones). Another 20 had assorted, unrelated physical abnormalities felt not to be the direct cause of their attacks. A careful psychosocial evaluation gave strong evidence of an emotional disturbance in 56 children and their families. Some investigators feel that, in addition to these genitourinary and gastrointestinal problems, a number of children with recurrent abdominal pain have a clinical picture resembling the "irritable bowel" syndrome of adults. Lactose intolerance has also been associated with abdominal pain in a high proportion of children and a trial of elimination may be merited although controlled studies do not confirm lactase deficiency as a major factor.

Since far and away the most common problems in these children are situational and emotional ones, it is well to have in mind the constellation of psychologic factors to be inquired about when interviewing the family. Four factors are commonly found in children whose conditon is on an emotional basis: (1) a "model" in the family; (2) a history of separation, such as a death in the family, impending divorce, or other perceived or threatened loss; (3) some clear psychologic gain for the child from the symptom; and (4) a compulsive, high-strung, fussy child (a "worrier") and an overprotective, excessively anxious family or one preoccupied with the child's complaints. While these factors may be present in children with organic disease as well, their *absence* should give the clinician pause. If such psychologic factors cannot be found, the search for an organic cause should be pursued.

The diagnostic evaluation of a child with recurrent abdominal pain should itself be a therapeutic process. It should convey to the family that the physician takes the problem seriously, understands the disruption and anguish it causes, and plans to explore it thoroughly, together with the family. It is essential that both psychologic and organic factors be considered together, rather than sequentially. "Ruling out organic problems" first can be an extensive task that avoids and unnecessarily delays addressing the common emotional etiology. Moreover, organic and emotional causes are not mutually exclusive, and a sensitive understanding of the emotional climate in the family is vital in dealing with any organic problems identified. This dual approach also tells the family that the physician is considering the influence of emotional factors from the outset—an important message for parents who might have difficulty accepting an emotional basis for their child's problem should it be introduced as an afterthought.

The most useful initial diagnostic step is the recognition that this patient indeed *has* recurrent abdominal pain. The child may have been seen repeatedly in the office or clinic for individual episodes and been given an antispasmodic or sedative or just reassured that nothing urgent was occurring. In fact, although the entity under consideration is a common one, only a minority of children who are seen by the physician for acute abdominal pain have a recurrent problem, and the physician may therefore fail to identify it as such. When the parent or clinician recognizes that the problem is a long-standing one, the child should be scheduled for a longer assessment. It may be helpful to tell the parents that this problem is too important to be handled in the usual brief office visit, and that a longer session will be necessary to begin a careful assessment. In particular, unless an organic lesion is immediately apparent, the physician should resist the impulse to order a battery of laboratory studies.

The next step is a thorough history and physical examination (valuable even if the patient has been previously seen in the practice), paying particular attention to the presence or absence of the psychologic factors mentioned. The physician should inquire about what the parents and child think is wrong—are they worried about some lethal condition (e.g., cancer, leukemia) because of prior family experience? It is helpful at some point to interview parents and child separately as well as together to provide varied insights about family interactions and individual fears. The character and timing of the abdominal pain itself are not as useful as might be hoped. In Apley's series, neither description nor severity (sharp or dull, excruciating and brief, or chronic and low-grade) helped to differentiate organic from nonorganic pain. In essence, the nonorganic pain was of any degree of severity from mild to incapacitating, and in some cases it awakened the patient from sleep. Associated phenomena, such as headache, pallor, and vomiting, were commonly found in children with pain from an emotional cause, perhaps relating to an autonomic imbalance. In general, the farther the pain is from the umbilicus, the more one should suspect an organic cause ("Apley's law").

Basic laboratory studies include urinalysis and several quantitative urine cultures, a total and differential white count, an erythrocyte sedimentation rate, and stool examination for occult blood.

It may take one or two visits to obtain all the necessary information, at which point the cases tend to fall into one of three categories:

1. Fairly definitely organic. Positive findings on history, physical examination, or baseline laboratory studies are suggestive of an organic lesion. As indicated, this will occur

perhaps 10 percent of the time. There may or may not be associated emotional aspects as well.

2. Fairly definitely functional. The family and personal history, the presence of a model, the identified secondary gain from the symptom, and the absence of any yield from the basic medical examination offer positive evidence for an emotional origin. About two-thirds of the patients are in this category.

3. Unclear. No strong positive evidence for either organic or functional diagnosis. Perhaps one-fourth of the patients are in this category.

Patients in whom an organic lesion seems evident require whatever further diagnostic or therapeutic maneuvers are appropriate for the disease in question. For children in whom an emotional cause appears likely, it is essential to meet with the family and inform them of that impression. It is most important that the physician convey to the parents that further organic studies are not indicated at that time and, indeed, can be counterproductive. To continue ordering "just one more test" prevents the family and physician from addressing the emotional problem directly. It delays resolution of the problem and also identifies the child as someone with a possible chronic physical difficulty, a label difficult to shed and one with potentially adverse effects on the child's future emotional development.

If a clear secondary gain has been identified, that must be eliminated; for example, the child must return promptly to school and, once in school, must not repeatedly be sent home. The child must not receive an inordinate amount of sympathy and attention for the symptom. The physician should then offer to see the child regularly for several visits (on a weekly or biweekly basis), using these visits to discuss the child's daily activities and to inquire further about any of the conflicts or fears identified earlier. This allows the physician to determine whether his advice has been followed and if there are more serious emotional problems in the family not previously appreciated that may require psychologic consultation. Once agreed on, these visits should not depend on the child's having abdominal pain as a "ticket of admission."

Several regularly scheduled visits are also useful for the child in whom neither an organic nor an emotional diagnosis is apparent. They provide the opportunity to learn more about the child and family. If, after further inquiry, emotional clues are not evident, the physician needs to consider more unusual organic diagnoses.

The majority, though not all, of the patients whose pain is on an emotional basis will respond to this management by a diminution in the frequency of—or at least in the turmoil accompanying—the episodes. The long-term prognosis may not be so optimistic, however; only one-third to one-half of patients are free from their pain in adulthood. There is some evidence that if the related emotional problems are identified and dealt with, the long-term prognosis for adequate psychologic functioning is improved. The physician's major contribution to the family may be to avoid or alter a pattern in which the child learns to use bodily symptoms to cope with problems rather than confronting and dealing with the problems directly.

Headaches are reported to occur at least several times per month in approximately 5 percent of 7 year olds (an equal number of boys and girls). The prevalence of headaches increases throughout childhood and by 15 years of age 20 percent of girls and 10 percent of boys report recurrent headaches.

Headache is produced by a limited number of mechanisms: pain-sensitive structures within the cranium include veins and arteries at the base of the skull, portions of the dura, and fifth, ninth, and tenth cranial nerves. The brain itself is insensitive to pain. The pain is a result of vasodilatation, inflammation, traction, or direct pressure by tumor or mass on these structures. Significant extracranial causes of headache include sustained contraction of scalp, face or neck muscles, or abnormalities within the sinuses or orbit, external and middle ear, and dental structures.

There are several patterns of headache that can be distinguished in children, including migraine, other vascular headache, muscle contraction ("tension") headache, headache associated with intracranial inflammation, and with other diseases of the head and neck structures.

Definitions of migraine headache vary but usually include a paroxysmal (in contrast to continuous) headache with at least two of the following criteria: unilateral pain, nausea, antecedent aura, and a positive family history. Migraine headache has several subcategories: classic migraine (an aura precedes the headache); common migraine (with a less well-defined aura but prominent autonomic features such as nausea and pallor); complicated migraine (with associated neurologic deficits); migraine variants (vertigo or cyclic vomiting); and cluster headache (several daily episodes of nonthrobbing "clusters" occurring each day for a period of weeks or months with interval remission). Perhaps one-third of recurrent headaches in childhood can be classified as migraine and two-thirds will fall into the other described categories. Approximately 15 percent of the latter group will have a single defined organic cause associated with eye, ear, dental, or sinus disease.

The medical history should define the location, frequency, character, time of day, and severity of the pain; associated symptoms; change in pattern over time; triggering (and ameliorating) factors; and family history (including the current psychologic milieu). Laboratory tests rarely yield a diagnosis not already suspected; computerized tomography (CT scan) should be reserved for cases where a mass lesion is suspected or a neurologic deficit identified. Skull films and EEG should be obtained only on specific indication. Lumbar puncture is indicated where central nervous system infection or bleeding is suspected but should be preceded by CT scan in the presence of papilledema or suspected mass lesion.

The treatment plan involves attention to precipitating stressful environmental factors; biofeedback and relaxation techniques are promising modalities of therapy. Simple analgesics are usually sufficient to control most childhood headaches, even in the majority of patients with migraine. Preadolescent children with migraine less often require abortive agents (e.g., ergotamine) or prophylactic agents (e.g., propranolol).

The prognosis of migraine and other chronic headache (where no organic lesion is identified) is generally favorable; two-thirds are significantly improved or symptom-free after a decade in follow-up studies. For migraine headaches, onset in early childhood has a better prognosis than does onset during adolescence.

Chest pain occurs less commonly than does headache or abdominal pain, but the perceived seriousness of the symptom often prompts a medical consultation. More than 650,000 office visits are made annually for chest pain in patients 10 to 21 years of age, and in one study one-fourth of adolescents reported more than three episodes in the prior year. The peak incidence in those less than 21 years of age occurs in early adolescence, a somewhat older age on average than the child with recurrent abdominal pain. In most series, one-third to one-half of patients have no defined etiology (an even higher proportion in those with symptoms for longer than 6 months). In approximately one-third of patients, a musculoskeletal cause is identified (e.g., costochondritis, anterior chest wall tenderness). A myriad of diagnoses account for the remaining cases, and several important ones may not immediately be evident: hyperventilation is a common adolescent syndrome, and the associated discomfort and anxiety may be perceived as chest pain; gynecomastia in males may be "painfully" embarrassing; occasionally depression may present as chest pain. Heart disease as a cause of anterior chest pain is extremely rare, although almost universally suspected by family and patient. An association of mitral valve prolapse with chest pain has been noted in some cases, but most authorities are skeptical that it accounts for the pain.

The diagnostic approach outlined for recurrent abdominal pain applies to this symptom as well, based on a very thorough history and physical examination both to identify the rare serious or urgent case and to reassure the family and patient. In the physical examination a full range of motion of upper extremities, neck, and trunk should be tested. An electrocardiogram and chest radiograph are often obtained but are rarely positive if cardiac disease is not suspected. The physician needs to deal with any functional impairment the symptom may have caused, and, as with abdominal pain, several visits may be required to sort out the problem.

Recurrent Abdominal Pain (RAP): General

1. Levine, M. (ed.). Recurrent pain in children. *Pediatr. Clin. North Am.* 31 (5) 1984.
   A useful collection of 10 articles on pain and common recurrent pain syndromes.
2. Apley, J. *The Child with Abdominal Pains* (2nd ed.). Oxford: Blackwell, 1975.
   The "compleat" reference: prevalence, differential diagnosis, psychologic management, prognosis—all in readable English. Start here by all means.

3. Green, M. Diagnosis and treatment: Psychogenic recurrent abdominal pain. *Pediatrics* 40:84, 1967.
   Helpful hints from an astute clinician. (Also see outline by the same author in Pediatric Diagnosis *(3rd ed.). Philadelphia: Saunders, 1980. Pp. 335–37.)*

RAP: Prevalence
4. Apley, J., and Naish, N. Recurrent abdominal pains: A field survey of 1000 school children. *Arch. Dis. Child.* 33:165, 1958.
   The first (and best) prevalence study. (For a more recent review of recurrent abdominal pain, headache, and limb pains, see Pediatrics *50:429, 1972.)*

RAP: Autonomic Dysfunction
5. Stone, R., and Barbero, G. Recurrent abdominal pain in childhood. *Pediatrics* 45:732, 1970.
   Protoscopic examination of children with recurrent abdominal pain revealed rectal dilatation, hyperemia, and pallor of the bowel wall in 88 of 90 studied.
6. Apley, J., Haslam, D., and Tullow, G. Pupillary reaction in children with recurrent abdominal pain. *Arch. Dis. Child.* 46:337, 1971.
   There is an altered pupillary response to stress (delayed return to normal constriction following stress-induced pupillary dilatation) in patients with recurrent abdominal pain. (Also see Psychosom. Med. *29:111, 1967.)*

RAP: Role of Lactase Deficiency
7. Barr, R., Levine, M., and Watkins, J. Recurrent abdominal pain of childhood due to lactase intolerance. *N. Engl. J. Med.* 300:1449, 1979.
   Lactose malabsorption in 40 percent of 80 schoolchildren with recurrent abdominal pain, but clinical history does not distinguish them from normal absorbers. Lactose-free diet was associated with improvement in malabsorbers. (Also see Pediatrics *64:43, 1979.) However, note the following:*
8. Lebenthal, E., et al. Recurrent abdominal pain and lactose absorption in children. *Pediatrics* 67:828, 1981.
   Lactase deficiency as prevalent in control group as in those with recurrent abdominal pain (26 versus 30%). Moreover, recovery rate from recurrent pain similar in lactose absorbers and nonabsorbers independent of dietary restriction. (Confirmed: J. Pediatr. *100:65, 1982.)*

RAP: Management
9. Berger, H., Honig, P., and Liebman, R. Recurrent abdominal pain: Gaining control of the symptom. *Am. J. Dis. Child.* 131:1340, 1977.
   A practical approach is presented, emphasizing the value of a family conference.

RAP: Prognosis
10. Apley, J., and Hale, B. Children with recurrent abdominal pain: How do they grow up? *Br. Med. J.* 3:7, 1973.
    Not as well as we would wish; better with counseling.
11. Christensen, J., and Mortonson, O. Long term prognosis in children with recurrent abdominal pain. *Arch. Dis. Child.* 50:110, 1975.
    An attempt at a long-term controlled (retrospectively) study. Abdominal pain in adults begets abdominal pain in children.
12. Stickler, G., and Murphy, D. Recurrent abdominal pain. *Am. J. Dis. Child.* 133:486, 1979.
    After 5 years, 75 percent of 161 patients free of pain episodes.

Headache
13. Bille, B. Migraine in schoolchildren. *Acta Paediatr. Scand. [Suppl.]* 136, 1962.
    Of 8993 children questioned, 10.6 percent reported "frequent" (more than monthly) headaches. The pattern suggested migraine in 2 percent of 7 year olds, and in 4 percent of boys, and 6.4 percent of girls at 13 to 15 years.

14. Egermark-Erikson, I. Prevalence of headache in Swedish schoolchildren. *Acta Paediatr. Scand.* 71:135, 1982.
    In 402 children 5 percent of 7 year olds and 14 percent of 15 year olds have headaches "at least once weekly."

15. Del Bene, E. Multiple aspects of headache risk in children. *Adv. Neurol.* 33:187, 1982.
    Autonomic and recurrent pain symptoms (e.g., cyclic vomiting, dizziness, abdominal and limb pain) are more prevalent among headache sufferers than among controls.

16. Congden, P., and Forsyth, W. Migraine in childhood: A study of 300 children. *Dev. Med. Child Neurol.* 21:209, 1979.
    Spontaneous annual remission rate of 3 to 14 percent was noted in follow-up of 300 children; 37 of 108 followed for 12 years were free of headache.

17. Shinnar, S., and D'Souza, B. The diagnosis and management of headaches in children. *Pediatr. Clin. North Am.* 29:79, 1981.
    A concise and practical approach with a useful list of questions for patient and family; 52 references. (For a more complete review of migraine in children and adolescents by the same authors, see Pediatr. Rev. 3:257, 1982.)

18. Thompson, J. Diagnosis and treatment of headache in the pediatric patient. *Curr. Probl. Pediatr.* 10(10), 1980.
    Another good discussion of etiology, classification, pathophysiology and therapy; 70 references. (For another general review, see Pediatr. Ann. 12:806, 1983.)

19. Honig, P., and Charney, E. Children with brain tumor headaches: Distinguishing features. *Am. J. Dis. Child.* 136:121, 1982.
    Diagnosis of brain tumor was strongly suggested by specific abnormalities in physical examination or history within 4 months of onset of headaches in 69 of 72 cases.

Chest Pain

20. Driscoll, D., Glicklich, L., and Gallen, W. Chest pain in children: A prospective study. *Pediatrics* 57:648, 1976.
    In 43 consecutive patients one-half had no identifiable etiology. Cardiac disease was often feared—but not found—in this series.

21. Pantell, R., and Goodman, B. Adolescent chest pain: A prospective study. *Pediatrics* 71:881, 1983.
    In 100 patients musculoskeletal problems found in 31 percent and hyperventilation in 20 percent; symptoms caused considerable anxiety and dysfunction. (Also by the same authors: Chest Pain in Adolescents: A Strategy for Evaluation and Management. In A. Moss (ed.), Pediatrics Update. New York: Elsevier, 1985.) For cardiologist's perspective, see Pediatr. Clin. North Am. 31:1241, 1984.

22. Brown, R. Costochondritis in adolescents. *J. Adol. Health Care* 1:198, 1981.
    Another series of 100 adolescents with chest or upper abdominal pain; costochondritis particularly sought for (and found) in 79.

30. SEXUAL DEVELOPMENT
Margaret E. Mohrmann and John T. Hayford, Jr.

Sexual development encompasses both the biologic processes of differentiation and maturation and the psychologic concept of sexuality.

Normal sexual *differentiation* of the human fetus depends on both the sex chromosome complement and the presence or absence of substances produced by the fetal testis. The sex genome governs the intrauterine differentiation of bipotential gonadal tissue into testes (XY) or ovaries (XX). The normal fetal testis produces müllerian inhibiting factor (MIF) and testosterone. MIF is necessary for the regression of the anlage of female internal genitalia; testosterone is required for development of male internal genital structures from the embryonic Wolffian duct system and for differentiation of male external genitalia. Female internal reproductive organs develop if MIF is absent, whether because of normal ovarian differentiation or testicular dysfunction; female external genitalia differentiate in the absence of systemic androgens. Defective activity of any of the independent organizing factors—chromosomes, MIF, androgens—can lead to discordant sexual differentiation.

Gonadal dysgenesis is a term encompassing a wide range of anomalies in ovarian development due to abnormal sex chromatin. Complete gonadal aplasia is the expression of the XO karyotype, while variable degrees of ovarian dysfunction result from sex chromosome mosaicism. Internal and external genital structures are always female, but secondary sexual maturation fails to occur because of absent or inadequate estrogen production. Most patients with gonadal dysgenesis, especially those with the XO karyotype, have other characteristic features (Turner syndrome), such as short stature, low hairline, webbed neck, shieldlike chest, cubitus valgus, multiple nevi, or coarctation of the aorta. The diagnosis of gonadal dysgenesis, which is confirmed by documentation of an abnormal karyotype, must be considered in any female with nonfamilial short stature, or failure of secondary sexual development, or both, even in the absence of the classic physical findings of Turner syndrome. Treatment includes estrogen replacement and psychologic counseling.

Klinefelter syndrome (seminiferous tubule dysgenesis) occurs in males with XXY karyotypes. Testes are present, but there is hyalinization and aplasia of the seminiferous tubules. Internal and external genitalia are male because adequate masculinizing factors are present in utero. Males with Klinefelter syndrome present in adolescence or adulthood with gynecomastia or occasionally with some degree of failure of secondary sexual development. Physical examination reveals a eunuchoid body habitus, female escutcheon of pubic hair, and small, firm testes. Therapy involves androgen supplementation, psychologic counseling, and bilateral mastectomy if the gynecomastia causes significant psychosocial problems.

Pseudohermaphroditism is a disorder in which the external genital phenotype is not consistent with the genotype. Female pseudohermaphrodites have XX karyotypes, normal ovaries, and female internal genital structures but have virilized external genitalia, with varying degrees of phallic development and fusion of labioscrotal folds. Virilization is the result of excessive levels of androgens, usually due to congenital adrenal hyperplasia (see Chap. 74), but occasionally secondary to androgen-producing adrenal or ovarian tumors, exogenous androgens, or maternal virilizing disorders. Male pseudohermaphrodites have XY karyotypes, testes, and male internal genital structures but have incompletely masculinized external genitalia. The degree of failure of masculinization ranges from mild hypospadias to unequivocally female genitalia, as in the syndrome of androgen insensitivity ("testicular feminization"). Male pseudohermaphroditism is the result of one or more of numerous possible defects in testosterone synthesis or activation or in the responsiveness of target-cell receptors.

In *true hermaphroditism,* the least common of the "intersex" disorders, both testicular and ovarian tissues are present. The ambiguity of the external genitalia is variable, and there may be no evidence of anomalous sexual differentiation until discordant secondary sexual development occurs at the time of puberty. Most true hermaphrodites have XX karytoypes, but sex chromatin mosaicism is not uncommon. The diagnosis, which is confirmed by histologic study of gonadal tissue, must be considered in any patient with ambiguous genitalia and a XX karyotype in whom the adrenals are not the source of the increased androgens.

Management of the infant with ambiguous sexual development requires careful attention to the many psychologic and social factors involved. In general, a female pseudohermaphrodite would be reared as a female, since suppression or elimination of the androgen source and surgical correction of the virilized genitalia result in a normally functioning, often fertile female. On the other hand, a male pseudohermaphrodite with marked failure of masculinization of the genitalia may never have normal male sexual function, despite hormonal or surgical therapy, or both. Early consideration must be given to rearing such a child as a female, since surgical procedures and estrogen supplementation can enable the patient to function sexually as a female. Although gender-specific behavior is probably influenced to some degree by prenatal hormone levels, *gender identity* (the experience of oneself as male or female) is determined by the gender of rearing and is probably fixed by 3 or 4 years of age. Sex reassignment and correction of discordant external genitalia are most likely to be successful, in terms of achieving unambiguous gender identity, if accomplished before the age of 18 to 24 months.

During the period between birth and the time of sexual *maturation* (puberty), the pituitary-gonadal axis operates at a low level, with very small amounts of hormones produced. The initiation of puberty is dependent on a disruption of this balance by a decrease in hypothalamic sensitivity to circulating levels of gonadal steroids, such that higher levels of androgen or estrogen are required for feedback inhibition of gonadotropin secretion. The factors effecting the "resetting" of the axis are not clearly defined, but probably include body mass and degree of skeletal maturation.

Sexual maturation at puberty (development of secondary sexual characteristics and the capacity for fertility) normally progresses in an orderly pattern, often described in terms of the "Tanner stages" of growth of pubic hair in both sexes and of breast in the female, genitalia in the male. (Tanner stage I is prepubertal; Tanner stage V is mature adult.) Testicular enlargement and the appearance of pubic hair herald the onset of puberty in the male. The growth spurt is considered the final male pubertal milestone, although maturation of external genitalia may not be completed until after the peak height velocity is attained. In the female, puberty begins with appearance of breast buds and pubic hair and culminates in menarche; the growth spurt occurs near the midpoint of female puberty. In both sexes, the average time from beginning to end of puberty is about 3 years, although there is considerable variation.

Delayed puberty is defined as the absence of secondary sexual characteristics by the age of 13 years in a female or 14 years in a male, or as failure to reach the final milestone of puberty within 5 years of the first sign of maturation. Constitutional delay of growth and adolescence, a normal variant of somatic and sexual development, is the most common cause (see p. 62). Chronic systemic diseases may also result in delayed sexual development. Persistent failure of sexual maturation is due to deficient production of gonadotropins or to primary gonadal failure. Hypogonadotropic hypogonadism is usually idiopathic but may be the result of a hypothalamic or pituitary lesion; the diagnosis is substantiated by a poor gonadotropin response to provocative testing. Primary gonadal failure, characterized by markedly increased levels of gonadotropins (hypergonadotropic hypogonadism), is due to gonadal agenesis or dysgenesis or to a postnatal process, such as infection or trauma, that has destroyed the gonads. The treatment of failure of sexual maturation consists of the administration of gonadal hormones to produce and maintain secondary sexual characteristics.

Sexual maturation is considered precocious if secondary sexual characteristics appear before the age of 10 years in males or 8 years in females. *True isosexual precocious puberty* implies early maturation of the hypothalamic-pituitary-gonadal axis or, rarely, the autonomous production of gonadotropins by an extracranial tumor (e.g., hepatoblastoma in males). True precocity is idiopathic in 80 percent of females but in less than 40 percent of males. The usual cause of nonidiopathic precocious puberty is disease involving the hypothalamus or pituitary or both, a category that includes such diverse disorders as hamartoma, craniopharyngioma, hydrocephalus, tuberous sclerosis, and postinflammatory or posttraumatic lesions.

The precocious appearance of secondary sexual characteristics in the absence of gonadotropin-stimulated gonadal maturation is termed *precocious pseudopuberty* and is usually due to autonomous production of sex steroids by gonadal tumors (e.g., ovarian granulosa cell tumors, testicular Leydig cell tumors). Precocious pseudopuberty may result from functional adrenal tumors or congenital adrenal hyperplasia in males and from ingestion of birth control pills in females.

Sexual precocity must be differentiated from premature adrenarche (pubarche) and premature thelarche, benign variants in which early sexual hair growth or breast development is the only finding. This distinction can often be made by careful history and physical examination, measurements of growth, and observation for evidence of further sexual development during the ensuing months. In some cases, however, it may be necessary to assess skeletal maturation and hormone levels to confirm the benign nature of the physical finding.

Treatment of early sexual development is directed at the cause. In general, hormone suppression of gonadotropins retards further sexual development but does not prevent accelerated growth. Psychologic counseling is often needed; it is important to recognize that the psychosexual orientation of the precociously mature child is age-appropriate rather than appropriate for the stages of sexual maturation.

The development of *sexuality*, although usually discussed in the context of adolescence, is a lifelong process, involving the development of gender identity, an understanding of modes of sexual expression, and an acceptance of the role of the body in interpersonal relationships. The task of the physician in helping patients develop a healthy sexuality involves not only counseling about intercourse and contraception but also anticipatory guidance and reassurance, especially concerning secondary sexual characteristics, sexual fantasies, sexual orientation, and the importance of nonsexual physical contact in loving human relationships.

Reviews

1. Wilson, J. Sexual differentiation. *Annu. Rev. Physiol.* 40:279, 1978.
   A detailed, scholarly review (20 pages, 178 references).
2. Saenger, P. Abnormal sex differentiation. *J. Pediatr.* 104:1, 1984.
   Thorough and readable.
3. Stempfel, R. Introduction to Abnormalities of Sexual Differentiation. In L. Gardner (ed.), *Endocrine and Genetic Diseases of Childhood and Adolescence* (2nd ed.). Philadelphia: Saunders, 1975.
   This and the subsequent chapter are excellent, detailed textbook reviews of normal and abnormal differentiation.
4. Parks, J. Intersex. In S. Kaplan (ed.), *Clinical Pediatric and Adolescent Endocrinology.* Philadelphia: Saunders, 1982.
   A thorough, succinct chapter including a good brief review of normal sexual differentiation.
5. Baker, S. Psychosexual differentiation in the human. *Biol. Reprod.* 22:61, 1980.
   A lucid exposition of factors governing development of gender identity, gender role, and sexual orientation.

Abnormalities of Sex Chromatin

6. Gerald, P. Sex chromosome disorders. *N. Engl. J. Med.* 294:706, 1976.
   A brief review of the sex chromosome disorders of phenotypic males and females.
7. Lemli, L., and Smith, D. The XO syndrome: A study of the differentiated phenotype in 25 patients. *J. Pediatr.* 63:577, 1963.
   A review of the spectrum of clinical stigmata observed in Turner syndrome.
8. Davidoff, F., and Federman, D. Mixed gonadal dysgenesis. *Pediatrics* 52:725, 1973.
   A comprehensive review of the syndrome of XO/XY mosaicism. (For a discussion of the rare syndrome of XY gonadal dysgenesis, see Pediatrics 59:569, 1977; emphasizes prophylactic gonadectomy to prevent neoplasia.)
9. Becker, K., et al., Klinefelter syndrome. *Arch. Intern. Med.* 118:314, 1966.
   An analysis of the clinical and biochemical characteristics of XXY patients.

Pseudohermaphroditism, True Hermaphroditism

10. Lippe, B. Ambiguous genitalia and pseudohermaphroditism. *Pediatr. Clin. North Am.* 26:91, 1979.
    An excellent review of the differential diagnosis with a helpful introductory section on normal intrauterine development; see Pediatr. Clin. North Am. 23:361, 1976, for the same topic from the surgeon's viewpoint.
11. Imperato-McGinley, J., and Petersen, R. Male pseudohermaphroditism: The complexities of male phenotype development. *Am. J. Med.* 61:251, 1976.
    An extensive review of disordered male sexual development. (Also see Pediatr. Ann. 10:330, 1981; and Pediatr. Rev.3:273, 1982.)
12. Van Niekerk, W. True hermaphroditism: An analytical review with a report of 3 new cases. *Am. J. Obstet. Gynecol.*126:890, 1976.
    A review of the literature.
13. Feldman, K., and Smith, D. Fetal phallic growth and penile standards for newborn male infants. *J. Pediatr.* 86:395, 1975.
    A presentation of important normative data for the decision about sex of rearing in male pseudohermaphrodites.

Puberty, Normal and Abnormal: Reviews

14. Rosenfeld, R. Evaluation of growth and maturation in adolescence. *Pediatr. Rev.* 4:175, 1982.
    An organized approach.

15. Marshall, W., and Tanner, J. Variations in pattern of pubertal change in girls. *Arch. Dis. Child.* 44:291, 1969. Marshall, W., and Tanner, J. Variations in the pattern of pubertal changes in boys. *Arch. Dis. Child.* 45:13, 1970.
    Two major papers on the sequence and timing of normal pubertal sexual development; source of Tanner stages. (Also see J. Pediatr. 95:293, 1979, and 96:1074, 1980.)
16. Root, A. Endocrinology of puberty. *J. Pediatr.* 83:1, 187, 1973.
    A comprehensive, lucid two-part review of normal and abnormal puberty.
17. Ducharme, J., and Collu, R. Pubertal development: Normal, precocious and delayed. *Clin. Endocrinol. Metab.* 11:57, 1982.
    Well-organized, well-referenced, and thorough. (Also see Pediatr. Clin. North Am. 26:107, 123, 1979, for separate discussions of male and female development.)

Delayed Adolescence

18. Barnes, H. The problem of delayed puberty. *Med. Clin. North Am.* 59:1337, 1975.
    A review of etiology, diagnosis, and treatment.
19. Root, A., and Reiter, E. Evaluation and management of the child with delayed pubertal development. *Fertil. Steril.* 27:745, 1976.
    A comprehensive review in 10 pages, emphasizing the workup; Pediatr. Ann. 7:605, 1978, is another practical, well-reasoned approach to delayed puberty and short stature in adolescence.

Precocious Puberty

20. Bierich, J. Sexual precocity. *Clin. Endocrinol. Metabol.* 4:107, 1975.
    An extensive review of accelerated sexual maturation. (For a brief review of tumors known to cause sexual procacity, see Ann. N.Y. Acad. Sci. 230:195, 1974.)
21. Rosenfield, R. Androgen disorders in children: Too much, too early, too little, or too late. *Pediatr. Rev.* 5:147, 1983.
    Includes a concise, practical approach to precocious puberty and premature pubarche.
22. Rosenfield, R., Rich, B., and Lucky, A. Adrenarche as a cause of benign pseudo-puberty in boys. *J. Pediatr.* 101:1005, 1982.
    Clinical and hormonal profiles of males with premature pubarche. (Also see Clin. Pediatr. [Phila.] 7:29, 1968.)
23. Mills, J., et al. Premature thelarche. *Am. J. Dis. Child.* 135:743, 1981.
    Description of 46 cases with a practical approach to evaluation; discussion of the role of free estradiol in the pathogenesis of premature thelarche may be found in J. Pediatr. 89:719, 1976.

Sexuality

24. Silber, T. (ed.). Normal adolescent sexuality. *Pediatr. Ann.* 11(9), 1982.
    A collection of six articles covering specific aspects such as menarche and masturbation.
25. Litt, I., and Cohen, M. Adolescent sexuality. *Adv. Pediatr.* 26:119, 1979.
    An excellent overview of physical and psychologic aspects. (For a discussion of developmental factors resulting in sexual dysfunction, see Curr. Probl. Pediatr. 1(4), 1971.)
26. Duke, P. Adolescent sexuality. *Pediatr. Rev.* 4:44, 1982.
    Important aspects of the history, physical examination, and counseling at various stages of puberty.

III. THE NEONATE

31. ASSESSMENT OF THE NEWBORN
Robert D. White

The physician's first contact with a neonate is usually in the newborn nursery, after an uneventful labor and delivery; ideally, the relationship with the parents has begun prenatally, with a conference during the third trimester. The prenatal visit serves to initiate communication between physician and parents, permits a mutual assessment of child-rearing styles, and affords the physician the opportunity to elicit a personal and family history in an unpressured setting. Parental fears and concerns, if any, can be aired, and the physician can then give specific attention to these when assessing the newborn.

Evaluation of the neonate properly begins with a review of the pregnancy, labor, delivery, and immediate neonatal period, as well as the mother's medical history and the family history. The physical examination of a newborn requires patience and gentleness and is most successful when unpleasant procedures such as examining the ears and hips are performed last. While the infant is resting quietly, one should inspect the color, activity, and respiratory effort, then determine the vital signs and listen to the heart sounds. An estimate of gestational age should be made and the weight, length, and head circumference measured; these can be used to determine whether the physical measurements are appropriate, large, or small for gestational age. The remainder of the physical examination is directed to detection of congenital malformations or signs and symptoms of potentially serious disease.

The importance of this examination cannot be overemphasized. Many findings, such as the clouded cornea of congenital glaucoma or the hip "click" of congenital hip dislocation, may be the only clue to potentially disabling disorders; if the early, subtle signs are overlooked, the disorders are likely not to be discovered until permanent damage has occurred.

The neurologic examination of a neonate is largely accomplished during the general physical examination and gestational age assessment, which provide a reasonable impression of muscle tone, alertness, and irritability; the Moro, suck, grasp, and deep tendon reflexes should also be tested.

The data from the history and physical examination are combined to form an initial health profile of the infant: genetic endowment, exposure to potentially harmful factors in utero, and physical well-being. The health profile is not complete, however, until a clear impression of the child's future home environment is obtained. The first postpartum meeting should consist of two-way communication: the parents learn the results of the initial assessment and have an opportunity to ask questions; the physician learns the mother's plans for feeding the baby, and what preparations have been made for the infant's general care.

Occasionally, the physician's first contact with a newborn follows an emergency call to the delivery room. Even then, a history is essential to interpret the infant's physical condition properly. Obstetric complications, maternal medications, and notable events during labor and delivery must rapidly be ascertained. In some cases the situation is so emergent that history taking is interspersed with the first few minutes of active resuscitation and physical examination, but it cannot be safely omitted.

At the moment of birth, the integrity of a neonate's respiratory, cardiovascular, and neurologic systems must be established to permit a healthy transition from fetal to extrauterine life; the initial physical examination therefore considers these first. The Apgar score permits rapid assessment by grading the infant's heart rate, respiratory effort, color, tone, and reflex irritability, each on a scale of 0 to 2 points. Infants whose score is 4 to 7 of the possible 10 points at 1 minute of life have generally been depressed in utero by hypoxia or maternal medications and require assistance in the form of oxygen and gentle stimulation. An Apgar score of less than 4 at 1 minute of age indicates that the infant is profoundly depressed and must be given immediate respiratory assistance and, in many cases, cardiovascular and metabolic support as well. A second determination of Apgar score at 5 minutes of age reflects the success of resuscitative efforts and correlates with the infant's ultimate prognosis. While in the delivery room, an abbreviated physical examination is performed to rule out life-threatening congenital malformations, and the obstetrician and parents are briefly apprised of the infant's condition. The neonate is transferred to an intensive care nursery if seriously ill or at high risk of becoming ill; many initially depressed infants require only a period of observation in a transitional nursery prior to routine care in the healthy newborn nursery.

During the baby's stay in the nursery, further assessments and action on the part of the infant's physician depend largely on whether or not problems are detected in the initial health profile. A healthy, full-term infant with a good home setting needs only a daily reassessment of feeding, urine and stooling patterns, extent of jaundice, and body weight, and visits with the parents to discuss new questions or problems. A second, abbreviated physical examination prior to discharge is necessary, since heart murmurs, decreased femoral pulses, hip clicks, increasing head circumference, and other signs of significant disease frequently do not become apparent until after the first day of life; in addition, a minor abnormality present on the initial assessment often requires further assessment on following days. With this in mind, infants should only be discharged "early" (i.e., on the first day of life) if appropriate arrangements are made for follow-up, particularly during the critical next few days. All parents should be alerted to signs that require prompt communication with the physician (e.g., marked jaundice, poor feeding, lethargy, fever).

A discharge conference serves several purposes: arrangements for well-baby care are confirmed; feeding plans are discussed (if the infant will be breast-fed, vitamin D supplementation should be considered; if bottle feeding is planned, a formula fortified with vitamins A, C, and D and iron should be selected); and the parents are instructed in umbilical cord, circumcision, and skin care; in normal patterns of sleep, crying, and stooling; and about normal events that might be alarming to new parents, such as transient vaginal bleeding. This is also an appropriate time to emphasize that a significant reduction in accidental injuries (the leading cause of childhood mortality) is possible through early establishment of safety habits, such as use of an infant car seat.

Fetal Monitoring

1. Petrie, R. Fetal monitoring. *Clin. Perinatol.* 9:229, 1982.
   A full issue devoted to this topic. (Also see Semin. Perinatol. *3:105, 1981.)*

Initial Assessment and Resuscitation

2. Nelson, K., and Ellenberg, J. Apgar scores as predictions of chronic neurologic disability. *Pediatrics* 68:36, 1981.
   Low Apgar scores constitute a risk factor for later disability but are neither very specific nor sensitive.
3. Advanced cardiac life support for neonates. *J.A.M.A.* 244:495, 1980.
   Many details of ABCs worthy of study.

Extensive Assessment

4. Philip, A., et al. Neonatal mortality risk for the eighties: The importance of birth weight/gestational age groups. *Pediatrics* 68:122, 1983.
   Valuable for predicting mortality risk in premature infants. (Also see J. Pediatr. *101:969, 1982.)*
5. Robertson, A. Gestational age. *J. Pediatr.* 95:732, 1979.
   Reviews the various methods of estimating gestational age, including the Dubowitz examination and more recent modifications.
6. Desmond, M., et al. The clinical behavior of the newly born. *J. Pediatr.* 62:307, 1963.
   Observation in the first 6 hours of life showed a relatively constant pattern of behavior: alertness, followed by somnolence, then reawakening.
7. Brazelton, T., Parker, W., and Zuckerman, B. Importance of behavioral assessment of the neonate. *Curr. Probl. Pediatr.* 7(2), 1976.
   A review of the remarkable complexity and capacity of neonatal behavior. (Also see Pediatrics *64:548, 1979.)*
8. Lozoff, B., et al. The mother-newborn relationship: Limits of adaptability. *J. Pediatr.* 91:1, 1977.
   Review of mother-infant bonding in the first days of life; comment on how current hospital practices interfere.

9. Siegel, E. Early and extended maternal-infant contact: A critical review. *Am. J. Dis. Child.* 136:251, 1982.
   An attempt to put early maternal-infant bonding into perspective.
10. Charney, E. Counseling of parents around the birth of a baby. *Pediatr. Rev.* 4:167, 1982.
    For more wisdom, this time from the other side of the Atlantic, see Arch. Dis. Child. *59:380, 1984. These two papers should be read by every pediatrician.*
11. Lozoff, B., and Brittenham, G. Infant care: Cache or carry. *J. Pediatr.* 95:478, 1979.
    Many patterns developed by our society for infant care have convenience of the parents in mind, rather than the well-being of the infant.
12. Thompson, H. The value of neonatal circumcision. *Am. J. Dis. Child.* 137:939, 1983.
    The author's annotation: "An unanswered and perhaps unanswerable question."

Normal and Abnormal Findings
13. Solomon, L., and Esterly, N. Neonatal dermatology: I. The newborn skin. *J. Pediatr.* 77:888, 1970.
    Helpful in deciding whether skin lesions are pathologic or normal variants. (For more by these authors, see Neonatal Dermatology. *Philadelphia: Saunders, 1973; for more on birthmarks with serious medical significance, see* J. Pediatr. *95:696, 1979, and* Pediatr. Rev. *1:21, 47, 1979.)*
14. Clark, D. Times of first void and first stool in 500 newborns. *Pediatrics* 60:457, 1977.
    Tabulation includes full-term, premature, and postmature infants.
15. Jorgenson, R., et al. Intraoral findings and anomalies in neonates. *Pediatrics* 69:577, 1982.
    Common and uncommon features of the oral examination.
16. Miller, H. Intrauterine growth retardation. *Am. J. Dis. Child.* 135:944, 1981.
    The author emphasizes the need to distinguish between different types of growth retardation.

32. RESPIRATORY DISTRESS SYNDROME
Robert D. White

The respiratory distress syndrome (RDS) is the most common cause of death among premature infants. It is caused by immaturity of the lungs and occurs in approximately 20 percent of infants weighing less than 1500 gm, but in less than 1 percent of those whose birth weight is over 2500 gm. Males, infants of diabetic mothers, infants delivered by cesarean section, and infants born to a mother who has had a previous child with RDS have a particularly high incidence of this disorder. Asphyxia during labor or delivery also seems to predispose the neonate to RDS. Conditions that may lessen the risk of RDS include prolonged rupture of the membranes and maternal heroin addiction.

The primary abnormality in RDS appears to be deficient synthesis or release of pulmonary surfactant. This material lines the alveoli of the mature lung and lowers the surface tension required to keep the alveolus open during expiration. When surfactant is deficient, diffuse alveolar atelectasis ensues, resulting in pulmonary insufficiency. Surfactant production is normally very low in utero until the third trimester of pregnancy; it then increases slowly until 33 to 36 weeks' gestation, when there is an abrupt rise to near-term levels. Respiratory distress often develops in infants born prior to this "surge" and does not improve until surfactant production "turns on" at 48 to 72 hours after birth. Those who die during the acute stage of respiratory insufficiency have profound, generalized atelectasis on autopsy. Often, an eosinophilic material composed of fibrin, hemoglobin products, and cellular debris coats the terminal bronchioles; this is the classically described "hyaline membrane," but it is not present in all cases, nor is it specific for RDS.

Respiratory distress syndrome produces characteristic clinical and radiographic findings. Tachypnea, nasal flaring, and retractions are usually present within the first 4 hours of life and may even be noted at birth. As the infant becomes progressively distressed, cyanosis is evident, and an expiratory grunt or cry is audible. Auscultation reveals poor breath sounds throughout the chest, often with fine, scattered rales. The chest roentgenogram shows a diffuse granular opacification of the lung fields, with prominent air bronchograms; the heart border and diaphragms are often obscured. Blood gas analysis demonstrates hypoxemia, and, in severe cases, hypercapnea and acidosis. Signs and symptoms usually worsen through the first 3 days of life, after which improvement and recovery are the rule, unless complications of RDS such as patent ductus arteriosus or bronchopulmonary dysplasia have developed.

Conditions that must be differentiated from RDS include meconium aspiration, pneumonia, pneumothorax, airway obstruction, congenital heart disease, hypoglycemia, and sepsis. A particularly difficult disease to distinguish from RDS is pneumonia and sepsis due to the group B streptococcus, which clinically and radiographically may be identical to RDS, but runs a rapidly progressive and frequently fatal course (see Neonatal Sepsis, Chap. 44).

Management of RDS is dependent on the severity of respiratory insufficiency. In milder cases, administration of supplemental oxygen provides adequate respiratory support through the 4- to 5-day course of the disease. When oxygen alone is insufficient, continuous distending pressure may aid in preventing alveolar collapse and thus improve respiratory function; distending pressure during spontaneous breathing may be delivered as continuous positive airway pressure (CPAP) by means of an endotracheal tube, nasal prongs, or face mask. Many infants with RDS require controlled mechanical ventilation during the most severe stage of their illness; this is the group most susceptible to complications of RDS.

High arterial oxygen concentrations during therapy can produce retinal damage (retrolental fibroplasia), while periods of hypoxemia may lead to neurologic damage; the goal of respiratory assistance, therefore, is to maintain arterial PO_2 between 50 and 70 mm Hg, a range that minimizes the incidence of these complications. Continuous distending pressure and positive-pressure ventilation produce pneumothorax in approximately 5 to 20 percent of cases; this complication usually causes sudden deterioration in respiratory function and can be diagnosed clinically by reduction of breath sounds over the affected lung and by transillumination. Use of high inspired oxygen concentrations during positive pressure ventilation can also cause bronchopulmonary dysplasia, a form of chronic pulmonary disease that is described more fully in the next section.

Many problems can complicate the course of RDS. Hypoglycemia, hypocalcemia, anemia, and acidosis are common and may seriously worsen respiratory function if untreated. In severely ill patients, disseminated intravascular coagulation, intracranial hemorrhage, and pulmonary hemorrhage are common and often fatal complications. Respiratory insufficiency can also be exacerbated by hypothermia or hyperthermia, which increases oxygen demands in the tissues. Hyperbilirubinemia is often severe in infants with RDS and is more likely to cause kernicterus when acidosis or hypoxemia is present. Feeding a severely distressed infant is difficult but essential, because of high energy requirements and minimal glycogen and fat reserves. Usually, this necessitates special feeding techniques, such as nasogastric gavage or intravenous alimentation. Renal function is compromised in infants with RDS, and fluid administration must be adjusted accordingly. This is especially true because patent ductus arteriosus (PDA) is also a complication of RDS, and signs and symptoms of heart failure may be exacerbated by excessive fluid administration.

Recovery from RDS usually begins on the third or fourth day of life and is complete by 1 week of age. Deviation from this course may be caused by a PDA, bronchopulmonary dysplasia, pneumonia, intracranial hemorrhage, or apnea of prematurity. The long-term outlook for survivors of RDS is good; permanent pulmonary or neurologic damage is uncommon.

Prevention of RDS in some infants have been achieved in the past decade. Amniocentesis permits analysis of the state of fetal lung maturation through measurement of the concentration of surfactant components in the amniotic fluid. As a result of this information, many semielective deliveries may be delayed until lung maturation is ensured. The discovery that corticosteroids induce the synthesis of surfactant has been utilized in some centers to decrease the incidence of RDS by prenatal administration of steroids to the mother, but the value of this treatment appears to be limited to fetuses of less than 32 weeks' gestation who have had more than 24 hours exposure to therapy. Several promising approaches remain in the experimental stage; these include newer drugs to inhibit premature labor, administration of natural or artificial surfactants, ventilation using fluorocarbon liquids, and extracorporeal oxygenation.

Books

1. Avery, M., Fletcher, B., and Williams, R. *The Lung and Its Disorders in the Newborn Infant* (4th ed.). Philadelphia: Saunders, 1981.
   Concise, easily read section on RDS.
2. Farrell, P. (ed.). *Lung Development: Biological and Clinical Perspectives. Vol. II: Neonatal Respiratory Distress.* New York: Academic Press, 1982.
   Basic science orientation.

Reviews

3. Fawcett, W., and Gluck, L. Respiratory distress syndrome in the tiny baby. *Clin. Perinatol.* 4:411, 1977.
   A good general review, with consideration of the special problems of babies weighing less than 1200 gm.
4. Hallman, M., and Gluck, L. Respiratory distress syndrome: Update 1982. *Pediatr. Clin. North Am.* 29:1057, 1982.
   For another thorough, current review, see Adv. Pediatr. 30:93, 1983.

Contributing Factors

5. Usher, R., McLean, F., and Maighan, G. Respiratory distress in infants delivered by caesarian section. *Am. J. Obstet. Gynecol.* 88:806, 1964.
   The risk of RDS is increased, independent of indications for section.
6. Graven, S., and Misenjeimer, H. Respiratory distress syndrome and the high risk mother. *Am. J. Dis. Child.* 109:489, 1965.
   Is there a genetic predisposition to prematurity and RDS in some families?
7. Bauer, C., Stern, L., and Colle, E. Prolonged rupture of membranes associated with decreased incidence of respiratory distress syndrome. *Pediatrics* 53:7, 1974.
   Prolonged ruptured of the membranes raised fetal steroid production and reduced the incidence of RDS.
8. Glass, L., Rajegowda, R., and Evans, H. Absence of respiratory distress syndrome in premature infants of heroin-addicted mothers. *Lancet* 2:685, 1971.
   The title is the message.
9. Jacob, J., et al. The contribution of PDA in the neonate with severe RDS. *J. Pediatr.* 96:79, 1980.
   Very-low-birth-weight infants routinely had respiratory compromise secondary to a PDA.
10. Ikegami, M., Jacobs, H., and Jobe, A. Surfactant function in respiratory distress syndrome. *J. Pediatr.* 102:443, 1983.
    Infants with RDS have proteins present in the alveolar space that inhibit surfactant.

Diagnosis

11. Rudolph, A., Desmond, M., and Pineda, R. Clinical diagnosis of respiratory difficulty in the newborn. *Pediatr. Clin. North Am.* 13:669, 1966.
    An excellent discussion of the clinical findings.
12. Torday, J., Carson, L., and Lawson, E. Saturated phosphatidylcholine in amniotic fluid and prediction of the respiratory distress syndrome. *N. Engl. J. Med.* 301:1013, 1979.
    Phosphatidylglycerol is now also routinely analyzed to assist in estimation of fetal lung maturity. (Also see Clin. Perinatol. 9:297, 1982.)

Management

13. Scopes, J. Management of respiratory distress syndrome. *Br. J. Anaesth.* 49:35, 1977.
    The rationale for and methods of respiratory assistance are briefly reviewed.
14. Krouskop, R., Brown, E., and Sweet, A. The early use of continuous positive airway pressure in the treatment of idiopathic respiratory distress syndrome. *J. Pediatr.* 87:263, 1975.
    Early use may diminish the severity of RDS.
15. James, L., and Lanham, J. History of oxygen therapy and retrolental fibroplasia.

Pediatrics 57:591, 1976.
An excellent review of this complication serves as cogent reminder to monitor arterial
PO₂ carefully.

16. Pasnick, M., and Lucey, J. Practical uses of continuous transcutaneous oxygen monitoring. *Pediatr. Rev.* 5:5, 1983.
    Also reviewed in Adv. Pediatr. *28:27, 1981, and* J. Pediatr. *103:837, 1983.*

17. Stevenson, J. Fluid administration in the association of patent ductus arteriosus complicating respiratory distress syndrome. *J. Pediatr.* 90:257, 1977.
    Less weight loss than expected in the first days of life may be a clue to excessive fluid administration.

18. Heaf, D., et al. Changes in pulmonary function during the diuretic phase of respiratory distress syndrome. *J. Pediatr.* 101:103, 1982.
    Spontaneous diuresis heralds improvement in respiratory symptoms; ventilatory assistance should be reduced at this time, if possible, to avoid air leak problems.

19. Delivoria-Papadopoulos, M., et al. The role of exchange transfusion in the management of low-birth-weight infants with and without severe RDS. *J. Pediatr.* 89:273, 1976.
    Exchange may improve oxygenation, for reasons still unknown.

20. Wagaman, M., et al. Improved oxygenation and lung compliance with prone positioning of neonates. *J. Pediatr.* 94:787, 1979.
    Positioning has a significant effect on pulmonary function in ill newborns.

21. Kuhns, L., et al. Diagnosis of pneumothorax or pneumomediastinum in the neonate by transillumination. *Pediatrics* 56:355, 1975.
    The technique is most useful in very small prematures, who also benefit most from early diagnosis and treatment.

Prevention

22. Farrell, P., and Kotas, R. The prevention of hyaline membrane disease: New concepts and approaches to therapy. *Adv. Pediatr.* 23:213, 1976.
    An excellent review that also discusses surfactant metabolism and conventional therapy of RDS.

23. Ambrus, C., et al. Prevention of hyaline membrane disease with plasminogen. *J.A.M.A.* 237:1837, 1977.
    A single dose of plasminogen at birth was effective in reducing the severity of RDS.

24. Ballard, P., and Ballard, R. Corticosteroids and respiratory distress syndrome: Status 1979. *Pediatrics* 63:163, 1979.
    Accompanies two articles in same issue documenting risks and benefits of steroid therapy.

25. Morley, C. Will exogenous surfactant treat respiratory distress syndrome? *Arch. Dis. Child.* 58:321, 1983.
    The author suggests since surfactant deficiency is only one of the biochemical abnormalities associated with RDS, exogenous surfactant is likely only to ameliorate the disease, rather than provide a cure.

Long-Term Follow-Up

26. Mayes, L., and Stahlman, M. Effect of hyaline membrane disease on outcome of premature infants. *Am. J. Dis. Child.* 136:885, 1982.
    Outlines the questions; does not provide the answers.

27. Field, T., et al. Respiratory distress syndrome: Perinatal prediction of one year developmental outcome. *Semin. Perinatol.* 6:288, 1982.
    Gestational age is a more predictive variable than respiratory distress.

33. CHRONIC PULMONARY DISEASE
Robert D. White

Respiratory insufficiency is a common complication of prematurity, due to immaturity of the lungs. The course may be acute, as in the respiratory distress syndrome (RDS) (see Chap. 32), or chronic, as in the Wilson-Mikity syndrome. Attempts to support pulmonary function in affected infants produce additional problems, among them bronchopulmonary dysplasia. The chronic pulmonary diseases that originate in the neonatal period share certain characteristics, the most encouraging of which is that infants who survive the first year of life usually have little or no residual symptomatic pulmonary disability.

Bronchopulmonary dysplasia (BPD) occurs in some infants who have received high concentrations of oxygen for several days. In most cases an endotracheal tube and intermittent positive pressure ventilation have also been used for at least 24 hours. These observations implicate both oxygen and pressure in the pathogenesis of BPD. It is most commonly seen in infants recovering from RDS, since this is by far the most common disease requiring intensive respiratory support.

The clinical course of BPD has been divided into four stages. In the first days of life (stage I), severe RDS is present. Late in the first week of life (stage II), there is clinical improvement, but the infant never becomes totally asymptomatic. In the second week of life (stage III), a clear departure from the natural history of RDS occurs: there is clinical deterioration, with increasing hypoxemia, hypercapnea, and acidosis, and additional respiratory support is required. The lungs at this point are diffusely opacified on chest roentgenograms; small cystic areas and streaky infiltrates appear shortly thereafter. The clinical picture is often very similar to that of patent ductus arteriosus, which often coexists with BPD in premature infants recovering from RDS. Histologically, there is evidence of intense inflammation, with edema, exudate, and macrophages filling the alveoli. This inflammatory response is strikingly similar to that described in experimental oxygen toxicity of the lung. Frequently, there is also disruption of the bronchiolar tissue, progressing to the cystic lesions noted on x-ray study. Deterioration continues for several weeks; pneumonia may also supervene and cause additional respiratory compromise.

Stage IV, the chronic healing phase of BPD, occurs after 1 month of age. Clinically, respiratory distress, cyanosis, and rales are present; radiographs and histologic examination reveal larger cystic lesions and progression of the fibroplasia. Approximately 25 percent of affected infants die during this stage, usually from superimposed pneumonia or heart failure.

The extent of healing in BPD is evidence of the tremendous regenerative capacity of an infant's lungs. In even the most severe cases, symptoms usually resolve by 2 years of age, although abnormalities in pulmonary function tests and ECG evidence of right ventricular hypertrophy may persist for several years.

The Wilson-Mikity syndrome differs from BPD in that RDS is mild or absent at birth, and oxygen requirements initially are minimal. It occurs almost exclusively in premature infants whose birth weight is less than 1500 gm. Many are moderately depressed at birth, but respiratory problems and oxygen administration are minimal. They then usually have a interval of several days with mild symptoms, followed by the insidious onset of respiratory insufficiency. Blood gases reveal hypoxemia, hypercarbia, and acidosis, with severe (30–80%) intrapulmonary shunting of blood. The radiograph demonstrates small cystic lesions scattered throughout the lungs, accompanied by a fine, lacy infiltrate; often, these changes precede clinical symptoms. Respiratory insufficiency may progress for 1 to 2 months, with a mortality approximated at 10%. The survivors of this stage often have no clinical or radiographic evidence of disease at 2 years of age, but exercise intolerance and pulmonary function test abnormalities may persist.

The etiology of the Wilson-Mikity syndrome is uncertain; histologically, it is characterized by cystic changes and mild scarring and is distinguished from BPD by the relative absence of inflammation.

A third chronic pulmonary disease of the premature infant, which may in fact be a mild form of the Wilson-Mikity syndrome, has also been described. This disease has been termed *chronic pulmonary insufficiency of prematurity;* the clinical syndrome is virtually identical to that of Wilson-Mikity, except that radiographic changes, when present, consist of a fine generalized opacification without cystic changes. Because mortality is rare, histologic characterization is lacking at present.

Because of the improved survival of premature infants, the incidence of chronic pulmonary disease in infancy is increasing. At present, only supportive therapy is available. Good nutrition is essential to lung healing; infants with chronic lung disease present a challenge because their caloric requirements are increased by the work of breathing, yet fluid tolerance is low due to cor pulmonale. Chest percussion and drainage are usually helpful in mobilizing the increased respiratory tract secretions. Diuretics are also frequently used to ameliorate fluid retention and pulmonary edema associated with cor pulmonale. The emotional and developmental needs of the patients and their parents should not be overlooked; the chronic, unstable course of BPD in particular requires close contact with a stable group of sympathetic and helpful caretakers for optimal support.

Bronchopulmonary Dysplasia: Etiology

1. Edwards, D., Dyer, W., and Northway, W. Twelve years experience with bronchopulmonary dysplasia. *Pediatrics* 59:839, 1977.
   Also see the original description: N. Engl. J. Med. *276:357, 1967.*
2. Watts, J., Ariagno, R., and Brady, J. Chronic pulmonary disease in neonates after artificial ventilation: Distribution of ventilation and pulmonary interstitial emphysema. *Pediatrics* 60:273, 1977.
   Pulmonary interstitial emphysema is a common prelude to BPD.
3. Brown, E., et al. Bronchopulmonary dysplasia: Possible relationship to pulmonary edema. *J. Pediatr.* 92:982, 1978.
   Authors propose that fluid overload in the first days of life increases risk of BPD.
4. Workshop on bronchopulmonary dysplasia. *J. Pediatr.* 95:815, 1979.
   An entire supplement devoted to this topic.

Bronchopulmonary Dysplasia: Management and Follow-Up

5. Bryan, M., et al. Pulmonary function studies during the first year of life in infants recovering from the respiratory distress syndrome. *Pediatrics* 52:169, 1973.
   A follow-up study describing the natural history through the first year of life.
6. Smith, J., Reynolds, E., and Taghizadeh, A. Brain maturation and damage in infants dying from chronic pulmonary insufficiency in the postneonatal period. *Arch. Dis. Child.* 49:359, 1974.
   Localized CNS lesions were found in this autopsy study of babies dying of BPD.
7. Kao, L., et al. Effect of oral diuretics on pulmonary mechanics in infants with chronic bronchopulmonary dysplasia: Results of a double-blind crossover sequential trial. *Pediatrics* 74:37, 1984.
   For a cautionary note, see Am. J. Dis. Child. *137:1145, 1983.*
8. Koops, B., Abman, S., and Accurso, F. Outpatient management and follow-up of bronchopulmonary dysplasia. *Clin. Perinatol.* 11:101, 1984.
   Extensive discussion of long-term management problems.
9. Yu, V., et al. Growth and development of very low birth weight infants recovering from bronchopulmonary dysplasia. *Arch. Dis. Child.* 58:791, 1983.
   For additional follow-up studies, see Am. J. Dis. Child. *136:443, 1982, and* Acta Paediatr. Scand. *72:225, 1983, and* Pediatrics *68:336; 1981.*

Wilson-Mikity Syndrome

10. Hodgman, J., et al. Chronic respiratory distress in the premature infant: The Wilson-Mikity syndrome. *Pediatrics* 44:179, 1969.
    A large series.
11. Coates, A., et al. Long-term pulmonary sequelae of the Wilson-Mikity syndrome. *J. Pediatr.* 92:247, 1978.
    Follow-up of 5 children for 8–10 years.

Chronic Pulmonary Insufficiency of Prematurity

12. Krauss, A., Klain, D., and Auld, P. Chronic pulmonary insufficiency of prematurity (CPIP). *Pediatrics* 55:55, 1975.
    Pulmonary function testing was used to document abnormalities in this syndrome.

34. CYANOTIC HEART DISEASE
Robert D. White and Jean S. Kan

Introduction of the Blalock-Taussig operation four decades ago for palliation of cyanotic congenital heart disease opened the modern era of pediatric cardiology and cardiovascular surgery. In the intervening years, diagnostic techniques have become highly sophisticated, and corrective or palliative surgery is now available for most cardiac lesions associated with cyanosis in the newborn.

Cyanosis occurs in a multitude of disorders. *Central* cyanosis is caused by disorders that permit unoxygenated blood to enter the arterial circulation and is only clinically apparent when at least 5 gm/dl of hemoglobin is desaturated. Congenital heart disease produces cyanosis by allowing venous blood to enter the systemic circulation through cardiac or vascular malformations; parenchymal lung disease, congenital anomalies of the lung or airways, and methemoglobinemia cause cyanosis by preventing oxygenation of blood as it passes through the pulmonary circulation. *Peripheral* cyanosis occurs in patients whose blood flow to the extremities is markedly diminished; arterial PO_2 is normal in these patients, but oxygen is extracted from the blood to an unusually high degree by underperfused tissues. Hypovolemia, heart failure, hypoglycemia, polycythemia, sepsis, acidosis, and hypothermia are common causes of peripheral cyanosis.

Cyanotic heart disease can be distinguished from other causes of cyanosis by several clinical and laboratory observations. Infants with peripheral cyanosis usually have pink mucous membranes and (by definition) normal arterial PO_2. Methemoglobinemia is also easily recognized; blood from a patient with this disorder will remain dark when exposed to oxygen in vitro, whereas that from infants with cyanosis from other causes becomes pink. Distinguishing heart disease from pulmonary problems is more difficult. A history of prematurity, prolonged rupture of the membranes, meconium-stained amniotic fluid, or other obstetric complications favors the diagnosis of lung disease. Pulmonary disorders cause severe dyspnea, whereas most infants with cyanotic heart disease seem relatively undistressed in proportion to their cyanosis. Auscultation may be useful if a murmur or gallop is detected, but these occur in only a minority of newborns with cyanotic heart defects. A normal heart size with increased pulmonary markings on chest x-ray examination suggests lung disease; some cyanotic heart lesions may also produce increased pulmonary vascular markings, but cardiomegaly is usually present in these patients. Diminished pulmonary markings on roentgenograms are highly suggestive of heart disease. Pulmonary problems can produce right axis deviation and right ventricular strain, but other electrocardiographic abnormalities suggest the presence of a cardiac malformation. Perhaps the most useful test is the hyperoxia test: after the infant breathes 100% oxygen for approximately 15 minutes, arterial PO_2 is measured. The PO_2 will usually rise above 150 mm Hg with lung disease, while it remains consistently below this level in cyanotic heart disease. An elevated PCO_2 is also strong evidence of lung disease. Echocardiography is very helpful in documenting certain cardiac malformations, but normal findings do not completely exclude heart disease.

These historical, clinical, and laboratory observations nearly always permit differentiation of lung disease from cyanotic heart disease. However, there is one notable exception: persistence of the fetal circulation (PFC), so-called because systemic-pulmonary communications (the ductus arteriosus and the foramen ovale) that normally close at birth remain open, and pulmonary vascular resistance remains higher than systemic resistance. The combination of high pulmonary resistance and an open communication to the systemic circulation permits unoxygenated venous blood to enter the arterial circulation. This disorder is frequently present in neonates with severe lung disease and may also be associated with asphyxia, polycythemia, intrauterine growth retardation, or hypoglycemia. Many of the clinical and laboratory findings mimic those of cyanotic heart disease; cyanosis is severe, and the PO_2 does not usually rise above 100 mm Hg during the hyperoxia test. Acidosis is common, disproportionate to the degree of hypoxia. Pulmonary blood flow is diminished, but pulmonary markings on the x-ray film may be decreased or increased, depending on the degree of associated lung disease. Some infants even have murmurs and heart failure due to insufficiency of the tricuspid valve induced by severe strain on the right side of the heart. The ECG, as in lung disease, usually shows right axis deviation and right ventricular strain. The echocardiogram is very useful; findings include normal pulmonary valve and outflow tract but abnormal right-sided systolic time intervals, indicative of severe pulmonary artery hypertension.

The clinical and laboratory observations that permit the distinction of heart from lung disease are also helpful in establishing the specific nature of the cardiac lesion. In the first week of life, transposition of the great arteries (see Chap. 52) and obstructions to pulmonary outflow (including pulmonary atresia and severe pulmonic stenosis) are the most common cardiac causes of cyanosis; these may be distinguished by the chest roentgenogram and echocardiogram. In the former, pulmonary blood flow appears slightly to moderately increased with transposition, but diminished in pulmonary stenosis or atresia. Echocardiography is usually diagnostic of transposition when it demonstrates an abnormally positioned pulmonary valve (leftward and posterior of its normal site), directly adjacent to the mitral valve.

Tricuspid atresia, Ebstein's anomaly (displacement of the tricuspid annulus into the right ventricle), and total anomalous pulmonary venous return are occasional causes of cyanosis in the first week of life. Tricuspid atresia, which often is associated with pulmonary valve stenosis or atresia, is characterized electrocardiographically by left axis deviation and left ventricular hypertrophy. Ebstein's anomaly produces large P waves and intraventricular conduction defects; the Wolff-Parkinson-White syndrome may occur with Ebstein's anomaly. Total anomalous pulmonary venous return is very difficult to diagnose, but should be suspected in an infant with cyanosis, increased pulmonary vascular markings, and a small left atrium. Hypoplastic left heart and truncus arteriosus more commonly cause heart failure in the neonatal period but may also occasionally present with cyanosis.

Tetralogy of Fallot (see Chap. 51) and other complex forms of pulmonary outflow obstruction are the only common causes of the cyanosis that appears later in the neonatal period.

Infants with cyanotic heart disease, and those with profound cyanosis in whom heart disease cannot be excluded, should be transferred to a center where cardiac catheterization can be performed to provide definitive information on the type and severity of cardiac malformation. Catheterization may also provide an opportunity for palliative treatment; in transposition of the great vessels, a balloon septostomy (Rashkind procedure) can be of immediate benefit, and balloon valvuloplasty may be effective in relieving the symptoms of critical pulmonic stenosis.

Good medical management of a newborn with cyanotic heart disease is crucial to survival. The oxygen requirements of the body should be minimized by keeping the infant warm and by foregoing unnecessary stressful procedures. Oxygen administration usually produces only a slight improvement in the PO_2, but the resultant increase in oxygen content of the blood may be significant, due to the configuration of the fetal oxygen-hemoglobin dissociation curve. Acidosis and hypoglycemia can cause rapid deterioration, so that monitoring for these complications must be frequent and the therapy aggressive. Prostaglandin E1 is useful in infants whose cyanosis is a result of reduced pulmonary blood flow; the resulting dilatation of the ductus arteriosus allows flow of blood from the aorta to the lungs, where it is oxygenated and returned to the systemic circulation. In some cases, such supportive care allows operation to be deferred until the infant is older, larger, and a better operative risk; in the others, it ensures that the infant is in the best possible preoperative condition.

An emergency operation may be necessary in many neonates with cyanotic heart disease. Infants with decreased pulmonary blood flow benefit from creation of a systemic-to-pulmonary shunt. In transposition of the great arteries, an atrial septostomy is palliative, but definitive repair is becoming an accepted procedure for young infants. Repair of total anomalous venous return is difficult but feasible if the diagnosis is made early. Surgery is almost never necessary for Ebstein's anomaly during the neonatal period, since cyanosis tends to improve with time as the pulmonary vascular resistance drops and right ventricular function improves.

Emotional support of the parents is an integral part of medical and surgical therapy. The prognosis of a neonate with cyanotic heart disease continues to improve as medical and surgical techniques become increasingly sophisticated. Most advances are too recent for adequate evaluation, but survival rates now seem to exceed 50 percent for infants with common malformations other than anomalous pulmonary venous return.

Reviews

1. Kitterman, J. Cyanosis in the newborn infant. *Pediatr. Rev.* 4:13, 1982.
   Current diagnostic and therapeutic modalities are described.
2. Lees, M. Cyanosis of the newborn infant. *J. Pediatr.* 77:484, 1970.
   A highly readable, clinically oriented discussion.
3. Engle, M. Cyanotic congenital heart disease. *Am. J. Cardiol.* 37:283, 1976.
   Thorough review (25 pages, 271 references).

4. Rowe, R. Serious congenital heart disease in the newborn infant: Diagnosis and management. *Pediatr. Clin. North Am.* 17:967, 1970.
   Helpful diagnostic approach uses probabilities based on incidence and age at diagnosis.

Specific Lesions
5. Rowe, R., Freedom, R., Mehrizi, A., and Bloom, K. *The Neonate with Congenital Heart Disease* (2nd ed.). Philadelphia: Saunders, 1981.
   Most comprehensive.
6. Fyler, D., et al. Report of the New England Regional Infant Cardiac Program. *Pediatrics* 65:377, 1980.
   Large series for each lesion.
7. Williams, W., et al. Tricuspid atresia: Results of treatment in 160 children. *Am. J. Cardiol.* 38:235, 1976.
   Many permutations of this malformation affect the natural history. (For another large series, see J. Thorac. Cardiovasc. Surg. 85:440, 647, 1983.)
8. Giuliani, E., et al. The clinical features and natural history of Ebstein's anomaly of the tricuspid valve. *Mayo Clin. Proc.* 54:163, 1979.
   The first of six articles (and an editorial) on various aspects of Ebstein's anomaly.
9. Cole, R., et al. Pulmonary atresia with intact ventricular septum. *Am. J. Cardiol.* 21:23, 1968.
   The ECG commonly shows that right ventricular forces are absent. (For a recent surgical series, see Circulation 67:1318, 1983.)
10. Awariefe, S., Clarke, D., and Pappas, G. Surgical approach to critical pulmonary valve stenosis in infants less than six months of age. *J. Thorac. Cardiovasc. Surg.* 85:375, 1983.
    Closed procedures gain favor, although reoperation is sometimes necessary.
11. Delisle, G., et al. Total anomalous pulmonary venous connection: Report of 93 autopsied cases with emphasis on diagnostic and surgical considerations. *Am. Heart J.* 91:99, 1976.
    An in-depth discussion of embryology and varying clinical manifestations. (Also see Br. Heart J. 39:436, 1977, and Circulation 66[Suppl I]:I-208, 1982.)
    Also see Tetralogy of Fallot (Chap. 51) and Transposition of the Great Arteries (Chap. 52).

Persistence of the Fetal Circulation
12. Rowe, R. Abnormal pulmonary vasoconstriction in the newborn. *Pediatrics* 59:318, 1977.
    An excellent brief review.
13. Drummond, W. Persistent pulmonary hypertension of the neonate (persistent fetal circulation syndrome). *Adv. Pediatr.* 30:61, 1983.
    Another extensive clinical review: Clin. Perinatol. 11(3), 1984.
14. Linday, L., et al. Noninvasive diagnosis of persistent fetal circulation versus congenital cardiovascular defects. *Am. J. Cardiol.* 52:847, 1983.
    ECG found to be most sensitive, while 2-D echo was most specific. Total anomalous pulmonary venous return continues to be the most difficult cardiac lesion to exclude.
15. Levin, D., et al. Persistent pulmonary hypertension of the newborn infant. *J. Pediatr.* 89:626, 1976.
    Tolazoline or curare may be effective in reducing hypoxemia. (Also see p. 617 of the same issue, and J. Pediatr. 95:550, 573, 1979, and 103:505, 1983.)

Diagnostic Techniques
16. Sahn, D., and Friedman, W. Difficulties in distinguishing cardiac from pulmonary disease in the neonate. *Pediatr. Clin. North Am.* 20:293, 1973.
    A good discussion of the pathophysiology of various diseases.
17. Jones, R., et al. Arterial oxygen tension and response to oxygen breathing in differential diagnosis of congenital heart disease in infancy. *Arch. Dis. Child.* 51:667, 1976.
    The hyperoxia test is described.

18. Elliott, L., and Schiebler, G. A roentgenologic-electrocardiographic approach to cyanotic forms of heart disease. *Pediatr. Clin. North Am.* 18:1133, 1971.
   A gold mine of diagnostic clues.

Management
19. Olley, P., Coceani, F., and Bodach, E. E-type prostaglandins: A new emergency therapy for certain cyanotic congenital heart malformations. *Circulation* 53:728, 1976.
   This experimental drug improved oxygenation by keeping the ductus arteriosus patent until surgical palliation could be performed. (Also see J. Pediatr. 93:481, 1978.)
20. Rudolph, A., et al. Formalin infiltration of the ductus arteriosus. *N. Engl. J. Med.* 292:1263, 1975.
   A means of keeping the ductus patent for prolonged periods in infants with complex cyanotic heart disease for whom an operation is not feasible.
21. Kan, J., et al. Percutaneous transluminal balloon valvuloplasty for pulmonary valve stenosis. *Circulation* 69:554, 1984.
   A major advance in therapy for selected infants.
22. Engle, M., and Diaz, S. Long-term results of surgery for congenital heart disease: I. Surgery of specific anomalies. *Circulation* 65:415, 1982.
   Multiple surgical follow-up series referenced for each anomaly.
23. Moss, A. What every primary physician should know about the postoperative cardiac patient. *Pediatrics* 63:320, 1979.
   Very lucid discussion of postoperative problems with each specific lesion.

35. HEART FAILURE IN THE NEONATE
Robert D. White and Jean S. Kan

Congestive heart failure (CHF) is manifested by tachypnea, cardiomegaly, and hepatomegaly in the newborn; tachycardia, a gallop, rales, rhonchi, or wheezes may also be present. Heart failure is usually due to congenital heart disease, but the cause of failure may also be noncardiac; hypoglycemia, anemia, sepsis, and pulmonary disease compromise cardiac function and should be considered in any neonate with CHF, since each is amenable to early treatment.

The differential diagnosis of cardiac causes of heart failure is made somewhat easier by the limited number of common malformations that produce CHF in the newborn period. In the first week of life, only obstructions of left ventricular outflow (the hypoplastic left heart syndrome, mitral atresia, critical aortic stenosis or atresia, and coarctation of the aorta) are common. In this group, peripheral pulses are poor, the precordium is hyperactive, and murmurs are absent or nonspecific. The ECG usually shows right ventricular hypertrophy, and the chest roentgenogram demonstrates cardiomegaly and pulmonary congestion. Distinguishing one disorder from another in this group is often difficult; frequently, two or more lesions are present. The pulses and blood pressure in the arms and legs are the most useful diagnostic signs; if a difference is found between the upper and lower pulses or blood pressure, coarctation of the aorta (often in association with other anomalies of the left side of the heart) is the probable diagnosis. Coarctation of the aorta or aortic stenosis should also be suspected in the infant with heart failure and signs suggestive of a ventricular septal defect in the first week of life.

Other causes of CHF in the first week of life include dysrhythmias, endocardial fibroelastosis (which has features very similar to those of the hypoplastic left heart syndrome except that left ventricular hypertrophy is present on the ECG), arteriovenous fistulas (which may produce a continuous murmur audible over the affected organ [brain, lung, liver, or heart]), and metabolic disorders, such as renal or adrenal insufficiency, hyperthyroidism, or hypertension.

Congestive heart failure that begins after 1 week of age is usually caused by a left-to-right (systemic-to-pulmonary) shunt. Ventricular septal defect (VSD) (see Chap. 50), patent ductus arteriosus (PDA) (see Chap. 53), and truncus arteriosus are the common malformations within this group. In each lesion, the ECG usually reflects right or combined ventricular hypertrophy, and the chest roentgenogram shows cardiomegaly and increased pulmonary vascularity. Auscultation is often helpful in distinguishing these lesions from one another. Ventricular septal defect is associated with a loud systolic murmur at the lower left sternal border that begins with the first heart sound and radiates to the right sternal border; PDA produces a systolic murmur at the left sternal border that radiates upward and laterally into the left chest and may extend through the second heart sound into diastole. In addition, the peripheral pulses may be "bounding". Infants with truncus arteriosus also have loud systolic murmurs, with a single second heart sound and, in some, an ejection click and an early diastolic insufficiency murmur of the truncus valve; 30 percent have a right aortic arch, and many have mild cyanosis or bounding pulses. Additional causes of heart failure occurring after the first week of life include coronary artery anomalies and endocardial cushion defect (AV canal).

The echocardiogram provides additional information of particular value in the diagnosis and evaluation of the hypoplastic left heart syndrome, PDA, and truncus arteriosus. In the hypoplastic left heart syndrome, it delineates the left ventricular chamber size; in PDA, it shows the degree of enlargement of the left atrium (which is related to the magnitude of the left-to-right shunt); and in truncus arteriosus, it demonstrates the large, single great vessel overriding the ventricular septum. Cardiac catheterization is indicated if specific physiologic data are necessary to make a decision about surgical intervention.

Medical management of CHF in a neonate consists of inotropic stimulation of the myocardium with digoxin, reduction in congestion of the pulmonary and systemic circulations with diuretics, and general supportive care. The use of digoxin requires considerable care because of its low toxic-therapeutic ratio and its variable excretion in newborns. Furosemide and chlorothiazide are commonly used diuretics; their use requires attention to serum electrolyte concentrations, since hypokalemia and hyponatremia are frequent complications that may predispose to digitalis toxicity. Supportive care includes reduction of metabolic requirements by keeping the infant warm and undistressed. Administration of oxygen will often decrease the respiratory effort, and gavage feedings lessen energy expenditure during feedings. The head of the infant's bed may be raised 10 to 20 degrees to reduce venous return of blood to the heart. Acidosis and hypoglycemia must be avoided. Infants with coarctation of the aorta may benefit from prostaglandin E1 infusion, which provides temporary symptomatic relief by causing dilatation of the stenotic segment and the ductus arteriosus.

The success of medical management of CHF is determined primarily by the infant's ability to grow and gain weight. Infants who present with heart failure in the first week of life rarely respond to medical therapy, however. Hypoplasia of the left side of the heart usually causes rapid deterioration and death; no surgical therapy has yet been introduced that clearly improves this prognosis. Infants with aortic stenosis or atresia and coarctation of the aorta also have a poor outlook when signs and symptoms are present in the first week of life, although surgical correction allows survival of up to 50 percent of patients. The prognosis is much better when heart failure is caused by a VSD or PDA; in many cases, spontaneous closure occurs during medical therapy, and in the remainder, surgical correction is usually successful. In truncus arteriosus, early corrective surgery is now advocated with the outcome largely dependent on the adequacy of the pulmonary circulation.

Reviews
1. Artman, M., and Graham, T. Congestive heart failure in infancy: Recognition and management. *Am. Heart J.* 103:1040, 1982.
   A general review; very comprehensive.
2. Rudolph, A. The changes in the circulation after birth: Their importance in congenital heart disease. *Circulation* 41:343, 1970.
   A classic description of the physiologic basis for symptoms.
3. Rheuban, K. The infant with congenital heart disease: Guidelines for care in the first year of life. *Clin. Perinatol.* 11:199, 1984.
   Practical guidelines, especially for postoperative patients.
4. Talner, N. Congestive heart failure in the infant: A functional approach. *Pediatr. Clin. North Am.* 18:1011, 1971.
   Emphasizes pathophysiology.
5. Rowe, R. Serious congenital heart disease in the newborn infant: Diagnosis and management. *Pediatr. Clin. North Am.* 17:967, 1970.
   An excellent discussion of diagnostic clues.

Specific Lesions

6. Noonan, J., and Nadas, A. The hypoplastic left heart syndrome: An analysis of 101 cases. *Pediatr. Clin. North Am.* 5:1029, 1958.
   Still the best clinical discussion of this anomaly.
7. Benzing, G., et al. Simultaneous hypoglycemia and acute congestive heart failure. *Circulation.* 40:209, 1969.
   Hypoglycemia is extremely common in infants with a hypoplastic left heart.
8. Norwood, W., Lang, P., and Hansen, D. Physiologic repair of aortic atresia–hypoplastic left heart syndrome. *N. Engl. J. Med.* 308:23, 1983.
   For hemodynamic follow-up data from this group, see Circulation *68:104, 1983.*
9. Lakier, J., et al. Isolated aortic stenosis in the neonate: Natural history and hemodynamic considerations. *Circulation* 50:801, 1974.
   A good description of typical clinical findings.
10. Shinebourne, E., et al. Coarctation of the aorta in infancy and childhood. *Br. Heart J.* 38:375, 1976.
    Over half of infants who were symptomatic as neonates had an associated VSD or PDA.
11. Talner, N., and Berman, M. Postnatal development of obstruction in coarctation of the aorta. *Pediatrics* 56:562, 1975.
    Explains the frequent delay in clinical signs of coarctation until several days after birth.
12. Hesslein, P., Gutgesell, H., and McNamara, D. Prognosis of symptomatic coarctation in infancy. *Am. J. Cardiol.* 51:299, 1983.
    For another recent series, see J. Thorac. Cardiovasc. Surg. *86:9, 1983; for a recent brief commentary, see* J. Pediatr. *102:253, 1983.*
13. Collins-Nakai, R., et al. Interrupted aortic arch in infancy. *J. Pediatr.* 88:959, 1976.
    In nearly all patients with interrupted arch, VSD and PDA are associated anomalies. (For a recent surgical perspective, see J. Thorac. Cardiovasc. Surg. *86:37, 1983.)*
14. Calder, L., et al. Truncus arteriosus communis: Clinical, angiocardiographic, and pathologic findings in 100 patients. *Am. Heart J.* 99:23, 1976.
    The median survival was only 5 weeks.
    Also see Ventricular Septal Defect (Chap. 50) and Patent Ductus Arteriosus (Chap. 53).

36. TRANSIENT METABOLIC DISTURBANCES
Robert D. White

Profound metabolic changes may occur at birth when the neonate assumes independent control of his or her homeostasis. The transition from fetal to newborn life does not always proceed smoothly; three of the more common and dramatic examples of transient neonatal metabolic disturbances are discussed in this chapter.

Hypoglycemia (see also Chap. 76) is defined as blood glucose of less than 30 mg/dl in full-term infants or less than 20 mg/dl in prematures; it occurs in 0.2 to 0.5 percent of newborns. There are many causes, including disorders in which inadequate substrate is available (reduced carbohydrate stores in premature and dysmature infants, galactosemia, glycogen storage disease I), in which utilization of glucose is increased (as with virtually any severe neonatal stress), or in which circulating levels of insulin are increased (maternal diabetes, erythroblastosis fetalis, insulin-producing tumor).

Most infants with hypoglycemia are asymptomatic. In symptomatic patients, the most common sign is jitteriness; some babies, however, present with more serious manifestations, such as convulsions, lethargy, apnea, or cyanosis. Any of these signs should prompt an immediate determination of blood glucose, even if other explanations are available, since hypoglycemia often coexists with sepsis, asphyxia, hypothermia, hypocalcemia, or congenital heart disease.

Hypoglycemia is treated by providing sufficient glucose to the neonate and correcting underlying diseases when possible. Some symptomatic infants require intravenous infusion of more than 10 mg/kg/minute of dextrose to maintain a normal blood glucose, but oral feeding of dextrose solution of formula is usually sufficient for asymptomatic infants. Most full-term infants with hypoglycemia due to perinatal asphyxia or intra-uterine malnutrition will need glucose supplementation for only 1 or 2 days; premature infants and those with erythroblastosis or whose mothers are diabetic often require a longer period of therapy. The duration of glucose supplementation needed in infants with sepsis, congestive heart failure, and other similar disorders depends on the severity and outcome of the underlying disease. Rarely, patients have profound hypoglycemia that persists much longer than expected; these infants require an extensive evaluation for hyperinsulinism or metabolic disease and may become normoglycemic only after therapy with ACTH or glucocorticoids.

The prognosis is guarded if severe symptoms have occurred; only 50 percent of this group develop normally. The outlook for asymptomatic hypoglycemia, or when only jitteriness is present, is much better; 90 percent or more of these children are normal or have only minimal sequelae on long-term follow-up. Prevention of hypoglycemia is possible in most cases by identification and early feeding of high-risk infants.

Like hypoglycemia, *hypocalcemia* is a manifestation common to several different dis-eases. "Early" hypocalcemia, which occurs during the first 72 hours of life, is particularly prevalent in prematures and in infants who have undergone stress, as in asphyxia or maternal toxemia; increasing evidence suggests that immature parathyroid function underlies the hypocalcemia in most such cases. "Late" hypocalcemia, occurring after several days of cow milk feedings in healthy full-term infants, results from the high renal phosphate load of cow milk; it has become rare since the resurgence in breast feeding and the introduction of commercial formulas with lower phosphate concentrations. Other rare causes of neonatal hypocalcemia include maternal hyperparathyroidism, congenital absence of the parathyroids, and exchange transfusion with citrated blood.

Hypocalcemia is also like hypoglycemia in that most affected neonates are asymp-tomatic; when signs do appear, twitching and convulsion are most common, although lethargy and apnea also occur. Carpopedal spasm is an infrequent but distinctive man-ifestation of hypocalcemia. Signs of hypocalcemia are rare unless the total serum calcium is below 6 mg/dl (or the ionized calcium less than 2.5 mg/dl) and the Q-T interval on the ECG is prolonged. Since hypoxemia, hypoglycemia, infection, or intracerebral hemor-rhage frequently coexists, it is not always clear to what extent nonspecific signs can be attributed to hypocalcemia; in these cases, calcium infusion may be both diagnostic and therapeutic. Hypomagnesemia is present in 40 to 50 percent of infants with hypo-calcemia; it is usually not necessary to administer magnesium, but, occasionally, hypo-calcemia and its symptoms will resolve only after correction of the hypomagnesemia.

The prognosis of hypocalcemia in neonates is similar to that of hypoglycemia. Asymp-tomatic or jittery infants have essentially normal development, while more than 50 percent of those with convulsions have permanent neurologic damage. Although it is not yet clear whether this morbidity is related to the hypocalcemia or to the associated disease often present, these figures emphasize the importance of frequent monitoring of high-risk infants to permit treatment prior to clinically apparent hypocalcemia and make prophylaxis an attractive consideration.

Heroin and methadone are responsible for the majority of serious neonatal *drug with-drawal reactions,* but more than a dozen other drugs are known to be addictive to the fetus, including the widely used barbiturates, antidepressants, and alcohol. The severity of fetal addiction and the subsequent withdrawal symptoms are dependent not only on the type of drug and the extent of its use during pregnancy, but also on the timing of the last dose prior to delivery, as well as on coexisting perinatal diseases.

Signs of drug withdrawal characteristically include tremors, irritability, increased muscle tone, diarrhea, and poorly coordinated sucking movements. Sneezing, sweating, and convulsions may also occur. Affected infants are unusually alert and cry frequently, behavior that may be particularly unpleasant to mothers who find it difficult to cope with stress. Symptoms generally appear on the first day of life in heroin-addicted infants but may be delayed 3 to 4 days or more in infants of methadone users.

Management of an infant with neonatal narcotic withdrawal is primarily supportive. Nursing in a quiet, darkened room and swaddling are often employed to reduce abrasions on the extremities caused by the nearly incessant activity; feeding requires patience and persistence. In many nurseries, paregoric, phenobarbital, or diazepam is used in symp-tomatic infants. Even without therapy, however, symptoms are self-limited and, except for the uncommon occurrence of convulsions or severe dehydration from diarrhea, are benign.

Although drug withdrawal is usually the most dramatic manifestation of fetal drug addiction, of equal or greater importance are the associated problems, such as prematurity, intrauterine growth retardation, meconium staining, and perinatal asphyxia. Beyond the neonatal period, sudden infant death, child abuse and neglect, and developmental delay are all more common in this group of infants than in the general population. Thus, maximal effort is indicated in discharge planning, with provision for regular follow-up of these infants, since few groups have a higher risk for subsequent problems.

Hypoglycemia: Reviews and Series

1. Haworth, J., and Vidyasagar, D. Hypoglycemia in the newborn. *Clin. Obstet. Gynecol.* 14:821, 1971.
   A good description of fetal and neonatal carbohydrate metabolism.
2. Gutberlet, R., and Cornblath, M. Neonatal hypoglycemia revisited, 1975. *Pediatrics* 58:10, 1976.
   Defines four categories of hypoglycemia on the basis of presentation and outcome.
3. Beard, A., et al. Neonatal hypoglycemia: A discussion. *J. Pediatr.* 79:314, 1971.
   Practical questions put to the experts.

Hypoglycemia: Causes

4. Perelman, R. The infant of the diabetic mother.*Primary Care* 10:751, 1983.
   For other reviews, see N. Engl. J. Med. 289:902, 1973; C.C.Q. 4:59, 1981; and Pediatr. Clin. North Am. 29:1213, 1982.
5. Lubchenco, L., and Bard, H. Incidence of hypoglycemia in newborn infants classified by birth weight and gestational age. *Pediatrics* 47:831, 1971.
   Intrauterine growth retardation (decreased energy stores) and birth asphyxia (increased energy demand) are found in most neonates with hypoglycemia.
6. Fisher, G., et al. Neonatal islet cell adenoma: Case report and literature review. *Pediatrics* 53:753, 1974.
   Subtotal pancreatectomy is the therapy of choice.
7. Cornblath, M., and Schwartz, R. *Disorders of Carbohydrate Metabolism in Infancy* (2nd ed.). Philadelphia: Saunders, 1976.
   A good review of all causes.

Hypoglycemia: Follow-up Studies

8. Pildes, R., et al. A prospective controlled study of neonatal hypoglycemia. *Pediatrics* 54:5, 1974.
   The frequent association of additional cerebral insults makes conclusions difficult, but absence of symptoms is documented as a favorable indicator.

Hypocalcemia: Reviews

9. Mizrahi, A., London, R., and Gribertz, D. Neonatal hypocalcemia: Its causes and treatment. *N. Engl. J. Med.* 278:1163, 1968.
   Brief and practical.
10. Forfar, J. Normal and abnormal calcium, phosphorus and magnesium metabolism in the perinatal period. *Clin. Endocrinol. Metabol.* 5:123, 1976.
    A more extensive review (130 references) investigates the complex biochemistry of calcium metabolism.

Hypocalcemia: Causes

11. Tsang, R., et al. Possible pathogenetic factors in neonatal hypocalcemia of prematurity. *J. Pediatr.* 82:423, 1973.
    Patients with early-onset disease respond to parathyroid hormone.
12. Bergman, L. Studies on early neonatal hypocalcemia. *Acta Paediatr. Scand. [Suppl.]* 248, 1974.
    Implicates elevated levels of growth hormone and calcitonin in the functional hypoparathyroid of early-onset hypocalcemia.

13. Cockburn, F., et al. Neonatal convulsions associated with primary disturbance of calcium, phosphorus, and magnesium metabolism. *Arch. Dis. Child.* 48:99, 1973.
    A large series of late-onset disease.

Hypocalcemia: Diagnosis
14. Sorrell, M., and Rosen, J. Ionized calcium: Serum levels during symptomatic hypocalcemia. *J. Pediatr.* 87:67, 1975.
    Ionized calcium correlates poorly with total calcium, even when serum albumin is considered.
15. Colleti, R., et al. Detection of hypocalcemia in susceptible neonates: The Q-oTc interval. *N. Engl. J. Med.* 290:931, 1974.
    A highly sensitive and simple means of identifying hypocalcemia.

Hypocalcemia: Prophylaxis
16. Brown, D., Tsang, R., and Chen, I. Oral calcium supplementation in premature and asphyxiated neonates. *J. Pediatr.* 89:973, 1976.
    Low-dose oral supplementation was found effective in high-risk infants.
17. Brown, D., Steranka, B., and Taylor, F. Treatment of early-onset neonatal hypocalcemia. *Am. J. Dis. Child.* 135:24, 1981.
    Low-dose parenteral prophylaxis is also effective.

Drug Withdrawal: Reviews
18. Blinick, G., et al. Drug addiction in pregnancy and the neonate. *Am. J. Obstet. Gynecol.* 125:135, 1976.
    Pragmatic and thorough. (Also see Pediatr. Rev. *3:285, 1982.)*
19. Committee on Drugs, American Academy of Pediatrics. Neonatal drug withdrawal. *Pediatrics* 72:895, 1983.
    Exhaustive review of the many drugs that produce symptoms of withdrawal or intoxication in the fetus.
20. Finnegan, L. The effects of narcotics and alcohol on pregnancy and the newborn. *Ann. N. Y. Acad. Sci.* 362:136, 1981.
    Lengthy, with nearly 100 references.

Drug Withdrawal: Therapy
21. Kron, R., et al. Neonatal narcotic abstinence: Effects of pharmacotherapeutic agents and maternal drug usage on nutritive sucking behavior. *J. Pediatr.* 88:637, 1976.
    Methadone addiction depressed infants more than did heroin; therapy with diazepam eliminated attempts to suck, while paregoric had a favorable effect. (For additional support of paregoric as the drug of choice, see Am. J. Dis. Child. *137:378, 1983.)*
22. Treatment of neonatal withdrawal syndrome. *Med. Lett. Drugs Ther.* 15:46, 1973.
    A brief review of available drugs.

Drug Withdrawal: Follow-Up
23. Sardemann, H., Madsen, K., and Friis-Hansen, B. Follow-up of children of drug-addicted mothers. *Arch. Dis. Child.* 51:131, 1976.
    Describes problems after discharge from the nursery; 14 of 17 infants required temporary or permanent placement in a foster home.

37. NEONATAL SEIZURES
Robert D. White

Seizures are a manifestation of many diseases in the newborn. Neonatal convulsions are different from those in older age groups, in that well-characterized grand mal movements are rarely seen; instead, there is a wide spectrum of clinical signs, ranging from brief apneic episodes to multifocal clonic spasms.

There are many causes for neonatal seizures, but most convulsions result from relatively few disorders, which can be distinguished by certain characteristic clinical features. One consideration is the age at onset of the seizure. Asphyxia and birth trauma (often accompanied by intracranial hemorrhage) are the most common causes of seizures in the first day of life, but are uncommon after 3 days of age. Hypoglycemic seizures follow a similar time course and usually occur in infants already ill with respiratory distress, heart failure, hypothermia, polycythemia, or sepsis. Hypocalcemic seizures have a bimodal chronologic distribution; "early" hypocalcemia occurs in the first 3 days of life in premature or ill infants, whereas "late" hypocalcemia is a disease of healthy, full-term infants that presents late in the first week of life. (The pathophysiology of abnormalities in glucose and calcium homeostasis is discussed in greater depth in the preceding section.) Seizures due to infection (usually meningitis) or congenital anomalies of the brain may present at any time.

Certain rare but potentially fatal causes of seizures also have a characteristic time of presentation. Pyridoxine dependency causes seizures shortly after birth; convulsions may even begin in utero. Aminoacidopathies, such as maple syrup urine disease or ketotic hyperglycinemia, are usually asymptomatic until several days after feedings have begun. The onset of drug withdrawal (heroin, methadone, barbiturates) and hyponatremic or hypernatremic seizures, on the other hand, may be at any time in the neonatal period.

The infant's clinical status and the nature of the convulsion may also provide a clue to the cause. Seizures caused by asphyxia or birth trauma are usually preceded by lethargy for several hours after birth, followed by increasing alertness and even jitteriness later in the first day of life, culminating in the seizure. Convulsions due to hypoglycemia or early hypocalcemia usually occur in very ill infants, while neonates with late hypocalcemia are generally vigorous, appear completely well between seizures, and may even seem alert and undisturbed during the convulsion.

Further clues to the cause of a neonatal seizure may be obtained during the early stages of active management, which frequently cannot await a definitive diagnosis. Estimation of the blood glucose is rapidly available, but the exact value should also be determined, along with serum levels of electrolytes, calcium, and magnesium. Sequential infusions of calcium and pyridoxine are both diagnostic and therapeutic, since rapid improvement will occur if a specific deficiency is present, although calcium may suppress seizures resulting from a variety of causes.

Control of seizures refractory to these interventions may be accomplished with diazepam, phenobarbital, or phenytoin. A spinal tap should be performed as soon as the infant is stable, to detect meningitis or intracranial hemorrhage. A CT scan provides valuable information regarding the presence and location of an intracranial hemorrhage, CNS malformation, or hydrocephalus, and may also show evidence of cerebral edema or ischemia. These tests, coupled with the infant's history and the clinical characteristics, permit determination of a cause in more than 75 percent of newborns with seizures. Subsequent therapy in these infants can then be directed toward correction of the underlying disorder, where possible.

The prognosis of convulsions in a neonate is determined primarily by the cause of the seizure. Infants with seizures caused by asphyxia, intraventricular hemorrhage, meningitis, or central nervous system anomalies have less than a 25 percent chance for normal development, whereas those with subarachnoid hemorrhage or late hypocalcemia have a 90 percent chance for subsequent normal development. Seizures due to hypoglycemia or hypocalcemia in the first 3 days of life are associated with a 50 percent risk of brain damage. The interictal electroencephalogram also provides a valuable indication of the prognosis for full-term infants; in this group, a normal tracing is associated with an 80 percent chance of normal development; grossly abnormal recordings are associated with a 20 percent chance, and "borderline" or unifocal abnormalities, with a 50 percent chance.

Reviews

1. Volpe, J. Neonatal seizures. *N. Engl. J. Med.* 289:413, 1973.
   Concise and comprehensive; ideal for an initial overview.

2. Freeman, J., and Lietman, P. A basic approach to the understanding of seizures and the mechanism of action and metabolism of anticonvulsants. *Adv. Pediatr.* 20:291, 1973.
   Insight into the pathogenesis of seizures and the pharmacology of anticonvulsants.
3. Myers, G., and Cassady, G. Neonatal seizures. *Pediatr. Rev.* 5:67, 1983.
   Also reviewed in Semin. Perinatol. 6:54, 1982, along with articles on asphyxia, hemorrhage, trauma, and meningitis.

Large Series

4. Rose, A., and Lombroso, C. Neonatal seizure states: A study of clinical, pathological, and electroencephalographic features in 137 full-term babies with long-term follow-up. *Pediatrics* 45:404, 1970.
   This prospective study found the electroencephalogram more valuable than the neurologic examination in establishing prognosis.
5. Dennis, J. Neonatal convulsions: Aetiology, late neonatal status and long-term outcome. *Dev. Med. Child Neurol.* 20:143, 1978.
   Infants considered to be "definitely normal" or "definitely abnormal" at the time of discharge from nursery were similarly considered 4 years later.
6. Keen, J., and Lee, D. Sequelae of neonatal convulsions: Study of 112 infants. *Arch. Dis. Child.* 48:542, 1973.
   A prospective study documenting the lower incidence of complications and a better prognosis than reported in previous retrospective studies.
7. Holden, K., Mellits, D., and Freeman, J. Neonatal seizures: I. Correlation of prenatal and perinatal events with outcomes. *Pediatrics* 70:165, 1982.
   Most survivors from this large collaborative study did well; 70 percent were entirely normal. Poor prognostic features are defined. (For additional series, see Dev. Med. Child Neurol. 19:719, 1977, and Arch. Dis. Child. 58:976, 1983.)

Specific Etiologies

8. Koivisto, M., Blanco-Sequeiros, M., and Krause, U. Neonatal symptomatic and asymptomatic hypoglycemia: A follow-up study of 151 children. *Dev. Med. Child Neurol.* 14:603, 1972.
   Only infants of diabetic mothers did well in this series. It is postulated that neurologic damage in most other infants was caused by coexisting illnesses rather than by hypoglycemia.
9. Forfar, J. Biochemical fits in the newborn. *Proc. R. Soc. Med.* 67:375, 1974.
   Of infants with neonatal seizures, 80 percent have low blood levels of glucose or calcium, even when the seizure is clearly due to other causes.
10. Bejsovec, M., Kulenda, Z., and Ponca, E. Familial intrauterine convulsions in pyridoxine dependency. *Arch. Dis. Child.* 42:201, 1967.
    This rare condition is lethal if untreated. Rapid alternation between lethargy and irritability and "lightninglike" spasms in a newborn suggest the diagnosis. (Also see Arch. Dis. Child. 58:415, 1983.)
11. Herzlinger, R. A., Kandall, S. R., and Vaughan, H. G., Jr. Neonatal seizures associated with narcotic withdrawal. *J. Pediatr.* 91:638, 1977.
    Seizures are more common in withdrawal from methadone than from heroin; the electroencephalogram is usually normal. Paregoric is more effective than diazepam in management.
12. Goldberg, H., and Sheehy, E. Fifth day fits: An acute zinc deficiency syndrome? *Arch. Dis. Child.* 57:633, 1982.
    A syndrome not yet described in the United States.
13. Watanabe, K., et al. Apneic seizures in the newborn. *Am. J. Dis. Child.* 136:980, 1982.
    Another difficult diagnosis, requiring a high index of suspicion.
    Also see Transient Metabolic Disturbances (Chap. 36).

Electroencephalography

14. Tibbles, J., and Prichard, J. The prognostic value of the electroencephalogram in neonatal convulsions. *Pediatrics* 35:778, 1965.

The EEG correlates well with subsequent development, but the association is not perfect, and a third of all records are equivocal.

15. Sokol, R., et al. Abnormal electrical activity of the fetal brain and seizures of the infant. *Am. J. Dis. Child.* 127:477, 1974.
    Fetal EEG may be diagnostic of severe hypoxic damage in utero prior to the onset of seizures in the newborn.
16. Eyre, J., Oozeer, R., and Wilkinson, A. Diagnosis of neonatal seizure by continuous recording and rapid analysis of the electroencephalogram. *Arch. Dis. Child.* 58:785, 1983.
    Incidence of seizures appears much higher when continuous recordings are done.

Management

17. Smith, B., and Masotti, R. Intravenous diazepam in the treatment of prolonged seizure activity in neonates and infants. *Dev. Med. Child Neurol.* 13:630, 1970.
    Neonates responded to small doses of diazepam initially, but recurrent seizures in 2 of 4 required much higher doses for control.
18. Painter, M., et al. Phenobarbital and phenytoin in neonatal seizures: Metabolism and tissue distribution. *Neurology* (Minneap.) 31:1107, 1981.
    A study in Arch. Dis. Child. *57:653, 1982, reached similar conclusions regarding optimal loading (15–20mg/kg) and maintenance (3–6 mg/kg/day) doses of phenobarbital.*
19. Gal, P., and Boer, H. Early discontinuation of anticonvulsants after neonatal seizures: A preliminary report. *South. Med. J.* 75:298, 1982.
    Only a minority of infants required chronic therapy with anticonvulsants.
20. Ellison, P., Largent, J., and Bahr, J. A scoring system to predict outcome following neonatal seizures. *J. Pediatr.* 99:455, 1981.
    An attempt to predict those infants who will require long-term anticonvulsants.

38. HYPERBILIRUBINEMIA
Robert D. White

Jaundice is a common occurrence in the newborn nursery; about 10 percent of full-term and over 50 percent of premature infants become clinically jaundiced during the first week of life. Many of these infants require some form of intervention to prevent more severe jaundice, since high levels of unconjugated bilirubin exceed the binding capacity of albumin, permitting bilirubin staining of the basal ganglia (kernicterus), which may result in cerebral palsy or death. A mild and transient elevation of serum bilirubin, on the other hand, is benign and occurs in virtually every newborn.

Bilirubin is a normal product of catabolism, primarily of hemoglobin, but with a contribution from other body proteins (collectively termed *shunt bilirubin*). In its unconjugated form (indirect bilirubin), it is fat-soluble, carried in the bloodstream bound to albumin. Unconjugated bilirubin is removed from the circulation by the liver, where conjugation into a water-soluble diglucuronide occurs. Hepatic conjugation involves at least three phases: (1) uptake by the hepatocyte, requiring the so-called Y and Z carrier proteins; (2) conjugation, which requires an enzyme (glucuronyl transferase), a glucuronic acid donor, and an energy source; and (3) excretion into the bile. Conjugated (direct) bilirubin is then carried with the bile to the intestine, where it is excreted from the body, except for a variable portion that is deconjugated by β-glucuronidase in the intestinal mucosa and then reabsorbed (the latter process is referred to as the enterohepatic recirculation of bilirubin).

In the first days of life, a mild degree of jaundice (physiologic jaundice) develops in most infants, probably related to several factors: increased hemolysis from trauma inherent in the birth process; immature uptake, or conjugation in the liver, or both; and enterohepatic recirculation. Unconjugated bilirubin levels usually reach a peak of between 2 and 12 mg/dl at 2 to 3 days of age in healthy full-term infants; this peak is higher and occurs later in the first week of life with increasing degrees of prematurity. The conditions that exaggerate this normal jaundice and predispose an infant to kernicterus constitute an extensive list, involving every step in the metabolic pathway of bilirubin.

The first group of diseases that cause significant hyperbilirubinemia are those associated with increased red cell hemolysis. Sepsis, polycythemia, and bleeding into an enclosed space (bruising, cephalhematoma, or intracranial hemorrhage) cause hemolysis of normal red cells; congenital red cell abnormalities (congenital spherocytosis, glucose 6-phosphate dehydrogenase deficiency, pyruvate kinase deficiency, and others) may also increase hemolysis and bilirubin production. Isoimmune hemolytic disorders were, until recent years, the most common cause of severe jaundice; these have in common the formation and placental transfer of maternal antibodies against specific antigens on the fetal red cell, causing a Coombs-positive hemolytic anemia in the affected infant (see Chap. 39).

Hyperbilirubinemia can also be caused by impaired hepatic metabolism of bilirubin. Uptake of unconjugated bilirubin by the liver may be decreased by persistent patency of the ductus venosus (caused by hypoxemia or other stress), thus allowing blood to be shunted past the liver; or it may be hindered by organic anions that compete with bilirubin for uptake by the carrier proteins. Conjugation is reduced if the hepatocytes are deficient in glucuronyl transferase, or if they lack an energy source, as in hypoxemia or hypoglycemia. Hepatitis or inhibition of conjugation by factors present in maternal serum or breast milk may also be responsible for reduced clearance of bilirubin from the circulation. Delayed excretion of bilirubin is rarely a problem in the first week of life except with sepsis or hepatitis.

Finally, elevated levels of unconjugated bilirubin may be caused by increased enterohepatic recirculation of bilirubin. Any condition that delays bowel motility and passage of bile (intestinal obstruction, meconium ileus, delayed feedings, hypothyroidism) will allow large amounts of bilirubin to be deconjugated and reabsorbed.

A separate group of disorders cause kernicterus by interfering with the ability of albumin to bind bilirubin. These diseases require particular attention, because damage can occur at moderate bilirubin levels that are usually considered safe. Severe acidosis affects albumin binding directly, while many chemicals compete with bilirubin for binding sites on the albumin molecule. Agents responsible for displacement of bilirubin from albumin include drugs (sulfonamides, aspirin, and others), hematin (produced during red cell hemolysis), and free fatty acids, which are found during periods of stress or inadequate caloric intake. Premature infants have an additional disadvantage, in that their normal albumin level may be 1 to 2 gm/dl less than that of full-term infants. Conditions that affect the permeability of the blood-brain barrier to albumin and/or bilirubin may also be important in producing kernicterus at serum bilirubin levels usually considered safe; however, studies to document this theory are difficult to perform in humans.

In full-term newborns, bilirubin levels less than 20 mg/dl are considered safe, except in infants whose bilirubin-binding capacity is compromised by hypoproteinemia, acidosis, hemolysis, starvation, sepsis, or hypoxia. Jaundice is clinically apparent at much lower levels in Caucasian infants, but careful observation is necessary to detect jaundice in black or Oriental infants. Premature infants may be at risk if the serum bilirubin exceeds 15 mg/dl because of their lower serum albumin levels; however, they are also frequently hypoxic, acidotic, or otherwise distressed, placing them at risk for kernicterus at even lower bilirubin levels.

Treatment of hyperbilirubinemia is not yet standardized. Most cases of moderate jaundice will resolve after nothing more than general supportive measures to ensure adequate fluid and caloric intake and bowel function. Severe jaundice, particularly in the presence of a hemolytic process, may require exchange transfusion; this process removes approximately 80 percent of the fetal red cells and 50 percent of the serum bilirubin. Between these extremes are a large number of infants who can be treated with phototherapy, which increases the degradation and excretion of unconjugated bilirubin. Phototherapy has been proved effective in reducing the serum bilirubin level and in reducing the necessity for exchange transfusion. Some doubt remains about its safety, since it utilizes an intense form of energy with largely unknown biologic effects. At present, phototherapy is clearly indicated only when there is a significant risk that hyperbilirubinemia will become severe enough to require an exchange transfusion if untreated; it cannot be used as a substitute for the initial exchange in erythroblastosis, whose primary purpose is to remove sensitized red cells and to correct anemia. Jaundice of sufficient degree to require phototherapy must be evaluated to determine the cause of the hyperbilirubinemia, since the jaundice of infection, hemorrhage, hemolysis, or metabolic disorders may respond to phototherapy initially, causing a dangerous delay in reaching the basic diagnosis. Infants receiving phototherapy should be protected from the direct adverse effects of light by shielding their eyes and gonads, and from the many indirect effects (e.g., hyperthermia, dehydration) as well.

Reviews

1. Seligman, J. Recent and changing concepts of hyperbilirubinemia and its management in the newborn. *Pediatr. Clin. North Am.* 24:509, 1977.
   A practical, clinically oriented review. (Also see Pediatr. Clin. North Am. *29:1191, 1982, and* Pediatr. Rev. *3:305, 1982.)*
2. Lee, K., et al. Unconjugated hyperbilirubinemia in very low birth weight infants. *Clin. Perinatol.* 4:305, 1977.
   Another good, general review, emphasizing prematures.
3. Brodersen, R. Prevention of kernicterus, based on recent progress in bilirubin chemistry. *Acta Paediatr. Scand.* 66:625, 1977.
   Focuses on the biochemical interactions that determine bilirubin toxicity and provides an excellent foundation for planning therapy.
4. Oski, F., and Naiman, J. *Hematologic Problems in the Newborn* (3rd ed.). Philadelphia: Saunders, 1982.
   Lengthier, but a well-written review.
5. Levine, R. Bilirubin: Worked out years ago? *Pediatrics* 64:380, 1979.
   We remain tantalizingly close to understanding the physiology of kernicterus—but perhaps no closer than years ago.

Etiologic Factors

6. Odell, G. "Physiologic" hyperbilirubinemia in the neonatal period. *N. Engl. J. Med.* 277:193, 1967.
   A discussion of several factors, unique to newborns, that contribute to hyperbilirubinemia.
7. Gartner, L., et al. Development of bilirubin transport and metabolism in the newborn rhesus monkey. *J. Pediatr.* 90:513, 1977.
   Phenobarbital proved capable of enhancing maturation of glucuronyl transferase when started prior to birth.
8. Cashore, W., et al. Influence of gestational age and clinical status on bilirubin-binding capacity in newborn infants. *Am. J. Dis. Child.* 131:898, 1977.
   Ill infants have a reduced capacity for albumin binding of bilirubin, even when the effect of acidosis is taken into account.
9. Wennberg, R., Schwartz, R., and Sweet, A. Early versus delayed feedings of low birth weight infants: Effects on physiologic jaundice. *J. Pediatr.* 68:860, 1966.
   Peak bilirubin levels averaged 3 mg/dl higher in infants not fed for 48 hours, when compared with those fed at 4 hours of age.
10. Dahms, B., et al. Breast feeding and serum bilirubin values during the first 4 days of life. *J. Pediatr.* 83:1049, 1973.
    Breast feeding did not increase bilirubin levels in a large, well-controlled study.
11. Poland, R. Breast-milk jaundice. *J. Pediatr.* 99:86, 1981.
    A succinct description of current understanding.
12. Oski, F. Oxytocin and neonatal hyperbilirubinemia. *Am. J. Dis. Child.* 129:1137, 1975.
    Reviews evidence implicating labor induction as cause of hyperbilirubinemia. Also see Erythroblastosis (Chap. 39).

Kernicterus

13. Van Praagh, R. Diagnosis of kernicterus in the neonatal period. *Pediatrics* 28:870, 1961.
    A superb clinical description of bilirubin toxicity.
14. Odell, G., Storey, G., and Rosenberg, L. Studies in kernicterus: III. The saturation of serum proteins with bilirubin during neonatal life and its relationship to brain damage at five years. *J. Pediatr.* 76:12, 1970.
    Bilirubin toxicity encompasses a wide spectrum of neurologic damage, including sometimes subtle learning disorders and high-frequency hearing loss.
15. Scheidt, P., et al. Toxicity to bilirubin in neonates: Infant development during the

first year in relation to maximum neonatal serum bilirubin concentration. *J. Pediatr.* 91:292, 1977.
Data from the Collaborative Perinatal Project implicate bilirubin levels greater than 12 mg/dl in neurologic damage.

16. Karp, W. Biochemical alterations in neonatal hyperbilirubinemia and bilirubin encephalopathy: A review. *Pediatrics* 64:361, 1979.
Review of the abundant literature, with no clear conclusions. (Also see Pediatrics 69:381, 1982, and, J. Pediatr. 96:349, 1980. For a humorous means of reaching the same conclusion, read Pediatrics 71:660, 1983.)

17. Pearlman, M., et al. The association of kernicterus with bacterial infection in the newborn. *Pediatrics* 65:26, 1980.
Good evidence for at least one clear predisposing factor for kernicterus.

18. Cashore, W., et al. Clinical application of neonatal bilirubin-binding determinations: Current status. *J. Pediatr.* 93:827, 1978.
Tests based on an uncertain principle remain uncertain in value. (Also see Pediatrics 64:375, 1979.)

Phototherapy

19. Lucey, J. Neonatal jaundice and phototherapy. *Pediatr. Clin. North Am.* 19:827, 1972.
Brief and straightforward, with 121 references.

20. Behrman, R., et al. Preliminary report of the committee on phototherapy in the newborn infant. *J. Pediatr.* 84:135, 1974.
A review of the effects of light on living systems; official recommendations for the use of phototherapy.

21. Lund, H., and Jacobsen, J. Influence of phototherapy on the biliary bilirubin excretion pattern in newborn infants with hyperbilirubinemia. *J. Pediatr.* 85:262, 1974.
Phototherapy increased excretion of bilirubin degradation products and possibly of bilirubin itself.

22. Drew, J., et al. Phototherapy: Short and long-term complications. *Arch. Dis. Child.* 51:454, 1976.
Of infants receiving phototherapy, 50 percent became hyperthermic, and a sizable minority had diarrhea or rash or both. "Long-term" (15-month) follow-up disclosed no permanent adverse effects.

23. Bakken, A. Temporary intestinal lactase deficiency in light-treated jaundiced infants. *Acta Paediatr. Scand.* 66:91, 1977.
An extensive study (including intestinal biopsy) documented lactase deficiency during phototherapy.

24. Gromisch, D., et al. Light (phototherapy)-induced riboflavin deficiency in the neonate. *J. Pediatr.* 90:118, 1977.
All infants who received phototherapy for more than 48 hours became riboflavin-deficient.

25. Oh, W., and Karecki, H. Phototherapy and insensible water loss in the newborn infant. *Am. J. Dis. Child.* 124:230, 1972.
Insensible water losses may double or triple during phototherapy, especially in very-low-birth-weight infants.

26. Maurer, H., et al. Effects of phototherapy on platelet counts in low-birthweight infants and on platelet production and life-span in rabbits. *Pediatrics* 57:506, 1976.
Phototherapy increases platelet turnover, which is clinically most apparent in infants with initially low platelet counts.

27. Vogl, T., et al. Intermittent phototherapy in the treatment of jaundice in the premature infant. *J. Pediatr.* 92:627, 1978.
Intermittent phototherapy, done properly, appears as effective as continuous phototherapy.

28. Telzrow, R., et al. The behavior of jaundiced infants undergoing phototherapy. *Develop. Med. Child. Neurol.* 22:317, 1980.
Both jaundice and phototherapy affect infant behavior during an important period for parents and baby.

29. Brown, A., and McDonagh, A. Phototherapy for neonatal hyperbilirubinemia: Efficacy, mechanism and toxicity. *Adv. Pediatr.* 27:341, 1980.
A recent summary of a common but complex therapy.

Exchange Transfusion
30. Odell, G., Bryan, W., and Richmond, M. Exchange transfusion. *Pediatr. Clin. North Am.* 9:605, 1962.
A review of criteria for and techniques of exchange transfusion.
31. Weldon, V., and Odell, G. Mortality risk of exchange transfusion. *Pediatrics* 41:707, 1968.
Two deaths were attributed to the procedure in a series of 351 exchanges.
32. Chan, G., and Schiff, D. Variance in albumin loading in exchange transfusions. *J. Pediatr.* 88:609, 1976.
Albumin administration prior to exchange did not increase the amount of bilirubin removed during the exchange, but it did transiently augment the patients' bilirubin-binding capacity.

39. ERYTHROBLASTOSIS
Robert D. White

Erythroblastosis fetalis is a syndrome produced by severe hemolytic anemia in the fetus and newborn. By far, the most common cause is Rh isoimmunization, although sensitization to the ABO, Kell, or several other red cell antigens can occur. The natural history of isoimmunization of an Rh-negative mother and of erythroblastosis in her Rh-positive infant is vital to an understanding of the rationale for and limitations of current treatment. Prior to pregnancy, Rh-negative women usually possess no antibodies to the Rh(D) antigen (although there are several antigens in the Rh group, nearly all isoimmunizations occur to the D antigen). The first Rh-positive fetus usually escapes unaffected because of this lack of anti-Rh(D) antibodies, but a small fetal-maternal hemorrhage during labor and delivery, as is commonplace, allows Rh-positive cells from the fetus to enter the mother's circulation. An antibody response to these "foreign" cells occurs, and the mother is then "sensitized." Subsequent Rh-positive fetuses are exposed to the maternal anti-Rh(D) antibodies (which are of the IgG class and therefore transported across the placenta) and a severe hemolytic anemia may develop.

In approximately 25 percent of such fetuses, hemolysis is profound, leading to severe hypoproteinemia, edema, and hepatosplenomegaly (hydrops fetalis); death may occur in utero or shortly after birth. In another 25 percent of erythroblastotic infants, hemolysis is not severe enough to cause hydrops, but marked hyperbilirubinemia develops in the neonate, with the potential for producing kernicterus and its permanent sequelae. In the remaining 50 percent of infants born to Rh-sensitized mothers, hemolysis is mild and may be unrecognized.

The natural history can be altered in several ways. The most effective is prevention of isoimmunization of an Rh-negative mother, accomplished by administration of anti-Rh(D) antibody (RhoGAM) to the mother after the birth of each Rh-positive infant. These exogenous antibodies promote clearing of the fetal Rh-positive red cells from the mother's circulation before her immune system is stimulated to produce its own anti-Rh(D) antibodies. Routine administration of anti-Rh(D) immunoglobulin during the past decade has dramatically reduced the incidence of isoimmunization and the perinatal mortality resulting from erythroblastosis. Nevertheless, a few babies continue to be born with erythroblastosis; some of these are infants of mothers who were sensitized prior to the availability of anti-Rh(D) immunoglobulin, but some are born to women already sensitized at the time of their first pregnancy (during a previous abortion or at the time of their own birth to an Rh-positive mother); to women in whom a large fetal-maternal hemorrhage occurs, rendering the usual dose of anti-Rh(D) immunoglobulin ineffective; or to women sensitized by a fetal-maternal bleed prior to parturition, usually in the third trimester. These complications do not appear insurmountable, however, making eradication of this disease in the next decade seem a feasible goal.

Therapy of erythroblastosis is much more difficult than its prevention. Management must often begin in utero, since, without therapy, about 10 percent of Rh-positive fetuses with Rh-negative, sensitized mothers die prior to term, nearly all with profound anemia and hydrops. Fetuses at risk are identified by regular amniocentesis; high or rising levels of bilirubin in the amniotic fluid are an ominous sign. Intervention consists of one or more intrauterine transfusions (in which Rh-negative cells are injected into the fetus' abdominal cavity, where they are absorbed into the bloodstream) and early delivery, often at 32 or 33 weeks' gestation, since after this time the risks of intrauterine transfusion exceed those of prematurity.

The minutes surrounding delivery of an erythroblastotic infant are critical. During this period, the infant is under severe stress, often in excess of his limited cardiovascular capacity. Asphyxia is common; pallor is a more frequent sign than cyanosis, due to the severe anemia. A severely hydropic, anemic infant may require an immediate transfusion of packed red cells. Following resuscitation, other problems commonly associated with erythroblastosis may rapidly become apparent, such as hypoglycemia, respiratory distress, and hyperbilirubinemia.

The management of hyperbilirubinemia (also see the preceding section) is particularly important, since this is the most common cause of permanent morbidity in untreated erythroblastotic infants who survive the early neonatal period. Severe hemolysis causes a rapid rise in the serum level of bilirubin, which may reach toxic levels as early as 12 hours of age. A blood smear shows marked fragmentation of red cells, with an elevated reticulocyte count, and the Coombs' test is usually strongly positive, indicating the presence of antibody on the red cell membrane. Exchange transfusion, using a volume of donor blood that is approximately twice the infant's circulating blood volume ("two-volume exchange"), removes about 80 percent of the fetal red cells, 50 percent of the bilirubin, and some of the anti-Rh(D) antibody. Exchange is usually indicated when the cord bilirubin exceeds 4.0 mg/dl, or when serum bilirubin rises to a point (usually in excess of 15 to 18 mg/dl) at which kernicterus becomes a risk; multiple exchange transfusions are often necessary. Phototherapy has become an important adjunct to exchange transfusion and may be the only intervention necessary for milder cases of erythroblastosis.

The prognosis for infants born with erythroblastosis fetalis has improved dramatically in the last 25 years. Preventive measures have reduced the incidence of this disease by 90 percent, and aggressive therapeutic intervention by obstetricians and pediatricians has reduced mortality from 20 percent to less than 3 percent. Kernicterus has also been virtually eliminated, making the outlook for present-day survivors an optimistic one.

Reviews

1. Bowman, J. The management of Rh-isoimmunization. *Obstet. Gynecol.* 52:1, 1978.
   Emphasis on obstetric management and prevention.
2. Naiman, J. Current management of hemolytic disease of the newborn infant. *J. Pediatr.* 80:1049, 1972.
   Practical discussion of techniques and their rationale.
3. Oski, F., and Naiman, J. *Hematologic Problems in the Newborn* (3rd ed.). Philadelphia: Saunders, 1982.
   Emphasis on pathophysiology.
4. Weinstein, L. Irregular antibodies causing hemolytic disease of the newborn. *Obstet. Gynecol. Surv.* 31:581, 1976.
   Isoimmunization by antigens other than Rh(D).
5. Zlatnick, F. Non-Rh(D) hemolytic disease of the newborn: An obstetric viewpoint. *Semin. Perinatol.* 1:169, 1977.
   ABO hemolytic disease also reviewed in Clin. Obstet. Gynecol. *25:333, 1982.*

Intrauterine Management

6. Bock, J. Intrauterine transfusion in severe rhesus hemolytic disease. *Acta Obstet. Gynecol. Scand. [Suppl.]* 53, 1976.
   Indications, technique, and outcome.
7. Harman, C., et al. Severe Rh disease: Poor outcome is not inevitable. *Am. J. Obstet. Gynecol.* 145:823, 1983.
   Management skills continue to be refined; fetal loss is low, even in the hydropic fetus.

8. Fraser, I., et al. Intensive antenatal plasmapheresis in severe rhesus isommunization. *Lancet* 1:6, 1976.
   A less invasive alternative to intrauterine transfusion that reduces maternal levels of anti-Rh(D) IgG.

Postnatal Management

9. Diamond, L., Allen, F., and Thomas, W. Erythroblastosis fetalis: Treatment with exchange transfusion. *N. Engl. J. Med.* 244:39, 1951.
   The classic.
10. Moller, J., and Ebbesen, F. Phototherapy in newborn infants with severe rhesus hemolytic disease. *J. Pediatr.* 86:135, 1975.
    Phototherapy reduced the need for exchange transfusion, but over one-half the infants still required at least one exchange.

Complications

11. Phibbs, R., et al. Cardiorespiratory status of erythroblastotic newborn infants: III. Intravascular pressures during the first hours of life. *Pediatrics* 58:484, 1976.
    High pressures at birth dropped to normal or below after resuscitation.
12. Chessells, J., and Wigglesworth, J. Haemostatic failure in babies with rhesus isoimmunization. *Arch. Dis. Child.* 46:38, 1971.
    Disseminated intravascular coagulation is common if anemia is severe, and is exacerbated by hepatic dysfunction.
13. Barrett, C., and Oliver, T. Hypoglycemia and hyperinsulinism in infants with erythroblastosis fetalis. *N. Engl. J. Med.* 278:1260, 1968.
    Hyperplasia of the islets of Langerhans is common in hydrops.
14. Simmons, M., et al. Splenic rupture in neonates with erythroblastosis fetalis. *Am. J. Dis. Child.* 126:679, 1973.
    Stemming from trauma to the enlarged spleen, often unsuspected.

Prevention

15. Herman, M., and Kjellman, H. Rh-prophylaxis with immunoglobulin anti-D administered during pregnancy and after delivery. *Acta Obstet. Gynecol. Scand.* [Suppl.] 49, 1976.
    The current status is discussed.
16. Bowen, F., and Renfield, M. The detection of anti-D in Rh_o (D)-negative infants born of Rh_o (D)-positive mothers. *Pediatr. Res.* 10:213, 1976.
    Anti-D IgG may prevent sensitization of Rh-negative infants after their birth to Rh-positive mothers.
17. Freda, V., et al. The threat of Rh immunisation from abortion. *Lancet* 2:147, 1970.
    Sensitization occurred in 3 to 4 percent of Rh-negative mothers following abortion (nearly 10% of the abortions were performed during the second trimester).
18. Nusbacher, J., and Bove, J. Rh immunoprophylaxis: Is antepartum therapy desirable? *N. Engl. J. Med.* 303:935, 1980.
    A cost-benefit analysis of third trimester administration of Rh-immune globulin.

---

40. NUTRITION IN THE ILL NEONATE
Robert D. White

The unique metabolic requirements for maintenance and growth of sick infants often create a need for special fomulas or feeding techniques. Premature infants are the major group requiring specialized nutritional therapy; their management will be the focus of most of this chapter, with some attention also given to infants with congenital heart disease.

The nutritional needs of prematures are not yet fully defined, largely because of a debate concerning the yardstick by which to measure optimal growth. Many experts believe prematures should be fed so that they continue to grow at intrauterine rates

(20–40 gm/day), while others point out that this approach has not been proved superior to the more easily attained rate of 10 to 30 gm/day. In spite of this unresolved issue, several conclusions regarding specific nutritional therapy for premature infants can be made.

The caloric requirement of premature infants is initially less than that of full-term babies (because of a lower basal metabolic rate), but it rises to exceed that of full-term infants after the first week of life. For the "normal" growth of healthy prematures, 120 to 130 cal/kg/day are usually needed; sepsis, respiratory or heart disease, and heat or cold stress may elevate energy demands to as much as 180 cal/kg/day.

The protein need of premature infants is dependent in part on the food source. Human milk has only about 1.1 gm of protein per dl but is highly digestible; recent studies indicate that 1.7 to 2.0 gm/kg/day of human milk protein is adequate for growth in most healthy prematures. Most commercial cow milk formulas have 1.5 gm of protein per dl, but the concentrations of whey protein, cystine, and taurine are lower than those of human milk, and 2.5 to 3.0 gm/kg/day of formula protein is recommended for mainte-nance and growth of premature infants. Higher protein intakes, especially those in excess of 6 gm/kg/day, are associated with hyperammonemia, metabolic acidosis, and neurologic damage.

Premature infants do not appear to differ from full-term infants in their need for fat and carbohydrate, except in relation to total caloric requirements. Fat should ideally constitute approximately 40 to 50 percent of the caloric intake, with 3 percent of this as linoleic acid. Absorption of fat is somewhat impaired in prematures due to immature bile acid synthesis, but this difficulty can be partially circumvented by the use of medium-chain triglycerides, which are absorbed directly by the intestinal mucosa. Absorption is sometimes a factor in the choice of carbohydrate as well, since many prematures are lactase-deficient until the second week of life, resulting in a higher incidence of diarrhea and metabolic acidosis. Lactose appears to have a salutary effect on calcium absorption and the bacterial flora of the intestine, however, and for this reason it should probably be replaced in the diet only if diarrhea is a problem and then only temporarily until intestinal lactase production matures.

Premature infants require large quantities of vitamins and minerals in their feedings. Both human milk and cow milk contain adequate quantities of potassium, chloride, magnesium, and most trace minerals. Neither human nor cow milk seems ideal with respect to calcium and phosphorus content. Human milk contains both in relatively low concentrations, at a ratio of 2:1, while formulas based on cow milk have somewhat higher concentrations, usually in a calcium-phosphorus ratio of approximately 1.3:1.0. Cow milk formulas promote better bone mineralization but may produce hyper-phosphatemia and secondary hypocalcemia. Iron supplementation is probably not neces-sary in the first month of life and may actually be detrimental to prematures who are deficient in vitamin E. Reports of hyponatremia and copper deficiency in premature infants nourished on human milk indicate that supplementation of these minerals might be beneficial.

Although premature infants are smaller than full-term babies and take less volume of feedings daily, their absolute vitamin requirements are equal to that of full-term infants—or greater, in the case of vitamin E. Vitamin E is poorly absorbed in pre-matures, and the requirement is further increased by dietary polyunsaturated fat and iron. Vitamin D, folate, and B_{12} deficiencies also occur in premature infants; rickets is especially common in breast-fed prematures, since human milk has an extremely low concentration of vitamin D and, as noted earlier, is also low in calcium and phosphorus. Thus, the vitamin needs of premature infants seem to be best met by daily adminis-tration of a multivitamin preparation, with special attention to the delivery of vitamin D (no less than 200 units/day) and vitamin E (no less than 5 IU/day).

From the preceding discussion, it is apparent that a healthy premature infant fed 170 to 200 ml/kg/day of human milk or a cow milk-based formula receives an adequate quantity of calories, protein, fat, carbohydrate, minerals, and vitamins (provided that a multivitamin preparation is given). This goal is not always easily met, however. Illness may elevate the caloric requirement at the same time that fluid intake must be re-stricted. The suck and swallow reflexes are immature in prematures, gastric emptying is often slow, and gastric distention is poorly tolerated, especially in infants with respi-ratory disease. These factors often combine to make adequate intake of calories and nutrients impossible without the use of special formulas, or special feeding techniques, or both.

The provision of adequate caloric intake when fluid consumption must be limited may be accomplished by adding a calorie-rich, easily absorbed substance to the feedings (such as medium-chain triglycerides) or by using a more concentrated formula (which provides more calories per unit volume, but also more protein, minerals, and so on). Each approach has disadvantages. Medium-chain triglycerides in large quantities can produce diarrhea and may exceed the recommended proportion of calories provided as fat, resulting in enough calories but inadequate protein for proper growth. Concentrated formulas have high osmolalities, which may contribute to the development of necrotizing enterocolitis; they also create a high renal solute load. In moderation, however, both approaches have proved useful for large numbers of prematures.

Nipple feedings are often taken poorly by small or ill prematures. Alternatives include feeding by gavage tube, or by intravenous solution, or both. Gavage feedings, which are usually given into the stomach, permit frequent small feedings (or continuous, if desired) without requiring the infant to expend energy by sucking. An additional advantage is that regurgitation of gastric contents can usually be avoided by leaving the gavage tube in place and open to the air. Occasionally, even gavage feedings are poorly tolerated; recent work suggests that feedings may also be successfully given in some premature infants through a Silastic tube passed into the duodenum or jejunum.

Parenteral alimentation may be a valuable adjunct to oral feedings, or it may be used as the total food source for weeks or months when oral feedings are impossible, as in infants with catastrophic intestinal disease. Water-soluble preparations of amino acids, carbohydrate, minerals, and vitamins are available, as is a lipid-containing emulsion of vegetable oil; these can be administered by intravenous infusion in amounts necessary to meet the infant's needs for maintenance and growth. Complications are common; most are mild biochemical abnormalities, but serious problems, such as sepsis, liver disease, and rickets, also occur.

Infants with congestive heart failure pose special feeding problems, some of which have been alluded to previously. Tachypnea and tachycardia, cardinal signs of heart failure, cause increased metabolic demands; at the same time, fluid and sodium tolerance are often markedly diminished. Tachypnea also interferes with nipple feedings, resulting in the dilemma of a child with very high energy requirements who can take only limited amounts. Low-sodium formulas are commercially available that can be prepared in concentrated form and supplemented by medium-chain triglycerides in order to meet these special needs. Occasionally, infants with congestive heart failure also have severe, persistent vomiting induced by digitalis or by heart failure itself and can only be given adequate calories and protein by intravenous alimentation.

Nutrition of ill infants further requires that supportive measures to minimize energy demands be fully utilized. Cold and heat stress should be avoided and underlying diseases treated aggressively. Gavage feedings may be indicated to diminish the energy expenditure of infants who are sucking poorly. Complications associated with feeding must also be monitored, especially diarrhea, acidosis, hyponatremia or hypernatremia, and hypocalcemia. The ultimate success of a feeding regimen is measured primarily by weight gain and increases in body length and head circumference; the latter two measures are probably the most useful, because they more nearly reflect lean body mass than does weight gain.

Reviews

1. Dweck, H. Feeding the prematurely born infant. *Clin. Perinatol.* 2:183, 1975.
   A good discussion of the physiologic basis for current feeding practices.
2. Barness, L., et al. Nutritional needs of low-birth-weight infants. *Pediatrics* 60:519, 1977.
   Recommendations of the American Academy of Pediatrics Committee on Nutrition. Includes a listing of the composition of infant formulas and human milk; 111 references.
3. Barness, L. Nutrition in the tiny baby; Update and problems. *Clin. Perinatol.* 4:377, 1977.
   A summary of current controversies. This author also edited the symposium on perinatal nutrition in Clin. Perinatol. *2(2), 1975.*

Protein Requirements

4. Raiha, N. Biochemical basis for nutritional management of preterm infants. *Pediatrics* 53:147, 1974.
   An excellent review of amino acid metabolism in the fetus and newborn.
5. Raiha, N., et al. Milk protein quantity and quality in low-birthweight infants: I. Metabolic responses and effects on growth. *Pediatrics* 57:659, 1976.
   A controlled study compared the beneficial and harmful effects of human milk and four different cow milk formulas with differing protein content and composition.
6. Fomon, S., and Ziegler, E. Protein intake of premature infants: Interpretation of data. *J. Pediatr.* 90:504, 1977.
   This commentary and the reply from Raiha's group (p. 507 in the same issue) summarize the current debate on the proper measure of the "optimal growth" of prematures.

Vitamin and Mineral Requirements

7. Dallman, P. Iron, vitamin E, and folate in the preterm infant. *J. Pediatr.* 85:742, 1974.
   A review of the dietary limits for these vitamins, with a good description of the antagonistic interaction between iron and vitamin E.
8. Lewin, P., et al. Iatrogenic rickets in low-birth-weight infants. *J. Pediatr.* 78:207, 1971.
   Four cases of rickets in infants who did not receive vitamin supplementation are discussed.
9. Phelps, D. Vitamin E: Where do we stand? *Pediatrics* 63:933, 1979.
   The "vitamin without a disease" is gaining respectability.

Human Milk Versus Formula

10. Fomon, S., Ziegler, E., and Vazquez, H. Human milk and the small premature infant. *Am. J. Dis. Child.* 131:463, 1977, Heird, W. Feeding the premature infant: Human milk or an artificial formula? *Am. J. Dis. Child.* 131:468, 1977.
    This debate about the adequacy of human milk for prematures considers both nutritional and nonnutritional factors.
11. Gross, S., Geller, J., and Tomarelli, R. Composition of breast milk from mothers of preterm infants. *Pediatrics* 68:490, 1981.
    Preterm delivery causes secretion of human milk more appropriate for preterm infants.
12. Bose, C., et al. Relactation by mothers of sick and premature infants. *Pediatrics* 67:565, 1981.
    With proper support and patience, relactation can be successful in a majority of mothers.

Special Feeding Techniques

13. Pereira, G., and Lemons, J. Controlled study of transpyloric and intermittent gavage feeding in the small preterm infant. *Pediatrics* 67:68, 1981.
    No benefit from routine use of transpyloric route.
14. Tantibhedhyangkul, P., and Hashim, S. Medium-chain triglyceride feeding in premature infants: Effects on fat and nitrogen absorption. *Pediatrics* 55:359, 1975.
    Administration of medium-chain triglycerides improved both weight gain and nitrogen retention.

Parenteral Nutrition

15. Mauer, A., et al. Commentary on parenteral nutrition. *Pediatrics* 71:547, 1983.
    For more extensive reviews, see Curr. Probl. Pediatr. *13(5):24, 1983;* Clin. Perinatol. *9:637, 1982;* Pediatr. Clin. North Am. *29:1171, 1982;* Surg. Clin. North Am. *61:1089, 1981; and* Pediatr. Rev. *2:99, 1980.*
16. Pereira, G., et al. Hyperalimentation-induced cholestasis. *Am. J. Dis. Child.* 135:842, 1981.
    A large clinical series. (For histopathologic correlation, see J. Pediatr. Surg. *17:463, 1982.)*
17. Zlotkin, S., and Buchanan, B. Meeting zinc and copper intake requirements in the parenterally fed preterm and full-term infant. *J. Pediatr.* 103:441, 1983.

Prematures easily become deficient in these minerals. (Also see J. Pediatr. *102:304, 1983, and* J. Pediatr. Surg. *19:126, 1984.)*

Congenital Heart Disease

18. Fomon, S., and Ziegler, E. Nutritional management of infants with congenital heart disease. *Am. Heart J.* 83:581, 1972.
    Specific recommendations for choosing a diet and defining its adequacy are given.
19. Rickard, K., Brady, M., and Gresham, E. Nutritional management of the chronically ill child: Congenital heart disease and myelomeningocele. *Pediatr. Clin. North Am.* 24:157, 1977.
    The authors recommend limited use of semisolid foods in children with heart disease and failure to thrive during the first 6 to 8 months of life.

41. NECROTIZING ENTEROCOLITIS
Robert D. White

Necrotizing enterocolitis (NEC) is the most common serious intestinal problem in the neonate. It occurs in approximately 5 percent of prematures and in a much smaller proportion of full-term babies. In a minority of affected infants, necrosis progresses to perforation of the intestine, necessitating emergency surgery; mortality in this group is 30 to 40 percent.

The cause of NEC is unclear. The disorder is associated with a large number of conditions and interventions and has a fluctuating incidence, with a tendency to epidemics within a nursery. One hypothesis to account for both observations is that there are two distinct events in the pathogenesis of NEC: the first is hypoxic injury to the intestine; the second is bacterial invasion of the necrotic bowel wall. Considering hypoxic injury a prerequisite explains why apparently diverse conditions are associated with NEC: they share the complication of reduced oxygen supply to the gastrointestinal tract. Included among these conditions are: disorders that cause generalized hypoxemia (e.g., intrauterine asphyxia, respiratory distress syndrome, prolonged apnea); hypoperfusion of the descending aorta (e.g., patent ductus arteriosus, coarctation of the aorta); obstruction or thrombosis of the mesenteric arteries (e.g., umbilical artery catheter); hyperviscosity (e.g., polycythemia); and venous congestion of the portal system causing reduced intestinal capillary perfusion (e.g., exchange transfusion into the portal system). The postulate that bacterial invasion is another necessary component explains the episodic nature and the sepsislike early symptoms of NEC. Commercial formulas may play a permissive role in the latter event, perhaps by supporting bacterial multiplication; NEC is rare in infants who have not been fed, or in those fed fresh human milk, which contains numerous bacteriostatic factors.

The early signs of NEC are often nonspecific. Apnea, lethargy, poor feeding, lactose malabsorption, and thrombocytopenia all may suggest an infectious disorder. Ileus, abdominal distention, bilious vomiting, erythema of the abdominal wall, and bloody stools are later, more specific signs of NEC but are highly variable from one case to another. One or more of the latter signs indicate the need for an abdominal radiograph; gas in the bowel wall (pneumatosis intestinalis) or in the portal vein is highly suggestive of NEC, and free air in the abdominal cavity is evidence of perforation of the bowel.

Several regimens have been proposed for medical treatment of NEC in infants whose intestine is not perforated. Most protocols include systemic antibiotics, continuous nasogastric drainage, and frequent monitoring of the physical examination and abdominal roentgenograms to detect progression of the disease or the development of complications. With aggressive medical treatment of NEC, most cases resolve without perforation. Oral feedings can be restarted several days after symptoms, thrombocytopenia, and radiographic abnormalities have resolved, but relapses are common, and some infants require prolonged periods of intravenous alimentation before oral feedings are tolerated.

The complications of NEC are perforation of the bowel, generalized sepsis, disseminated intravascular coagulation, and intestinal strictures. Perforation is an absolute indication for surgery; persistent dilatation of an individual loop of bowel may also indicate the presence of nonviable intestine. At surgery, necrotic sections of bowel are removed, and the proximal intestinal end is brought to the skin as an ostomy. These infants then require parenteral alimentation, and their course is often complicated and prolonged. In most cases, continuity of the intestine can be reestablished by a second operation prior to discharge. Contrast x-ray studies of the bowel may reveal strictures even in infants successfully managed without surgical intervention.

A better understanding of NEC is essential for eventual prevention of this disease. Its sporadic nature and the lack of good criteria for early diagnosis have hampered efforts to establish a firm scientific understanding through controlled trials. In the absence of definitive studies, good neonatal care and a high index of suspicion remain the most important means of reducing the mortality and morbidity of this disease.

Reviews and Series

1. O'Neill, J., Neonatal necrotizing enterocolitis. *Surg. Clin. North Am.* 61:1013, 1981.
   Also reviewed recently in Pediatr. Clin. North Am. *29:1149, 1982,* Clin. Perinatol. *5:29, 1978; and* N. Engl. J. Med. *310:1093, 1984.*

2. Schullinger, J., et al. Neonatal necrotizing enterocolitis. *Am. J. Dis. Child.* 135:612, 1981.
   Two other articles in same issue provide experience totaling more than 200 cases.

Etiologic Factors

3. Touloukian, R., Posch, J., and Spencer, R. The pathogenesis of ischemic gastroenterocolitis of the neonate: Selective gut mucosal ischemia in asphyxiated neonatal piglets. *J. Pediatr. Surg.* 7:194, 1972.
   Asphyxia causes both hypoxemia and reduced perfusion of the gut, particularly in the stomach, ileum, and colon.

4. Touloukian, R., Kadar, A., and Spencer, R. The gastrointestinal complications of neonatal venous exchange transfusion: A clinical and experimental study. *Pediatrics* 51:36, 1973.
   Transfusions in or below the portal system caused a fivefold increase in portal venous pressure.

5. Willis, D., et al. Unsuspected hyperosmolality of oral solutions contributing to necrotizing enterocolitis in very-low-birth-weight infants. *Pediatrics* 60:535, 1977.
   Oral administration of undiluted calcium lactate solution was implicated in this study as a possible cause of NEC.

6. Pitt, J., Barlow, B., and Heird, W. Protection against experimental necrotizing enterocolitis by maternal milk: I. Role of milk leukocytes. *Pediatr. Res.* 11:906, 1977.
   In rats, mononuclear phagocytes from maternal milk protected against NEC, whereas frozen milk was not protective.

7. Book. L., et al. Clustering of necrotizing enterocolitis: Interruption by infection-control measures. *N. Engl. J. Med.* 297:984, 1977.
   An epidemic of NEC was interrupted by strict hand washing, isolation, and exclusion of staff with symptoms of gastroenteritis.

8. Rotbart, J., and Levin, M. How contagious is necrotizing enterocolitis? *Pediatr. Infect. Dis.* 2:406, 1983.
   Extensive review of epidemiologic and bacteriologic evidence for infectious cause of NEC.

9. Marchildon, M., Buck, F., and Abdenour, G. Necrotizing enterocolitis in the unfed infant. *J. Pediatr. Surg.* 17:620, 1982.
   Demonstrates the true heterogeneity of this syndrome.

10. Stoll, B., et al. Epidemiology of necrotizing enterocolitis: A case control study. *J. Pediatr.* 96:447, 1980.
    This study, along with one in Am. J. Dis. Child. *136:814, 1982, documents the delayed onset of NEC in very premature infants.*

11. Kliegman, R., et al. *Clostridia* as pathogens in neonatal necrotizing enterocolitis, *J. Pediatr.* 95:287, 1979.
    Pathogen or innocent bystander? Also see Am. J. Dis. Child. *138:686, 1984.*

Diagnosis

12. Yu, V., Tudehope, D., and Gill, G. Neonatal necrotizing enterocolitis: Radiological manifestations. *Aust. Paediatr. J.* 13:200. 1977.
    A "foamy" or asymmetric gas pattern may accompany or precede intramural air. (Also see Pediatr. Radiol. *7:70. 1978.)*

13. Cohen, M., et al. Evaluation of the gasless abdomen in the newborn and young infant with metrizamide. *AJR* 142:393, 1984.
    When typical radiographic findings are absent but clinical suspicion is high, this technique may be very useful.

14. German, J., et al. Prospective application of an index of neonatal necrotizing enterocolitis. *J. Pediatr. Surg.* 14:364, 1979.
    For those who like to keep score, this appears to be a reasonable system for determining the severity of NEC.

15. Hutter, J., Hathaway, W., and Wayne, E. Hematologic abnormalities in severe neonatal necrotizing enterocolitis. *J. Pediatr.* 88:1026, 1976.
    Thrombocytopenia is a sensitive index of severity, and neutropenia indicates a poor prognosis. (Also see Pediatr. Clin. North Am. *24:579, 1977.)*

16. Book. L., Herbst, J., and Jung, A. Carbohydrate malabsorption in necrotizing enterocolitis. *Pediatrics* 57:201, 1976.
    Significant quantities of reducing substance in the stool may be an early sign of NEC.

Surgical Management and Complications

17. Kosloske, A., Papile, L., and Burstein, J. Indications for operation in acute necrotizing enterocolitis of the neonate. *Surgery* 87:502, 1980.
    Analysis of diagnostic criteria, with support for paracentesis as a useful diagnostic procedure.

18. Harberg, F., et al. Resection with primary anastomosis for necrotizing enterocolitis. *J. Pediatr. Surg.* 18:743, 1983.
    Authors encourage use of this procedure whenever possible, to avoid stoma problems.

19. Tejani, A., et al. Growth, health, and development after neonatal gut surgery: A long-term follow-up. *Pediatrics* 61:685, 1978.
    High incidence of neurologic defects in this small series.

20. Clark, J. Management of short bowel syndrome in the high-risk infant. *Clin. Perinatol.* 11:189, 1984.
    Current thoughts about the most difficult chronic management problem in the postoperative infant.

42. SURGICAL EMERGENCIES
Robert D. White

Life-threatening congenital anomalies occur in more than 1 percent of newborns. Some are extremely complex and incompatible with life, but most are localized to a specific organ system and are surgically remediable. The most common surgical emergencies in the newborn involve the gastrointestinal tract; these are discussed in this section, as are two causes of acute respiratory distress (diaphragmatic hernia and choanal atresia) and exstrophy of the bladder.

Five anatomic variants of *esophageal atresia with tracheoesophageal fistula* exist, but by far the most common (87%) is atresia of the proximal esophagus, with a fistula between the trachea and distal esophagus. The lesion probably occurs during septation of the trachea and esophagus, which begin embryologically as a single structure. Polyhydramnios and low birth weight commonly accompany esophageal atresia, and there is a high incidence of associated anomalies, including vertebral, cardiac, and renal defects and imperforate anus (the VATER syndrome). Excessive salivation, regurgitation of feedings with consequent aspiration pneumonia, and gaseous distention of the stomach generally appear in the first day of life. The diagnosis can be established by failure of a nasogastric tube to reach the stomach; a radiograph confirms that the tip of the catheter is in a distended proximal esophageal pouch. The catheter should be connected to suction to remove secretions, and feedings should be discontinued. Until the tracheoesophageal fistula is repaired, the infant should be kept in a semiupright position, and respiratory assistance, if needed, should be with minimal pressure.

Immediate operative intervention usually consists of gastrostomy and division of the fistula. In some infants, anastomosis of the proximal and distal esophagus is also possible in the first days of life, but in most, the definitive procedure must be delayed for weeks or months. Postoperatively, skilled, constant nursing attention is required; with such care, a survival rate of better than 90 percent can be anticipated.

Duodenal obstruction is most frequently due to atresia, less commonly to stenosis, webs, or extrinsic compression by an annular pancreas or peritoneal bands. Low birth weight, Down syndrome, and cardiac defects are frequently associated problems. The characteristic clinical manifestation is bilious vomiting on the first day of life; the diagnosis is supported by the radiographic appearance of the "double bubble" caused by the gas-filled, distended stomach and proximal duodenum. If obstruction or atresia of the duodenum is complete, no air is present in the intestine distal to the double bubble.

Dehydration and electrolyte imbalance secondary to persistent emesis are frequently present at the time of diagnosis and should be corrected prior to operation. Other metabolic problems are common, especially in the premature infant; hyperbilirubinemia is particularly difficult to control, since bile cannot be excreted normally. The operation for duodenal obstruction is usually straightforward; the prognosis depends largely on the presence of associated anomalies.

Jejunoileal atresia probably occurs as the result of a mesenteric vascular accident in utero. Atresia may occur at any point in the small bowel; multiple atresias are not uncommon, but associated nonintestinal anomalies are rare. Bilious vomiting, abdominal distention, and delay or failure in passing meconium are present in most patients. Radiographically, distended loops of small bowel with air-fluid levels are characteristic but not pathognomonic; a barium enema is performed to rule out associated colonic obstruction distal to the atretic area.

Initial supportive management is decompression of the stomach and intravenous replacement of fluid and electrolyte losses from vomiting. Following operative repair, parenteral alimentation is often necessary for prolonged periods until small-bowel function has been restored. Sepsis and pneumonia are common problems in these infants and largely account for the mortality of 25 percent.

Imperforate anus ranges from a thin membrane obstructing the anus to complete anorectal atresia. For ease of discussion, this spectrum is usually divided into "low" and "high" obstructions: in low obstructions, the colon and rectum are patent distal to the levator sling, whereas in high obstructions, the bowel ends above the sling. In low obstructions other than those caused by a thin membrane, the anus is anteriorly displaced, connected to the rectum by fistula. In high obstructions, a fistula is usually present from the rectum into the lower urinary tract or vagina. The location of the obstruction and the fistula can be determined radiographically. The estimated frequency of associated anomalies (the VATER syndrome previously mentioned) varies from 25 to 75 percent of cases.

Low obstructions can usually be corrected primarily; in high obstructions, a colostomy is usually performed initially and definitive repair is delayed until late in the first year of life. Associated anomalies, particularly cardiac and renal anomalies, are responsible for most of the deaths of infants with imperforate anus; the survival rate exceeds 90 percent in those without associated life-threatening malformations. The most notable morbidity of this anomaly is permanent incontinence; this complication occurs in less than 5 percent of infants with low obstructions, but it occurs in 25 to 50 percent of those with high obstructions.

In *omphalocele* and *gastroschisis* the intestines protrude through the abdominal wall. An omphalocele is a protrusion of the bowel through the umbilicus; this has been attributed to an arrest of development in utero when the intestines are still in the yolk sac, outside the abdomen. The bowel in most omphaloceles is covered by a sac of peritoneum, although in some infants the sac ruptures prior to birth. Gastroschisis is herniation of the bowel through a defect in the abdominal musculature next to the umbilicus; there is no covering membrane. A feature helpful in differentiating omphalocele from gastroschisis, besides the presence of a covering membrane, is the point of insertion of the umbilical cord: in omphalocele, the cord inserts into the sac containing the bowel, whereas in gastroschisis, it inserts normally into the abdominal wall. With either anomaly, associated malformations are frequent, particularly intestinal malrotation; renal and cardiac anomalies and low birth weight also may be features.

Initial management is crucial: the exposed intestine must be kept clean, moist, and untraumatized to prevent infection and necrosis. Sterile "bowel bags" filled with warm saline are ideal for this purpose. A nasogastric tube is placed to prevent vomiting and aspiration pneumonia. Primary repair of the defect is possible in a limited number of patients; in the remainder, the bowel is enclosed in a plastic sheath and gradually returned to the abdominal cavity over a 1- to 2-week period (or longer). Parenteral nutrition is required during this time and usually for several weeks thereafter; infants with gastroschisis and "ruptured" omphalocele are particularly likely to need prolonged therapy, due to thickening and inflammation of the bowel caused by exposure to amniotic fluid in utero. Survival rates of 75 percent are currently reported.

Malrotation of the bowel may be unsuspected in a healthy neonate for days or weeks and then cause acute bilious vomiting and abdominal distention. The abnormal position of the intestines is not dangerous per se (many patients with malrotation never become symptomatic), but the bowel is poorly fixed to a narrow vascular pedicle, permitting it to twist (*volvulus*), occluding the superior mesenteric artery and producing extensive bowel necrosis. Volvulus is a true surgical emergency, since the viability of large portions of the bowel is dependent on the prompt return of the blood supply; bloody stools are particularly ominous. Plain x-ray films of the abdomen will often suggest the diagnosis by demonstrating an anomalous position of the cecum, but a barium study is usually necessary for confirmation. Repair consists of mobilization and repositioning of the bowel; if frankly necrotic intestine is present, it must be removed and the proximal end of viable intestine exteriorized as an ostomy, although in some cases an end-to-end anastomosis is possible.

Hirschsprung's disease (congenital aganglionic megacolon) produces a spectrum of disability ranging from acute obstruction in the neonate to chronic constipation in older infants and children. It is caused by an absence of parasympathetic innervation of the internal anal sphincter and varying portions of the colon and terminal ileum. Peristalsis does not occur in the aganglionic segment, which is spastic and contracted, impairing fecal passage. In infants, obstruction and distention often alternate with bouts of diarrhea and periods when the abdominal findings are normal, but virtually all neonates with this anomaly fail to pass meconium in the first 24 hours of life. Diagnostic evaluation consists initially of a barium enema, followed in some centers by anorectal manometrics, or electromyographic study, or both; confirmation of Hirschsprung's disease requires histologic demonstration that ganglion cells are absent.

In ill newborns, initial surgery is colostomy; unnecessary delay in undertaking this procedure puts the infant at risk for toxic megacolon, a highly dangerous condition. Later, the aganglionic segment of colon may be removed and a more definitive procedure performed (Soave, Swenson, Duhamel). Myectomy, with incision of the internal anal sphincter, may be all that is required in children with involvement limited to a short segment of colon, but colostomy is preferred for severely affected neonates. Some patients experience significant complications from surgery, including abscess formation, stricture, and damage to the pelvic nerves. However, provided that toxic megacolon does not occur, the survival rate is very high (95% or better).

Of infants born with cystic fibrosis 10 to 20 percent have intestinal obstruction due to their extremely thick, almost solid meconium (*meconium ileus*). This is their first manifestation of abnormal exocrine gland function, and it may be life-threatening if perforation occurs, causing an intense chemical peritonitis. The triad of abdominal distention, bilious vomiting, and failure to pass meconium is common, but does not permit distinction from other causes of intestinal obstruction. Radiographic studies are more helpful; intraperitoneal calcifications suggest the diagnosis.

The surgical approach in these patients depends on the extent of obstruction and whether or not an associated perforation, volvulus, or atresia is present. The postoperative course is often difficult because of the predisposition to pneumonia.

Diaphragmatic hernia results from a failure of complete formation of the diaphragm early in fetal life. The defect is usually unilateral and involves the left side in 75 percent of cases. The presence of abdominal contents in the thorax throughout most of gestation does not permit normal development of the ipsilateral lung and thus is an important cause of respiratory distress following birth.

Successful management of infants with diaphragmatic hernia requires prompt diagnosis and intensive management of respiratory problems. A chest radiograph in the neonate with respiratory distress will establish the diagnosis; the physical findings of a scaphoid abdomen, bowel sounds in the left chest, and prominent heart sounds in the right chest are diagnostic but not sufficiently common to be generally useful. Hypoxia, hypercapnea, and acidosis are generally present, and respiratory assistance is often of only moderate benefit. Severe hypoplasia of a lung may increase pulmonary vascular resistance, promoting extensive right-to-left shunting of blood through the ductus arteriosus and foramen ovale. Prior to operation or transport to a neonatal center, it is important that a nasogastric tube be placed for decompression, so as to minimize respiratory compromise, and acidosis should be vigorously corrected. Intubation is also indicated in any infant with respiratory symptoms, however mild.

Operative repair consists of removing the bowel from the thorax, closing the hernia, and correcting malrotation, if present. Immediately after operation most patients experience significant improvement in their respiratory status, but deterioration over the next 24 hours often occurs, especially in infants who had severe cyanosis and distress in the first hours of life. In these infants, attempts to reduce pulmonary vascular resistance pharmacologically have been made, with some success. Patients asymptomatic in the first day of life do well following operation, whereas survival in those with distress of earlier onset is only slightly better than 50 percent.

Choanal atresia is the persistence of a fetal membrane between the anterior and posterior choanae that results in obstruction of one or both nares. The obstruction may remain membranous but is usually bony (in 85–90%); bilateral atresia is slightly more common than unilateral atresia, and it virtually always causes severe respiratory distress within minutes of birth. Two-thirds of affected neonates are female.

Since newborns are obligate nose breathers, bilateral choanal atresia produces cyanosis and severe retractions as the infant attempts to inspire. Not until the mouth is opened to cry can air exchange occur, resulting in a dramatic and characteristic syndrome of intermittent cyanosis relieved by crying. Infants who survive the neonatal period without treatment usually learn to breathe through the mouth, becoming symptomatic only when attempting to nurse. The diagnosis is easily established when a catheter cannot be passed into the pharynx through either nares. Immediate treatment consists of placement of an oropharyngeal airway; feedings, if any, are given through an orogastric tube. A palliative operation may then be performed electively, although definitive correction is not usually undertaken until after 6 months of age.

In *exstrophy of the bladder* the walls of the urinary bladder fail to fuse anteriorly and are open to the abdominal wall. Exstrophy is more common in boys (70% of cases) and is part of a malformation complex that includes a caudally placed umbilicus, a widely separated symphysis pubis, external rotation of the hips, and epispadias (or, in girls, a bifid clitoris). Malformations of the upper urinary tract and kidneys are uncommon. There is usually no distress at birth, but immediate intervention is necessary to reduce the risk of chronic urinary tract infection and its sequelae. The defect should be covered with sterile dressings initially, and antibiotics are often administered prophylactically. Primary closure is recommended in the first week of life. Nearly all infants survive, although many have chronic urinary tract infections and incontinence.

General Reviews

1. Rowe, M. (ed.). Neonatal surgery. *Clin. Perinatol.* 5(1), 1978.
   The volume is a collection of reviews of several surgical emergencies.
2. Grosfeld, J. (ed.). Symposium on pediatric surgery. *Surg. Clin. North Am.* 61:995, 1981.
   Includes papers on each of the common neonatal emergencies.
3. Lister, J. Surgical emergencies in the newborn. *Br. J. Anaesth.* 49:43, 1977.
   A brief review, followed in the same issue by an article on supportive and intraoperative care (p. 51).

Intestinal Anomalies

4. Holder, T., and Leape, L. The acute surgical abdomen in the neonate. *N. Engl. J. Med.* 278:605, 1968.
   A very brief, general review.
5. Talbert, J., Felman, A., and DeBusk, F. Gastrointestinal surgical emergencies in the newborn infant. *J. Pediatr.* 76:783, 1970.
   A more extensive review, with a good discussion of differential diagnosis.
6. Temtamy, S., and Miller, J. Extending the scope of the VATER association: Definition of the VATER syndrome. *J. Pediatr.* 85:345, 1974.
   A review of the literature, updating the spectrum of anomalies.
7. Greenwood, R. Patterns of gastrointestinal and cardiac malformations. *J. Pediatr. Surg.* 11:1023, 1976.
   The incidence and types of heart defects associated with intestinal atresias.
8. Rowe, M., and Arango, A. Colloid vs. crystalloid resuscitation in experimental bowel obstruction. *J. Pediatr. Surg.* 11:635, 1976.
   Colloid therapy may be detrimental.
9. Koop, C., Schnaufer, L., and Broennle, A. Esophageal atresia and tracheoesophageal fistula: Supportive measures that affect survival. *Pediatrics* 54:558, 1974.
   Early diagnosis and transport improve survival.
10. Jouhimo, I., and Lindahl, H. Esophageal atresia: Primary results of 500 consecutively treated patients. *J. Pediatr. Surg.* 18:217, 1983.
    A 30-year perspective, with encouraging results in the most recent cases.
11. Gourevitch, A. Duodenal atresia in the newborn. *Ann. R. Coll. Surg. Engl.* 48:141, 1971.
    An interesting discussion of possible causes.
12. Nixon, H., and Tawes, R. Etiology and treatment of small intestinal atresia: Analysis of a series of 127 jejunoileal atresias and comparison with 62 duodenal atresias. *Surgery* 69:41, 1971.
    As described in the title.
13. Grosfeld, J., and Weber, T. Congenital abdominal wall defects: Gastroschisis and omphalocele. *Curr. Probl. Surg.* 19:158, 1982.
    Especially valuable for detailed description of surgical techniques.
14. Colombani, P., and Cunningham, M. Perinatal aspects of omphalocele and gastroschisis. *Am. J. Dis. Child.* 131:1386, 1977.
    Additional malformations were found in 70 percent of patients with omphalocele and 20 percent of those with gastroschisis.
15. Swenson, O., Sherman, J., and Fisher, J. Diagnosis of congenital megacolon: An analysis of 501 patients. *J. Pediatr. Surg.* 8:587, 1973.
    A large series. Also see J. Pediatr. Surg. 19:370, 1984.
16. O'Neill, J., et al. Surgical treatment of meconium ileus. *Am. J. Surg.* 119:99, 1970.
    Includes a useful outline of postoperative management.

Diaphragmatic Hernia

17. Bloss, R., Aranda, J., and Beardmore, H. Congenital diaphragmatic hernia: pathophysiology and pharmacologic support. *Surgery* 89:518, 1981.
    Review of management options for symptomatic infants.
18. Cloutier, R., Fournier, L., and Levasseur, L. Reversion to fetal circulation in congenital diaphragmatic hernia: a preventable postoperative complication. *J. Pediatr. Surg.* 18:551, 1983.
    Suggests that the most difficult postoperative management problem may be avoided by changing the surgical and ventilatory techniques used.

Choanal Atresia

19. Trail, M., Creely, J., and Landrum, C. Congenital choanal atresia. *South. Med. J.* 66:460, 1973.
    Suggests delaying operation for 6 months or more in selected cases.
20. Winther, L. Congenital choanal atresia. *Arch. Dis. Child.* 53:338, 1978.
    The author's personal experience with 15 cases.

Exstrophy of the Bladder

21. Glasson, M. Extrophy of the urinary bladder. *Aust. Paediatr. J.* 11:204, 1975.
    An extensive review.
22. Feinberg, T., et al. Questions that worry children with exstrophy. *Pediatrics* 53:242, 1974.
    The same questions worry parents, too. A strong psychologic rationale is presented for urinary diversion at an early age if incontinence is encountered.

43. CONGENITAL INFECTIONS
Robert D. White

Chronic fetal and neonatal infections by nonbacterial agents comprise a clinical spectrum of disease known as the TORCHES syndrome. The acronym is derived from the most common organisms responsible for this entity: *to*xoplasmosis, *r*ubella, *c*ytomegalovirus, *he*rpes simplex, and *s*yphilis. The incidence of disease caused by this group of agents is uncertain and changing. In the last decade, for example, the incidence of rubella has been reduced by large-scale immunization, syphilis and herpes simplex type 2 have become more common, and appreciation of the usually subtle nature of cytomegalovirus infection has altered earlier beliefs that it was relatively uncommon. At present, it is likely that fetal or neonatal infection with one of these organisms occurs in about 1 percent of all births, with serious disease in perhaps 10 percent of infected infants.

The classic syndrome of fetal infection by one of the various TORCHES agents was initially characterized as prematurity, intrauterine growth retardation, microcephaly, hepatosplenomegaly with jaundice, thrombocytopenia, hemolytic anemia, chorioretinitis, adenopathy, and rash; the diagnosis was supported by elevated IgM levels in the neonate and by persistently high antibody titers to the offending organism during early infancy. This generalized approach to congenital infection has been improved by the recent recognition of specific syndromes, improved diagnostic tests, and a better understanding of the natural history and prognosis of disease caused by each organism.

Toxoplasma is a protozoal parasite common in domestic animals such as cats, swine, and sheep. In the United States, infection is probably most frequently transmitted by oocysts in cat feces. Acute infection is usually unrecognized; symptoms, if present, include a nonspecific lymphadenopathy, malaise, and fever. Antibodies to this organism are present in 20 to 40 percent of the adult population in the United States.

Infection occurring in pregnant women is transmitted to the fetus in approximately 40 percent of cases. The severity of fetal disease depends strongly on the time during gestation at which the mother acquires toxoplasmosis; acquisition in the first two trimesters may cause stillbirth, severe neurologic damage, or subclinical disease; infection in the last trimester is associated only with subclinical symptoms. Overall, only one-third of infected infants have clinically apparent disease at birth, and in 40 percent of these, evidence of involvement is limited to the frequently overlooked but characteristic chorioretinitis. The rest of the affected infants generally have central nervous system involvement (hydrocephalus, microcephaly, or intracranial calcifications) in addition to chorioretinitis, while only a few exhibit the classic TORCHES syndrome of hepatosplenomegaly, lymphadenopathy, and anemia. Some infants with infection that is not apparent at birth may become symptomatic weeks or months later, but most remain apparently normal.

The diagnosis of congenital toxoplasmosis should be suspected in any infant with chorioretinitis or intracranial calcifications, as well as in those with nonspecific symptoms of congenital infection. Persistently elevated antibody titers, using the Sabin-Feldman dye test, the IgM-specific fluorescent antibody test, or the IgM-specific ELISA test establish the diagnosis. Sulfadiazine and pyrimethamine may be useful in controlling *Toxoplasma* infection; it is not clear whether or not their use improves the prognosis. The outlook for symptomatic infants is poor. Mental retardation and convulsions occur in most, and cerebral palsy, blindness, deafness, and hydrocephalus are also common;

only 10 to 15 percent are normal. The prognosis of infants with subclinical disease is less certain; most appear to be normal, but vision and hearing defects, learning disabilities, and epilepsy occur in some.

Rubella is an RNA virus that usually causes mild or inapparent disease in children, but it may be devastating to the fetus. Primary infection of susceptible pregnant women results in viremia that persists for 2 to 3 weeks until maternal antibodies reach appreciable levels. During this time, which is prior to the onset of symptoms in the mother, placental and fetal invasion may occur. Maternal infection during the first 8 weeks of gestation is transmitted to the fetus in more than 50 percent of cases, whereas infection beginning in the second or third trimester is transmitted to the fetus less frequently.

Fetal infection during the first trimester may cause stillbirth or, more commonly, a constellation of findings that includes growth retardation, cataracts, a characteristic "salt-and-pepper" retinitis, and peripheral pulmonary artery stenosis. The nonspecific signs of adenopathy, hepatosplenomegaly, and thrombocytopenia are also frequent; patent ductus arteriosus, myocardial necrosis, bony radiolucencies, and a "blueberry-muffin" appearance of the skin caused by intradermal erythropoiesis are all less common, but highly suggestive of rubella. Infection later in gestation may cause prematurity or result in mild or no disease in the fetus.

The diagnosis of rubella should be considered in the presence of one or more of the characteristic clinical signs. Antibody titers to rubella in affected infants are persistently elevated, but more immediate evidence is usually available in the form of isolation of virus from the nasopharynx, or occasionally from conjunctival secretions, urine, or feces.

Signs of congenital rubella may also appear after the neonatal period. Pneumonitis, encephalitis, and hypogammaglobulinemia may be progressive during infancy, while sensorineural hearing loss (the single most common manifestation of congenital rubella), dental, renal, and urinary defects, and diabetes are often not appreciated until later in childhood. Mental retardation of mild to moderate severity is present in 10 to 20 percent of affected patients; learning disabilities or cerebral palsy may also occur.

Although relatively little can be accomplished therapeutically at present in the management of an infant with congenital rubella, eradication of this disease is now conceivable with the introduction of mass immunization; no major epidemics have occurred in the United States since 1964-1965. It is not yet clear, however, whether the immunity conferred by the administration of attenuated viral vaccine to young children will persist through the childbearing age 20 to 40 years hence.

Cytomegalovirus belongs to the herpesvirus family of organisms. Transmission to the fetus is usually by contact with infected maternal secretions; between 5 and 10 percent of pregnant women excrete virus in the urine or cervical secretions. The mother is usually asymptomatic and may harbor the virus for years, even in the presence of "adequate" antibody titers; consequently, it is possible for a woman to infect her offspring in several pregnancies.

Screening programs have demonstrated cytomegalovirus in the urine of 0.5 to 1.0 percent of newborns, making it the most common of all perinatal infections. Chronic intrauterine infection classically produces cerebral calcifications (distinguished from those of toxoplasmosis by their periventricular location) and microcephaly, although the nonspecific sign of hepatosplenomegaly is actually more common. Intrauterine transmission of virus appears to be the exception with this organism, however; most infants are infected at the time of birth and are asymptomatic. Infants with "silent" infection at birth later exhibit sensorineural hearing loss, minimal cerebral dysfunction, or mental retardation in 10% of cases or more.

Virus isolated from the urine or throat of a neonate is diagnostic; antibody titers are also useful, but complement-fixing antibody may disappear within months of birth, even though viral excretion by the infant continues. Prevention of cytomegalovirus disease in the newborn using mass vaccination is currently being investigated, but may be hampered by the previously noted ability of women to harbor this organism even in the presence of circulating antibody. Some infants are infected with cytomegalovirus through transfusions: this complication appears to be largely preventable, however, by using blood from cytomegalovirus-negative donors or by maneuvers that remove white blood cells from the transfused blood (washing, irradiating, or filtering).

Herpes simplex is a DNA virus with two distinct subtypes that produce disease in humans. Herpes simplex type 1, or labial herpesvirus, infects primarily nongenital areas and is the etiologic agent of many cold sores. Herpes simplex type 2, or genital herpes, appears to be venereally transmitted and is present in the cervical secretions of up to 1 percent of pregnant women and is the predominant cause of neonatal disease. Unlike rubella, but like the related cytomegalovirus, viremia and transplacental transmission of herpesvirus is uncommon, and most fetuses are infected after rupture of the fetal membranes or during vaginal delivery through an infected birth canal. When a primary maternal infection occurs prior to 32 weeks' gestation, the risk to a full-term infant is low; it increases to a 10 percent risk of infection if maternal colonization begins after the thirty-second week, and to 40 percent if the virus is present at the time of vaginal delivery.

Neonatal herpesvirus infection may produce systemic or localized disease; asymptomatic patients are thought to be rare. Signs of systemic disease may be present at birth or delayed for as much as 3 weeks; usually, however, signs become apparent late in the first week of life. Lethargy, vomiting, and fever are the most common initial manifestations and suggest neonatal sepsis; with central nervous system involvement, irritability and convulsions also occur. Hepatomegaly, jaundice, and skin vesicles occur in only a minority of infants with disseminated herpesvirus. Shock and disseminated intravascular coagulation are frequent as terminal events; only 20 percent survive this illness, one-half with permanent sequelae, although this prognosis may be improving with the introduction of newer antiviral drugs.

The prognosis is better for the 30 to 50 percent of infants with neonatal herpesvirus infection whose disease is localized. Meningoencephalitis, keratoconjunctivitis, and herpetic vesicles of the skin or mouth may occur together or as isolated findings. The central nervous system disease has a 40 percent mortality, with permanent sequelae in an additional 40 percent; disease limited to the eye, or skin, or both is not fatal, but 30 percent have sequelae. It should be noted that central nervous system or disseminated disease subsequently develops in one-half the infants who initially have only skin vesicles, with a marked change in prognosis.

Herpesvirus infection in the neonate is difficult to diagnose in the absence of the characteristic (but uncommon) vesicular eruption, unless suspicion has been raised by the finding of active herpetic lesions in the mother. Rapid confirmation of the presumptive diagnosis is possible by demonstration of multinucleated giant cells and intranuclear inclusions in cell scrapings from mother and infant; subsequent isolation of virus from infected organs is usually possible. Antibody titers are sometimes helpful, although the majority of infected infants succumb before results are available.

Neonatal herpesvirus infection is, in large part, a preventable disease. Delivery by cesarean section within 4 hours following rupture of the membranes in mothers with active cervical lesions will usually protect the fetus; strict rules prohibiting medical staff or visitors with cold sores from contact with newborns may interrupt another mode of transmission. Therapy with the antiviral drugs, adenine arabinoside and acyclovir is currently under investigation.

Congenital syphilis is a disease with many manifestations, which extend from birth to adulthood. It was extensively studied in the early 1900s, then became virtually extinct with the introduction of penicillin. Its resurgence in this decade parallels the increase in venereal disease.

Treponema pallidum is a spirochete with almost exclusively venereal transmission. If untreated, maternal disease persists for years, resulting in the birth of many affected infants. The fetus is infected transplacentally; if maternal infection begins or becomes active during pregnancy, virtually 100 percent of fetuses will be damaged, one-half being stillborn or dying in the neonatal period. When the maternal infection is acquired prior to, and is latent during, pregnancy, the risk of perinatal death falls to 10 to 20 percent, but an additional 10 to 40 percent of infants bear permanent stigmata of the disease.

The clinical syndrome of congenital syphilis has few specific signs in the neonate. Usually, the infant is considered normal at birth, or prematurity and intrauterine growth retardation are attributed to other causes. Persistent rhinitis ("snuffles"), hepatosplenomegaly, hemolytic anemia, or skin rash appears later in the neonatal period and suggests the diagnosis; a thorough physical examination may also disclose lymphadenopathy and chorioretinitis. Later in childhood, Hutchinson's teeth (peg-shaped, notched permanent incisors), "mulberry molars," interstitial keratitis, saddlenose, rhagades (linear scars around the mouth and nose), central nervous system involvement, and periostitis ("saber shins") may become evident, although the natural history is usually altered markedly by early treatment.

Radiography is particularly useful in the early diagnosis of congenital syphilis. Metaphyseal involvement of the long bones is the earliest and most characteristic sign of this disease, progressing to diffuse osteitis in many cases. Serologic identification of antitreponemal antibodies in the neonate confirms maternal infection, but is not diagnostic of fetal involvement unless the antibodies are of the IgM class or persist after passively acquired maternal antibodies are no longer present. The spinal fluid should be examined in all infants suspected of having a congenital infection, regardless of the etiologic agent, but is especially important in the evaluation of congenital syphilis, since silent neurosyphilis is not uncommon and, if untreated, may be devastating later in life.

Unlike most of the other forms of congenital infection, congenital syphilis is treatable. Serologic screening of mothers during the first and third trimester of pregnancy and treatment of those found to be infected can minimize fetal damage; affected infants are treated with penicillin and observed carefully during the first year of life to ensure that control of the infection and its sequelae has been achieved.

Recently it has become clear that a number of infectious agents can be transmitted from mother to baby during labor, delivery, and the neonatal period, including hepatitis B virus, *Chlamydia trachomatis*, enteroviruses, and rotavirus. The time and severity of the disease produced by these organisms depend on the incubation period, the magnitude of the inoculum, and the time of infection.

Reviews

1. Remington, J., and Klein, J. (eds.). *Infectious Diseases of the Fetus and Newborn Infant*. Philadelphia: Saunders, 1976.
   Authoritative (and lengthy, well-referenced) reviews.
2. Hanshaw, J., and Dudgeon, J. *Viral Diseases of the Fetus and Newborn*. Philadelphia: Saunders, 1978.
   For a shorter review, see J. Pediatr. 77:315, 1970, or Clin. Obstet. Gynecol. 1:17, 1974.

Diagnosis and Sequelae

3. Alford, C., Stagno, S., and Reynolds, D. Diagnosis of chronic perinatal infections. *Am. J. Dis. Child.* 129:455, 1975.
   A review of the usefulness and limitations of diagnostic techniques.
4. Griffith, J. Nonbacterial infections of the fetus and newborn. *Clin. Perinatol.* 4:117, 1977.
   Pathogenesis, signs, and pathologic features as they relate to the central nervous system; long-term neurologic follow-up is reviewed.
5. Overall, J. Intrauterine virus infections and congenital heart disease. *Am. Heart J.* 84:823, 1972.
   Rubella, Coxsackie, and perhaps others.

Toxoplasmosis

6. Desmonts, G., and Couvreur, J. Congenital toxoplasmosis: A prospective study of 378 pregnancies. *N. Engl. J. Med.* 290:1110, 1974.
   The prospective study and the accompanying editorial (p. 1138) summarize current understanding of the spectrum of disease.
7. Stagno, S. Congenital toxoplasmosis. *Am. J. Dis. Child.* 134:635, 1980.
   A brief review. (Also see Arch. Dis. Child. 56:494, 1981.)
8. Naot, Y., Desmonts, G., and Remington, J. IgM enzyme-linked immunosorbent assay test for the diagnosis of congenital *Toxoplasma* infection. *J. Pediatr.* 98:32, 1981.
   Latest addition to the diagnostic armamentarium. (For an update on older methods, see Am. J. Dis. Child. 131:21, 1977.)
9. Remington, J., and Desmonts, G. Congenital toxoplasmosis: Variability in the IgM-fluorescent antibody response and some pitfalls in diagnosis. *J. Pediatr.* 83:27, 1973.
   Negative test results do not rule out congenitally acquired infection.

10. Wilson, C., et al. Development of adverse sequelae in children born with subclinical congenital *Toxoplasma* infection. *Pediatrics* 66:767, 1980.
    Chorioretinitis occurs in nearly all infected children.

Rubella
11. Dudgeon, J. Congenital rubella. *J. Pediatr.* 87:1078, 1975.
    A short review, with particular attention to advances in control by active immunization.
12. Modlin, J., et al. Risk of congenital abnormality after inadvertent rubella vaccination of pregnant women. *N. Engl. J. Med.* 294:972, 1976.
    Vaccine virus was recovered from several abortuses of mothers inadvertently vaccinated, but infants carried to term showed no evidence of disease.
13. Miller, E., Cradock-Watson, J., and Pollack, T. Consequences of confirmed maternal rubella at successive stages of pregnancy. *Lancet* 2:781, 1982.
    Further delineation of the many sequelae of the congenital rubella syndrome. (Also see J. Pediatr. 93:584 and 699, 1978.)
    Also see Immunizations and Vaccine-Preventable Diseases, Chapter 100.

Cytomegalovirus
14. Granstrom, M., et al. Perinatal cytomegalovirus infection in man. *Arch. Dis. Child.* 52:354, 1977.
    Cesarean section does not appear to protect an infant from acquiring cytomegalovirus at birth, as is the case with the related herpesvirus.
15. Hanshaw, J., et al. School failure and deafness after "silent" congenital cytomegalovirus infection. *N. Engl. J. Med.* 295:468, 1976.
    Intrauterine infection (asymptomatic at birth in nearly all patients) produced bilateral hearing loss in 10 percent of patients and learning problems later in childhood in approximately 20 percent.
16. Congenital cytomegalovirus infection. *Lancet* 1:801, 1983.
    For additional reviews, see J. Infect. Dis. 143:618, 1981, and Pediatr. Rev. 2:245, 1981.
17. Hanshaw, J. A new cytomegalovirus syndrome? *Am. J. Dis. Child.* 133:475, 1979.
    Outlines the syndrome of acquired cytomegalovirus infection in premature infants.
18. Medearis, D. CMV immunity: Imperfect but protective. *N. Engl. J. Med.* 306:985, 1982.
    Discusses the peculiar features of CMV immunity and its impact on reinfection and vaccination. (For another perspective on prevention of CMV disease, see Pediatr. Infect. Dis. 3:1, 1984.)
19. Stagno, S., et al. Comparative study of diagnostic procedures for congenital cytomegalovirus infection. *Pediatrics* 65:251, 1980.
    Accuracy of several methods compared; electron microscopy of the urine found most useful.

Herpes
20. Nahmias, A., and Tomeh, M. Herpes simplex virus infection. *Curr. Probl. Pediatr.* 4(4), 1974.
    An extensive review, based largely on the authors' experience.
21. Hanshaw, J. Herpesvirus hominis infections in the fetus and the newborn. *Am. J. Dis. Child.* 126:546, 1973.
    Somewhat shorter but thorough review, with a complete list of references.
22. Whitley, R., et al. Neonatal herpes simplex virus infection: Follow-up evaluation of vidarabine therapy. *Pediatrics* 72:778, 1983.
    Outcome has improved with therapy, but 80 percent of symptomatic newborns still die or have some long-term damage. (For a cautionary note on the use of antiviral drugs, see J. Pediatr. 86:317, 1975—and watch for coming studies on acyclovir.)
23. Brunell, P. Fetal and neonatal varicella-zoster infections. *Semin. Perinatol.* 7:47, 1983.
    This entire issue is devoted to infections caused by herpesviruses, including varicella-zoster, CMV, and herpes simplex. Also see Pediatr. Infect. Dis. 3:193, 1984.

Syphilis

24. Oppenheimer, E., and Hardy, J. Congenital syphilis in the newborn infant: Clinical and pathological observations in recent cases. *Johns Hopkins Med. J.* 129:63, 1971.
Sixteen cases from the "penicillin era" are compared with those from the prepenicillin era.

25. McCracken, G., and Kaplan, J. Penicillin treatment for congenital syphilis: A critical reappraisal. *J.A.M.A.* 228:855, 1974.
Dosage schedules of penicillin are evaluated with regard to the adequacy of central nervous system levels for the treatment of syphilis; recommendations are given.

26. Srinivasan, G., et al. Congenital syphilis: A diagnostic and therapeutic dilemma. *Pediatr. Infect. Dis.* 2:436, 1983.
The incidence of CNS involvement was quite low in this series.

Hepatitis B

27. Chin, J. Prevention of chronic hepatitis B virus infection from mothers to infants in the United States. *Pediatrics* 71:289, 1983.
Treatment plan utilizing passive and active immunization is outlined.

28. Hepatitis B vaccine. *Med. Lett. Drugs Ther.* 24:75, 1982.
Presents rationale, indications, and adverse reactions to vaccine.

Chlamydia

29. Nichols, R. Infections with *Chlamydia trachomatis*. *Pediatrics* 64:269, 1979.
Treatment summary.

30. Hammerschlag, M., et al. Prospective study of maternal and infantile infection with *Chlamydia trachomatis*. *Pediatrics* 64:142, 1979.
Conjunctivitis and pneumonitis are common symptoms in neonatally acquired Chlamydia *infection. (Also see J. Pediatr. 95:28, 1979, and Pediatr. Rev. 3:77, 1981.)*

44. NEONATAL SEPSIS
Robert D. White

Infections are a major cause of morbidity and mortality among newborns, and their significance continues to grow as modern neonatal care permits survival of increasing numbers of neonates at high risk. Newborns differ from older children and adults in virtually every aspect of infectious disease: their immunologic defenses are immature; they are susceptible to a unique spectrum of organisms; symptoms of infection may be subtle and nonspecific; and antibiotic pharmacokinetics differ.

In the first 2 months of gestation, the fetus is virtually defenseless against invading organisms. The placenta and amniotic sac are highly effective barriers to infection, but transplacental passage of certain viruses, such as rubella, can occur. During the third month of gestation, differentiation and maturation of cellular and humoral immune factors begin, and continue up to and after birth.

At birth, the newborn loses the protection afforded in utero and is exposed to a multitude of virulent organisms. Secretory immunoglobulin (IgA), normally the first line of defense against infection entering through the mucous membranes, is virtually absent at birth. (Fresh human milk contains IgA, but appreciable IgA levels do not develop in formula-fed infants until several weeks after birth.) Infection may also enter the body through aspiration of infected material, through a break in the skin, or by iatrogenic means (umbilical catheter, endotracheal tube).

With the onset of infection, several immunologic defenses respond. IgG immunoglobulins transported from mother to fetus in the third trimester of pregnancy provide the newborn with passive immunity against many organisms. The infant can produce IgM and small amounts of IgG, but their effectiveness is limited because opsonization, phagocytosis, and intracellular killing of virulent organisms are not yet mature. Prematures are at greater risk, since they are born before receiving the full maternal transfer of IgG, their own immmunologic responses are immature, their nutrition may be inadequate for days or weeks following birth, and they are more frequently subjected to invasive procedures. Other factors associated with neonatal sepsis include being male, prolonged rupture of the membranes with active labor, maternal intrapartum infection, and certain congenital anomalies.

In most infants the onset of neonatal sepsis is heralded by nonspecific signs such as lethargy and poor feeding; fever or hypothermia may occur (with the latter more common), but either can be obscured by incubators or warmers that maintain constant body temperature. Because of the newborn's reduced capacity to control infection, any localized signs of infection (e.g., omphalitis, abscess) should be considered part of a systemic infection until proved otherwise.

Laboratory clues to the diagnosis of neonatal infection are often scanty. Cultures are definitive and vital in planning therapy after the infection is brought under control, but are not helpful in the initial evaluation. Hematologic studies may show an increased band count, leukocytosis, or occasionally neutropenia (a poor prognostic sign); thrombocytopenia and toxic granulation of the neutrophils may also be seen, but these hematologic changes often do not reach diagnostic significance until several hours after the onset of symptoms. More valuable is examination and gram stain of body fluids; demonstration of organisms by gram stain of the buffy coat is uncommon but of great value in the diagnosis of bacteremia. Cerebrospinal fluid should be examined whenever sepsis is suspected, since up to one-third of infants with sepsis also have meningitis, and bacteria may be easily identified in the cerebrospinal fluid. Specimens of urine and fluid from any localized area of infection should be examined and a chest radiograph obtained. Although any of these tests may be extremely useful in an individual case, their yield is relatively low, and the decision to treat a neonate for sepsis is usually based on the nonspecific clinical signs of illness.

Certain pathogens cause identifiable syndromes of disease in neonates. The group B beta-hemolytic streptococcus (GBS), which is the leading cause of neonatal sepsis, produces two distinct patterns of disease. "Early-onset" disease occurs in the first 24 hours of life; its incidence is 2 to 3 per 1000 live births and is highest in prematures and infants born after prolonged rupture of the membranes. Infants are colonized with GBS during labor or delivery if the organism is present in the maternal vaginal flora; the incidence of maternal colonization varies from 1 to 30 percent, depending on the culture technique used and the population studied. Of colonized infants, only 1 percent become infected. Full-term infants with early-onset GBS infection usually appear healthy at birth, then become lethargic and distressed, with irregular or rapid respirations. Shock, pneumonia, and acidosis occur in most cases; neutropenia is also present in about one-half of the infants and is highly suggestive of GBS sepsis and pneumonia. Premature infants may have a similar course, but often GBS sepsis in this group is indistinguishable from the respiratory distress syndrome (see Chap. 32). Clinically, tachypnea and dyspnea are prominent with both disorders; radiographically, generalized opacification of the lung fields is a consistent finding. Severe apnea in the first 24 hours, relatively good pulmonary compliance in spite of severe hypoxemia, neutropenia, gram-positive cocci in the gastric aspirate, or prolonged rupture of the membranes should suggest GBS sepsis in a premature infant initially believed to have respiratory distress syndrome; differentiating between these two diseases is nevertheless extremely difficult in many cases. The prognosis of early-onset GBS sepsis is poor; only 25 to 40 percent of symptomatic infants survive, and many of these have permanent neurologic damage.

"Late-onset" GBS infection occurs between 1 and 12 weeks of age. Colonization probably occurs in the newborn nursery, and meningitis is the usual form of infection. The type III serotype is responsible for over 90 percent of late-onset infections, whereas Ia is the most common serotype in early-onset sepsis. The clinical signs are less fulminant and the prognosis better in this group than in early-onset disease; nearly all infants with late-onset GBS infection survive, and only 15 to 20 percent sustain neurologic damage.

The choice of antibiotics in the therapy of neonatal infection is usually made in the absence of information about the specific organism responsible and its sensitivities. Drugs must be chosen that provide coverage against the common pathogens, with recognition that no antibiotic regimen that will protect against every organism is practical. Infections that occur shortly after birth are usually caused by organisms acquired from the mother; GBS and coliforms are the most common pathogens in this group. Infections later in the neonatal period are often due to hospital-acquired organisms; GBS, penicillinase-producing staphylococci, and gram-negative bacilli (sometimes resistant to several antibiotics) must then be considered. Bacteria of relatively low virulence, such as *Listeria* and *Pseudomonas*, can also produce serious infections in neonates, and anaerobic organisms have recently been implicated as well.

Intensive supportive care is important for neonates with life-threatening infections. Shock, respiratory failure, hypothermia, hypoglycemia, and disseminated intravascular coagulation are complications of sepsis that must be anticipated and treated vigorously. Renal and hepatic function should be monitored, since impairment in these functions requires adjustment of antibiotic dosage. The duration of treatment must be individualized on the basis of the site of infection and the response to antibiotics; the prognosis also depends on these factors, as well as on the presence of associated diseases and the type of organism responsible for the infection. White cell transfusion (still experimental) may offer improved survival for septic infants with profound neutropenia.

Prevention of neonatal infection is possible in many cases. Hand washing by nursery personnel prior to each infant contact, sterilization of equipment, and restraint in the use of invasive procedures are of obvious importance but are often neglected. Cesarean section in mothers who become febrile during labor or who have had prolonged rupture of membranes may prevent some intrapartum infections, especially pneumonia. Efforts to prevent early-onset GBS sepsis by treatment of colonized mothers or prophylaxis of newborns have not yet been successful, but studies continue in several centers.

Reviews

1. Siegel, J. and McCracken, G. Sepsis neonatorum. *N. Engl. J. Med.* 304:642, 1981.
   Strong pathophysiologic orientation.
2. Harris, M., and Polin, R. Neonatal septicemia. *Pediatr. Clin. North Am.* 30:243, 1983.
   Predominant focus is on therapy. (Also see Adv. Pediatr. *31:405, 1984.)*
3. Freedman, R., et al. A half century of neonatal sepsis at Yale. *Am. J. Dis. Child.* 135:140, 1981.
   Large series reflects on the changing spectrum of organisms in neonatal sepsis.

The Immune System

4. Cates, K., Rowe, J., and Ballow, M. The premature infant as a compromised host. *Curr. Probl. Pediatr.* 13(8), 1983.
   For a symposium on host defenses in the fetus and newborn, see Pediatrics *64:705, 1979 (19 articles, 128 pages).*

Infectious Agents: Group B Streptococcus

5. Feigin, R. The perinatal group B streptococcal problem: More questions than answers. *N. Engl. J. Med.* 294: 106, 1976.
   A brief review. (Another article in this issue compares signs and symptoms of GBS with those of respiratory distress syndrome: p. 65.)
6. Manroe, B., et al. The differential leukocyte count in the assessment and outcome of early-onset neonatal group B streptococcal disease. *J. Pediatr.* 91:632, 1977.
   An absolute neutrophil count and ratio of juvenile to mature forms may distinguish between GBS and other causes of respiratory distress.
7. McCracken, G., and Feldman, W. Editorial comment. *J. Pediatr.* 89:203, 1976.
   Antibiotic regimen recommended for GBS meningitis is also appropriate for sepsis. There are several articles on various aspects of GBS in the same issue.
8. Baker, C. Group B streptococcal infections in neonates. *Pediatr. Rev.* 1:5, 1979.
   Good section on prospects for prevention. (For summary of current research efforts, see J. Infect. Dis. *148:163, 1983.)*

Infectious Agents: Other

9. Ray, C., and Wedgewood, R. Neonatal listeriosis: Six cases and a review of the literature. *Pediatrics* 34:378, 1964.
   Late-onset Listeria *meningitis was characterized by mononuclear pleocytosis.*
10. Chow, A., et al. The significance of anaerobes in neonatal bacteremia: Analysis of 23 cases and review of the literature. *Pediatrics* 54:736, 1974.

Anaerobes comprised 25 percent of isolates when special culture techniques were used, but their significance is uncertain.

11. Baumgart, S., et al. Sepsis with coagulase-negative staphylococci in critically ill newborns. *Am. J. Dis. Child.* 137:461, 1983.
    No longer safe to disregard this organism, especially in patients with indwelling vascular catheters.

12. Siegel, J., and McCracken, G. Group D streptococcal infections. *J. Pediatr.* 93:542, 1978.
    Now a more common pathogen in newborns than E. coli in some hospitals.

Sites of Infection: Meningitis

13. Berman, P., and Banker, B. Neonatal meningitis. *Pediatrics* 38:6, 1966.
    A classic study that established meningitis in neonates as a disease with minimal signs, high mortality, and frequent sequelae.

14. Overall, J. Neonatal bacterial meningitis. *J. Pediatr.* 76:499, 1970.
    A prospective study that outlines the natural history of this disease.

15. Sarff, L., Platt, L., and McCracken, G. Cerebrospinal fluid evaluation in neonates: Comparison of high-risk infants with and without meningitis. *J. Pediatr.* 88:473, 1976.
    Lists normal cerebrospinal fluid values. Of infants with meningitis, 99 percent had at least one abnormality (by gram stain, cell count, chemistries).

16. McCracken, G., et al. Moxalactam therapy for neonatal meningitis due to gram-negative enteric bacilli. *J.A.M.A.* 252:1427, 1984.
    Ampicillin/amikacin and ampicillin/moxalactam gave similar cure rates in this large collaborative study.

17. Chang, M., et al. Kanamycin and gentamicin treatment of neonatal sepsis and meningitis. *Pediatrics* 56:695, 1975.
    Chloramphenicol may be a reasonable alternative to the aminoglycosides.

18. Fulginiti, V. Treatment of meningitis in the very young infant. *Am. J. Dis. Child.* 137:1043, 1983.
    Recommendations for drug therapy.

19. Baumgartner, E., Augustine, A., and Steele, R. Bacterial meningitis in older neonates. *Am. J. Dis. Child.* 137:1052, 1983.
    A different clinical and microbiologic picture emerges when onset of meningitis occurs late in the neonatal period.

Sites of Infection: Other

20. Pittard, W., Thullen, J., and Fanaroff, A. Neonatal septic arthritis. *J. Pediatr.* 88:621, 1976.
    Of nine infants, eight previously had had umbilical catheters. In all, the same organism was present in the joint and on the umbilicus.

21. Weissberg, E., Smith, A., and Smith, D. Clinical features of neonatal osteomyelitis. *Pediatrics* 53:505, 1974.
    Of 17 with osteomyelitis, 12 also had arthritis, and in 7 of these, multiple joints were involved.

22. Bergstrom, T., et al. Studies of urinary tract infections in infancy and childhood: XII. Eighty consecutive patients with neonatal infections. *J. Pediatr.* 80:858, 1972.
    Congenital anomalies and permanent sequelae found in less than 5 percent.

23. Bland, R. Otitis media in the first six weeks of life: Diagnosis, bacteriology, and management. *Pediatrics* 49:187, 1972.
    Frequently overlooked but common site of infection; 40 percent of organisms were resistant to ampicillin. (Also see Pediatrics 62:198, 1978.)

Diagnostic Aids

24. Manroe, B., et al. The neonatal blood count in health and disease: I. Reference values for neutrophilic cells. *J. Pediatr.* 95:89, 1979.
    Normal range for neutrophil counts changes markedly during the first 72 hours of life.

25. Christensen, R., Bradley, P., and Rothstein, G., The leukocyte left shift in clinical and experimental neonatal sepsis. *J. Pediatr.* 98:101, 1981.

Greatly elevated immature to total neutrophil ratio shown to be good marker for bone marrow depletion and, consequently, for death from sepsis.

26. Philip, A. and Hewitt, J. Early diagnosis of neonatal sepsis. *Pediatrics* 65:1036, 1980.
    A panel of tests allowed sepsis to be excluded with 99 percent certainty in many patients. (Also see J. Pediatr. *98:795, 1981, and* Clin. Pediatr. *[Phila.] 20:385, 1981.)*

27. Faden, H. Early diagnosis of neonatal bacteremia by buffy-coat examination. *J. Pediatr.* 88:1032, 1976.
    The only test that was diagnostic for sepsis during the initial workup, but there were many false-negatives. (Also see J. Pediatr. *105:419, 1984.)*

28. Visser, V., and Hall, R. Lumbar puncture in the evaluation of suspected neonatal sepsis. *J. Pediatr.* 96:1063, 1980.
    Found LP to be of value in workup of suspected sepsis in the first 72 hours of life. (Urine culture is low yield, however: J. Pediatr. *94:635, 1979.)*

Management

29. McCracken, G., and Nelson, J. *Antimicrobial Therapy for Newborns* (2nd ed.). New York: Grune & Stratton, 1983.
    For an additional in-depth discussion of aminoglycosides, see Semin. Perinatol. *6:155, 1982.*

30. Christensen, R., et al. Granulocyte tranfusions in neonates with bacterial infection, neutropenia, and depletion of mature marrow neutrophils. *Pediatrics* 70:1, 1982.
    The dawn of a new era? (Also see J. Pediatr. *98:118, 1981,* Arch. Dis. Child. *58:1003, 1983, and* Pediatrics, *74:887, 1984.)*

31. Ellner, J. Septic shock. *Pediatr. Clin. North Am.* 30:365, 1983.
    Current therapy for a difficult management problem.

32. Wasserman, R. Unconventional therapies for neonatal sepsis. *Pediatr. Infect. Dis.* 2:421, 1983.
    Briefly summarizes exchange transfusion, granulocyte transfusion, and fresh-frozen plasma therapy.

33. Roberts, K. Management of young febrile infants. *Am. J. Dis. Child.* 137:1143, 1983.
    Also see Pediatrics *69:40, 1982, for pointers on diagnosis and management of newborns with fever.*

45. BLEEDING
Robert D. White

Normal neonatal hemostasis differs from that of the older child or adult in several areas. Capillary fragility is often increased, especially in premature infants. Platelet counts are the same in newborns as in adults, but platelet aggregation appears to be impaired. Levels of vitamin K-dependent clotting factors are lower than adult norms, and the level of circulating anticoagulant activity also seems to be reduced. As a result of the differences, the neonate's prothrombin time (PT) and activated partial thromboplastin time (PTT) are moderately prolonged, the bleeding time is normal, and whole blood clotting time is more rapid than in the adult.

When abnormalities of hemostasis occur, the cause can usually be established by a careful history and physical examination and a relatively few laboratory tests. Two considerations are particularly helpful in categorizing the cause of bleeding: (1) Aside from the bleeding, does the infant appear healthy, or are other serious diseases also present (e.g., respiratory distress, sepsis)? (2) Is the platelet count normal or diminished?

Bleeding in a healthy neonate with a normal platelet count is usually caused by a hereditary clotting factor deficiency; hemophilia A (factor VIII deficiency) and Christmas disease (factor IX deficiency) account for nearly all such cases (see Hemophilia, Chap. 89). It is not common, however, for infants with these disorders to have excessive bleeding in the neonatal period, and when it does occur, it is rarely life-threatening; prolonged oozing following circumcision is the most frequent manifestation. Hemophilia and Christmas disease are X-linked recessive disorders, and a history of bleeding diatheses in male relatives of the mother supports the diagnosis. The platelet count and PT are normal, but the PTT is prolonged; specific clotting factor assay is diagnostic. Acquired deficiency of the vitamin K-dependent clotting factors (hemorrhagic disease of the newborn) may occur in healthy neonates but is now rare, since vitamin K is administered prophylactically at birth. Bleeding in healthy newborns with normal platelet counts may also be caused by maternal drug therapy; the synthesis of clotting factors is depressed in utero by anticonvulsants and warfarin; aspirin crosses the placenta and may interfere with platelet function.

In some healthy infants with bloody stools or vomitus or both in the first days of life, the history, physical findings, and laboratory test results are normal. In this group, an Apt test (alkali denaturation of the hemoglobin) often demonstrates that the blood is of maternal origin, swallowed by the infant during delivery. Alternatively, this bleeding may be due to gastric ulceration, occasionally present in newborns. Not all infants with this syndrome are asymptomatic, however; in some cases, blood is also aspirated, causing an intense chemical pneumonitis.

Bleeding in healthy neonates with low platelet counts is usually caused by congenital platelet deficiencies; these include autoimmune and isoimmune thrombocytopenias and the thrombocytopenia-absent radius (TAR) syndrome. Autoimmune thrombocytopenia in a newborn reflects a disorder in the mother, such as idiopathic thrombocytopenic purpura or systemic lupus erythematosus; in these diseases, autoantibodies against maternal platelets cross the placenta and react with similar antigens on the fetal platelets, causing their destruction. In isoimmune thrombocytopenia, on the other hand, fetal platelets contain an antigen not present in the mother, which stimulates production of maternal antibody directed specifically against the fetal platelets, in a manner analogous to Rhesus factor isoimmunization of the red cell (erythroblastosis fetalis). Immune thrombocytopenias may cause petechiae, bruising, and mucosal bleeding beginning in the first 2 days of life; some neonates sustain intracranial hemorrhage during vaginal delivery. The PT and PTT are normal in these disorders; the platelet count is usually less than 25,000 when bleeding is present. The two diseases can be distinguished from one another by the maternal platelet count, which is markedly diminished in autoimmune thrombocytopenia and normal in isoimmune disease. Both disorders are self-limited; platelet counts rise as maternal antibody is catabolized, and usually become normal by 2 months of age. Ingestion of thiazide diuretics by the mother during pregnancy has been implicated but not proved as a cause of neonatal thrombocytopenia.

In ill neonates, bleeding is usually a manifestation of disseminated intravascular coagulation (DIC), a disorder in which clotting factors and platelets are rapidly consumed in response to a variety of stresses, such as hypoxia, acidosis, sepsis, or necrotizing enterocolitis. Infants with DIC may have diffuse bleeding from needle-puncture sites, mucous membranes, and the gastrointestinal tract; in some cases, pulmonary or intracranial hemorrhage occurs and may be fatal. The platelet count is markedly reduced, the PT and PTT are prolonged, and fibrinogen concentration is reduced; the red blood cells appear fragmented ("microangiopathic") on smear. Some infants, especially those with sepsis or necrotizing enterocolitis, may have abnormal consumption only of platelets. Severe hepatitis is another cause of bleeding in ill neonates; synthesis of clotting factors is impaired, and platelets may be sequestered in an enlarged spleen. Hepatomegaly and direct-reacting or mixed hyperbilirubinemia suggest the diagnosis.

Management of bleeding in an otherwise healthy infant can usually await specific diagnosis; in most cases active intervention is unnecessary. Bleeding in infants with hemophilia or Christmas disease can usually be managed with local therapy, although transfusion of fresh-frozen plasma or factor concentrate occasionally is needed. In severe bleeding caused by isoimmune thrombocytopenia, transfusion of platelets that do not carry the offending antigen is helpful; the best source of these is the mother. Platelet transfusions are of little value to infants with autoimmune thrombocytopenia, however, since virtually all donor platelets carry the offending antigen and will be destroyed by antibody. Steroids may be useful in these infants until the catabolism of antibody is complete.

In seriously ill infants, therapy often must begin before a firm diagnosis is established. Fresh-frozen plasma and vitamin K may be given empirically; if the hematocrit is low or platelets are reduced on smear, transfusion of needed components is indicated. When DIC is the cause of bleeding, exchange transfusion may be helpful. Of crucial importance in the management of DIC is correction of the underlying disease; occult infection, thrombosis, or necrotizing enterocolitis must be considered, and any source of metabolic stress (e.g., hypoglycemia, hypocalcemia, hypothermia) must be vigorously treated. The role of heparin in the management of DIC remains controversial. Ill infants with bleeding due to liver disease should also be given vitamin K; transfusion of fresh-frozen plasma may transiently improve circulating levels of clotting factors, but these patients are among the most difficult to treat because of their protracted and complicated course.

Intracranial hemorrhage (ICH) is a form of bleeding in the newborn that presents special problems in diagnosis, management, and prevention. Subarachnoid hemorrhage primarily occurs in full-term infants; seizures, lethargy, and jaundice are frequent concomitants, but long-term complications are rare. In preterm infants, ICH is predominantly peri- or intraventricular, with incidences as high as 30 to 70 percent reported in infants less than 32 weeks' gestation. Prematures appear to be particularly susceptible for the following reasons: the vessels in the germinal matrix are fragile and poorly supported; the capacity to modulate cerebral blood flow changes occurring in response to stress is limited; and stresses are common. Most hemorrhages are thought to occur when stress (or recovery from stress) causes increased cerebral blood flow and subsequent rupture of vessels within the germinal matrix. (Other causes have been proposed for some cases of ICH in prematures: e.g., compression of the soft premature skull by the maternal cervix during labor, hemorrhage into ischemic tissue, or impaired cerebral venous return during pneumothorax/pneumopericardium.) Hemorrhage may be limited to the germinal matrix (also known as subependymal, periventricular, or grade I hemorrhage) or may extend into the lateral ventricle (grade II hemorrhage; grade III if ventricular dilatation is present). Hemorrhage that extends into the adjacent cerebral tissue is considered grade IV. Such bleeding usually occurs in the first 72 hours of life and rarely after 14 days of age. Diagnosis is established by ultrasonography or CT scan. Management of hemorrhage and its early complications (anemia, jaundice, lethargy, apnea, seizures, and cardiovascular instability) is strictly supportive at present. Death and serious long-term complications (especially progressive hydrocephalus or cerebral palsy) occur in a majority of infants with grade IV hemorrhage and in approximately 25 percent of those with grade III but are rare in those with grade I or II hemorrhage. Prevention of ICH in the near future will probably depend largely on avoiding stress in the preterm fetus and newborn during labor and the first days of life.

Reviews
1. Oski, F., and Naiman, J. *Hematologic Problems in the Newborn* (3rd ed.). Philadelphia: Saunders, 1982.
   A more thorough discussion of most disease entities than in the articles that follow.
2. Bleeding in the newborn. *Br. Med. J.* 2:915, 1977.
   A concise summary.
3. Glader, B., and Buchanan, O. The bleeding neonate. *Pediatrics* 58:548, 1976.
   A straightforward approach to diagnosis. (Also see Pediatr. Rev. 1:271, 1980.)
4. Gross, S., and Stuart, M. Hemostasis in the premature infant. *Clin. Perinatol.* 4:259, 1977.
   An extensive review (over 200 references) of normal and abnormal hemostasis in prematures, with special emphasis on DIC.
5. Bleyer, W., Hakami, N., and Shepard, T. The development of hemostasis in the human fetus and newborn infant. *J. Pediatr.* 79:838, 1971.
   An outline of the ontogeny of hemostasis through fetal life and the neonatal period.
6. McDonald, M., and Hathaway, W. Neonatal hemorrhage and thrombosis. *Semin. Perinatol.* 7:213, 1983.
   Discussion of thrombosis makes this review especially useful.

Platelet Disorders
7. Mull, M., and Hathaway, W. Altered platelet function in newborns. *Pediatr. Res.* 4:229, 1970.
   Platelets from newborns demonstrate relative thrombasthenia in vitro, but it is not clear whether this contributes to or protects from hemorrhagic disorders.

8. Corby, D., and Schulman, I. The effects of antenatal drug administration on aggregation of platelets of newborn infants. *J. Pediatr.* 79:307, 1971.
   Platelets of neonates are more susceptible to drug-induced dysfunction than are those of their mothers.
9. Pochedly, C. Thrombocytopenic purpura of the newborn. *Obstet. Gynecol. Surv.* 26:63, 1971.
   An encyclopedic review (40 pages, 355 references) of all bleeding disorders associated with thrombocytopenia.
10. Handin, R. Neonatal immune thrombocytopenia: The doctor's dilemma. *N. Engl. J. Med.* 305:951, 1981.
    Discusses prediction and manipulation of the fetal platelet count to permit a safe delivery—with more questions than answers. (Also see Am. J. Obstet. Gynecol. *144:449, 1982.)*

Clotting Factor Disorders

11. Baehner, R., and Strauss, H. Hemophilia in the first year of life. *N. Engl. J. Med.* 275:524, 1966.
    Only 17 of 192 patients with hemophilia or Christmas disease had serious hemorrhage in the first month of life.
12. Haemorrhage in the newborn. *Br. Med. J.* 4:1, 1971.
    A short review of hemorrhagic disease of the newborn.
13. Vitamin K and the newborn. *Lancet* 1:755, 1978.
    Suggests that vitamin K prophylaxis be used selectively for high-risk infants, rather than universally for all newborns.

Disseminated Intravascular Coagulation

14. Hathaway, W., Mull, M., and Pichet, G. Disseminated intravascular coagulation in the newborn. *Pediatrics* 43:233, 1969.
    Assay of factors V and VIII is advocated as the definitive diagnostic test for DIC.
15. Favara, B., Franciosi, R., and Butterfield, L. Disseminated intravascular and cardiac thrombosis of the neonate. *Am. J. Dis. Child.* 127:197, 1974.
    In a neonatal autopsy series, 8 percent showed intracardiac thromboses, previously thought to be a rare complication of DIC.

Intracranial Hemorrhage

16. Volpe, J. Neonatal intraventricular hemorrhage. *N. Engl. J. Med.* 304:886, 1981.
    Oriented toward explanation of pathophysiology. (Also see Pediatr. Clin. North Am. *29:1077, 1982, and* Semin. Perinatol. *6:42, 1982.)*
17. McDonald, M., et al. Role of coagulopathy in newborn intracranial hemorrhage. *Pediatrics* 74:26, 1984.
    Hypocoagulability was associated with a higher incidence of hemorrhage. (Also see article from same group on p. 32.)
18. Whitelaw, A., et al. Phenobarbitone for prevention of periventricular haemorrhage in very low birth-weight infants. *Lancet* 2:1168, 1983.
    Phenobarbital may reduce the severity—but not the incidence—of intraventricular hemorrhage. (For a study of ethamsylate, which may decrease the incidence of hemorrhage, see Arch. Dis. Child. *59:82, 1984.)*

46. CONGENITAL ANOMALIES
Robert D. White

Four common congenital malformations are discussed in this section. Much of the definitive therapy for each is surgical, but emotional support and genetic counseling are vital for optimal management. The pediatrician's role also includes referral for operation at the proper time, management of the long-term medical and surgical complications, and ongoing support of the parents.

Cleft lip, with or without cleft palate, occurs in 0.1 percent of live births, with a higher incidence in males. The incidence of 4 percent in siblings of affected patients clearly indicates the familial clustering of this disorder. It is also found as a component of over 50 syndromes of multiple malformations. Embryologically, cleft lip has been considered a defect of lip fusion during the second month of gestation.

The clinical spectrum of lip deformity ranges from almost imperceptible defects to bilateral clefts extending into the nostrils. Clefts may be unilateral or midline; the single most common abnormality is a unilateral left–sided cleft. Surgical repair of an uncomplicated cleft lip may be undertaken within days of birth, but many surgeons believe that both cosmetic results and parental satisfaction are improved if the operation is delayed until the infant is 2 to 3 months of age.

Management is much more difficult when a cleft palate is present. As with cleft lip, defects may be unilateral, bilateral, or midline, and they may be isolated, be associated with a cleft lip, or occur as a component of many syndromes. Complications prior to repair (at approximately 18 months of age) are common; especially common are feeding difficulties and otitis media. Even after palatal repair, dental and speech difficulties demand continued attention. Early feeding problems may be eased by the use of a special nipple, a medicine dropper, or a temporary orthodontic device that occludes the palatal defect. Comprehensive management of cleft palate is best accomplished by the combined efforts of a pediatrician and a multidisciplinary team that includes a plastic surgeon, orthodontist, oral surgeon, otolaryngologist, hearing and speech therapist, psychologist, social worker, and parents of other children with the anomaly.

Congenital dislocation of the hip (CDH) occurs in nearly 1 percent of newborn females, but in less than 0.2 percent of males. The incidence of siblings of affected infants approaches 10 percent, suggesting a genetic origin, but "environmental" influences may also be important, since almost 20 percent of infants with CDH are born in the breech position. Underdevelopment of the acetabulum and laxity of the hip ligaments have been postulated as the abnormalities that predispose to CDH.

Early diagnosis of the instability of the hip joint is necessary to prevent long-term morbidity. The Ortolani procedure permits diagnosis of more than 90 percent of cases during the neonatal period; most are actually subluxation or "dislocatable" hips, since frank dislocations are uncommon in neonates. The yield of this maneuver is maximized by performing it not only at birth but also at several days of age and at the first well-baby visit, as well as by recognizing that limitation of abduction to less than 180 degrees is equivalent to the classic "click" as a pathologic sign and by remembering that most hip dislocations are unilateral. The anomaly should also be suspected in infants with asymmetric leg lengths or thigh creases. Radiographs should be reserved for doubtful cases; routine x-ray confirmation of the clinical diagnosis is discouraged by many authors because it results in high gonadal radiation.

Hip dislocation diagnosed in the neonatal period can be successfully managed by application of splints designed to maintain the hip joints in abduction for 2 to 3 months. Splinting is not without complications, however; ischemic necrosis of the femoral head occasionally occurs. When diagnosis and treatment are delayed until later in infancy, splinting must be prolonged and an operation is sometimes required.

In *hypospadias,* the urethral orifice is located proximally on the ventral surface of the penis, apparently due to defective fusion of the urogenital groove. In the most severe form of this defect, the urethral opening is at the base of the penis or on the perineum; in milder forms, it may be on the shaft of the penis or at the base of the glans. Chordee nearly always accompanies hypospadias; meatal stenosis, cryptorchidism, urinary tract anomalies, and pseudohermaphroditism also coexist in a small percentage of affected infants. The incidence of hypospadias is approximately 0.3 percent in male infants, and most cases appear to occur sporadically.

Diagnosis of hypospadias and most of the associated anomalies is not difficult. Urinary tract anomalies may be detected by ultrasonography or intravenous pyelography, but the yield of functionally significant abnormalities is less than 4 percent. In patients whose urethral orifice is located on the perineum or the base of the penis and who also have cryptorchidism, a karyotype should be obtained to exclude pseudohermaphroditism.

Repair of hypospadias may be a single or multistaged procedure, depending on the severity of the defect and the preference of the surgeon. In most cases, the operation is performed between the first and fifth birthdays. Complications include formation of fistulas, strictures, or diverticula; these may require further operative procedures and can permanently limit function. Medical complications include urinary tract infection and renal damage, especially in patients with urinary tract anomalies.

Cryptorchidism, or undescended testis, is the result of an interruption in the normal descent of the testis from the abdomen into the scrotum at a point proximal to the external iliac ring. Since descent of the testis is not always complete at birth, the incidence of this disorder depends on age: in premature (male) infants the incidence is 30 percent, in full-term infants it is 4 percent, and by 1 year of age it is less than 1 percent; spontaneous descent after 1 year of age is rare. True cryptorchidism must be differentiated from retractile testes, which are only intermittently absent from the scrotum, and from ectopic testes, which are located distal to the inguinal ring, but outside the scrotum. Cryptorchidism is bilateral in 20 percent of cases; total absence of the testes suggests the possibility of intersexuality. Cryptorchidism is associated with inguinal hernia, urinary tract anomalies, hypospadias, and several syndromes.

Dysgenesis and susceptibility to malignancy in the undescended testis appear to be progressive with age. Some authors have suggested that the contralateral "normal" testis is also subject to dysmorphic changes, malignancy, and decreased fertility. Testicular torsion, presenting as lower abdominal pain, is another complication of cryptorchidism and is especially treacherous, since the diagnosis is often not considered.

The ideal therapy for cryptorchidism is not clear, since no treatment yet proposed provides entirely satisfactory results. Medical therapy with injections of human chorionic gonadotropin or luteinizing hormone-releasing hormone is under investigaton and appears to produce testicular descent in some patients. Surgical orchiopexy is still the standard therapy and is most commonly performed by 4 to 5 years of age. Delay of therapy beyond this time carries the risk of the progressive changes noted earlier, as well as the risk of serious psychologic problems.

General

1. Holmes, L. Inborn errors of morphogenesis: A review of localized hereditary malformations. *N. Engl. J. Med.* 291:763, 1974.
   Explores the genetics of a long list of congenital anomalies.

Cleft Lip and Cleft Palate

2. Hogan, V. (ed.). Cleft lip and palate. *Clin. Plast. Surg.* 2(2), 1975.
   Contains 150 pages on embryology, physiology, surgery and long-term management but is easy to read and well indexed.
3. Spriestersbach, D., et al. Clinical research in cleft lip and cleft palate: The state of the art. *Cleft Palate J.* 10:113, 1973.
   A general review, oriented primarily toward future research needs.
4. Fraser, F. The genetics of cleft lip and palate. *Am. J. Hum. Genet.* 22:336, 1970.
   Summary of a workshop.
5. Dar, H., Winter, S., and Tal, Y. Families of children with cleft lips and palates: Concerns and counseling. *Dev. Med. Child Neurol.* 16:513, 1974.
   Essential reading for those who treat a child with a cleft.
6. Paradise, J., and Bluestone, C. Early treatment of the universal otitis media of infants with cleft palate. *Pediatrics* 53:48, 1974.
   This complication requires nearly constant attention in order to preserve middle ear function.
7. Kelts, D., and Jones, E. The infant with cleft lip and/or palate. *Curr. Probl. Pediatr.* 13(5):17, 1983.
   Several useful nutritional ideas for breast-fed, bottle-fed, and postoperative babies.

Congenital Dislocation of the Hip

8. Stanisavljevic, S. (ed.). Congenital dislocation of the hip. *Clin. Orthop.* 119:2, 1976.
   A collection of papers on all aspects.
9. Congenital dislocation of the hip. *Br. Med. J.* 1:1303, 1977.
   A quick, one-page review.
10. Harrole, A. Problems in congenital dislocation of the hip. *Br. Med. J.* 1:1071, 1977.
    A short discussion of specific management difficulties.

11. Cyvin, K. Congenital dislocation of the hip joint. *Acta Paediatr. Scand. [Supp.]* 263, 1977.
    A study of etiologic factors in almost 400 cases.
12. Sherk, H., Pasquariello, P., and Watters, W. Congenital dislocation of the hip. *Clin. Pediatr.* (Phila.) 20:513, 1981.
    Well-organized and illustrated review.

Hypospadias

13. Horton, C., and Devine, C., Jr. Hypospadias and epispadias. *Clin. Symp.* 24(3), 1972.
    Easy reading; beautifully illustrated by Frank Netter.
14. Lutzker, L., Kogan, S., and Levitt, S. Is routine intravenous pyelography indicated in patients with hypospadias? *Pediatrics* 59:630, 1977.
    Sonography may obviate the need for an intravenous pyelogram in most patients.
15. Kelalis, P., et al. The timing of elective surgery on the genitalia of male children with particular reference to undescended testes and hypospadias. *Pediatrics* 56:479, 1975.
    An attempt to balance physiologic and psychologic considerations related to surgery.
16. Mills, C., et al. Analysis of different techniques for distal hypospadias repair: Price of perfection. *J. Urol.* 125:701, 1981.
    One of a group of articles in this issue on current surgical techniques.

Cryptorchidism

17. Waaler, P. Clinical and cytogenetic studies in undescended testes. *Acta Paediatr. Scand.* 65:553, 1976.
    Large series; accompanying article (p. 559) demonstrates abnormalities of gonadotropin secretion beginning in early childhood.
18. Allen, T. Cryptorchidism. *Pediatr. Rev.* 5:317, 1984.
    A short review.
19. Section on Urology, American Academy of Pediatrics. 49th annual meeting, Oct. 24–26, 1980. *Pediatrics* 69:100, 1982.
    Summary of the annual meeting, including a discussion of surgical and hormonal therapies for cryptorchidism.
20. Gilhooly, P., Meyers, F., and Lattimer, J. Fertility prospects for children with cryptorchidism. *Am. J. Dis. Child.* 138:940, 1984.
    Long (up to 48 years) and large (145 patients) retrospective study; fertility demonstrated following surgical repair in 80% with unilateral cryptorchidism, in 35% with bilateral.

Hernias

21. Avery, G., Berg, R., and Widmann, W. The clinical value of pediatric herniography. *Am. J. Dis. Child.* 131:1255, 1977.
    For conflicting thoughts on the risks and benefits of radiography and of surgical exploration of the contralateral side, see p. 1206 of the same issue and J. Pediatr. Surg. 15:313, 1980.
22. Hall, D., Roberts, K., and Charney, E. Umbilical hernia: What happens after age 5 years? *J. Pediatr.* 98:415, 1981.
    Documents continued spontaneous closure in black children after 5 years of age.

IV. CARDIOVASCULAR DISORDERS

Robert D. White and Jean S. Kan

The conduction system of the heart comprises five distinct segments: (1) the sinoatrial (SA) node, which usually functions as the cardiac pacemaker; (2) the atria, which contain specialized conduction tissue; (3) the atrioventricular (AV) node; (4) the bundle of His; and (5) the ventricular myocardium. Anomalous development or injury to any segment of the conduction system may result in abnormal initiation or propagation of electrical activity within the heart—a dysrhythmia. (Technically, *arrhythmia* means absence of rhythm; *dysrhythmia* means disorder of rhythm.) In practice, dysrhythmias are divided into supraventricular disorders (involving the SA node, atria, or AV node), ventricular disorders (involving the bundle of His or the ventricular myocardium), and heart block. In infants and children, supraventricular dysrhythmias are much more common than ventricular dysrhythmias or heart block.

The most common supraventricular dysrhythmia is paroxysmal supraventricular tachycardia (SVT, also called PAT for paroxysmal atrial tachycardia). This dysrhythmia may be associated with the Wolff-Parkinson-White (WPW) syndrome, congenital heart disease (especially Ebstein anomaly), cardiac surgery digitalis toxicity, viral myocarditis, or hypothyroidism, but in most cases no underlying disease is found. Its incidence is approximately 1 in 25,000 live births.

Children with SVT may be divided into two groups; the first comprises infants under four months of age at their initial presentation. There is a 2 : 1 male predominance in this group, and very few have underlying heart disease. These infants are usually in good health until shortly before coming to medical attention. Pallor, dyspnea, and malaise are early signs; congestive heart failure, when present, indicates that tachycardia has been present for at least 24 hours. Cardiomegaly and pulmonary congestion are frequently apparent on the initial chest roentgenogram and may lead to an initial impression of congenital heart disease. The ECG is diagnostic, however; the cardiac rate may be 180 to 300 but is extremely constant in each infant, being only minimally affected by respiration, activity, or vagal stimulation. P waves are often hidden within the T waves, and the QRS complexes are usually normal.

In infants who are moribund, the dysrhythmia should be converted immediately by electric countershock (0.25–1.0 watts/second per kg). Overdrive pacing may also be carried out by placing an electrode catheter in the right atrium and pacing at a rate faster than the SVT rate. Infants who are only moderately distressed can be converted by invoking the "diving reflex" (by placing an ice-cold wet cloth over the face) or by medication. Digoxin is usually effective in converting SVT but may take 6 hours or longer to control the dysrhythmia. Other medications with a more rapid onset of action include phenylephrine, Tensilon, and ipecac, all of which have direct or indirect vagal effects, and propranolol, which has a direct effect on the cardiac conducting system. Verapamil is effective in older children with SVT but may cause severe hypotension in infants and is therefore contraindicated in any child less than 1 year of age. Vagal stimulation by direct eyeball pressure is usually unsuccessful in young children and can be dangerous; other vagal maneuvers such as carotid massage or induction of vomiting are less reliable than induction of the diving reflex and therefore are now used infrequently. In the absence of underlying heart disease the prognosis for infants with SVT is excellent. Generally digoxin is continued for the first year of life, then stopped. The incidence of recurrent attacks of SVT is low.

The second group of children with SVT become symptomatic after infancy; they differ from those with the infantile form in that many more have underlying heart disease. Males and females are equally affected. Congestive heart failure is uncommon in this group; palpitations and syncope are more common complaints. The ECG is often bizarre during an attack, with conduction blocks at the atrial or ventricular level. Conversion to sinus rhythm and prevention of recurrences are more difficult than in infants; quinidine or propranolol may be required to control dysrhythmias refractory to digoxin.

One cause of SVT, the Wolff-Parkinson-White (WPW) syndrome, deserves special attention because it is the only cause of SVT for which the basic pathologic mechanism is known. In the WPW syndrome, there is a "short circuit" between the atria and ventricles through a collection of fibers called the bundle of Kent. These fibers connect the atria directly to either left (type A WPW) or right (type B WPW) ventricular tissue, bypassing the AV node. In normal sinus rhythm, electrical activity reaches the ventricular myocardium sooner through the bundle of Kent than through the AV node and bundle of His, causing a shortened P–R interval and broadening of the QRS complex. During the paroxysms of tachycardia, however, a loop of electrical activity is established between the atria and ventricles. The pathway of electrical activation is usually antegrade through the AV node and retrograde through the accessory electrical pathway. Therefore, the QRS complex is narrow with no delta wave during the tachycardia. Because the loop is relatively short, rapid ventricular rates result; because it is independent of the sinus node and its autonomic innervation, the rate is extremely constant. The diagnosis of WPW can be established by recording an electrocardiogram after the tachycardia has been converted to a sinus rhythm. The prognosis for SVT secondary to the WPW syndrome is less optimistic than when the SVT is idiopathic. The rate of recurrence remains high. Although many pediatric cardiologists continue to use digoxin for treatment of SVT whether or not there is underlying WPW, digoxin may decrease the refractoriness of the accessory pathway, thereby allowing the rapid firing of the ventricle if atrial fibrillation should occur.

Other supraventricular disorders of rhythm are much less common than SVT. Supraventricular tachycardias secondary to ectopic atrial pacemakers or junctional ectopic tachycardia may be extremely difficult to treat. Chronic supraventricular tachycardia may occur; in this condition, there are no intervening periods of normal sinus rhythm, but affected children are usually asymptomatic. Atrial flutter is similar to the infantile form of SVT in its epidemiology and management, while atrial fibrillation is nearly always associated with massively enlarged atria secondary to severe congenital or rheumatic heart disease. Premature atrial contractions occasionally indicate underlying heart disease but are an isolated and benign phenomenon. Premature infants frequently have severe sinus bradycardia, which is probably due to immaturity of the sinus node or its autonomic innervation. The sick sinus syndrome, which may develop spontaneously or as a complication of cardiac surgery, frequently presents with bradycardia or syncope. The natural history of this disorder is not clear, but in many patients the disease progresses to complete nonfunction of the sinus node. Sudden death may occur in affected persons and, for this reason, permanent pacemakers are used in symptomatic patients.

Ventricular arrhythmias are rare in childhood. Occasional premature ventricular contractions (PVCs) occur in many normal individuals and rarely require therapy in the absence of underlying heart disease. The presence of symptoms (chest pain, syncope), long runs of ventricular tachycardia, or exacerbation of the dysrhythmia with exercise would alert the physician to the possibility of underlying heart disease. Paroxysmal and chronic ventricular tachycardia have been described in children; these disorders may complicate myocarditis or cardiomyopathies and may be difficult to control. Lidocaine and electric countershock are effective as acute therapy. However, long-term treatment may require the use of new antidysrhythmic agents. Ventricular fibrillation may occur as a terminal event in patients with or without heart disease. Electric countershock is the treatment of choice for this disorder.

A rare disorder of ventricular repolarization, characterized by prolongation of the Q–T interval, has been the subject of recent interest. Initially described as a syndrome that includes deaf-mutism, the ECG abnormality is now reported in otherwise normal patients who present with syncopal attacks. The baseline resting ECG may have a normal Q–T interval and Q–T prolongation may occur only during periods of exercise. Therefore, a patient who presents with syncope of uncertain etiology should have a stress electrocardiogram to evaluate the Q–T interval. Pathogenesis of this syndrome may be related to an asymmetry of sympathetic innervation to the heart; its significance lies in the high incidence of sudden death in untreated patients. Propranolol is effective in preventing syncope and sudden death, even though the Q–T interval remains prolonged during treatment.

Complete heart block in children may be congenital, acquired as a complication of myocardial disease, or iatrogenic—the result of cardiac surgery or digitalis toxicity. Congenital heart block in most cases is a benign disorder, but associated heart disease must be excluded (especially corrected transposition of the great vessels). In a few children, syncopal attacks may be life-threatening, and implantation of a permanent pacemaker is indicated. Acquired heart block may be temporary or permanent; the prognosis in most cases is dependent on progression of the underlying myocarditis. Heart block secondary to cardiac surgery may be transient, with problems only in the immediate postoperative period, or permanent.

The diagnosis of a rhythm disorder in a child may be difficult, since the rhythm abnormality may be intermittent. Electrocardiogram findings may be subtle, as in the short P–R interval of WPW syndrome, the long Q–T syndrome, or variable P–P interval in the sick sinus syndrome. In some cases dysrhythmias not apparent on a routine ECG can be detected by a 24-hour Holter monitor ECG recording. Small portable event recorders are available that permit recording of a brief period of the electrocardiogram during periods of symptoms. Conduction studies using several intracardiac electrodes during cardiac catheterization delineate specific conduction abnormalities and provide a rational basis for drug therapy. In addition, ablation by electric shock delivered through the catheter to the offending pathologic conduction tissue may abolish the rhythm disorder.

Reviews

1. Gillette, P., and   Garson, A. (eds.). *Pediatric Cardiac Dysrhythmias*. New York: Grune & Stratton, 1981.
   The *comprehensive text on the subject. (For an overview by the first author, see* Pediatr. Rev. *3:190, 1981.)*

2. Guntheroth, W. Disorders of heart rate and rhythm. *Pediatr. Clin. North Am.* 25:869, 1978.
   Good explanation of the electrophysiologic basis for dysrhythmias.

3. James, T. Order and disorder in the rhythm of the heart. *Circulation* 47:362, 1973.
   An elegant monograph on the cellular control of electrical activity in the heart.

4. Schamroth, L. How to approach an arrhythmia. *Circulation* 47:420, 1973.
   It is probably easier than you thought.

5. Guntheroth, W. Arrhythmias in children. *Circulation* 64:647, 1981.
   A list of more than 170 "key references" in 12 categories, from general reviews to treatment. (Also in the Circulation *"key reference" series: pediatric electrophysiology, 61:1266, 1980; sick sinus syndrome, 60:1422, 1979; digitalis, 59:838, 1979.)*

Supraventricular Disorders of Rhythm: Paroxysmal Supraventricular Tachycardia

6. Paroxysmal tachycardia in children. *Br. Med. J.* 4:248, 1973.
   A concise summary.

7. Andersen, E., et al. Paroxysmal tachycardia in infancy and childhood: I. Paroxysmal supraventricular tachycardia. *Acta Paediatr. Scand.* 62:341, 1973.
   The natural history. (Also see Pediatrics *51:26, 1973;* J. Pediatr. *98:875, 1981; and* Pediatrics *70:638, 1982.)*

8 Radford, D., Izukawa, T., and Rowe, R. Congenital paroxysmal atrial tachycardia. *Arch. Dis. Child.* 51:613, 1976.
   Hydrops fetalis is a common finding when PST is present prior to birth.

9. Roelandt, J., and Roos, J. On the mechanism of paroxysmal tachycardias in neonates. *Am. Heart J.* 81:842, 1971.
   An intriguing hypothesis links the infantile form of supraventricular tachycardia to a transient WPW-like phenomenon.

Supraventricular Disorders of Rhythm: Wolff-Parkinson-White Syndrome

10. Giardina, A., Ehlers, K., and Engle, M. Wolff-Parkinson-White in infants and children: A long-term follow-up study. *Br. Heart J.* 34:839, 1972.
    One-third of the patients had additional heart disease, but only 10 percent of the patients presented severe management difficulties.

11. Benson, D., and Gallagher, J. Electrophysiologic evaluation and surgical correction of Wolff-Parkinson-White syndrome in children. *Clin. Pediatr.* (Phila.) 19:575, 1980.
    Intracardiac catheter studies permit precise localization of the accessory pathway when surgery is indicated for refractory or life-threatening dysrhythmias.

Supraventricular Disorders of Rhythm: Other

12. Jacobsen, J., et al. Chronic supraventricular tachycardia in infancy and childhood. *Acta Paediatr. Scand.* 64:597, 1975.

Digitalis was of little benefit in asymptomatic patients. See also the series by Keane et al., Am. Heart J. *84:748, 1972.*

13. Church, S., et al. Cardiac arrhythmias in premature infants: An indication of autonomic immaturity? *J. Pediatr.* 71:542, 1967.
    Of infants weighing under 1500 gm, 90 percent had notable arrhythmias.
14. Yabek, S., and Jarmakani, J. Sinus node dysfunction in children, adolescents, and young adults. *Pediatrics* 61:593, 1978.
    Describes the "sick sinus syndrome."
15. Radford, D., and Izukawa, T. Atrial fibrillation in children. *Pediatrics* 59:250, 1977.
    Of 35 patients with this arrhythmia, 3 had cerebral emboli.
16. Martin, T., and Hernandez, A. Atrial flutter in infancy. *J. Pediatr.* 100:239, 1982.
    Series of 10 infants; 1 died of underlying heart disease, but the remainder did well.

Ventricular Disorders of Rhythm
17. Hernandez, A., et al. Idiopathic paroxysmal ventricular tachycardia in infants and children. *J. Pediatr.* 86:182, 1975.
    The clinical presentation may be extremely variable. See also series by Videbaek, J., al., Acta Paediatr. Scand. *62:349, 1973.*
18. Radford, D. Izukawa, T., and Rowe, R. Evaluation of children with ventricular arrythmias. *Arch. Dis. Child.* 52:345, 1977.
    Syncope is a common symptom, and sudden death occurred in one child despite therapy.
19. Schwartz, P., Periti, M., and Malliani, A. The long Q-T syndrome. *Am. Heart J.* 89:378, 1975.
    A review, with good sections on causes and treatment.
20. Stevens, D., et al. Fetal and neonatal ventricular arrhythmia. *Pediatrics* 63:771, 1979.
    More than 90 percent of the dysrhythmias were limited to the neonatal period.

Congenital Heart Block
21. Ayers, C., Boineau, J., and Spach, M. Congenital complete heart block in children. *Am. Heart J.* 72:381, 1966.
    A review, with emphasis on developmental aspects.
22. Pinsky, W., et al. Diagnosis, management, and long-term results of patients with congenital complete atrioventricular block. *Pediatrics* 69:728, 1982.
    Diagnostic evaluation of a neonate with heart block should include screening of the mother for connective tissue disorders.

Postoperative Dysrhythmias
23. Clark, D., et al. Electrocardiographic changes following surgical treatment of congenital cardiac malformations. *Prog. Cardiovasc. Dis.* 17:451, 1975.
    An extensive review of transient and permanent ECG changes following surgery, discussed according to specific cardiac lesion.
24. Krongrad, E. Prognosis for patients with congenital heart disease and postoperative intraventricular conduction defects. *Circulation* 57:867, 1978.
    The prognosis is discussed according to the site of the conduction block.

Management
25. Gelband, H., and Rosen, M. Pharmacologic basis for the treatment of cardiac arrhythmias. *Pediatrics* 55:59, 1975.
    A good general overview.
26. Atkinson, A., and Davison, R. Diphenylhydantoin as an antiarrhythmic drug. *Annu. Rev. Med.* 25:99, 1974.
    Most useful for the treatment of digitalis toxicity.
27. Porter, C., Garson, A., and Gillette, P. Verapamil: An effective calcium blocking agent for pediatric patients. *Pediatrics* 71:748, 1983.
    For a discussion of the use of this drug in the treatment of PST, see J. Pediatr. *98:323, 1981.*
28. Gillette, P., et al. Oral propranolol treatment in infants and children. *J. Pediatr.* 92:141, 1978.

For a discussion of the antiarrhythmic effects of acute beta-blockage with atenolol on supraventricular tachycardias, see Klin. Wochenschr. *2:123, 1981.*

29. Coumel, P., and Fidelle, J. Amiodarone in the treatment of arrhythmias in children: One hundred thirty-five cases. *Am. Heart J.* 100:1063, 1980.
    For a discussion of amiodarone in children with WPW syndrome, see Pediatrics *72:813, 1983; for a cautionary comment, see* Pediatrics *72:817, 1983.*
30. Gillette, P. Advances in the diagnosis and treatment of tachydysrhythmias in children. *Am. Heart J.* 102:111, 1981.
    A succinct description of the more recent medical, surgical, and pacemaker modes of therapy.
31. Sperandeo, V., et al. Supraventricular tachycardia in infants: Use of the "diving reflex." *Am. J. Cardiol.* 51:286, 1983.
    Twice as much fun to do when you understand the physiology!
32. Resnekov, L. Present status of electroversion in the management of cardiac dysrhythmias. *Circulation* 47:1356, 1973.
    Read this before you need to use electroversion! (For specific aspects in children, see Circulation *56:502A, 1977, and* Pediatrics *58:898, 1976.)*
33. Benrey, J., et al. Permanent pacemaker implantation in infants, children, and adolescents. *Circulation* 53:245, 1976.
    Improvements in recent years have made pacemakers practical and safe.

48. MYOPERICARDITIS

Margaret E. Mohrmann

Inflammatory diseases of the heart are often difficult to diagnose in children; myocarditis and pericarditis are relatively uncommon problems in childhood and may present with nonspecific or misleading symptoms. The diagnosis is often made on the basis of an unexpected radiologic finding or as the clinical course evolves. Moreover, although myocarditis and pericarditis are discussed as distinct diseases in this section, they probably seldom exist as isolated entities. Since infection of the pericardium usually involves the myocardium, and vice versa, the term *myopericarditis* is most descriptive.

Nonrheumatic myocarditis, classically associated with the exotoxin of diphtheria, is now probably caused most often in the United States by Coxsackie group B viruses. There are also reports of myocarditis as a complication of mumps, measles, varicella, rubella, influenza, infectious mononucleosis, certain congenital infections, and in association with elevated titers of antibody to *Chlamydia trachomatis*.

Clinically, myocarditis covers a broad spectrum ranging from incidental ECG changes during an infectious illness to refractory, rapidly fatal cardiac failure. Most children with significant disease have fever and malaise; abdominal pain, with or without nausea and vomiting, may be present and may suggest the diagnosis of acute appendicitis. More specific signs and symptoms are referable to the presence of dysrhythmias (bradycardia, syncope) or heart failure (fatigue, dyspnea, tachypnea, tachycardia), or both.

Examination of the heart often reveals cardiomegaly, muffled heart sounds, gallop rhythms, and an absence of significant murmurs. Usually, although not invariably, the heart appears enlarged on a chest roentgenogram, and an echocardiogram affirms that the enlargement is one of dilatation rather than hypertrophy. A triad of nonspecific changes may be seen on the ECG: low voltages, flattened or inverted T waves, and S-T segment depression. The sedimentation rate is usually elevated; "cardiac enzymes" (LDH, SGOT) may or may not be increased.

Acute infectious myocarditis may be differentiated from the carditis of rheumatic fever by the presence of murmurs in the latter condition. The finding of a rash, hepatosplenomegaly, or arthritis is suggestive of juvenile rheumatoid arthritis or systemic lupus erythematosus as the cause of myocarditis. Other differential diagnostic possibilities include a multitude of diseases that primarily or secondarily affect the myocardium: the cardiomyopathies. A thorough history and physical examination should suffice to exclude malnutrition, hypothyroidism or hyperthyroidism, muscular dystrophy, and Friedreich ataxia. Metabolic disorders, such as glycogen storage disease type II (Pompe disease) and mucopolysaccharidosis type I (Hurler syndrome), and idiopathic hypertrophic cardiomyopathy may be ruled out in the presence of low voltages and ventricular dilatation. In the neonate the major diagnostic alternative is endocardial fibroelastosis, a disease that some consider a chronic or end-stage form of viral carditis.

The treatment of acute viral myocarditis is primarily supportive. Several animal studies have demonstrated a markedly detrimental effect of exercise on survival, and bed rest or at least a significant decrease in activity therefore is recommended. Heart failure may respond to digitalis and diuretics, but it must be emphasized that the inflamed myocardium is often sensitive to the effects of digitalis, and signs of toxicity must be watched for closely. Administration of digitalis, using a short-acting preparation (e.g., digoxin), is often started at one-half the usual dose. The use of corticosteroids has been advocated but should be limited to patients who are severely ill and refractory to supportive therapy, since there is suggestive evidence that viral infections may be exacerbated by these drugs. Dysrhythmias should be treated appropriately.

The symptomatic myocarditis of diphtheria has a very high mortality, as does Coxsackie virus myocarditis in the neonate. In contrast, mortality for viral myocarditis in children beyond infancy is less than 5 percent, and sequelae are uncommon; occasionally, a child will suffer recurrences of disease or will succumb to chronic myocarditis.

With the decline in incidence of acute rheumatic fever, infectious agents are now probably the most common cause of acute pericarditis in childhood. The infecting organism is usually bacterial; a viral etiology has occasionally been documented, and it is assumed that many cases of so-called benign idiopathic pericarditis are viral in origin. Types of pericardial inflammation other than that caused by infection include: uremic pericarditis, an often hemorrhagic inflammation of unknown pathogenesis; the postpericardiotomy syndrome, a self-limited, possibly immunologically mediated pericarditis seen in the first few weeks to months following cardiac surgery; and the often asymptomatic pericarditis associated with juvenile rheumatoid arthritis.

Bacterial, or purulent, pericarditis is usually found in association with other foci of infection, such as pneumonia, meningitis, osteomyelitis, and skin infections, but may occur as an isolated disease. *Staphylococcus aureus* is the most frequent agent, followed in frequency by *Haemophilus influenzae* and *Neisseria meningitidis;* the pneumococcus has been implicated only infrequently since the beginning of the antibiotic era, and tuberculous pericarditis is uncommon in developed countries. Pericarditis in neonates and in immunocompromised children may be caused by gram-negative bacilli.

Infectious pericarditis is characterized by chest pain or pressure; pain may also be referred to the neck, trapezius ridge, or epigastric area, or all these areas. Symptoms of an upper respiratory tract infection and fever are usually present, and the majority of patients show signs of congestive heart failure. A pericardial friction rub is present in only 35 percent, and approximately the same percentage exhibits paradoxical pulse. Heart sounds are usually muffled and murmurs are absent.

The chest roentgenogram often shows an enlarged, globular heart, and fluoroscopy may reveal decreased pulsation, as in myocarditis. The ECG findings are nonspecific for the most part, but may reveal a typical progression from ST-T segment elevation to T wave inversion over several days. The echocardiogram is the most useful noninvasive diagnostic tool available and may show accurately both the size and the location of a pericardial effusion. Pericardiocentesis may be considered both a diagnostic and a therapeutic maneuver; it should be carried out in all cases of suspected purulent pericarditis.

Treatment of infectious pericarditis has two essential components: antibiotics and drainage. Appropriate antibiotics are administered intravenously for 2 to 6 weeks, depending on response. Pericardiectomy is usually required for adequate drainage of pus, especially when the infecting organism is *Haemophilus influenzae;* occasionally a child with mild disease, caused by another organism, can be treated successfully with one or several pericardiocenteses. Prognosis is directly related to the adequacy of therapy: mortality is 100 percent in untreated patients, 70 to 90 percent in patients treated with antibiotics or drainage alone, and 0 to 20 percent in those treated with both therapeutic modalities.

Cardiac tamponade may occur at any time during the acute phase of pericarditis and must be anticipated; any evidence of increasing heart failure or hypotension is an indication for emergency therapeutic pericardiocentesis. Constrictive pericarditis occasionally occurs as an early, acute complication of purulent pericarditis and must be considered in a clinical situation resembling tamponade; therapy is immediate circulatory support and emergency pericardiectomy. There is little evidence for the development of constrictive pericarditis as a late sequela of acute, nontuberculous infection or as a manifestation of chronic infection, although it is suspected that "idiopathic" constrictive pericarditis is, in many instances, the result of an unrecognized viral inflammation. Chronic constrictive pericarditis may be associated with intestinal lymphangiectasia, ascites, failure to thrive, or a specific syndrome of growth failure known as mulibrey nanism; surgical removal of the pericardium often relieves the associated problems.

General

1. Noren, G., Kaplan, E., and Staley, N. Nonrheumatic Inflammatory Cardiovascular Diseases. In F. Adams and G. Emmanouilides (eds.), *Heart Disease in Infants, Children and Adolescents* (3rd ed.). Baltimore: Williams & Wilkins, 1983.
   An excellent, well-referenced textbook discussion.

2. Burch, G., and Giles, T. The role of viruses in the production of heart disease. *Am. J. Cardiol.* 29:231, 1972.
   Clinical and experimental evidence of viral etiologies of myocarditis, pericarditis, and endocarditis.

3. Woodruff, J. Viral myocarditis: A review. *Am. J. Pathol.* 101:427, 1980.
   A well-written detailed review of what is known and speculated about Coxsackie B viral myopericarditis (38 pages, 306 references); an earlier review, in Am. J. Cardiol. *34:224, 1974, emphasizes the properties of the Coxsackie virus and problems of diagnosis.*

Myocarditis: Etiology

4. Morgan, B. Cardiac complications of diphtheria. *Pediatrics* 32:549, 1963.
   Among 95 children with diphtheria there were 4 cases of myocarditis, with 3 deaths; description of clinical and ECG findings.

5. Wagner, H. Cardiac disease in congenital infections. *Clin. Perinatol.* 8:481, 1981.
   A discussion of both structural and inflammatory heart disease caused by intrauterine rubella, cytomegalovirus, and enterovirus infections.

6. Grayston, J., Mordhorst, C., and Wang, S. Childhood myocarditis associated with *Chlamydia trachomatis* infection. *JAMA* 246:2823, 1981.
   Antibodies to Chlamydia *were found (fortuitously) in the serum of 4 children (aged 1–6 years) with acute myocarditis. (Also see* Pediatrics *70:54, 1982.)*

7. Miller, J., and French, J. Myocarditis in juvenile rheumatoid arthritis. *Am. J. Dis. Child.* 131:205, 1977.
   Three case reports; emphasis on distinction from pericarditis and heightened sensitivity to digitalis.

Myocarditis: Diagnosis and Outcome

8. Harris. L., Powell, G., and Brown, O. Primary myocardial disease. *Pediatr. Clin. North Am.* 25:847, 1978.
   Concise discussions of myocarditis, cardiomyopathies, and endocardial fibroelastosis. (For a description of cardiac abnormalities in hypothyroidism and the response to hormone replacement, see Am. J. Dis. Child. *137:65, 1983.)*

9. Boles, E., and Hosier, D. Abdominal pain in acute myocarditis and pericarditis. *Am. J. Dis. Child.* 105:104, 1963.
   Among 26 children with myocarditis and 15 with pericarditis, 5 in each group presented with abdominal pain as the most prominent symptom; 4 of the 10 were initially thought to have acute surgical abdominal disease.

10. Sanner, E., et al. Acute myopericarditis: A long-term follow-up study. *Ups. J. Med. Sci.* 81:167, 1976.
    Only 1 of 29 patients (followed for a mean of 6 years) had functional impairment.

Pericarditis: Reviews

11. Spodick, D. The normal and diseased pericardium: Current concepts of pericardial physiology, diagnosis, and treatment. *J. Am. Coll. Cardiol.* 1:240, 1983.

A superb review that gives the information promised in the title in just 10 pages (100 references).

12. Gersony, W., and Hordof, A. Infective endocarditis and diseases of the pericardium. *Pediatr. Clin. North Am.* 25:831, 1978.
    A concise, accessible review.

Pericarditis: Etiology

13. Feldman, W. Bacterial etiology and mortality of purulent pericarditis in pediatric patients. *Am. J. Dis. Child.* 133:641, 1979.
    In this well-referenced review of 163 cases (1950–1977), Staphylococcus aureus *was the infecting organism in 44 percent,* Haemophilus influenzae *in 22 percent; apparent prognostic factors are discussed.*

14. Okoroma, E., et al. Acute bacterial pericarditis in children: Report of 25 cases. *Am. Heart J.* 90:709, 1975.
    Mortality in the period 1962–1967 was 77 percent versus 25 percent in the period 1968–1973; 90 percent of those treated with antibiotics plus drainage survived. (For other series, see Am. J. Med. *59:68, 1975;* J. Pediatr. *85:165, 1974; and* Pediatrics *40:224, 1967.)*

15. Echeverria, P., et al. *Hemophilus influenzae* b pericarditis in children. *Pediatrics* 56:808, 1975.
    Includes 5 cases (no deaths) plus 28 from the literature; discusses the use of countercurrent immunoelectrophoresis (CIE) on pericardial fluid; advocates pericardiectomy (not pericardotomy) on all patients after initial diagnostic pericardiocentesis.

16. Comty, C., et al. Uremic pericarditis. *Cardiovasc. Clin.* 7(3):219, 1976.
    Discusses all aspects, emphasizing possible causes and therapy.

17. Engle, M., et al. The postpericardiotomy and similar syndromes. *Cardiovasc. Clin.* 7(3):211, 1976.
    A good, brief discussion, primarily concerning children who have undergone surgical correction of congenital heart disease. The development of symptoms was correlated with the appearance of antiheart and antiviral antibodies. Steroid therapy is advocated.

18. Brewer, E. Juvenile rheumatoid arthritis: Cardiac involvement. *Arthritis Rheum.* 20:231, 1977.
    A good, brief review, primarily concerned with pericarditis. (The classic discussion is in Pediatrics *32:855, 1963.)*

Pericarditis: Diagnosis

19. Dunn, M., and Rinkenberger, R. Clinical aspects of acute pericarditis. *Cardiovasc. Clin.* 7(3):131, 1976.
    Symptoms, ECG, and echo findings in pericarditis, effusions, and tamponade. (For an explanation of the phenomenon of paradoxical pulse, see N. Engl. J. Med. *301:480, 1979.)*

20. Stolz, J., Borns, P., and Schwade, J. The pediatric pericardium. *Radiology* 112:159, 1974.
    Radiologic findings; straightening of the left heart border was an early sign of pericardial effusion in 73 percent.

21. Engel, P. Echocardiography in pericardial disease. *Cardiovasc. Clin.* 13(3):181, 1983.
    A detailed and technical review. (Computed tomography is helpful when the ultrasound examination is technically unsatisfactory: Ann. Intern. Med. *97:473, 1982.)*

Pericarditis: Management

22. Morgan, R., et al. Surgical treatment of purulent pericarditis in children. *J. Thorac. Cardiovasc. Surg.* 85:527, 1983.
    Of 15 children with pericarditis, the 7 with Haemophilus influenzae *as the etiologic agent all required pericardiectomy; in only 4 of the other patients did pericardiocentesis alone suffice for drainage. (Need for extensive anterior pericardiectomy with* H. influenzae *pericarditis also emphasized in* J. Pediatr. Surg. *17:285, 1982.)*

Constrictive Pericarditis

23. Fowler, N. Constrictive pericarditis: New aspects. *Am. J. Cardiol.* 50:1014, 1982.
    A concise (four pages) review of physical and electrocardiographic findings, hemodynamics, and therapy.
24. Strauss, A., et al. Constrictive pericarditis in children. *Am. J. Dis. Child.* 129:822, 1975.
    There were three deaths among five patients. The chronic presentation is differentiated from acute, posteffusive constriction.
25. Greenwood, R., et al. Constrictive pericarditis in childhood due to mediastinal irradiation. *Circulation* 50:1033, 1974.
    Disease occurred in 7 percent of 86 irradiated children and was the cause of death in three children. Symptoms appeared 15 months (mean) after radiation. The development of disease was related to dose and technique (all cases occurred after orthovoltage, none after supravoltage).
26. Voorhees, M., et al. Growth failure with pericardial constriction: The syndrome of mulibrey nanism. *Am. J. Dis. Child.* 130:1146, 1976.
    A case report and discussion of clinical features in other reported cases of this rare recessive syndrome. (Also see J. Pediatr. 88:569, 1976.)

49. BACTERIAL ENDOCARDITIS
Kenneth B. Roberts

Because bacterial endocarditis (BE) is a uniformly fatal disease in children when not treated, the clinician who cares for children with heart disease must remain alert to this diagnostic possibility. Today, the underlying heart defect is more likely to be congenital than rheumatic, with tetralogy of Fallot the malformation most frequently associated with infection and ventricular septal defect a close second. Notably, secundum-type atrial septal defects are rarely associated with infection. Children under 2 years of age seem relatively protected from bacterial endocarditis, but when it occurs in this age group, it is usually a devastating illness.

The pathogenesis of bacterial endocarditis begins with a platelet-fibrin thrombus on a damaged valve or in an area of low pressure that has been traumatized by a jet effect of rapid flow. When bacteremia occurs, such as following dental manipulation, the bacteria aggregate the platelets, host antibody agglutinates the bacteria, and the entrapped platelets and bacteria stick to the propagating thrombus. Although parts of the infected mass may break off, embolization appears to be less frequent than previously thought. Phenomena once considered embolic are now felt to be due to immune complexes: glomerulonephritis, Janeway lesions, Roth spots, splinter hemorrhages, and possibly Osler nodes. The immune complexes are reflected in many patients by the appearance of rheumatoid factor and a decrease in the levels of complement in the serum after a few weeks of disease; there is a return to normal values with successful treatment.

Traditionally, bacterial endocarditis has been thought of as acute and fulminant (ABE), or subacute (SBE) with more subtle signs, such as unexplained fever and lethargy, as the principal complaints. *Staphylococcus aureus* is usually the pathogen in ABE and streptococci of the viridans group, the pathogen in SBE. Children who have had cardiac surgery may pursue an intermediate course, with fever and lethargy months after their operation and with *S. aureus* as the offending organism.

The clinical challenge in the management of SBE in children is to establish the diagnosis early. A high index of clinical suspicion is essential. Fever and malaise may be the only symptoms; splenomegaly and hematuria may not appear until late in the course; and splinter hemorrhages and petechiae, especially in the cyanotic child, are only of modest diagnostic benefit. The other lesions of the hands (Janeway lesions, Osler nodes) are rare. An increased sedimentation rate is usually present but is nonspecific. The white blood cell count is normal, and anemia, when present early, is usually mild. Congestive heart failure and changing murmurs develop only after the infection is well established;

for the best outcome, the diagnosis must be made and treatment instituted before these two signs develop.

The first blood culture reveals the pathogen in most cases of SBE, but the yield can be increased by culturing six specimens of blood; some authors propose as many as 10. Although bacteremia is continuous, the number of organisms circulating in the blood varies, so that, for practical purposes, the bacteremia may be considered intermittent. The exact timing of blood specimens with relation to fever is less critical than obtaining multiple separate specimens to "catch" the bacteremia. In up to 20 percent of patients who appear to have BE clinically, multiple, repeated blood cultures are sterile. One explanation given is that in right-sided SBE, such as occurs with ventricular septal defects in children, organisms are shed into the pulmonary circulation, and the lungs remove the bacteria from the bloodstream, so that venous specimens are sterile although infection persists. Two additional causes for "blood-culture-negative SBE" are laboratory related: (1) discarding specimens prematurely (2 weeks of incubation may be required before growth is recognized) and (2) the inability of the usual media to support the growth of nutritionally deficient—but pathogenic—streptococci.

Antibiotics are selected for initial treatment that are effective against the organisms usually responsible for the patient's clinical syndrome. Streptococci of the viridans group are exquisitely sensitive to penicillin in vitro, but the old clinical observation that penicillin plus streptomycin might be more effective than penicillin alone has recently been confirmed, both in vitro and in vivo. Many authors now recommend penicillin plus an aminoglycoside for patients with viridans group streptococcal endocarditis as well as for those with disease caused by the enterococcus; the latter is an infrequent cause of SBE in children, but one to be thought of when endocarditis follows manipulation of the genitourinary tract. If staphylococcal infection is likely, a penicillinase-resistant antibiotic is used in place of penicillin. Prolonged therapy (4–6 weeks) is necessary to eliminate "persisters." Operative intervention must be considered in the child who progresses to cardiac failure despite medical therapy.

Prophylaxis against endocarditis with penicillin for dental procedures and penicillin plus an aminoglycoside for genitourinary manipulation has been recommended by the American Heart Association for many years; recent investigations suggest that penicillin plus an aminoglycoside may be preferable for all procedures. The specific regimen may not be the limiting factor in prophylaxis, however: in a survey at one cardiac clinic, only half the families knew to take endocarditis prophylaxis precautions, and even fewer knew why.

The prognosis of bacterial endocarditis is not related clearly to either the organism or the mode of presentation, but, rather, to a combination of the two. Infants do not fare as well as older children, and the prognosis is guarded if signs and symptoms progress while the child is on therapy. The apparent key to a good prognosis is clinical suspicion of the diagnosis aroused early enough for the institution of appropriate therapy before irreversible damage occurs.

Reviews

1. Kaplan, E., and Taranta, A. (eds.). *Infective Endocarditis (Monograph 52)*. Dallas: American Heart Association, 1977.
   Contains 23 articles, covering epidemiology, microbiology, pathology, pathogenesis, clinical problems, therapy, prophylaxis, and prevention, and an overview of endocarditis in children (p. 51).
2. Newburger, J., and Nadas, A. Infective endocarditis. *Pediatr. Rev.* 3:226, 1982.
   Brief, readable review. (Another review: Pediatr. Clin. North Am. 25:831, 1978.)

Pathophysiology

3. Weinstein, L., and Schlesinger, J. Pathoanatomic, pathophysiologic and clinical correlations in endocarditis. *N. Engl. J. Med.* 291:832, 1122, 1974.
   Delivers what the title promises in a succinct, simplified manner (two parts).

Clinical Series

4. Johnson, D., Rosenthal, A., and Nadas, A. A forty-year review of bacterial endocarditis in infancy and children. *Circulation* 51:581, 1975.
   Covers 149 cases, 1933–1972. (The 1970s: Am. J. Dis. Child. 138:720, 1984.)

5. Gersony, W., and Hayes, C. Bacterial endocarditis in patients with pulmonary stenosis, aortic stenosis or ventricular septal defect. *Circulation* 56 [Suppl. I] :I–84, 1977.
  From the Natural History Study. The risk of BE with a ventricular septal defect is 1.5 per 1000 patient-years; with aortic stenosis, 1.8 per 1000 patient-years; and with pulmonary stenosis, 0.2 per 1000 patient-years. Mortality was 25 percent. Operative closure of ventricular septal defects reduced the risk.
6. Clemens, J., et al. A controlled evaluation of the risk of bacterial endocarditis in persons with mitral-valve prolapse. *N. Eng. J. Med.* 307:776, 1982.
  Mitral valve prolapse presents greater risk than normal mitral valve.
7. Johnson, D., Rosenthal, A., and Nadas, A. Bacterial endocarditis in children under 2 years of age. *Am. J. Dis. Child.* 129:183, 1975.
  Uncommon but devastating in this age group; occurs in high-risk neonates, too: Pediatrics 71:392, 1983.

Bacteriologic Confirmation

8. Washington, J. Blood cultures, principles and techniques. *Mayo Clin. Proc.* 50:91. 1975.
  An excellent review, including practical aspects (78 references).
9. Belli, J., and Waisbren, B. The number of blood cultures necessary to diagnose most cases of bacterial endocarditis. *Am. J. Med. Sci.* 232:284, 1956.
  In patients with positive cultures, the first culture was positive in 60.5 percent; six cultures were required to identify 95 percent and ten cultures to identify 100 percent.
10. Werner, A., et al. Studies on the bacteremia of bacterial endocarditis. *JAMA* 202:199, 1967.
  The first culture was positive in 95 percent, and more than 98 percent of patients who had positive cultures were identified with two cultures. A higher percentage of first cultures was positive in those with streptococcal infections than in those with non-streptococcal infections. Bacteremia was continuous and of low magnitude.
11. Roberts, K., and Sidlak, M. Satellite streptococci: A major cause of "negative" blood cultures in bacterial endocarditis? *JAMA* 241:2293, 1979.
  A brief report with recommendations for clinicians and microbiologists.

Immune Complexes

12. Gutman, R., et al. The immune complex glomerulonephritis of bacterial endocarditis. *Medicine* (Baltimore) 51:1, 1972.
  A small number of patients thoroughly studied; 25 pages, 91 references.
13. Alpert, J., et al. Pathogenesis of Osler's nodes. *Ann. Intern. Med.* 85:471, 1976.
  Immune complex or microemboli? (Includes Osler's description, p. 470.)

Management

14. Bisno, A., et al. Treatment of infective endocarditis due to viridans streptococci. *Circulation* 63:730A, 1981.
  Report of the Subcommittee on Treatment of Bacterial Endocarditis of the American Heart Association Council on Cardiovascular Disease in the Young, detailing diagnosis and treatment.
15. Sande, M., and Shelb, W. Combination antibiotic therapy of bacterial endocarditis. *Ann. Intern. Med.* 92:390, 1980.
  Reviews penicillin-aminoglycoside regimen not only for enterococcal endocarditis but for disease caused by other organisms as well.
16. Cleary, T., and Kohl, S. Anti-infective therapy of infective endocarditis. *Pediatr. Clin. North Am.* 30:349, 1983.
  In addition to discussing antimicrobials, the authors provide an overview of the problem and discuss indications for surgery.
17. Kavey, R., et al. Two-dimensional echocardiographic assessment of infective endocarditis in children. *Am. J. Dis. Child.* 137:851, 1983.
  May be helpful in diagnosis and, serially, in management.

Prophylaxis
18. Shulman, S., et al. Prevention of bacterial endocarditis. *Pediatrics* 75:603, 1985.
    American Heart Association review and recommendations.
19. Durack, D., and Petersdorf, R. Chemotherapy of experimental streptococcal
    endocarditis. *J. Clin. Invest.* 52:592, 1973.
    *Uses an animal model to test various regimens for prophylaxis; penicillin plus
    aminoglycoside won. High-dose procaine penicillin also worked but high-dose
    penicillin G did not (needed high blood levels early and for more than 9 hours).*
20. Everett, E., and Hirschmann, J. Transient bacteremia and endocarditis prophylaxis:
    A review. *Medicine* (Baltimore) 56:61, 1977.
    Assessment of the risks of bacteremia following various procedures.
21. Caldwell, R., Hurwitz, R., and Girod, D. Subacute bacterial endocarditis in children.
    Am. J. Dis. Child. 122:312, 1971.
    *Less than 50 percent of families knew of SBE precautions and even fewer understood
    why prophylaxis was needed.*
22. Hess, J., Holloway, Y., and Dankert, J. Incidence of postextraction bacteremia under
    penicillin cover in children with cardiac disease. *Pediatrics* 71:554, 1983
    *Raises questions about the enterprise of endocarditis prophylaxis. (For an analysis of
    52 cases of "apparent failures of endocarditis prophylaxis," see* JAMA *250:2318,
    1983.)*

50. VENTRICULAR SEPTAL DEFECT
Robert D. White and Jean S. Kan

Ventricular septal defect (VSD) is the most common congenital cardiac malformation. Of
all cardiac defects, 30 percent are isolated VSDs, and an additional 15 percent are VSDs
associated with other malformations (tetralogy of Fallot, truncus arteriosus, and others).
The overall incidence of VSD at birth is 3 to 4 per 1000 live births.

The cause of VSD is unclear. Most defects occur in the membranous portion of the
ventricular septum, which is the final area of the septum to form in utero, at approximately 7 weeks' gestation. Genetic predisposition probably plays a role in some cases,
since VSD is more common in certain families, in Down syndrome, in the Holt-Oram
syndrome, and in some inbred animals. Congenital infections and teratogenic agents
have also been implicated, as in the congenital rubella and fetal alcohol syndromes. The
great majority of VSDs, however, occur without apparent relationship to any of these
factors and must still be considered idiopathic.

Flow of blood through a VSD is dependent on the size of the defect and on pulmonary
vascular resistance. Shunting is minimal at birth, even with a very large defect, since
pulmonary and systemic resistances are balanced. As pulmonary resistance falls in the
first month of life, however, left-to-right shunting gradually increases. Because of this
large runoff into the pulmonary circulation, the left ventricle must pump large volumes
of blood to maintain adequate systemic blood flow. Congestive heart failure may supervene as early as the second week of life, but usually does not appear until after 1 month
of age. Small defects rarely cause heart failure, since the amount of blood shunted from
left to right is restricted.

Except in patients with very large VSDs, clinical improvement is the rule after the
sixth month of life. Spontaneous closure occurs in at least 25 percent of all defects in early
childhood, and in an additional 25 percent by age 50. Membranous defects may be
covered by the septal leaflet of the tricuspid valve or by fibrous tissue adherent to the
septum itself; muscular defects are occluded by continued growth of the muscle surrounding the VSD. Continued patency of the defect predisposes to bacterial endocarditis
and, in larger defects, to pulmonary vascular changes. Endocarditis (see the preceding
chapter) may occur even in very small defects; the incidence of this complication is
greatly reduced following successful closure—spontaneous or operative—of the septal
defect. Obstruction of the small pulmonary vessels develops with prolonged exposure of
the pulmonary circulation to increased blood flow and high pressure. It usually is not a

problem before 2 years of age, but may occur as early as the first year of life when a cleft mitral valve accompanies the VSD (this malformation complex is called an *endocardial cushion defect* and is especially common in children with Down syndrome).

The diagnosis of VSD is usually based on the characteristic heart murmur, which is coarse, holosystolic, and radiates well from the left to the right lower sternal borders. When the shunt is large, signs and symptoms of heart failure may be present along with a diastolic flow murmur at the apex. Examination of the precordium often yields a palpable thrill and "lift," and the pulmonary component of the second sound is loud. Chest radiographs demonstrate cardiomegaly with increased pulmonary vascularity, and the ECG usually reflects enlargement of the left atrium and one or both ventricles. In very small defects, the murmur may be abbreviated, ending well before the second sound, and the chest roentgenogram and ECG are usually normal. The 2-dimensional echocardiogram is extremely helpful in defining the size and location of the VSD, which may be in the membranous septum, the muscular septum (frequently as multiple defects), the inlet portion of the ventricle (AV canal), or the supracristal area just under the aortic valve.

Management of an infant with a VSD depends on the clinical symptoms. A baby who is in congestive heart failure with tachypnea and poor feeding may have some symptomatic improvement with diuretic therapy and salt restriction. The use of digoxin in infants with large left-to-right shunts is controversial, but evidence of left ventricular dysfunction is an accepted indication. If growth is poor, surgical closure of the VSD should be arranged promptly. A child with high pulmonary artery pressure should have the VSD closed by 6 months of age to avoid the risk of pulmonary vascular obstructive disease. An infant who improves with medical therapy may be managed without surgery for a period of time with careful follow-up. If clinical signs and cardiac catheterization document persistence of a left-to-right shunt with a pulmonary-systemic flow ratio greater than 2:1, the defect should be closed electively at around 4 years of age. Asymptomatic children in whom the pulmonary-systemic flow ratio is less than 2:1 do not require operative intervention; the VSD will close spontaneously in more than one-half of these children.

Large Series

1. Collins, G., et al. Ventricular septal defect: Clinical and hemodynamic changes in the first five years of life. *Am. Heart J.* 84:695, 1972.
   Provides a schema for classification by severity, with important therapeutic and prognostic implications.
2. Hoffman, J., and Rudolph, A. The natural history of ventricular septal defects in infancy. *Am. J. Cardiol.* 16:634, 1965.
   Heart failure developed in 40 percent of infants in this series and was controlled medically in two-thirds.
3. Campbell, M. Natural history of ventricular septal defect. *Br. Heart J.* 33:246, 1971.
   A follow-up into adulthood demonstrated continuing improvement in some patients through the fourth decade of life.
4. Weidman, W., et al. Clinical course in ventricular septal defect. *Circulation* 56 [Suppl. I]:I-56, 1977.
   This huge study had 1265 patients, most of whom had at least two cardiac catheterizations to document hemodynamic changes with age. (Also see Circulation 55:908, 1977, *and* Pediatrics 65:375, 1980.)

Additional Features of the Natural History

5. Alpert, B., et al. Spontaneous closure of small ventricular septal defects: Ten-year follow-up. *Pediatrics* 63:204, 1979.
   Improved detection of small defects probably accounts for part of the increased incidence of spontaneous closure in comparison to previous studies.
6. Anderson, R. A., et al. Rapidly progressing pulmonary vascular obstructive disease: Association with ventricular septal defects during early childhood. *Am. J. Cardiol.* 19:854, 1967.
   Clinical symptoms and signs are described, but serial cardiac catheterizations were a more effective means of detecting early changes.

7. Maron, B., Ferrans, V., and White, R., Jr. Unusual evolution of acquired infundibular stenosis in patients with ventricular septal defect. *Circulation* 48:1092, 1973.
   Hypertrophy of the right ventricular infundibulum converts some cases of VSD into tetralogy of Fallot.

Anatomic Variants

8. Goor, D., et al. Isolated ventricular septal defect: Developmental basis for various types and presentation of classification. *Chest* 58:468, 1970.
   Defects are classified by their location, and the embryology of each type is reviewed.
9. Towbin, R., and Schwartz, D. Endocardial cushion defects: Embryology, anatomy and angiography. *AJR* 136:157, 1981.
   For a description of pulmonary vascular disease in this group, see Am. J. Cardiol. *39:721, 1977.*

Endocarditis

10. Gersony, W., and Hayes, C. Bacterial endocarditis in patients with pulmonary stenosis, aortic stenosis, or ventricular septal defect. *Circulation* 56 [Suppl. I]:I-84, 1977.
    From the Natural History Study. The overall risk with VSD is 1.5 per 1000 patient-years; operative closure greatly reduces this risk.

---

51. TETRALOGY OF FALLOT
Robert D. White and Jean S. Kan

Tetralogy of Fallot is the most common of congenital heart defects that present with cyanosis after the first 2 weeks of life. Fallot described the association of infundibular and valvar pulmonic stenosis, ventricular septal defect (VSD), a large aorta overriding the ventricular septum, and right ventricular hypertrophy; occasionally, a fifth defect, patent foramen ovale or atrial septal defect, was present as well. There are many theories regarding the embryologic origin of this anomaly. Perhaps the most attractive hypothesis is that hypoplasia of the conus portion of the right ventricle early in fetal life is the primary defect, causing hemodynamic and anatomic alterations that result in the observed malformation complex. Both genetic and environmental factors have been implicated in tetralogy of Fallot, but in an individual patient, known risk factors can rarely be identified, even in retrospect.

Physiologically, obstruction to right ventricular outflow reduces pulmonary blood flow and diverts unoxygenated systemic venous blood through the VSD into the aorta. The extent of right-to-left shunting is dependent primarily on the degree of infundibular and pulmonary valve stenosis.

Physical examination reveals a child whose degree of cyanosis may vary from minimal to severe. The precordium is quiet, but with a predominately right ventricular impulse. The first heart sound is normal. The second heart sound is loud and single. The pulmonary component of the second heart sound is rarely heard. An aortic click may be present at the lower left sternal border due to ejection of blood from both ventricles into the dilated aorta. A grade III-IV systolic ejection murmur loudest at the mid-left sternal border is caused by turbulent blood flow through the narrowed right ventricular outflow tract. This murmur is much softer when blood flow is severely restricted as in infants with severe cyanosis or during a spell. Absence of the typical systolic murmur in a child who otherwise has typical features for tetralogy of Fallot suggests complete pulmonary atresia with pulmonary blood flow supplied by systemic collateral vessels. Right-to-left shunting through the ventricular septal defect does not produce any murmur.

Definite diagnosis is made by the 2-dimensional echocardiogram, which defines the large ventricular septal defect, a large aorta that overrides the interventricular septum and small pulmonary arteries. The chest x ray typically reveals decreased vascularity, a normal-sized heart with an uptilted apex, and a concave or absent pulmonary artery segment forming the "boot-shaped" heart. A right aortic arch is present in 25 percent of children with tetralogy of Fallot. The ECG demonstrates findings of right axis deviation and right ventricular hypertrophy. Cardiac catheterization is indicated prior to surgical correction to define the distribution of the coronary arteries, as coronary artery abnormalities are common in tetralogy of Fallot. Other structural features that need to be defined by cardiac catheterization include the structure of the pulmonary arteries (looking for branch pulmonary artery stenosis), and the anatomy of the interventricular septum including the presence of multiple ventricular septal defects.

The clinical manifestations of tetralogy constitute a spectrum. One-third of the patients are cyanotic as neonates, another third become cyanotic later in infancy, and the remainder—with so-called acyanotic tetralogy—are not cyanotic until later in childhood. Children in this last group often have signs of a left-to-right shunt through the VSD as infants.

Management is determined by the degree of hypoxia. Neonates with severe cyanosis require immediate intervention. Infusion of prostaglandin E1 provides transient palliation by dilating the ductus arteriosus. Infants presenting extremely early with severe hypoxia frequently have hypoplastic pulmonary arteries, which may be a contraindication to total correction. A surgical shunt may be constructed from the aorta to the pulmonary artery using the subclavian artery (Blalock-Taussig shunt) or by interposing a tubular piece of Gore-tex. The shunt procedure is only palliative and does not constitute complete correction; therefore, a subsequent surgical procedure is required to correct the cardiac abnormality. With improvement in surgical techniques, total correction of tetralogy of Fallot is now feasible in very small infants and in the absence of any major contraindications (e.g., coronary artery abnormality or extremely hypoplastic pulmonary arteries), and should be seriously considered as the first line surgical therapy.

In an infant whose cyanosis is less severe, the timing of surgical intervention is determined by the clinical course. Frequent measurements of the blood hematocrit provide an indication of the body's perception of oxygen deficit. Up to a point, an increase in hematocrit provides improved oxygen-carrying capacity and is beneficial. At hematocrits above 65, however, the blood viscosity increases markedly and the risk of neurologic sequelae (e.g., strokes and brain abscesses) outweighs the benefit of deferring surgical intervention. Spells may occur during periods of exercise or fever, or on arising in the morning. Clinically, a spell is expressed by hyperpnea and marked worsening of cyanosis, and is followed by a period of deep sleep. Although most spells are self-limited, they can be fatal. Recognition of a cyanotic spell requires an immediate response. Calming of the parents and child is always beneficial. The "knee-chest" position increases systemic resistance and increases then decreases systemic venous return. Additional treatment measures include administration of morphine, a beta-blocker (propranolol), an agent to increase systemic vascular resistance (phenylephrine, methoxamine), or sodium bicarbonate, if acidosis is demonstrated by blood gases. Administration of oxygen is probably of little benefit, since the pathophysiology is decreased pulmonary blood flow rather than pulmonary venous desaturation. Some children reach the age of 2 or 3 without encountering any of the clinical difficulties. In those children, elective surgical intervention should be scheduled after a complete cardiac catheterization to rule out any associated anomalies.

Review

1. Karp, R., and Kirklin, J. Tetralogy of Fallot. *Ann. Thorac. Surg.* 10:370, 1970.
   A lucid discussion of physiology and natural history.

Natural History

2. Van Praagh, R., et al. Tetralogy of Fallot: Underdevelopment of the pulmonary infundibulum and its sequelae. *Am. J. Cardiol.* 26:25, 1970.
   The "monology" theory.

3. Bonchek, L., et al. Natural history of tetralogy of Fallot in infancy: Clinical

classification and therapeutic implications. *Circulation* 48:392, 1973.
A system for classifying severity of right ventricular obstruction is presented.

4. Johnson, R., and Haworth, S. Pulmonary vascular and alveolar development in tetralogy of Fallot: A recommendation for early correction. *Thorax* 37:893, 1982.
Morphologic changes may be irreversible in symptomatic infants when surgery is delayed.

5. Maron, B., et al. Unusual evolution of acquired infundibular stenosis in patients with ventricular septal defect: Clinical and morphological observations. *Circulation* 48:1092, 1973.
Progressive infundibular hypertrophy microscopically similar to asymmetric septal hypertrophy in two cases of acyanotic tetralogy.

6. Naiman, J. Clotting and bleeding in cyanotic congenital heart disease. *J. Pediatr.* 76:333, 1970.
The nature of the coagulation defect is unclear.

7. Martelle, R., and Linde, L. Cerebrovascular accidents with tetralogy of Fallot. *Am. J. Dis. Child.* 101:206, 1961.
Cerebrovascular accidents in children under the age of 2 are related more to hypoxemia and episodes of dehydration than to polycythemia.

8. Clark, D. Brain abscess in congenital heart disease. *Clin. Neurosurg.* 14:274, 1966.
The differential diagnosis is outlined.

Medical Management

9. Garson, A., Gillette, P., and McNamara, D. Propranolol: The preferred palliation for tetralogy of Fallot. *Am. J. Cardiol.* 47:1098, 1981.
When successful relief of hypoxemic spells can be achieved, surgery can usually be postponed for a year or more.

10. Nudel, D., Berman, M., and Talner, N. Effects of acutely increasing systemic vascular resistance on oxygen tension in tetralogy of Fallot. *Pediatrics* 58:248, 1976.
The pharmacologic equivalent of squatting.

Surgical Management and Follow-up

11. Garson, A., et al. The surgical decision in tetralogy of Fallot: Weighing risks and benefits with decision analysis. *Am. J. Cardiol.* 45:108, 1980.
Discusses the rationale for avoiding palliative surgery.

12. McManus, B., et al. The case for preoperative coronary angiography in patients with tetralogy of Fallot and other complex congenital heart disease. *Am. Heart J.* 103:451, 1982.
Coronary anomalies are common and difficult to identify at surgery if not previously visualized at catheterization.

13. Kavey, R., Blackman, M., and Sondheimer, H. Incidence and severity of chronic ventricular dysrhythmias after repair of tetralogy of Fallot. *Am. Heart J.* 103:342, 1982.
Serious ventricular dysrhythmias seem to be common, but continuous monitoring or exercise testing may be required for detection. (For autopsy studies implicating ventricular dysrhythmias as cause of sudden death, see Circulation 67:626, 1983.)

14. Katz, N., et al. Late survival and symptoms after repair of tetralogy of Fallot. *Circulation* 65:403, 1982.
A series of more than 400 patients, showing acceptable surgical results in the great majority.

15. Taussig, H. Tetralogy of Fallot: Early history and late results. *AJR* 133:423, 1979.
The first survivors of surgical intervention reach middle age.

16. Garson, A., Williams, R., and Reckless, J. Long-term follow-up of patients with tetralogy of Fallot: Physical health and psychopathology. *J. Pediatr.* 85:429, 1974.
Like other children with chronic illness, those with tetralogy are subject to overprotection, frequent hospitalization, and social maladjustment.

52. TRANSPOSITION OF THE GREAT ARTERIES

Robert D. White and Jean S. Kan

Transposition of the great arteries is the most common congenital cardiac defect presenting with severe cyanosis in the newborn period. The structural abnormality is malposition of the aorta and pulmonary artery, with the aorta arising from the right ventricle and the pulmonary artery arising from the left ventricle. In contrast to the normal blood flow pattern in which the pulmonary and systemic circulation are in series, the two circulations are parallel to each other when the great arteries are transposed. Thus, unoxygenated blood flows from the systemic veins to the right atrium, to the right ventricle, and then back out to the systemic arteries through the aorta. Oxygenated pulmonary venous blood flows to the left atrium, left ventricle, and directly back to the lungs through the pulmonary artery. In the absence of some connection between the two circuits, this situation is incompatible with life. Two normal fetal structures—the foramen ovale and the ductus arteriosus—provide bidirectional shunting that is variably effective during the first few hours of life.

Severity of symptoms and the time of presentation may be modified by other coexisting cardiac defects. A ventricular septal defect, for example, provides a communication for mixing of systemic and pulmonary venous blood. In this situation cyanosis is less prominent, but if the ventricular septal defect is large, congestive heart failure is common. Pulmonic stenosis may be present along with the ventricular septal defect, preventing the development of congestive heart failure but exaggerating cyanosis because of limitation of pulmonary blood flow.

The association of ventricular inversion with transposition is referred to as "corrected transposition." This term implies a physiologically correct pathway for the blood flow rather than an anatomic correction. In this situation unoxygenated systemic venous return flows to the right atrium, which connects to the left ventricle and into the posteriorly positioned pulmonary artery. Oxygenated pulmonary venous return flows to the left atrium through the left sided tricuspid valve into the morphologic right ventricle and anteriorly into the aorta. The diagnosis of "corrected transposition" may not be suspected for several years unless there is an associated ventricular septal defect or insufficiency of the systemic AV valve related to an Ebstein malformation of the tricuspid valve.

Diagnosis of transposition of the great arteries is considered when an otherwise healthy well-developed newborn is cyanotic in the first 2 days of life. Respiratory systems may be completely absent or there may be mild tachypnea, but no dyspnea. Peripheral pulses are usually normal indicating a normal cardiac output. Diminished femoral pulses suggest the associated diagnosis of coarctation of the aorta, which occurs in 10 percent of infants with transposition and ventricular septal defect. Auscultation reveals a loud single second heart sound because of the anterior position of the aorta. The chest x ray may be normal in the immediate newborn period. As the pulmonary vascular resistance falls and the pulmonary blood flow increases, there is an increase in the pulmonary vascularity with a predominance of right-sided vascularity greater than on the left. The classic "egg-shaped" contour of the heart produced by absence of the pulmonary artery segment in the usual position is not uniformly seen. The electrocardiogram usually shows right ventricular hypertrophy; however, in the immediate newborn period this cannot always be distinguished from the normal right ventricular predominance. Two-dimensional echocardiography provides definitive diagnosis by identifying the anterior and rightward position of the aorta arising from the right ventricle. The posterior vessel arising from the left ventricle is shown to bifurcate to the right and left pulmonary artery branches.

Cardiac catheterization is both diagnostic and therapeutic for an infant with transposition. After diagnostic studies, a balloon-tipped catheter is introduced into the left atrium, and its position is confirmed by fluoroscopy. The balloon is inflated with dilute radiographic contrast media, then the catheter sharply tugged, resulting in rapid withdrawal of the inflated balloon from the left atrium to the junction of the right atrium and inferior vena cava. This procedure results in a tear in the atrial septum enlarging the foramen ovale into an atrial septal defect and allowing improved mixing of oxygenated and unoxygenated blood. In infants older than 1 month of age the Rashkind procedure is modified by initiating a cut in the atrial septum using a Sang Park knife-blade–tipped catheter, followed by the standard Rashkind balloon pull-through. Alternatively, surgical creation of an atrial septal defect (Blalock-Hanlon procedure) can be performed as a closed heart procedure.

Definitive surgical therapy should be anticipated early to avoid the long-term complications of hypoxia. For simple transposition without a ventricular septal defect, the standard surgical approach is redirection of the atrial blood by an intraatrial baffle, which directs systemic venous blood through the mitral valve and into the left ventricle and pulmonary venous blood into the tricuspid valve and right ventricle. The two surgical procedures for the atrial redirection are the Mustard procedure and the Senning procedure; the surgical techniques vary but not the ultimate physiology. Anatomic correction (arterial switch) is gaining in popularity. The Jatene procedure switches the connection of the aorta and pulmonary artery to the appropriate ventricles. Major limitations of the Jatene procedure are difficulties with reanastomosis of the coronary arteries to the newly created origin of the aorta and the need to prepare the left ventricle to be at a high pressure at the time of the surgery. In the presence of a large ventricular septal defect and pulmonary stenosis, the Rastelli operation is an alternative anatomic correction in which the blood from the left ventricle is directed through the ventricular septal defect and into the root of aorta, and a conduit is placed from the right ventricle into the main pulmonary artery.

The prognosis for an infant with transposition of the great arteries is improving with improved surgical techniques in small infants. Introduction of the Rashkind procedure in the mid-1960s resulted in an improvement in the 1-month survival from 10 to 95 percent. The surgical mortality at the time of the definitive surgical procedure is now in the range of 5 percent or less.

Natural History

1. Goor, D., and Edwards, J. The spectrum of transposition of the great arteries: With special reference to developmental anatomy of the conus. *Circulation* 48:406, 1973.
   An attempt to decipher the embryology.
2. Gallaher, M., Fyler, D., and Lindesmith, G. Transposition with intact ventricular septum: Its diagnosis and management in the small infant. *Am. J. Dis. Child.* 111:248, 1966.
   Cyanosis was present within 24 hours of life in 35 of 39.
3. Liebman, J., Cullman, L., and Belloc, N. Natural history of transposition of the great arteries: Anatomy and birth and death characteristics. *Circulation* 40:237, 1969.
   Before the introduction of corrective surgery, 90 percent of infants with this defect died in the first year. (For a more recent series, see Pediatrics *65:422, 1980.)*
4. Landtman, B., et al. Causes of death in transposition of the great arteries. *Acta Paediatr. Scand.* 64:785, 1975.
   An autopsy study that outlines many complications of transposition.
5. Newfeld, E., et al. Pulmonary vascular disease in complete transposition of the great arteries: A study of 200 patients. *Am. J. Cardiol.* 34:75, 1974.
   A large ventricular septal defect or patent ductus arteriosus reduces cyanosis but leads to serious pulmonary vascular disease, often in the first year.
6. Shaher, R., and Deuchar, D. Hematogenous brain abscess in cyanotic congenital heart disease. *Am. J. Med.* 52:349, 1972.
   This may become more common as a complication of transposition of the great vessels as longevity is increased.
7. Taylor, J. Transposition of the great arteries. *Arch. Dis. Child.* 59:4, 1984.
   A succinct, current review.

Atrial Septostomy

8. Rashkind, W., and Miller, W. Transposition of the great arteries: Results of palliation by balloon atrioseptostomy in thirty-one infants. *Circulation* 38:453, 1968.
   The Rashkind procedure described.

9. Park, S., et al. Blade atrial septostomy: Collaborative study. *Circulation* 66:258, 1982.
   Produced successful palliation for at least 6 months in 50 percent of infants.

Surgical Management and Follow-up
10. Pacifico, A., Stewart, R., and Bargeron, L. Repair of transposition of the great arteries with ventricular septal defect by an arterial switch operation. *Circulation* 68[Suppl. II]:49, 1983.
    Also described in Lancet 2:39, 1983.
11. Weldon, C., Hartman, A., and Kelly, J. Current management of transposition of the great arteries: Immediate septostomy, occasional prostaglandin infusion, and early Senning operations. *Ann. Thorac. Surg.* 36:10, 1983.
    Good description of management from diagnosis through correction.
12. Beerman, L., et al. Arrhythmias in transposition of the great arteries after the Mustard operation. *Am. J. Cardiol.* 51:1530, 1983.
    Seventy percent of children had evidence of dysrhythmia, but few were symptomatic.
13. Marx, G., et al. Transposition of the great arteries with intact ventricular septum: Results of Mustard and Senning operations in 123 consecutive patients. *J. Am. Coll. Cardiol.* 1:476, 1983.
    Early repair now compares very favorably with previous "staging" approach.
14. Graham. T. Hemodynamic residua and sequelae following intraatrial repair of transposition of the great arteries: A review. *Pediatr. Cardiol.* 2:203, 1982.
    Sequelae prevent these procedures from living up to their original billing as "total corrections."

53. PATENT DUCTUS ARTERIOSUS

Robert D. White and Jean S. Kan

The ductus arteriosus is an important structure in fetal life. Originating as part of the sixth aortic arch, it is a muscular conduit between the pulmonary artery and descending aorta and is equal in size to these vessels. Over 90 percent of the blood ejected by the right ventricle bypasses the fluid-filled lungs of the fetus, passing through the ductus arteriosus into the descending aorta. When the placental supply of oxygen is removed at birth, however, the ductus arteriosus constricts, permitting all the right ventricular output to perfuse the lungs for oxygen uptake.

The mechanisms responsible for constriction of the ductus arteriosus at birth are not fully understood. It is clear that the ductus is highly sensitive to changes in oxygen tension; the increase in arterial PO_2 that normally occurs after birth probably serves as the stimulus for ductal closure. How this response is mediated is less certain; it is likely that it is attributable to a complex interaction involving autonomic chemical mediators and nerves, prostaglandins, and the ductal musculature.

In most full-term infants the ductus is functionally closed within hours after birth, but anatomic obliteration does not occur until after the first week of life, and the ductus may reopen during this period. Failure of the ductus to close after birth (patent ductus arteriosus, or PDA) allows shunting of blood between the pulmonary and systemic circulations. Blood usually flows preferentially into the pulmonary circuit after birth because of its lower vascular resistance. The ductus may remain patent for a variety of reasons; hypoxia is probably the most common cause and accounts for the frequent association of PDA with the respiratory distress syndrome. Premature infants have a 15 to 20 percent incidence of PDA, and patients with intracardiac defects or the congenital rubella syndrome also have an increased incidence. Patent ductus arteriosus occurs in full-term infants without underlying heart or lung disease, but the incidence is low. Some of these cases are familial, caused by a defect in the ductus musculature or in its ability to respond to appropriate stimuli, but most are idiopathic.

Patent ductus arteriosus is usually diagnosed on the basis of a systolic ejection murmur at the lower left sternal border that radiates upward and laterally to the left chest. This murmur characteristically builds in a crescendo to the second heart sound and has a peculiar rough quality, referred to as "machinery-type" or "crunching." Infants with a widely patent ductus arteriosus and low pulmonary resistance have murmurs that "spill over" into diastole, in some cases becoming continuous. The runoff of blood from the aorta is considerable in such cases, producing jerky or "bounding" femoral pulses. Most full-term infants with PDA are asymptomatic, and the ECG, chest radiograph, and echocardiogram are frequently normal. Some infants in this group (the incidence is not clear) will experience spontaneous closure of the PDA, usually by 4 months of age; in the remainder, surgical ligation is indicated before 2 years of age, when the risks of pulmonary vascular disease, endocarditis, and the emotional sequelae of a surgical procedure begin to mount. A minority of full-term infants with PDA—perhaps 30 percent—become symptomatic, usually presenting after the first week of life with congestive heart failure. Chest radiographs in this group reveal cardiomegaly with prominent pulmonary vasculature, and the ECG and echocardiogram reflect right or biventricular hypertrophy with left atrial enlargement. Treatment with digitalis and diuretics often provides satisfactory improvement in the symptoms of congestive failure, but since spontaneous closure of the ductus is uncommon in full-term infants with heart failure, medical management in most cases is a prelude to surgical ligation.

The classic findings of PDA are frequently obscured by other medical problems. Premature infants, as mentioned earlier, have a 15 to 20 percent incidence of PDA; in this group, the murmur is usually confined to systole, and the rate of spontaneous closure approaches 80 percent in infants who survive the neonatal period. Prematures with respiratory distress syndrome (RDS) present special problems in diagnosis and management; the cardiac murmur may be soft or absent, and the only discernible symptom may be worsening of respiratory distress or failure to improve after the third day of life, expected with uncomplicated RDS. The diagnosis of PDA should be suspected when there is cardiomegaly on the chest roentgenogram or left atrial enlargement by echocardiogram; bounding pulses are also a valuable sign that PDA is present. Management of these critically ill infants with RDS and PDA is not yet satisfactory, as underscored by disagreement over the timing of and criteria for intervention. Vigorous but careful fluid restriction is essential, and some infants may also benefit from continuous positive airway pressure (CPAP) or assisted ventilation. Definitive therapy to close the ductus, either by surgery or the administration of indomethacin (a prostaglandin inhibitor), should be employed if clinical improvement is not rapid and sustained.

An additional source of diagnostic difficulty may be the presence of other congenital cardiac defects. The management and prognosis in these infants depends to a great extent on the nature of the associated defects; for example, the sytemic-pulmonary shunt of PDA may exacerbate congestive heart failure in an infant who already has increased pulmonary blood flow (e.g., because of ventricular septal defect), but it is essential for life in a cyanotic infant whose pulmonary blood flow is markedly diminished (e.g., because of pulmonary atresia), or in an infant with obstruction of the left side of the heart (e.g., hypoplastic left heart, aortic stenosis, coarctation of the aorta), in whom the systemic circulation depends on flow from the pulmonary artery through the ductus. Patency of the ductus in these newborns may be maintained by infusion of prostaglandin E1 until surgical intervention is possible.

Etiologic Factors

1. Jones, R., and Pickering, D. Persistent ductus arteriosus complicating the respiratory distress syndrome. *Arch. Dis. Child.* 52:274, 1977.
   For more of the natural history in prematures with RDS, see Pediatrics *57:347, 1976, and* N. Engl. J. Med. *287:473, 1972.*
2. Rudolph, A., et al. Hemodynamic basis for clinical manifestations of patent ductus arteriosus. *Am. Heart J.* 68:447, 1974.
   An excellent description of the pathophysiology.
3. Stevenson, J. Fluid administration in the association of patent ductus arteriosus complicating respiratory distress syndrome. *J. Pediatr.* 90:257, 1977.
   Excessive fluid administration was associated with the development of clinical signs of PDA. (Also see the commentary in the same issue, p. 262.)
4. Green, T., et al. Furosemide promotes patent ductus arteriosus in premature infants

with the respiratory distress syndrome. *N. Engl. J. Med.* 308:743, 1983.
Effect mediated by prostaglandins.

Diagnostic Aids

5. McGrath, R., et al. The silent ductus arteriosus. *J. Pediatr.* 93:110, 1978.
   Echocardiographic changes may precede the murmur by more than 24 hours.
6. Baden, M., and Kirks, D. Transient dilatation of the ductus arteriosus: The "ductus bump." *J. Pediatr.* 84:858, 1974.
   A radiographic "pearl," but more often seen as a normal variant than in infants with hemodynamically significant shunts.
7. Ellison, R., et al. Evaluation of the preterm infant for patent ductus arteriosus. *Pediatrics* 71:364, 1983.
   Outline of diagnostic scheme for infants without a murmur.
8. Allen, H., et al. Use of echocardiography in newborns with patent ductus arteriosus: A review. *Pediatr. Cardiol.* 3:65, 1982.
   Noninvasive studies now leave little to the imagination. (For echocardiographic series, see Pediatrics 72:864, 1983, and Arch. Dis. Child. 59:341, 1984.)

Management

9. Gersony, W., et al. Effects of indomethacin in premature infants with patent ductus arteriosus: Results of a collaborative study. *J. Pediatr.* 102:895, 1983.
   Control group had a 35 percent spontaneous closure rate; supportive care is often the only therapy needed.
10. Neal, W., and Mullett, M. Patent ductus arteriosus in premature infants: A review of current management. *Pediatr. Cardiol.* 3:59, 1982.
    Outlines the pros and cons of surgical and medical intervention. (Also see Pediatr. Clin. North Am. 29:1117, 1982.)
11. Zerella, J., et al. Indomethacin versus immediate ligation in the treatment of 82 newborns with patent ductus arteriosus. *J. Pediatr. Surg.* 18:835, 1983.
    The debate continues. (Also see Am. J. Dis. Child. 136:1005, 1982.)

54. RHEUMATIC FEVER
Kenneth B. Roberts

The incidence of rheumatic fever has declined over the past century in this country, but it has not been eliminated as a source of morbidity and mortality. Several authors have cautioned against complacency, pointing out that the major factors in the decrease appear to have been social and hygienic improvements and the prevention of recurrences.

Acute rheumatic fever is a nonsuppurative sequela of group A beta-hemolytic streptococcal pharyngitis, with onset 2–4 weeks after the acute infection; rheumatic fever does not develop following streptococcal skin infection (impetigo) (see Chap. 105). The incidence of rheumatic fever following untreated exudative streptococcal pharyngitis is 3 percent during epidemics, but under usual conditions in the community is much lower, 0.3 percent or less. School-age children are most frequently affected; the disorder is uncommon in infants under 3 years of age and exceedingly rare under the age of 18 months. Rheumatic fever is more common in the lower socioeconomic groups; this may be due largely to poorer access to medical care. Certain families seem to be at particular risk for the development of rheumatic fever, and patients who have had one bout of the disease are at great risk for another.

The exact pathogenesis of rheumatic fever is unknown, but persistence of streptococci appears to be necessary; eradication of the organism (as with penicillin therapy) greatly reduces the incidence.

Rheumatic fever generally presents in one of three ways: with the insidious development of carditis; with an acute, explosive onset of polyarthritis; or, least commonly, with chorea. The clinical findings may suggest a number of alternative diagnoses, including juvenile rheumatoid arthritis, systemic lupus erythematosus, serum sickness, sickle cell disease, viral pericarditis or myocarditis, leukemia, Henoch-Schönlein syndrome, or bacterial endocarditis.

Since there is no laboratory test specific for acute rheumatic fever, the diagnosis is based on guidelines proposed by T. Duckett Jones. The Jones criteria require evidence of a preceding streptococcal infection together with the presence either of two major criteria or of one major criterion and two minor criteria. The five major criteria are carditis, polyarthritis, erythema marginatum, subcutaneous nodules, and chorea. Evidence of carditis is provided by new murmurs, cardiomegaly (by physical examination or roentgenogram), pericarditis, or frank congestive heart failure; prolongation of the P-R interval by itself is not sufficient evidence and is considered a minor criterion. The polyarthritis of acute rheumatic fever is nearly always migratory and is objective arth*ritis*; arthralgia is not a major criterion. Erythema marginatum is an evanescent, pink rash with round margins and clear centers, without pruritus or induration; it is said not to occur on the face. Subcutaneous nodules develop on extensor surfaces of the limbs and in the occipital region; they are nontender and freely movable, and do not elicit a reaction in the overlying skin. Erythema marginatum and subcutaneous nodules are not specific for rheumatic fever and usually are not present unless the patient has carditis. Chorea is a feature of rheumatic fever that may occur up to 6 months after the initiating streptococcal infection and in the absence of other major manifestations of the disease.

The minor criteria are of two types, clinical and laboratory. The clinical criteria include arthralgia, fever, and a history of rheumatic fever or evidence of preexisting rheumatic heart disease. Laboratory criteria are increased erythrocyte sedimentation rate and the presence of C-reactive protein. Electrocardiographic changes, such as the P-R interval prolongation, are also minor criteria and, as noted, should not be used as the sole evidence for carditis.

Demonstration of the streptococcal infection is usually accomplished serologically, since most cases of rheumatic fever occur 2 to 4 weeks after acute infection, by which time the throat culture may be "negative." Antistreptolysin O (ASO) antibody titers are elevated in 80 to 85 percent of patients; measurement of antibodies against two additional extracellular products of the streptococcus (e.g., antihyaluronidase, anti-DNAase) permits identification of 95 percent of patients who have had a previous streptococcal infection.

Treatment is empirical and consists of the following: rest, to decrease demands on the myocardium and relieve joint pain; pharmacologic agents, to control inflammation; and antibiotics, to prevent the recurrence of streptococcal infections. Bed rest has not been studied scientifically but is recommended for children with severe carditis (by some authors for periods of up to 6 months); children with arthritis limit their activity themselves, according to the degree of joint inflammation. The anti-inflammatory agent used frequently is aspirin, with steroids reserved for patients with acute severe carditis. Treatment with penicillin should begin with the diagnosis and should be continued in a prophylactic regimen of monthly injections of benzathine penicillin; or, if compliance can be ensured, penicillin may be given twice daily by mouth.

It is said that rheumatic fever either "bites the heart and licks the joints" or the reverse. The prognosis for future heart disease is worse in patients with carditis during the initial episode, with a family history of rheumatic heart disease, or with repeated attacks, particularly in the first year after the acute disease. Chronic arthritis is not a sequela of rheumatic fever.

Prevention of rheumatic fever by antibiotic treatment of streptococcal pharyngitis is a limited approach, since in only one-third of patients in whom rheumatic fever develops is the preceding sore throat of sufficient symptomatic magnitude to cause the parents or the patient to seek medical attention. More specific strategies do not appear possible at present, however, since the pathogenesis of rheumatic fever remains obscure. Efforts to develop an effective streptococcal vaccine (that will not itself cause rheumatic fever) are in progress.

General

1. Markowitz, M., and Gordis, L. *Rheumatic Fever* (2nd ed.). Philadelphia: Saunders, 1972.
   Still the place to go for information about rheumatic fever.
2. Kaplan, E. Acute rheumatic fever. *Pediat. Clin. North Am.* 25:817, 1978.
   Good overview.
   Also see Streptococcal Infections, Chapter 105.

Diagnosis and Clinical Features

3. Jones criteria (revised) for guidance in the diagnosis of rheumatic fever. *Circulation* 32:664, 1954.
   The modification of the revision of the Jones criteria by a committee of the American Heart Association.
4. Burke, J. Erythema marginatum. *Arch. Dis. Child.* 30:359, 1955.
   Not specific for rheumatic fever, but when present in rheumatic fever, carditis is, too.
5. Aron, A., Freeman, J., and Carter, S. The natural history of Sydenham's chorea: Review of the literature and long-term evaluation with emphasis on cardiac sequelae. *Am. J. Med.* 38:83, 1965.
   In a long-term follow-up, 27 percent were found to have heart disease.
6. Feinstein, A., and Spagnuolo, M. The clinical patterns of acute rheumatic fever: A reappraisal. *Medicine* (Baltimore) 41:279, 1962.
   The frequency of various findings alone and in combination.
7. Mayer, F., et al. Declining severity of first attack of rheumatic fever. *Am. J. Dis. Child.* 105:146, 1963.
   The key observation is in the title; less severe disease or effect of treatment?
8. Taranta, A., and Moody, M. Diagnosis of streptococcal pharyngitis and rheumatic fever. *Pediatr. Clin. North Am.* 18:125, 1971.
   Discusses throat culture, serologic demonstration of streptococcal infection, tests of inflammatory state, heart antibody tests, and lymphocyte stimulation (78 references).
9. Vardi, P., et al. Clinical-echocardiographic correlations in acute rheumatic fever. *Pediatrics* 71:830, 1983.
   Echocardiography distinguishes valvular incompetence from myocardial failure.

Epidemiology

10. Rosenthal, A., Czoniczer, G., and Massell, B. Rheumatic fever under 3 years of age. *Pediatrics* 41:612, 1968.
    Rare in infants (the youngest patient of 1926 seen by this group was 18 months old).
11. Denny, F., et al. Prevention of rheumatic fever: Treatment of the preceding streptococcal infection. *J.A.M.A.* 143:151, 1950.
    The classic; a 3 percent attack rate under epidemic conditions was reduced by penicillin treatment of pharyngitis.
12. Seigel, A., Johnson, E., and Stollerman, G. Controlled studies of streptococcal pharyngitis in a pediatric population: 1. Factors related to the attack rate of rheumatic fever. *N. Engl. J. Med.* 265:559, 1961.
    The attack rate was much less than 3 percent in a pediatric walk-in clinic. However, the attack rate was 3 percent when the authors retrospectively identified the group comparable to that in reference 11. The attack rate was even lower in untreated asymptomatic children (Public Health Rep. 71:745, 1956).
13. Land, M., and Bisno, A. Acute rheumatic fever. *J.A.M.A.* 249:895, 1983.
    Survey in Memphis, 1977–1981, justifies subtitle, "A vanishing disease in suburbia"; implications discussed.

Pathogenesis

14. Wannamaker, L. Differences between streptococcal infections of the throat and of the skin. *N. Engl. J. Med.* 282:23,78, 1970.
    Rheumatic fever results only from throat infection.
15. Wannamaker, L. The chain that links the heart to the throat. *Circulation* 48:9, 1973.
    A discussion of what is—and what is not—known about the pathogenesis. (Also see Rev. Infect. Dis. 1:988, 1979.*)*

Prevention

16. Kaplan, E., et al. Prevention of rheumatic fever. *Circulation* 55:S-1, 1977.
    American Heart Association review and recommendations.
17. Catanzaro, F., et al. The role of the streptococcus in the pathogenesis of rheumatic fever. *Am. J. Med.* 17:749, 1954.
    The persistence of the streptococcus is the key factor; rheumatic fever can still be prevented even if the onset of penicillin therapy is delayed 9 days.
18. Krause, R. Prevention of streptococcal sequelae by penicillin prophylaxis: A reas-

sessment *J. Infect. Dis.* 131:592, 1975.
A thoughtful review of the data.
19. Markowitz, M. Eradication of rheumatic fever: An unfulfilled hope. *Circulation* 41:1077, 1970.
    The obstacles to eradication are discussed.
20. Spagnuolo, M., Pasternack, B., and Taranta, A. Risk of rheumatic-fever recurrences after streptococcal infections. *N. Engl. J. Med.* 285:641, 1971.
    The significant factors in this prospective study were symptomatic pharyngitis, young age, short interval since the preceding rheumatic attack, existing rheumatic heart disease, number of previous attacks, and oral (rather than parenteral) administration of drug prophylaxis. (Parenteral benzathine penicillin does not appear to provide protection for a full month: Pediatrics *69:452, 1982, and 73:530, 1984.)*

Treatment and Prognosis
21. Combined Rheumatic Fever Study Group. A comparison of short-term, intensive prednisone and acetyl-salicylic acid therapy in the treatment of acute rheumatic fever. *N. Engl. J. Med.* 272:63, 1965.
    Neither consistently terminated the clinical attack; no differences in 1-year follow-up. Recommends acetylsalicylic acid for the treatment of arthritis, but notes a clinical "impression . . . that steroids were useful in controlling the exudative phase of acute severe myocarditis in critically ill patients." (In a larger series, the same conclusions were reached: Circulation *11:343, 1955, or* Br. Med. J. *1:555, 1955; see reference 22.)*
22. Rheumatic Fever Working Party of the Medical Research Council of Great Britain and the Subcommittee of Principal Investigators of the American Council on Rheumatic Fever and Congenital Heart Disease, American Heart Association. The natural history of rheumatic fever and rheumatic heart disease: Ten-year report of a cooperative clinical trial of ACTH, cortisone and aspirin. *Circulation* 32:457, 1965.
    In this series of 497 patients, ACTH, cortisone, and aspirin were still equivalent. The most powerful predictor of rheumatic heart disease is the severity of heart involvement during the acute episode. (A shorter-term follow-up of patients receiving prophylaxis reached the same conclusion: Am. Heart. J. *68:817, 1964,* Circulation *45:543, 1972.)*

55. HYPERTENSION
Margaret E. Mohrmann

Although long recognized as a major cause of morbidity and mortality among adults, hypertension has often been overlooked by physicians who care for children, except in instances of severe blood pressure elevation associated with conditions such as renal disease. Increased attention to the preventive aspects of the therapy of adult hypertension has led to an awareness of the occurrence both of risk factors and of hypertension itself in children.

It is currently recommended that all children 3 years old and over have a blood pressure measurement annually; obtaining an accurate reading may be difficult, however, especially in the young child. The Doppler method most closely approximates true intraarterial pressure but requires relatively sophisticated equipment. Auscultation, using the sphygmomanometer, is the usual method and is the basis for tables of normal values. It is essential that the cuff be of an appropriate size for the child, with the width at least two-thirds the distance from elbow to axilla, and bladder length adequate to encircle the arm snugly. Cuff size must be given special attention when an obese child is examined; a cuff that is too narrow or too loose will give a falsely high pressure reading. The child being examined should be relaxed, and the pressure should be taken with the child seated with the arm raised to the level of the heart. In children in whom the blood pressure is elevated, readings should also be taken in the legs. The first Korotkoff sound is recorded as the systolic pressure; American Heart Association recommendations and most tables of normal values use the fourth sound (muffle) as the diastolic reading.

In adults, hypertension is usually defined as blood pressure over 140/90 mm Hg, a level that is too high for accurate detection of hypertension in children. Accordingly, hypertension in persons under the age of 18 years is defined as a blood pressure higher than the 95th percentile for age, observed on at least three separate occasions. By using this standard, studies have identified 1 to 3 percent of children in the United States as having persistent hypertension; there are no significant variations in incidence related to race or sex.

The relative incidence of primary and secondary hypertension in children vary both with the definition and with the severity of the hypertension. In studies that define hypertension as blood pressure higher than 140/90 mm Hg, or that are based on referred patients or on selected children with symptoms or signs of high blood pressure (headache, dizziness, nausea, fundal changes), it is usually found that over 80 percent of the study group have secondary hypertension. The great majority of these children (at least 80%) have renal or renovascular disease; the cause of hypertension in the remainder may be any of numerous disease states, such as coarctation of the aorta and Cushing syndrome.

In studies that define hypertension as three readings above the 95th percentile and that are based on routine screening of large numbers of unselected children, it is found that as many as 95 percent of affected children have primary (idiopathic, essential) hypertension, a proportion similar to that in hypertensive adults. In searching for factors related to the development of primary hypertension, epidemiologic surveys have shown marked familial and cultural influences on blood pressure. Some studies have attempted to link either high salt intake or obesity with primary hypertension, but no firm causal relationship has been proved for either.

The evaluation of the child with hypertension must include a thorough history; especially important points in the family history are the presence of parental hypertension and the occurrence of hypertension, stroke, myocardial infarction, or unexplained uremia in relatives less than 50 years old. A complete physical examination may disclose evidence of the cause of the hypertension (e.g., weak femoral pulses because of coarctation, abdominal bruit from renal artery stenosis) or signs of the chronicity and severity of the disease (target-organ damage, such as retinal vessel changes; growth disturbances).

There is much controversy concerning the extent to which further diagnostic studies should be carried out. It is generally agreed that a child who is hypertensive should have a urinalysis, and hemoglobin (or hematocrit), blood urea nitrogen, and serum creatinine should be determined. An echocardiogram is the most sensitive test available for detecting cardiac hypertrophy due to hypertension and should be performed both to assess existing target organ damage and to provide a baseline for monitoring the development of later changes. A decision to proceed beyond this point in the workup will depend on many factors. In general, an adolescent with a mild elevation of pressure and a positive family history probably needs no further investigation. On the other hand, a child with marked hypertension, or symptoms or signs of high pressure, or both, is more likely to have secondary hypertension and therefore should be evaluated extensively for a treatable cause. Some would include in the latter category any child less than 10 years old at the time of diagnosis. In the absence of clinical clues to the contrary, further investigation is primarily directed toward detection of a renal cause, with the initial step being rapid-sequence intravenous pyelography; additional studies may include a renal scan, arteriography, determination of peripheral or renal vein renin levels, and, in some cases, renal biopsy.

Assuming that a treatable cause, like coarctation of the aorta, is not found, the next questions are whether and how to institute treatment. There is little argument that the child or adolescent should be encouraged to lose weight if obese, decrease salt intake, exercise, and avoid substances that may exacerbate hypertension, such as contraceptives.

In debating the use of antihypertensive drugs, the presumed risk of vascular damage—a risk that depends on a myriad of known and unknown factors, including level and lability of pressure, age, sex, race, and family history—must be weighed against the toxic and psychological effects of chronic drug therapy in a child or adolescent. If the decision is made to use drug therapy, the current recommendation is that a diuretic be tried first; the second step is the addition of either propranolol or methyldopa (both of which are renin-lowering drugs), followed by the addition of a vasodilator, such as hydralazine, as needed. The child whose hypertension cannot be controlled by these measures may be treated successfully with more "potent" antihypertensive agents, such as minoxidil (a vasodilator) or captopril (an angiotensin II–converting enzyme inhibitor).

Acute hypertensive crises, which may occur either in the course of chronic hypertension or as the initial presentation of a disease such as acute glomerulonephritis, are life-threatening episodes characterized by the rapid development of signs of arteriolar spasm and resultant organ damage, including encephalopathy, retinopathy, renal failure, and left ventricular failure. Immediate treatment is essential. Intramuscular reserpine and hydralazine have been used but may take up to 3 hours to produce a hypotensive effect; intravenous vasodilators, specifically diazoxide and sodium nitroprusside, act within 1 to 2 minutes to effect a dramatic fall in blood pressure. A potentially serious side effect of frequent bolus administration of diazoxide is the development of marked hyperglycemia; cyanide poisoning may result from long-term use of nitroprusside.

There is little information available on the natural history of hypertension in children and adolescents; thus, a discussion of prognosis is necessarily limited. It is estimated that one-third of untreated hypertensive children will become normotensive, one-third will not change significantly, and one-third will have progression of disease, with increasing blood pressures and target-organ damage; it is by no means certain that these proportions are ultimately altered by present modes of therapy. Studies in adults have shown that drug therapy of significant hypertension (diastolic blood pressure of 105 mm Hg or greater) reduces the incidence of cardiovascular disease, including stroke. Whether or not treatment of hypertension in children will change the incidence of hypertension or its complications in adults remains to be seen. The pediatrician's role may well lie in the prevention of hypertension by manipulation of dietary and environmental factors in an identifiable at-risk population of children.

Reviews
1. Inglefinger, J. *Pediatric Hypertension*. Philadelphia: Saunders, 1982.
   Well-written, well-referenced, and complete.
2. Report of the Task Force on Blood Pressure in Children. National Heart, Lung, and Blood Institute. *Pediatrics* 59[Suppl.]:797, 1977.
   Information concerning screening, evaluation, and management that should be required reading for all involved in the primary health care of children. (For discussion of the controversy over "normal" BP values, see Pediatrics *68:268, 1981, and 70:143, 1982.)*
3. Goldring, D., and Hernandez, A. Hypertension in children. *Pediatr. Rev.* 3:235, 1982.
   A thorough, balanced review.
4. Loggie, J. (ed.). Symposium on hypertension in childhood and adolescence. *Pediatr. Clin. North Am.* 25(1), 1978.
   Both general and specific aspects are covered in 16 articles.
5. Loggie, J., New, M., and Robson, A. Hypertension in the pediatric patient: A reappraisal. *J. Pediatr.* 94:685, 1979.
   A thoughtful, detailed discussion of the many areas of controversy and inadequate knowledge concerning childhood hypertension. (For the summary of a recent state of the art conference, see J. Pediatr. *104:657, 1984.)*
6. Lieberman, E. Essential hypertension in children and youth: A pediatric perspective. *J. Pediatr.* 85:1, 1974.
   A good delineation of the problem; emphasis on early identification and prevention. (For a more detailed review by the same author, see Curr. Probl. Pediatr. *10(4), 1980.)*
7. Loggie, J., and Rauh, L. Persistent systemic hypertension in the adolescent. *Med. Clin. North Am.* 59:1371, 1975.
   A reasonable approach to hypertensive teenagers.
8. Steinfeld. L., et al. Sphygmomanometry in the pediatric patient. *J. Pediatr.* 92:934, 1978.
   A critical look at the problems in obtaining accurate blood pressure readings in children by indirect measurement.

Series

9. Londe, S. Blood pressure in children as determined under office conditions. *Clin. Pediatr.* (Phila.) 5:71, 1966.
   An important paper for two reasons: (1) It is the first study demonstrating the feasibility of blood pressure surveys in children, and (2) it presents the first set of normal blood pressure reference tables for children.
10. deSwiet, M., Fayers, P., and Shinebourne, E. Systolic blood pressure in a population of infants in the first year of life: The Brompton study. *Pediatrics* 65:1028, 1980.
    Normal values for infants; the percentile values at 6 weeks of age and older are similar to those at 2 years of age, as established by other studies.
11. Rames, L., et al. Normal blood pressures and the evaluation of sustained blood pressure elevation in childhood: The Muscatine study. *Pediatrics* 61:245, 1978.
    Of more than 6000 schoolchildren studied, fewer than 1 percent had persistent pressure elevation, a finding corroborated by the Minneapolis study (Am. Heart J. 105:316, 1983). The authors emphasize the importance of repeated measurements in the context of continuing pediatric care rather than mass screening efforts. (Similar conclusions from a more recent study: Pediatrics 72:459, 1983.)
12. Goldring, D., et al. Blood pressure in a high school population. *J. Pediatr.* 91:884, 1977.
    Normative data derived from examination of 7000 adolescents.
13. Voors, A., et al. Body height and body mass as determinants of basal blood pressure in children: The Bogalusa heart study. *Am. J. Epidemiol.* 106:101, 1977.
    Blood pressure norms correlate more closely with height and a weight/height index than with age.
14. Londe, S. Blood pressure in black and in white children. *J. Pediatr.* 90:93, 1977.
    Studies in large numbers of children (aged 3–14 years) revealed no racial differences in blood pressure.

Pathogenesis and Evaluation

15. Bailie, M., and Mattioli, L. Hypertension: Relationships between pathophysiology and therapy. *J. Pediatr.* 96:789, 1980.
    A lucid and concise explanation of current understanding of the pathogenesis and perpetuation of various types of hypertension.
16. Kaplan, M., and Hernandez, L. The pathogenesis and diagnosis of hypertension in children. *Pediatr. Ann.* 11:592, 1982.
    A well-written review of the physiology of blood pressure regulation and of a logical approach to evaluation of the hypertensive child.
17. Childs, B. Causes of essential hypertension. *Prog. Med. Genet.* 5:1, 1983.
    A very readable, detailed review of investigations to date into the factors predisposing persons to the development of primary hypertension.
18. Zinner, S., et al. Familial aggregation of blood pressure in childhood. *N. Engl. J. Med.* 284:401, 1971.
    Statistics showing definite familial influence, established early in life.
19. Gill, D., et al. Analysis of 100 children with severe and persistent hypertension. *Arch. Dis. Child.* 51:951, 1976.
    Renal disease was present in 83. (For information on the utility of various diagnostic studies in the detection of a renal or renovascular cause, see Pediatr. Clin. North Am. 23:795, 1976.)
20. Oberfield, S., Levine, L., and New, M. Childhood hypertension due to adrenocortical disorders. *Pediatr. Ann.* 11:623, 1982.
    Brief discussion of hyperaldosteronism and types of congenital adrenal hyperplasia associated with hypertension. (Pheochromocytoma: N. Engl. J. Med. 311:1298, 1984.)

Therapy

21. Gillum, R., et al. Nonpharmacologic therapy of hypertension: The independent effects of weight reduction and sodium restriction in overweight borderline hypertensive patients. *Am. Heart J.* 105:128, 1983.
    The effects are independent, additive, and significant.

22. Fixler, D., et al. Response of hypertensive adolescents to dynamic and isometric exercise stress. *Pediatrics* 64:579, 1979.
    This article and an accompanying editorial comment (p. 593) consider the risk of exercise for the hypertensive teenager and the possibility of assessing that risk in individual patients. (Exercise training can significantly reduce blood pressure in adolescents, although not to normal levels: Am. J. Cardiol. 52:763, 1983.)

23. Pruitt, A. Pharmacologic approach to the management of childhood hypertension. *Pediatr. Clin. North Am.* 28:135, 1981.
    Reviews several drugs. (Also see Pediatr. Ann. 11:604, 1982, for helpful, practical information about many of the antihypertensive agents used in children.)

24. Bailie, M., Linshaw, M., and Stygles, V. Diuretic pharmacology in infants and children. *Pediatr. Clin. North Am.* 28:217, 1981.
    A good general discussion.

25. Frishman, W. β-adrenoceptor antagonists: New drugs and new indications. *N. Engl. J. Med.* 305:500, 1981.
    A review of the similarities and differences among propranolol and five newer drugs.

26. Pettinger, W. Minoxidil and the treatment of severe hypertension. *N. Engl. J. Med.* 303:922, 1980.
    A review of the drug's pharmacologic properties. Its use in six children is reported in J. Pediatr. 90:813, 1977; the major problems were fluid retention and hirsutism.

27. Hymes, L., and Warshaw, B. Captopril. *Am. J. Dis. Child.* 137:263, 1983.
    A report of five patients and a brief discussion of the drug's characteristics (also see N. Engl. J. Med. 306:214, 1982) and utility in children; the references include other reports of its use in children and neonates.

28. Koch-Weser, J. Hypertensive emergencies. *N. Engl. J. Med.* 290:211, 1974.
    A brief review; drugs and warnings.

29. McLaine, P., and Drummond, K. Intravenous diazoxide for severe hypertension in childhood. *J. Pediatr.* 79:829, 1971.
    The drug was administered to 17 children (188 doses) with good results in all. The authors consider it the drug of choice in such cases.

30. Gordillo-Paniagua, G., et al. Sodium nitroprusside treatment of severe arterial hypertension in children. *J. Pediatr.* 87:799, 1975.
    The treatment produced good results in 20 children (all with renal disease), usually within 5 minutes and with no undesirable side effects. (For a good review of this drug, see Ann. Intern. Med. 91:752, 1979.)

V. RESPIRATORY DISORDERS

56. UPPER RESPIRATORY INFECTION
Kenneth B. Roberts

The upper respiratory tract is the most frequent site of infection in children. Thirty years ago, in a large study in Cleveland, Ohio, it was determined on the basis of weekly home visits that children in the first 5 years of life have between seven and nine upper respiratory tract infections (URIs) per year. Clinical illness after exposure is 2 to 3 times more likely to develop in infants than in older children or adults; this increased susceptibility is only partly explained by lack of previous exposure and immunity. Despite folklore to the contrary, chilling does not predispose to the development of disease. What is important is close contact with infected persons, specifically with their contaminated nasopharyngeal secretions. Although secretions rapidly lose their infectivity if permitted to dry or if trapped in a cotton handkerchief or paper tissue, they can remain infectious for hours or days on skin, nylon, and such surfaces as stainless steel and Formica. Once the fingers of a susceptible person are contaminated, virus is transferred to the nose or conjunctiva, resulting in infection and then disease. Illness occurs once per four to five exposures in older children and adults and once per one to two exposures in infants.

It is difficult to identify the onset of a URI, since the first symptom is often just a feeling of congestion or tightness in the upper part of the nose or a sensation of rawness in the nasopharynx; many people are convinced that a favorite remedy can abort a full-blown cold if taken during this early stage (lactose capsules used as placebos are so touted by 35% of experimental subjects). The infection is more easily recognized as sneezing and rhinorrhea become prominent. The volume of nasal secretions increases and may reach 100 times the normal quantity. The nasal secretions thicken, and the patient experiences malaise and, often, shivering, despite the absence of significant fever. Most people shed a large amount of virus early in the disease; symptoms persist, however, until the damaged nasal mucosa is "healed" by regeneration of cells.

The laboratory is of no help in establishing the diagnosis of URI acutely, although it may be possible to confirm the presence of rhinovirus. In the incubation period an increased number of lymphocytes may be present in the circulation, and during the illness the erythrocyte sedimentation rate is transiently elevated in approximately one-third of patients. The single most dependable indicator of URI is the presence of nasal discharge. In clinical practice it is often difficult to differentiate URI from allergy; the pattern of illness over time rather than the symptoms during any particular episode may help distinguish the two conditions. If rhinorrhea becomes chronic, particularly if it is purulent, the possibility of sinusitis should be considered.

Treatment is empirical—and inadequate—and folk remedies abound; $600 million is spent annually in the United States on medicines to alleviate the morbidity of URIs. After many studies it appears that vitamin C has neither prophylactic nor therapeutic value; the role of antihistamines, decongestants, and antitussives remains unclear. Antibiotics do not offer benefit in the uncomplicated viral URI; antiviral and immunologic approaches are currently under investigation.

The tonsils and adenoids are frequently (falsely) incriminated as responsible for the multiple episodes of upper respiratory tract illness in children. Tonsils and adenoids are part of the lymphoid system that surrounds the pharynx known collectively as Waldeyer's ring. The tonsils are involved in both humoral (IgA) and cell-mediated immunity and may play a role in immune surveillance against malignancy. Like other lymphoid tissue in the body, the growth rate of the tonsils and adenoids in the first 10 to 12 years of life exceeds that of general somatic growth; the tonsils and adenoids therefore appear particularly large in children. Rarely, the upper airway may be sufficiently obstructed to produce chronic pulmonary changes and cor pulmonale. Controlled studies have not demonstrated a reduction in total respiratory illness or upper respiratory tract infections associated with removal of tonsils and adenoids, but it does appear that the complaint of frequent sore throats is reduced (particularly if sore throat, tonsillitis, and cervical adenitis are lumped together). Children whose tonsils have been removed have fewer streptococcal infections of the oropharynx, but these children have a higher incidence of streptococcus-positive nasopharyngeal cultures than do nontonsillectomized children; attempting to document the presence of streptococci in children after the tonsils and adenoids are removed, then, may require both a nasopharyngeal and a throat culture.

189

Peritonsillar abscess, or quinsy, is commonly considered an indication for tonsillectomy; some otolaryngologists remove the tonsils only if quinsy is recurrent. Children with chronic otitis media and eustachian tube obstruction may benefit from adenoidectomy; tonsillectomy does not appear to contribute to the improvement, and at present it is not clear what the relative roles of tympanostomy tube insertion and adenoidectomy should be (see Chap. 57).

One million adenotonsillectomies are performed annually in the United States. Although adenotonsillectomy is generally considered a "benign procedure," the data suggest otherwise. The mortality is 1 per 16,000 operations; one-third of the deaths are due to hemorrhage, one-third to cardiopulmonary arrest, and one-third to a reaction to anesthesia. Bleeding sufficient to require carotid artery ligation or more than four transfusions occurs at a rate of 1 per 2400 operations. Currently, the indications commonly used to perform adenotonsillectomy are being questioned; studies are under way to provide guidelines for appropriate use of this operation.

Review
1. Andrewes, C. *The Common Cold.* London: Weidenfeld and Nicolson, 1965.
   A journalistic review of "colds" and the investigations of the Common Cold Research Unit, Salisbury, England (much the same ground in greater detail in D. Tyrell, Common Colds and Related Disease. *Baltimore: Williams & Wilkins, 1965).*

Epidemiology
2. Badger, G., et al. A study of illness in a group of Cleveland families: II. Incidence of the common respiratory diseases. *Am. J. Hyg.* 58:31, 1953.
   The epidemiology of over 4000 illnesses as ascertained by diaries and weekly home visits (more recent study, JAMA 227:164, 1974).
3. Fox, J., Cooney, M., and Hall, C. The Seattle Virus Watch: V. Epidemiologic observations of rhinovirus infections, 1965–1969, in families with young children. *Am. J. Epidemiol.* 101:122, 1975.
   The characteristics of a likely spreader: father with clinical illness, shedding viruses of certain strains; infants are likely recipients.
4. Monto, A. A community study of respiratory infections in the tropics: III. Introduction and transmission of infections within families. *Am. J. Epidemiol.* 88:69, 1968.
   Explores the cause for the increased frequency of infections in crowded households.
5. Strangert, K. Respiratory illness in preschool children with different forms of day care. *Pediatrics* 57:191, 1976.
   Exposing a child to other children is associated with an increased number of infections, but the maximal effect occurs with 4 to 6 children.

"Catching (a) Cold"
6. Dowling, H. Transmission of the common cold to volunteers under controlled conditions: III. The effect of chilling of the subjects upon susceptibility. *Am. J. Hyg.* 68:59, 1958.
   No effect using "infected secretions" (confirmed using rhinovirus: N. Engl. J. Med. 279:742, 1968); a good discussion of why colds are more prevalent in the cold months.
7. Hendley, J., Wenzel, R., and Gwaltney, J. Transmission of rhinovirus colds by self-inoculation. *N. Engl. J. Med.* 288:1361, 1973.
   Contains data on how often infected fingers enter the noses of grand round attendees!
8. Gwaltney, J., Moskalski, P., and Hendley, J. Hand-to-hand transmission of rhinovirus colds. *Ann. Intern. Med.* 88:463, 1978.
   Direct contact was more efficient than aerosols as means of transmitting rhinovirus.
9. Gwaltney, J., and Hendley, J. Rhinovirus transmission: One if by air, two if by hand. *Am. J. Epidemiol.* 107:357, 1978.
   Summarizes the work by this group and others regarding mode of transmission, aerosol versus contact.
10. D'Alessio, D., et al. Transmission of experimental rhinovirus colds in volunteer married couples. *J. Infect. Dis.* 133:28, 1976.
   It took prolonged exposure for a person with virus on the fingers to transmit a URI to the spouse.

Clinical Course

11. Jackson, G., et al. Transmission of the common cold to volunteers under controlled conditions: I. The common cold as a clinical entity. *Arch. Intern. Med.* 101:267, 1958.
    Clinical description and development of "symptom score."
12. Douglas, R. Pathogenesis of rhinovirus common cold in human volunteers. *Ann. Otol. Rhinol. Laryngol.* 79:563, 1970.
    An overview, based largely on the author's studies; relationship of symptoms to viral shedding and host responses.

Remedies

13. Stanley, E., et al. Increased virus shedding with aspirin treatment of rhinovirus infection. *JAMA* 231:1248, 1975.
    Acetylsalicylic acid given prior to inoculation; questions and answers in letters to the editor: JAMA 235:801, 1976.
14. Oral cold remedies. *Med. Lett. Drugs Ther.* 17:89, 1975.
    The Medical Letter does not sound impressed (table of ingredients in various preparations are given).
15. Soyka, L., et al. The misuse of antibiotics for treatment of upper respiratory tract infections in children. *Pediatrics* 55:552, 1975.
    A brief overview, exhorting against the use of antibiotics.
16. Laropert, R., Robinson, D., and Soyka, L. A critical look at oral decongestants, *Pediatrics* 55:550, 1975.
    Brief; more of a critical look than a critical analysis.
17. West, S., et al. A review of antihistamines and the common cold. *Pediatrics* 56:100, 1975.
    An analysis of 35 studies for scientific merit.
18. Randall, J., and Hendley, J. A decongestant antihistamine mixture in the prevention of otitis media in children with colds. *Pediatrics* 63:483, 1979.
    Didn't work.
19. Segal, S., et al. Use of codeine and dextromethorphan-containing cough syrups in pediatrics. *Pediatrics* 62:118, 1978.
    The AAP Committee on Drugs reviews cough as a sign, indications and contraindications to antitussive drugs, and the drugs themselves. (Expectorants briefly reviewed: JAMA 236:193, 1976.)
20. Chalmers, T. Effects of ascorbic acid on the common cold: An evaluation of the evidence. *Am. J. Med.* 58:532, 1975.
    A critical review of 14 trials, 1942–1974, with a note that one of the recent blind studies in favor of vitamin C turned out not to be so blind after all (JAMA 231:1038, 1975). For other therapeutic approaches, see Am. J. Epidemiol. 103:345, 1976 (rhinovirus vaccine); Lancet 1:382, 1976 (levamisole); Practitioner 216:341, 1976 (bacterial vaccine); N. Engl. J. Med. 291:57, 1974 (interferon); and—this one's for you, Mom—Chest 74:408, 1978 (chicken soup).

Differential Diagnosis/Complications

21. Furukawa, C., Shapiro, G., and Rachelefsky, G. Children with sinusitis. *Pediatrics* 71:133, 1983.
    A brief editorial: URI, allergy, or sinusitis?
22. Fagin, J., Friedman, R., and Fireman, P. Allergic rhinitis. *Pediatr. Clin. North Am.* 28:797, 1981.
    A consideration of allergic rhinitis, eosinophilic nonallergic rhinitis, and vasomotor rhinitis.
23. Wald, E., et al. Sinusitis and its complications in the pediatric patient. *Pediatr. Clin. North Am.* 28:777, 1981.
    An excellent review, from embryology to complications, including orbital and intracranial.
    Also see Otitis Media, Chapter 57.

Tonsils and Adenoids

24. Paradise, J., et al. Efficacy of tonsillectomy for recurrent throat infection in severely affected children. *N. Engl. J. Med.* 310:674, 1984.

With summary editorial (p. 717), "Tonsillectomy: justified but not mandated in special patients."

57. OTITIS MEDIA
Kenneth B. Roberts

Otitis media is one of the most common infections in infants and children. Although suppurative complications, such as mastoiditis and brain abscess, are no longer frequent, chronic middle ear disease with attendant hearing loss is a problem of considerable magnitude and importance and has recently begun to receive the research interest and attention it merits.

The functional state of the eustachian tube appears central in the development and in the resolution of middle ear disease. Normally, the eustachian tube (1) protects the middle ear from infected nasopharyngeal secretions, (2) permits drainage of fluid into the nasopharynx, and (3) ventilates and equilibrates pressure in the middle ear. If edema or perhaps lymphoid hyperplasia occludes the patency of the eustachian tube, negative pressure in the middle ear produces a transudation of fluid, resulting in serous otitis media. Nasopharyngeal flora, which colonizes the medial portion but does not normally reach the middle ear, may be "trapped" distal to the obstruction. If an organism is able to proliferate in the transudate despite the multiple defenses of the middle ear, acute suppurative otitis media results. Although the organisms originate in the nasopharynx, studies have failed to demonstrate a precise correlation between nasopharyngeal cultures and middle ear aspirates.

The pathogen most frequently responsible for acute suppurative otitis media after the neonatal period is the pneumococcus, accounting for approximately 40 percent of cases. The clinical correlates of pneumococcal infection are high fever and pronounced pain. Many otitis-prone children are noted to have had pneumococcal otitis in the first year of life. Under the age of 5 years, the second most common pathogen is untypable *Haemophilus influenzae;* thereafter, otitis is less frequently caused by this organism, but it remains a cause to consider when selecting treatment. During the school years, the group A streptococcus must also be considered. Fully one-fourth of the aspirates of middle ear exudates are sterile; attempts to demonstrate viruses or *Mycoplasma* have generally been unsuccessful.

The symptoms of acute suppurative otitis media are nonspecific. Fever and ear pain suggest the diagnosis but are present in less than half the patients. Older children may complain of a sense of fullness rather than, or in addition to, pain. The most frequent symptoms, irritability and rhinorrhea, are also the most nonspecific, and examination of the tympanic membranes is required to establish the diagnosis. Injection of the eardrum by itself is not a valid sign of otitis media; more valuable findings are the loss of the light reflex and landmarks, bulging of the pars tensa and pars flaccida, and impaired mobility of the tympanic membrane. Subjective impairment of mobility perceived by pneumatic otoscopy can now be confirmed by tympanometry, an objective mechanical means of recording data about the compliance of the tympanic membrane and pressure in the middle ear.

The goals of treatment are to provide clinical "cure" of symptomatic disease, to eradicate organisms and prevent suppurative complications, and to clear the fluid from the middle ear and prevent chronic serous otitis media. Clinical improvement within 48 hours may occur even without treatment (thus, in a child with chronic ear disease, the history of "no previous ear infections" may not always be accurate). Antibiotics effectively eradicate the offending organisms; treatment for 7 or 10 days is equally effective, and high-dose therapy does not seem to offer an advantage over the usual dosage. Many children still have fluid in the middle ear after antibiotic treatment: 70 percent at 2 weeks, 40 percent at 1 month, 20 percent at 2 months, and 10 percent at 3 months. In the majority of children, this fluid spontaneously clears, but some retain the fluid chronically. Regimens that include decongestants, antihistamines, and/or myringotomy have all been advocated, but none has been demonstrated repeatedly to reduce the incidence of "residual" serous otitis.

Frequent recurrences of acute suppurative otitis media develop in certain children. Eskimos, American Indians, premature and low-birth-weight infants, and infants with cleft palate, allergy, or a bout of pneumococcal otitis in the first year of life are at high risk and deserve particular attention. Prophylactic daily ampicillin or sulfonamides may decrease the frequency of recurrences and may be warranted for the otitis-prone patient.

Chronic serous otitis media (CSOM) may develop with or without (recognized) antecedent suppuration; it is particularly common in children with allergies. It appears that CSOM may cause sufficient hearing loss or distortion of sound (or both) to interfere with the development of receptive language skills in infants; in older children, fluctuating hearing loss may cause difficulties in school. The evaluation of children with CSOM includes quantification of hearing loss; a single determination may not be a valid assessment of impairment, however, since the deficit characteristically fluctuates. The role of decongestants, antihistamines, or combinations of these drugs in the treatment of CSOM remains uncertain; tympanostomy tubes and, in some cases, adenoidectomy may be required, particularly if the disorder is long-standing, bilateral, and associated with a significant hearing deficit. Chronic middle ear disease develops in almost 100 percent of children with cleft palate, and most centers advocate early insertion of tympanosotomy tubes for these patients. Adenoidectomy is contraindicated in these children, since they have velopalatine incompetence and need the "extra" nasopharyngeal tissue to assist in articulation. Chronic serous otitis media is not a valid indication for combined adenotonsillectomy in any child (see Chap. 56).

Reviews

1. Paradise, J. Otitis media in infants and children. *Pediatrics* 65:917, 1980.
   A 26-page tour de force (167 references).
2. Senturia, B., et al. (eds.). Recent advances in otitis media with effusion. *Ann. Otol. Rhinol. Laryngol.* 89:Suppl 68, 1980.
   Proceedings of an international symposium with 80 papers, more than 350 pages, on virtually all aspects: definition, classification, epidemiology, natural history, etiology and pathogenesis, diagnosis, sequelae, prevention, surgical and nonsurgical management.
3. Marchant, C., and Shurin, P. Therapy of otitis media. *Pediatr. Clin. North Am.* 30:281, 1983.
   More than just therapy; a readable review.
4. Bluestone, C. Recent advances in the pathogenesis, diagnosis, and management of otitis media. *Pediatr. Clin. North Am.* 28:727, 1981.
   Contains more on the pathophysiology of eustachian tube dysfunction than most reviews. (Same author, shorter review: N. Engl. J. Med. 306:1399, 1982.)

Natural History/Prevention

5. Teele, D., Klein, J., and Rosner, B. Epidemiology of otitis media in children. *Ann. Otol. Rhinol. Laryngol.* 89:Suppl 68, S5, 1980.
   Lays it all out in two pages.
6. Jaffe, B., Hurtado, F., and Hurtado, E. Tympanic membrane mobility in the newborn (with seven months' follow-up). *Laryngoscope* 30:36, 1970.
   Immobile drums early in life are associated with repeated ear disease.
7. Groothuis, J., et al. Otitis media in infancy: Tympanometric findings. *Pediatrics* 63:435, 1979.
   Abnormal tympanograms preceded the development of suppurative otitis media in normal children. (Tympanograms also of prognostic significance in acute otitis media: Am. J. Dis. Child. 135:233, 1981. For an "editorial retrospective" review of tympanometry, see N. Engl. J. Med. 307:1074, 1982.)
8. Shurin, P., et al. Persistence of middle-ear effusion after acute otitis media in children. *N. Engl. J. Med.* 300:1121, 1979.
   Most significant risk factors were age less than 24 months and white race (see also reference 5).
9. Schwartz, R. Prevention of otitis media: A multitude of yellow brick roads. *Pediatr. Infect. Dis.* 1:3, 1982.
   A review of various approaches, including drugs, pneumococcal vaccine, and surgery, with personal recommendations.

Also see reference 11.

Microbiology/Clinical

10. Berman, S., Balkany, T., and Simmons, M. Otitis media in infants less than 12 weeks of age: Differing bacteriology among in-patients and out-patients. *J. Pediatr.* 93:453, 1978.
    *This study helps to reconcile differences in previous reports (*Pediatrics *49:187, 1972;* J. Pediatr. *92:893, 1978;* Pediatrics *59:827, 1977).*
11. Halsted, C., et al. Otitis media: Clinical observations, microbiology, and evaluation of therapy. *Am. J. Dis. Child.* 115:542, 1968.
    Established impaired mobility as the most valid diagnostic sign; includes data on controls not given antibiotics.
12. Howie, V., Ploussard, J., and Lester, R. Otitis media: A clinical and bacteriological correlation. *Pediatrics* 45:29, 1970.
    The clinical illnesses caused by different pathogens are characterized.
13. Teele, D. Respiratory syncytial virus and otitis media with effusions. *J. Pediatr.* 101:61, 1982.
    An editorial review of attempts to implicate viruses and Mycoplasma *in otitis media; only RSV seems to play a role. (Role of* Mycoplasma *overstated even in bullous myringitis:* Pediatrics *65:761, 1980.)*
14. Teele, D., Pelton, S., and Klein, J. Bacteriology of acute otitis media unresponsive to initial antimicrobial therapy. *J. Pediatr.* 98:537, 1981.
    The results of tympanocentesis in 43 children who did not improve after at least 36 hours of therapy. (Note that in bilateral otitis, what is in one ear is not necessarily what is in the other: Am. J. Dis. Child. *134:951, 1980.)*
15. Riding, K., et al. Microbiology of recurrent and chronic otitis media with effusion. *J. Pediatr.* 93:739, 1978.
    Nonsuppurative middle ear effusions are not necessarily sterile. (Also see Pediatrics *63:915, 1979.)*

Complications/Sequelae

16. Ginsburg, C., Rudoy, R., and Nelson, J. Acute mastoiditis in infants and children. *Clin. Pediatr.* (Phila.) 19:549, 1980.
    Review of an infrequent complication.
17. Bluestone, C., et al. Workshop on effects of otitis media on the child. *Pediatrics* 71:639, 1983.
    Addresses issues such as complications and sequelae of management, effect on hearing, language development, cognitive development, articulation development, and an assessment of socioeconomic impact.
18. Paradise, J. Otitis media during early life: How hazardous to development? *Pediatrics* 68:869, 1981.
    A critical review of the evidence supports position of "relative conservatism" in management.

Chronic Serous Otitis Media

19. Bluestone, C. Chronic otitis media with effusion. *Pediatr. Infect. Dis.* 1:180, 1982.
    Thorough review, covering epidemiology, eustachian tube physiology, role of microorganisms, diagnosis, management, complications, and sequelae. Also in this volume are the proceedings of a symposium on diagnosis and management of the child with persistent middle ear effusion: Pediatr. Infect. Dis. *1(5), Suppl., 1982 (8 papers, 140 pages). Symposium update:* Pediatr. Infect. Dis. *3:377, 1984.*
20. Cantekin, E., et al. Lack of efficacy of a decongestant-antihistamine combination for otitis media with effusion ("secretory" otitis media) in children. *N. Engl. J. Med.* 308:297, 1983.
    A double-blind, randomized trial of 553 infants and children: the drug didn't work.
21. Kaleida, P., and Stool, S. Otitis media with effusion: An approach to the management of persistent symptoms and signs in the pediatric patient. *Pediatr. Rev.* 5:108, 1983.
    A step-by-step discussion of a proposed algorithm for management, accompanied by helpful diagrams and color photographs of illustrative tympanic membranes.

22. Paradise, J. On tympanostomy tubes: Rationale, results, reservations, and recommendations. *Pediatrics* 60:86, 1977.
    The state of the art. (Brief, editorial update: Pediatrics *74:292, 1984.)*

Other

23. Teele, D., et al. Middle ear disease in the practice of pediatrics: Burden during the first five years of life. *JAMA* 249:1026, 1983.
    The burden considered is on the workload of the pediatrician. (Also see Am. J. Dis. Child. *137:155, 1983.)*

58. BRONCHIOLITIS

Kenneth B. Roberts

As the term suggests, bronchiolitis is an inflammatory disease of the bronchioles. It is a common disorder in infants; the incidence is estimated at 6 to 7 cases per 100 infants under the age of 2 years, with one-half the cases occurring between 2 and 7 months of age. Males predominate 2 : 1, and there is a seasonal clustering of cases between December and March.

The small airways of affected infants are obstructed in two ways: the bronchiolar walls are thickened as a result of edema, lymphocytic infiltration, and, occasionally, proliferation of cells; and the lumens are plugged by mucus, cellular debris, and, in severe cases, desquamated bronchiolar epithelium. A reduction in the radius of the small airways causes a disproportionate increase in airflow resistance (since resistance is related to the radius raised to the fourth power), and the already small size of the lower airways in young infants may account for the age-related severity.

The distribution of involvement in bronchiolitis is patchy; thus, some areas are obstructed and some are not. Those that are completely obstructed become atelectatic; those that are partially obstructed become overinflated. The unaffected areas remain normal and "hyperventilate" in an attempt to maintain the normality of the arterial PO_2 and PCO_2.

The first clinical sign of bronchiolitis in an infant is an upper respiratory tract infection; usually, another family member is ill with a respiratory infection. After a few days the infant begins to cough and breathe more rapidly, often with feeding difficulty or vomiting. Wheezing and retractions may be prominent at this time, and the infant is irritable, although without much fever. Physical examination confirms the presence of agitation, retractions, wheezing, rales, and impaired air exchange. The liver and spleen may be palpable, usually due to air trapping with downward displacement of the diaphragm rather than to congestive heart failure. The temperature is below 38°C (100°F) in half the patients and is rarely over 39.5°C (103°F). The respiratory rate is usually increased and provides a good guide to arterial PO_2 and PCO_2. As the respiratory rate increases, the PO_2 falls in a linear fashion (from 80 mm Hg at a respiratory rate of 20, to 60 mm Hg at a respiratory rate of 60). The relationship between respiratory rate and PCO_2 is not linear, however; PCO_2 remains normal until a respiratory rate of 50 to 60 is reached and then rapidly rises with increasing tachypnea.

A radiograph of the chest reveals hyperinflation and small areas of collapse; it is often possible to see thickened bronchioles on end. Arterial blood gases indicate the patchy nature of the obstruction: the PO_2 is invariably reduced as a consequence of the obstructed and partially obstructed bronchioles, since normally ventilated areas cannot compensate for poorly ventilated but well-perfused areas unless oxygen is added to the inspired air. The PCO_2 is normal if the hypercapnea caused by affected areas can be balanced by the hyperventilation of normal areas; when compensation is not possible, respiratory failure supervenes.

Once the signs of bronchiolar obstruction appear, the course of the illness is usually brief, on the order of a few days. Following this severe period, during which approximately 5 percent of affected infants require hospitalization, gradual improvement is the rule, and by 2 weeks most infants have recovered. Complications such as pneumonia, pneumothorax, apnea, and respiratory failure are infrequent but occur; mortality is less than 1 percent.

Bronchiolitis is most commonly caused by respiratory syncytial virus (RSV). Disease may be a direct result of RSV infection of bronchiolar epithelium in an infant host, but it is also postulated that bronchiolitis may, at least in part, represent severe local interaction of RSV antigen and maternal, transplacentally acquired IgG. This theory proposes that local IgA is the important defense against RSV and that IgG in the absence of IgA may be harmful. Supporters point out that children immunized with killed RSV vaccine in trials in the 1960s were sensitized rather than protected and had worse disease when challenged with "wild" RSV.

During the acute event it may be impossible to distinguish bronchiolitis from asthma. The infant who seems to be at particular risk for asthma is one with a family history of atopy whose bronchiolitis is caused by a virus other than RSV (such as parainfluenza virus) and who has increased levels of IgE. It seems prudent, however, to follow all infants who have had bronchiolitis and reserve the diagnosis of asthma for those who demonstrate recurrent bouts of wheezing (see Asthma, Chap. 60).

The treatment of bronchiolitis is supportive, and simple measures generally suffice. The hypoxia, for example, usually responds well to increasing the inspired oxygen content. Weight loss should be expected during the acute stage, and the infants should be permitted small feedings while awake, not to meet caloric needs, but to relieve the agitation caused by hunger; if respiratory distress becomes severe, oral feedings are withheld. Intravenous fluids may be required but should not be excessive, since the combination of increased negative intrathoracic pressure during inspiration (caused by airway obstruction) and excessive fluid administration may lead to pulmonary edema. Mist therapy is commonly given, but there is little reason to expect added benefit over that provided by adequate hydration. Some clinicians prescribe sedatives, such as chloral hydrate, to alleviate anxiety and provide rest; it is important that respiratory drive not be depressed, since the defense against respiratory failure is in the infant's ability to maintain a twofold to threefold increase in minute ventilation. If respiratory failure does occur, it may be managed by a few days of controlled ventilation.

The prognosis of bronchiolitis is excellent, at least in the short term; recent investigations suggest a relationship between bronchiolitis in infancy and pulmonary disorders in later life, however. Other areas of current interest and effort are the use of antiviral medication and the development of an RSV vaccine.

Reviews

1. Wohl, M., and Chernick, V. Bronchiolitis. *Am. Rev. Resp. Dis.* 118:759, 1978.
   A 22-page, 140-reference state of the art review.
2. Workshop on bronchiolitis. *Pediatr. Res.* 11:209, 1977.
   Articles on anatomic, physiologic, and immunologic factors; on infectious agents; and on diagnosis, treatment, and prevention (22 articles, 60 pages).

Series

3. Leer, J., et al. Corticosteroid treatment in bronchiolitis. *Am. J. Dis. Child.* 117:495, 1969.
   A collaborative study of 297 infants with clinical features well displayed.
4. Hall, C., et al. Neonatal respiratory syncytial virus infection. *N. Engl. J. Med.* 300:393, 1979.
   Emphasizes role of staff in transmission and atypical nature of illness with apnea a prominent feature. (Apnea also a feature in hospitalized infants with RSV, particularly those with a history of prematurity or young postnatal age: Am. J. Dis. Child. 138:247, 1984.)
5. Tyeryar, F. Report of a workshop on respiratory syncytial virus and parainfluenza viruses. *J. Infec. Dis.* 148:588, 1983.
   An update of what is known about RSV and the epidemiology, natural history, pathogenesis, therapy, and immunoprophylaxis of RSV infection. (Also see Rev. Infect. Dis. 2:384, 1980.)
6. Parrott, R., et al. Epidemiology of respiratory syncytial virus infection in Washington, D.C. *Am. J. Epidemiol.* 98:289, 1973.

Infection and disease by age, immunologic status, race, and sex.

7. Henderson, F., et al. Respiratory-syncytial-virus infections, reinfections and immunity: A prospective, longitudinal study in young children. *N. Engl. J. Med.* 300:530, 1979.
   Repeated infections resulted in milder disease rather than in immunity to reinfection.
8. Hall, C., et al. Respiratory syncytial virus infections within families. *N. Engl. J. Med.* 294:414, 1976.
   Nearly one-half the members of one-half the families studied contracted RSV infection; the incidence was even higher in infants (nosocomial threat, too: N. Engl. J. Med. 293:1343, 1975).
9. Hall, C., and Douglas, R. Modes of transmission of respiratory syncytial virus. *J. Pediatr.* 99:100, 1981.
   Close contact is key; includes discussion of fomites.

Clinical and Laboratory Assessment
10. Krieger, I. Mechanics of respiration in bronchiolitis. *Pediatrics* 33:45, 1964.
    Low respiratory resistance and a short expiratory phase, explained by patchy involvement of disease.
11. Reynolds, E. Arterial blood gas tensions in acute disease of lower respiratory tract in infancy. *Br. Med. J.* 1:1192, 1963.
    Patterns of hypoxemia and carbon dioxide retention, explained again by patchy involvement of disease.
12. Reynolds, E. Recovery from bronchiolitis as judged by arterial blood gas tension measurements. *J. Pediatr.* 63:1182, 1963.
    The course of improvement is described.

Relationship to Asthma
13. Simon, G., and Jordan, W. Infectious and allergic aspects of bronchiolitis. *J. Pediatr.* 70:533, 1967.
    Bronchiolitis due to RSV was less likely than non-RSV bronchiolitis to "lead to" asthma.
14. Polmar, S., Robinson, L., and Minnefor, A. Immunoglobulin E in bronchiolitis. *Pediatrics* 49:279, 1972.
    IgE levels were higher in children with nonepidemic (?non-RSV) bronchiolitis; did these children have asthma rather than bronchiolitis?
15. Rooney, J., and Williams, H. The relationship between proved viral bronchiolitis and subsequent wheezing. *J. Pediatr.* 79:744, 1971.
    The family history may be helpful in sorting things out.

Treatment
16. Reynolds, E. The effect of breathing 40 per cent oxygen on the arterial blood gas tensions of babies with bronchiolitis. *J. Pediatr.* 63:1135, 1963.
    Found that 40 percent oxygen by mask was sufficient to increase PaO_2.
17. Yaffe, S., et al. Should steroids be used in treating bronchiolitis? *Pediatrics* 46:640, 1970.
    "No scientific basis for the routine administration . . . ." (See reference 3)
18. Avery, M., Galina, M., and Nachman, R. Mist therapy. *Pediatrics* 39:160, 1967.
    An excellent review, suggesting that mist offers little over humidity; clearly presented.
19. Lenney, W., and Milner, A. At what age do bronchodilator drugs work? *Arch. Dis. Child.* 53:532, 1978.
    Infants under 18 months of age were less responsive to bronchodilators than infants over 20 months; inhaled sympathomimetics are not effective in bronchiolitis (Pediatrics 44:493, 1969), nor is theophylline (Am. J. Dis. Child. 135:934, 1981).
20. Downes, J., et al. Acute respiratory failure in infants with bronchiolitis. *Anesthesiology* 29:426, 1968.
    Intubation, paralysis, and ventilation for approximately 3 days for PCO_2 greater than 65 mm Hg. (A particularly clear explanation of the rationale for the technique is given in S. Gellis, Yearbook of Pediatrics. Chicago: Year Book, 1970. P. 193.) Also see Am. J. Dis. Child. 138:1071, 1984.

21. Hall, C., et al. Aerosolized ribavirin treatment of infants with respiratory synctial viral infections. *N. Engl. J. Med.* 308:1443, 1983.
   A randomized, double-blind study of this new antiviral agent, demonstrating benefit. (Also see Pediatrics *72:613, 1983.)*

Sequelae
22. Kattan, M., et al. Pulmonary function abnormalities in symptom-free children after bronchiolitis. *Pediatrics* 59:683, 1977.
   One of many reports suggesting sequelae. (Also see J. Pediatr. *98:871, 1981;* Br. Med. J. *1:11, 1978.)*

59. PNEUMONIA
Kenneth B. Roberts

Pneumonia, defined as inflammation of lung parenchyma, can be caused by virtually every class of microorganism, and a specific etiologic diagnosis is often difficult, particularly in children. Viruses and *Mycoplasma pneumoniae* are the primary agents in pneumonia in infants and children, respectively; bacteria are much less frequently incriminated. *Streptococcus pneumoniae* (the pneumococcus) and *Haemophilus influenzae* are commonly recovered from cultures of the upper respiratory tract (in both well and sick children), but numerous studies have failed to correlate these findings with the isolates recovered from diseased lungs. Bacteremia occurs in children with pneumonia less often than in adults with pneumonia. The pneumococcus is the organism most likely to be isolated from the blood, with *H. influenzae* next in frequency; in infants, debilitated hosts, and adolescents with widely disseminated disease, *Staphylococcus aureus* may be isolated from the blood.

The most direct approach to bacteriologic diagnosis is needle aspiration of the affected area. This procedure has been used most often in children who are abnormal hosts (malnourished, immunosuppressed) or in those who have not responded to the usual therapy. As a result, the relative frequencies of various bacterial pathogens are difficult to assess: for example, the pneumococcus is the identified pathogen in 8 percent in some studies, in 54 percent in others; and *H. influenzae* is the identified pathogen in from 1 to 29 percent depending on the study. The studies do demonstrate the relative safety of the procedure: symptomatic pneumothorax occurs in fewer than 3 percent of patients, transient hemoptysis in about the same number, and more serious complications only rarely. Results from lung aspirates and blood cultures may be additive.

The clinical and radiographic findings may provide a clue to the etiologic agent, but pediatricians rarely see the classic clinical picture of pneumococcal pneumonia described in adults, with shaking chills, pleuritic pain, prostration, rusty sputum, and high mortality. In infants in particular, the only sign may be fever and tachypnea. Involvement is characteristically a lobar consolidation. Response to penicillin therapy is prompt, with marked improvement evident within 48 hours; radiographic resolution may take up to 6 weeks, however. The complications of concern are empyema formation and systemic dissemination with septicemia. Children with sickle cell disease are particularly susceptible to overwhelming infections with the pneumococcus.

H. influenzae may also cause a lobar consolidation, which is distinguished from pneumococcal pneumonia by its more indolent course and inadequate response to penicillin. Empyema is not rare, as it was once considered to be, and often the disease progresses while the child receives oral ampicillin, despite in vitro sensitivity of the organism to this antibiotic. A therapeutic response is obtained by parenteral administration of the same agent, or administration of chloramphenicol if the *Haemophilus* is resistant to ampicillin.

Staphylococcal pneumonia was much more frequent 25 years ago than it is today. It remains most common in the first year of life and characteristically is unilateral, with a peculiar predilection for the right hemithorax. Mortality as high as 50 percent has been recorded as a result of abscess formation, tissue destruction, and overwhelming septicemia. The two typical features of staphylococcal pneumonia are pneumatocele formation and rapid progression, with worsening detectable on chest roentgenograms taken hours apart. Empyema, with thick, purulent fluid, is a hallmark of the disease.

Recommendations for treatment of staphylococcal pneumonia have traditionally included instructions that the largest possible chest tube be inserted for drainage; triple antibiotic therapy has largely given way to the administration of a single penicillinase-resistant penicillin in large doses. Infants who recover from staphylococcal pneumonia when tested later in childhood do not have the marked diminution in respiratory function that one might expect.

Streptococcal pneumonia is much less common than are the other bacterial pneumonias. It may mimic the others but has some unique features: the onset simulates pneumococcal pneumonia, but the response to penicillin is much less dramatic. Empyema occurs, as in staphylococcal pneumonia, but the fluid is serosanguinous and thin at first, becoming purulent and thick as the disease progresses. Penicillin is the drug of choice.

Mycoplasma pneumoniae is said to account for 25 to 35 percent of pneumonias in late childhood and early adulthood. The incubation period is 2 to 3 weeks, considerably longer than with the bacterial agents. Symptoms such as headache, malaise, fever, and cough are more dramatic than are the signs of respiratory involvement. Unlike the pattern with the bacterial pneumonias, the white blood cell count and differential count are usually normal; "cold agglutinins" may be demonstrated by the end of the first week of illness (complement-fixing antibodies appear a week later). The x-ray characteristically has more extensive involvement than the physical examination would suggest and "looks worse than the patient." The disease is mild but prolonged, with cough in particular lasting several weeks in untreated patients. A tetracycline or erythromycin decreases the duration of clinical illness (with improvement evident on the chest radiograph) but does not shorten the period of shedding of the organism from the pharynx.

As noted above, viruses cause most bouts of pneumonia. Respiratory syncytial virus is the most frequent agent in infancy, followed by the parainfluenza viruses. Adenovirus may cause a destructive pneumonia; influenza (common in adults) infrequently causes severe pneumonia in children. Viral agents noted for their characteristic exanthems, such as measles and varicella (chickenpox), are also capable of causing serious or fatal pneumonias, particularly in immunosuppressed hosts. Other opportunistic organisms, such as cytomegalovirus and the protozoan *Pneumocystis carinii,* have become important causes of morbidity (and mortality) in children with cancer, in prematures, and in malnourished or immunosuppressed patients. Staphylococcal pneumonia may develop in children with cystic fibrosis early in their course, but it is not the devastating disease previously described. Once the lung disease is established, these children invariably become colonized with mucoid strains of *Pseudomonas,* leading to bronchiectasis but not to systemic disease (see Cystic Fibrosis, Chap. 61).

In 1977, a pneumonia syndrome with marked tachypnea and cough due to *Chlamydia trachomatis* was described in young infants. The relative role of other "new" pathogens (*Legionella pneumophila, Ureaplasma urealyticum*) is not yet clear. "Old" pathogens must also be remembered; for example, a "simple pneumonia" may represent a primary infection with *Mycobacterium tuberculosis.*

Infections of the upper respiratory tract are the most common infections of humans, and concern that a child with a cold will "catch pneumonia" is widespread; the true relationship between these two infections is obscure, however. When examining children with respiratory complaints for evidence of pneumonia, most clinicians depend as much on breathing patterns, particularly tachypnea and flaring of the alae nasi, as on auscultatory findings; rales may be heard, but signs of consolidation are infrequent. An elevated white blood cell count suggests a bacterial process; if the illness is persistent, although not necessarily progressive, evidence of *Mycoplasma* infection should be sought. A tuberculin test should be performed if encounter with *M. tuberculosis* has been at all likely. A chest radiograph may be helpful in identifying the presence and extent of pneumonia, but unless the child is severely ill or has a classic syndrome, the decision to treat with an antibiotic is usually made clinically. Expectorants have not been shown to be of benefit at recommended dosages, and mist therapy as commonly used is ineffective.

In some children pneumonias will be recurrent, and further investigation is then re quired; considerations include cystic fibrosis, anatomic disorders such as right middl lobe syndrome, and immunodeficiency.

General

1. Long, S. Treatment of acute pneumonia in infants and children. *Pediatr. Clin. Nort Am.* 30:297, 1983.
   An extensive (25 pages, 81 references), practical consideration of age, agent, an clinical syndrome in determining treatment.

2. Seto, D., and Heller, R. Acute respiratory infections. *Pediatr. Clin. North Am.* 21:683 1974.
   The characteristic x-ray appearance, together with a brief clinical description.

3. Murphy, T., et al. Pneumonia: An 11-year study in a pediatric practice. *Am. J Epidemiol.* 113:12, 1981.
   A catalogue of nearly 1500 cases of pneumonia, 1964–1975, by age and sex of patien and by etiologic agent.

Diagnosis

4. McCarthy, P., et al. Radiographic findings and etiologic diagnosis in ambulatory childhood pneumonias. *Clin. Pediatr.* (Phila.) 20:686, 1981.
   A general pediatrician, pediatric radiologist, and general radiologist did not agree on their interpretation of 128 chest x-rays; three are presented in this paper so the reader can participate. (Lateral decubitus films may help clarify ill-defined infiltrates. Pediatrics 71:192, 1983.)

5. Klein, J. Diagnostic lung puncture in the pneumonias of infants and children. *Pediatrics* 44:486, 1969.
   The same issue includes an editorial (p. 471) and a related article (p. 477); indications for the procedure are proposed. (Blood culture and lung tap are additive, no redundant: Clin. Pediatr. *[Phila.] 14:130, 1975.)*

6. McCarthy, P., Tomasso, L., and Dolan, T. Predicting fever response of children with pneumonia treated with antibiotics. *Clin. Pediatr.* (Phila.) 19:753, 1980.
   WBC > 15,000 and "positive" C-reactive protein slide tests were better predictors of rapid defervescence than sedimentation rates > 30 mm/hour or T > 40°C.

Specific Agents

7. Townsend, E., and Decancq, H. Pneumococcic segmental (lobar) pneumonia. *Clin. Pediatr.* (Phila.) 4:117, 1965.
   The clinical response to penicillin is dramatic, even to a small dose. (Radiographic resolution takes weeks, however: N. Engl. J. Med. *293:798, 1975.)*

8. Ginsburg, C., Howard, J., and Nelson, J. Report of 65 cases of *Haemophilus influenzae* b pneumonia. *Pediatrics* 64:283, 1979.
   Diagnosis by culture of blood, pleural fluid, or lung aspirate fluid or by detection of antigen in pleural fluid; consolidation present in 75 percent, pleural fluid in 75 percent. (Also see J. Pediatr. 93:389, 1978, for similar findings in 43 children.)

9. Chartrand, S., and McCracken, G. Staphylococcal pneumonia in infants and children. *Pediatr. Infect. Dis.* 1:19, 1982.
   A relatively modern series (1965–1978), with many echoes from the past (see JAMA 168:6, 1958). Review of empyema: Pediatr. Rev. *3:578, 1984.*

10. Ceruti, E., Contreras, J., and Neira, M. Staphylococcal pneumonia in childhood. *Am. J. Dis. Child.* 122:386, 1971.
    The results of pulmonary function tests to 2 to 4 years after the episode of staphylococcal pneumonia seem much better than one might expect.

11. Denny, F., Clyde, W., and Glezen, W. Mycoplasma pneumoniae disease: Clinical spectrum, pathophysiology, epidemiology, and control. *J. Pediatr. Dis.* 123:74, 1971.
    A thorough review (18 pages, 73 references).

12. Hall, C., and Douglas, R. Respiratory syncytial virus and influenza. *Am. J. Dis. Child.* 130:615, 1976.
    The former is more often a cause of lower respiratory tract infection in infants and children than is the latter.

13. Beem, N., and Saxon, E. Respiratory-tract colonization and a distinctive pneumonia syndrome in infants infected with *Chlamydia trachomatis*. *N. Engl. J. Med.* 296:306, 1977.

    The classic description of infants with tachypnea and a distinctive cough. (Also see Pediatrics 63:192, 1979, for more on the clinical features; AJR 137:703, 1981, for x-ray findings; and Pediatrics 63:198, 1979, for treatment.)

14. Dworsky, M., and Stagno, S. Newer agents causing pneumonitis in early infancy. *Pediatr. Infect. Dis.* 1:188, 1982.

    Reviews viruses, chlamydia, ureaplasma, and pneumocystis.

15. Orenstein, W., et al. The frequency of *Legionella* infection prospectively determined in children hospitalized with pneumonia. *J. Pediatr.* 99:403, 1981.

    Apparently, similar to adults, 0.3 to 5.0 percent; reviews of Legionnaires' disease: N. Engl. J. Med. 300:654, 1979, Ann. Intern. Med. 94:164, 1981, and Ann. Intern. Med. 90:491, 1979, the entire April issue (more than 200 pages of articles on the subject from an International Symposium).

    Also see Tuberculosis, Chapter 103.

Noninfectious Pneumonia

16. Bartlett, J., and Gorbach, S. The triple threat of aspiration pneumonia. *Chest* 68:560, 1975.

    A critical review.

17. Mellins, R., and Park, S. Respiratory complications of smoke inhalation in victims of fire. *J. Pediatr.* 87:1, 1975.

    Chemical or thermal injury, or both, usually apparent within 24 hours. (Also see JAMA 246:1694, 1981, and Pediatrics 68:215, 1981.)

18. Eade, N., Taussig, L., and Marks, M. Hydrocarbon pneumonitis. *Pediatrics* 54:351, 1974.

    A general review. (Criteria for hospitalizing children who have ingested products containing hydrocarbon: JAMA 246:840, 1981.)

19. Hilman, B. Interstitial and hypersensitivity pneumonitis and their variants. *Pediatr. Rev.* 1:229, 1980.

    A thorough review of the pathogenesis, diagnosis, and management of various forms of interstitial and hypersensitivity pneumonias.

Recurrent/Chronic Pneumonia

20. Eigen, H., Laughlin, J., and Homrighausen, J. Recurrent pneumonia in children and its relationship to bronchial hyperreactivity. *Pediatrics* 70:698, 1982.

    Asthma as a cause of recurrent pneumonia.

21. Berquist, W., et al. Gastroesophageal reflux–associated recurrent pneumonia and chronic asthma in children. *Pediatrics* 68:29, 1981.

    This group finds gastroesophageal reflux to be a frequent cause of recurrent pneumonia; accompanied by two editorials, pages 132 and 134.

22. Davis, P., et al. Familial bronchiectasis. *J. Pediatr.* 102:177, 1983.

    Considers immotile cilia syndrome, alpha-1-antitrypsin deficiency, immune deficiency, Williams-Campbell syndrome, and, for comparison, cystic fibrosis.

60. ASTHMA
Kenneth B. Roberts

Asthma is characterized by bronchial hyperreactivity to a multitude of stimuli causing airway constriction in the lower respiratory tract; the narrowing of the bronchi is reversible and is usually clinically manifested as wheezing.

Many authors choose to distinguish "extrinsic asthma," that provoked by external stimuli such as allergy, from "intrinsic" asthma, that not provoked by external stimuli; this classification is of limited usefulness in infancy, when wheezing is commonly associated with infection. It is useful to recognize, however, that allergy plays a prominent role in some children and should be considered in those with repeated episodes of wheezing.

Mortality from asthma in children under the age of 19 is low (about 2–3 per million population); the full impact of the disease is reflected by its wide incidence and morbidity. By household interview it is estimated that 5 percent of boys and 3 percent of girls under the age of 15 have asthma or hay fever, and that a fourth of all school days missed because of chronic conditions in children are missed because of asthma.

Many conditions are capable of producing wheezing, leading to the aphorism "All that wheezes isn't asthma." Congestive heart failure, foreign bodies, cystic fibrosis, aspirin intoxication, compression of the bronchi by lymph nodes or vessels, alpha-1-antitrypsin deficiency, and visceral larva migrans are a few of the entities to be differentiated from asthma, but the most frequent problem in differential diagnosis—and by far the hardest—is pulmonary infection, particularly bronchiolitis. There is no single diagnostic test to differentiate bronchiolitis from asthma; even isolation of the respiratory syncytial virus, the usual agent in bronchiolitis, does not eliminate the possibility of underlying asthmatic predisposition. A previous history of wheezing or family history of atopic conditions, including asthma, may be helpful. IgE levels are higher in children with asthma than in those with bronchiolitis, but the differentiation remains difficult. Many clinicians presume that the infant whose wheezing lessens following the administration of epinephrine has asthma, but this—and the converse—have many exceptions. The diagnosis is most often made by following the clinical course: repeated bouts of wheezing are usually called "asthma."

The goal of management of childhood asthma is normal growth, activity, and development. Attempts to normalized pulmonary function test results or to abolish wheezing totally may be futile and have therefore been abandoned as goals by most authorities. An important part of therapy is the use of pharmacologic agents. The two most commonly used classes of agents are the methylxanthines (e.g., theophylline) and beta-adrenergic agonists (e.g., epinephrine, isoproterenol, salbutamol). A theory that explains the benefit of these two classes of drugs proposes that beta-adrenergic activity is insufficient to block the release of mediators that cause bronchospasm and that the situation can be remedied by increasing adenosine 3':5'-cyclic phosphate (cyclic AMP). Beta agonists promote synthesis of cyclic AMP by stimulating the enzyme adenyl cyclase, and the methylxanthines maintain the accumulation of cyclic AMP by inhibiting the enzyme phosphodiesterase. Although many of the current drugs have been in use for over 50 years, widespread and enthusiastic interest in the pharmacology and pharmacokinetics of these agents is recent and has led to the development of new drugs and better ways of using the old ones.

Theophylline is presently the mainstay of outpatient pharmacologic management. Many forms are available for administration by various routes. Since plasma levels of theophylline can now be determined readily, the clinician can use any favorite theophylline preparation for a maximal therapeutic benefit and minimize the hazards of intoxication or of ineffectiveness due to inadequate levels. The pharmacokinetics have been well studied in children, but individual variation is so great that current dosage recommendations can be taken only as guidelines for initiating therapy.

Epinephrine has long been used in the treatment of asthma, but is available only by injection or inhalation. Isoproterenol administered by inhalation was popular in the 1960s, but the (ab)use of inhalers with high concentrations of isoproterenol seems to have resulted in many deaths; recognition of this problem led to a reluctance of pediatricians to prescribe inhaled medication. In recent years, the use of aerosolized bronchodilators has greatly increased. Agents with specific beta-2 activity, designed to avoid cardiostimulatory adrenergic effects, are now available, including oral preparations.

Corticosteroids do not appear to relieve bronchospasm, but they promote relief from hypoxia in status asthmaticus and appear to be of benefit in prophylaxis, perhaps by membrane stabilization. The usefulness of this group of drugs has been limited by the systemic side effects, including a cushingoid appearance and growth retardation. Beclomethasone, a steroid preparation for inhalation, offers steroid effect with minimal systemic toxicity.

Sodium cromoglycate is also available for the prevention of attacks and may permit a reduction in steroid dosage; it is not effective in the management of acute asthmatic episodes. Expectorants are often prescribed, but there is no documentation that they offer any additional benefits over adequate hydration. Postural drainage is also often included

n the treatment of an acute asthma attack. Antibiotics are useful for bacterial infection,
ut not in the uncomplicated asthmatic attack.

Treatment of children with asthma requires attention to more than medications.
:motional support is a major part of management. Many authors speak of an "asthmatic
ersonality," but controlled studies have revealed no differences between children with
sthma and children with other chronic diseases, such as congenital heart disease. It
ppears that recurrent bouts of dyspnea may be as much the cause as the effect of the
nxiety and neuroses in these children.

Because of the frequent association of allergy with childhood asthma, most clinicians
romote environmental control measures for their patients with repeated bouts of wheez-
ng. Skin testing and specific immunotherapy may be indicated for selected patients, but
voidance of the known precipitants of asthma is clearly indicated for all.

In more than half the patients the onset of childhood asthma is before age 5. Some
hildren have multiple bouts of status asthmaticus (see Chap. 5), while others experience
nly occasional mild wheezing, perhaps limited to episodes of respiratory infection.
)verall, one-half to two-thirds of children "outgrow" their asthma by adolescence. Un-
ortunately, it is not possible to predict the course in the individual child with asthma
vith certainty.

eviews and Natural History

1. Leffert, F. The management of chronic asthma. *J. Pediatr.* 97:875, 1980.
   Beautifully written, with due consideration to the history and to dialogue with patient and family, as well as to laboratory and therapeutic aspects.
2. Leffert, F. Asthma: A modern perspective. *Pediatrics* 62:1061, 1978.
   A review of basic concepts and theories about asthma.
3. Landau, L. Outpatient evaluation and management of asthma. *Pediatr. Clin. North Am.* 26:581, 1979.
   A useful review; recommends tailoring therapy according to frequency and severity of episodes (four patterns of disease illustrated).
4. Kuzemko, J. Natural history of childhood asthma. *J. Pediatr.* 97:886, 1980.
   "Will he grow out of it, doctor?" A review of the factors with favorable, unfavorable, and questionable impact on prognosis.
   Also see Respiratory Failure and Status Asthmaticus, Chapter 5.

iagnosis and Evaluation

5. Richards, W. Differential diagnosis of childhood asthma. *Curr. Probl. Pediatr.* 4(5), 1974.
   "All that wheezes . . . ."
6. Taussig, L., Smith, S., and Blumenfeld, R. Chronic bronchitis in children: What is it? *Pediatrics* 67:1, 1981.
   Chronic bronchitis, chronic cough (Pediatrics 67:6, 1981), "hidden asthma" (Am. J. Dis. Child. 135:1053, 1981), and, in some children, recurrent pneumonia (Pediatrics 70:698, 1982), may all be part of the spectrum of asthma, airway hyperreactivity without gross wheezing.
7. Commey, J., and Levinson, H. Physical signs in childhood asthma. *Pediatrics* 58:537, 1976.
   Only retraction of the sternocleidomastoid seems to correlate with the results of pulmonary function tests.
8. Hsu, K., et al. Ventilatory functions of normal children and young adults— Mexican-Americans, white, and black: I. Spirometry. II. Wright peak flowmeter, *J. Pediatr.* 95:14,168, 1979.
   Normal values, noting significant differences among races and between sexes. (Proposed standards for performance of PFTs in children: J. Pediatr. 97:668, 1980.)
9. Kravis, L. The complications of acute asthma in children. *Clin. Pediatr.* (Phila.) 12:538, 1973.
   What to be on the lookout for: atalectasis, pneumonia, mucous plugging, subcutaneous emphysema, pneumomediastinum, pneumothorax, bronchiectasis, and aspergillosis.

Pharmacologic Management: General

10. Weinberger, M., Hendeles, L., and Ahrens, R. Clinical pharmacology of drugs used for asthma. *Pediatr. Clin. North Am.* 28:47, 1981.
    A lengthy review by major contributors to the literature on drug therapy of asthma (2 pages, 135 references).

11. Rachelefsky, G. Pharmacologic management of childhood asthma. *Pediatr. Rev* 1:301, 1980.
    An intermediate length review. (For a brief summary, see Med. Lett. Drugs Ther 24:83, 1982.)

Theophylline

12. Weinberger, M., Hendeles, L., and Bighley, L. The relation of product formulation to absorption of oral theophylline. *N. Engl. J. Med.* 299:852, 1978.
    Liquid versus uncoated tablets versus coated tablets versus sustained-release tablet versus sustained-release capsules; adult volunteers. (Same group, similar but more limited study using children: J. Pediatr. 99:145, 1981; more information on sustained-release products: N. Engl. J. Med. 308:760, 1983, and Med. Lett. Drug Ther. 26:1, 1984.)

13. Bukowsky, M., Nakatsu, K., and Munt, P. Theophylline reassessed. *Ann. Intern Med.* 101:63, 1984.
    An update of interactions, kinetics, and newly discovered actions.

14. Gaudreault, T., Wason, S., and Lovejoy, F. Acute pediatric theophylline overdose: a summary of 28 cases. *J. Pediatr.* 102:474, 1983.
    There is a direct correlation between the serum theophylline concentration and the incidence of vomiting, seizures, and cardiac arrhythmias.
    Also see reference 10. (The place to start your reading about theophylline.)

Other Drugs

15. Lee, H., and Evans, H. Albuterol by aerosol and orally administered theophylline in asthmatic children. *J. Pediatr.* 101:632, 1982.
    Additive beneficial effects: the former peaked early and declined rapidly, the latter was more gradual and sustained the beneficial effect. (Aerosol as effective as injection: J. Pediatr. 102:465, 1983; also as effective as oral but with fewer side effects: J. Pediatr. 99:805, 1981. Proper inhalation techniques: Clin. Pediatr. [Phila.] 22:440, 1983.)

16. Williams, M. Beclomethasone dipropionate. *Ann. Intern. Med.* 95:464, 1981.
    A status report on aerosolized steroid, 5 years after licensure. (Brief editorial review of benefits and adverse effects in children, concluding that the suppressive effects on the hypothalamus-pituitary axis have been exaggerated: Pediatrics 72:130, 1983.)

17. Berman, B. Cromolyn: Past, present, and future. *Pediatr. Clin. North Am.* 30:915 1983.
    Reviews the use of cromolyn in asthma and other conditions.

Special Groups

18. Jones, R. Management of asthma in the child aged under 6 years. *Br. Med. J* 282:1914, 1981.
    Beyond "wheezy bronchitis": focus on the age group in which specific diagnosis and successful management are most difficult. (Adrenergic bronchodilator not as effective in children less than 18 months as in children over 20 months: Arch. Dis. Child 53:532, 1978; also, dose requirements of theophylline are affected by young age: J. Pediatr. 98:158, 1981, and, for sustained-release preparations, Am. J. Dis. Child 136:790, 1982.)

19. Turner, E., Greenberger, T., and Patterson, R. Management of the pregnant asthmatic patient. *Ann. Intern. Med.* 93:905, 1980.
    The effect of pregnancy on asthma, and the effect of asthma on pregnancy, including labor, delivery, and the baby.

20. Symposium on exercise and asthma. *Pediatrics* 56 (Suppl.):843, 1975.
    Multiple facets of this aspect of the asthma problem (28 articles, 114 pages); update of proposed mechanism of exercise-induced asthma: N. Engl. J. Med. 301:763, 1979.

Nonpharmacologic Management

1. Lichtenstein, L., Valentine, M., and Norman, P. A reevaluation of immunotherapy for asthma. *Am. Rev. Respir. Dis.* 129:657, 1984.
   *A brief update of a scholarly review (*Am. Rev. Respir. Dis. *117:191, 1978); there is reason to believe immunotherapy could be beneficial, but better studies are needed.*

2. Gortmaker, S., et al. Parental smoking and the risk of childhood asthma. *Am. J. Public Health* 72:574, 1982.
   Throw this at the next mother who lights up in your office: Between 18 and 34 percent of childhood asthma was found attributable to maternal smoking. (Dust also an important environmental factor; benefit of "dust-free bedrooms": Pediatrics *71:418, 1983.)*

3. Erskine-Milliss, J., and Schonell, M. Relaxation therapy in asthma: A critical review. *Psychosom. Med.* 43:365, 1981.
   Muscular relaxation therapy not effective but mental relaxation techniques of subjective and clinical benefit to some patients. Also see reference 1.

---

61. CYSTIC FIBROSIS
Dennis C. Stokes

Cystic fibrosis (CF) is an autosomal recessive inherited, generalized disorder of exocrine gland function that results in abnormal mucus production. Chronic obstructive pulmonary disease, pancreatic insufficiency, and an abnormally high electrolyte concentration in sweat are the hallmarks, but there is a remarkable variability in severity and expression among affected persons. It is a disease primarily of Caucasians and, with an estimated incidence of approximately 1 in 1800 to 1 in 2000 live births, is the most common lethal genetic disorder in this population. There are only very rare reported cases in native African blacks and an incidence of only 1 in 90,000 in Mongolians. There is at present no satisfactory explanation for the high carrier rate in Caucasians (about 5% of the general population); the frequency seems too high to be explained by new mutations alone and suggest a heterozygote reproductive advantage. Heterozygotes are completely normal clinically and cannot be detected by presently available tests.

Chronic, progressive pulmonary disease is the most serious manifestation of CF, responsible for most of the morbidity and the early death of these patients. Chronic cough, wheezing, hyperinflation, or lower respiratory tract infections are frequent initial pulmonary manifestations and may begin at any age, from weeks to months or years after birth.

The pathogenetic mechanism responsible for the pulmonary disease is presumed to be related to the abnormal character of the bronchial mucus or to the presence of a "factor" (or factors) in mucus or serum interfering with the efficient mucociliary transport elevator. Mucous gland morphology and distribution are normal.

Obstruction of small airways probably results from mucous plugging, and secondary bacterial infection then occurs, with bronchiolitis as the earliest lesion. Initial pulmonary infections are frequently with *Staphylococcus aureus* or *Haemophilus influenzae*, but *Pseudomonas* species are isolated after repeated antibiotic therapy eliminates other more susceptible organisms. "Mucoid" *Pseudomonas* strains, which are heavy "slime" producers and are unique to CF patients, are frequently isolated from the sputum and, once established, can only rarely and transiently be eliminated from the sputum flora. Although the exact role of *Pseudomonas* infection in contributing to the progressive pulmonary disease is uncertain, it has been suggested that circulating *Pseudomonas* antibodies may contribute to a hypersensitivity reaction in bronchial walls.

The early physiologic consequences of small airway obstruction are abnormalities in the ventilation-perfusion ratio distribution, hyperinflation, and focal atelectasis. Arterial PO_2 is the earliest pulmonary function test to become abnormal; later involvement leads to more severe obstruction, loss of lung elastic recoil, bronchiectasis, and multiple microabscesses. The result of this progressive pulmonary disease is larger airway ob-

TNT   Tobra
          Naf
          Ticar

struction, increased airway resistance, and profound hypoxemia and hypercapnea. The course of pulmonary function is highly variable, and some patients have normal lung function into the second decade of life. In most patients, however, there is an exponential decline in lung function of approximately 8 to 10 percent per year. Females appear to have accelerated decline in lung function, particularly after adolescence.

Right heart enlargement and strain (cor pulmonale) follow the development of hypoxic pulmonary vascular constriction and occur in up to 70 percent of patients dying with CF. The early clinical evaluation of cor pulmonale is complicated by the difficulty in appreciating the physical signs of right heart failure in these patients. The most reliable clinical indicators of the development of cor pulmonale include a PO_2 of less than 50 mm Hg and a PCO_2 above 45 mm Hg, with the changes of right ventricular enlargement by echocardiography or vectorcardiography; cardiac function can also be assessed non invasively using radionuclide angiography. Once this complication occurs, death usually ensues within 2 years despite vigorous medical management.

Other serious pulmonary complications of CF include abscesses, cysts, persistent atelectasis, recurrent pneumothorax, and massive—often fatal—hemoptysis. All are associated with advanced lung disease. Recurrent or persistent pneumothorax is best managed by closed thoracotomy drainage and instillation of a sclerosing agent such as quinacrine or by surgery and pleural abrasion. Hemoptysis can be managed successfully by embolization of hypertrophied bronchial arteries.

Clubbing as the result of hypoxemia becomes an invariable and often useful diagnostic finding as this disease progresses. Hypertrophic osteoarthropathy, with joint swelling, pain, and tenderness, is present occasionally.

Although chronic pulmonary infections are the rule in CF, systemic infections (sepsis, meningitis) are rare, even in severely debilitated patients. Cell-mediated immunity is not impaired, and immunoglobulin levels tend to be normal or elevated.

Many patients with CF show considerable reversibility in airway obstruction when bronchodilators are used. Respiratory allergy and CF clearly occur together, although the exact role of atopy in promoting bronchospasm or pulmonary damage is uncertain. Allergic bronchopulmonary aspergillosis, a type III (Arthus) reaction to noninvasive aspergillus colonization of mucous plugs, also occurs.

Approximately 20 percent of patients with cystic fibrosis have nasal polyps. Although symptomatic disease is rare, almost all have radiologic evidence of chronic sinusitis.

Gastrointestinal obstruction due to meconium ileus occurs in 10 to 15 percent of patients with CF and is the earliest presenting manifestation. Meconium ileus is produced by the abnormal character of the meconium, which has a higher protein content and is "stickier" and drier than normal meconium. Obstruction of the distal ileum may lead to perforation and meconium peritonitis (occasionally occurring in utero), atresias, or volvulus. Delayed passage of meconium—the so-called "meconium plug syndrome"—also occurs in newborns with CF. Patients who survive the complications of meconium ileus and the following months of recovery may not have a worse prognosis than patients without this complication. There is evidence for a risk of recurrence of meconium ileus in siblings.

So-called meconium ileus equivalent occurs in older children, adolescents, and adults with CF, due to the collection of abnormal fecal material in the cecum, ileum, and colon. The clinical presentation may be recurrent abdominal pain, abdominal masses, intestinal obstruction, or intussusception.

Pancreatic insufficiency with absent trypsin, chymotrypsin, lipases, and amylase leads to the characteristic fat- and protein-maldigestive stools—bulky, foul-smelling, and greasy. Treatment is effectively accomplished by pancreatic enzyme supplements and is not a major problem after the diagnosis is made.

Malabsorption secondary to pancreatic insufficiency was felt initially to be a sine qua non of cystic fibrosis, but 15 to 20 percent of patients have significant or normal pancreatic function; this group also appears to have milder clinical symptoms and less lung involvement. Patients with residual pancreatic function are at risk for recurrent bouts of acute pancreatitis. Abnormal pancreatic endocrine function may be found in older patients with CF as a result of the disturbance in pancreatic organization. Chemical diabetes (as manifested by glucose tolerance test abnormalities or elevated glycosylated hemoglobin levels) due to impaired insulin release occurs in 40 percent of patients and precedes the onset of clinical diabetes mellitus. There is evidence that the impaired insulin release is partly compensated for by increased peripheral tissue sensitivity to insulin in these patients, and ketoacidosis is rare.

In infants with CF fed soy-based formulas (perhaps as treatment for their diarrhea), a clinical picture characterized by hypoproteinemia, edema, and anemia may develop; this may also occur in breast-fed infants, because of the relatively low protein content of these diets compared with cow milk formulas. Affected infants with edema may have a falsely low sweat chloride determination that becomes diagnostic with proper nutritional management, such as the use of an elemental formula or enzyme replacement.

Although clinical expression is rare, fat-soluble vitamins A, E, and K are deficient in these patients when there is malabsorption and are usually supplemented

Other common kinds of gastrointestinal involvement with CF include rectal prolapse (20% of patients, related to chronic cough, the passage of large stools, or malnutrition) and cirrhosis, with the development of portal hypertension, esophageal varices, and hypersplenism (2–5% of patients); cirrhosis may occur in patients with very mild pulmonary disease and may even be the presenting manifestation. The mechanism leading to the cirrhosis involves abnormalities in bile character and plugging of the intrahepatic bile ducts.

The sweat glands are morphologically normal in CF, but produce sweat with excessive amounts of Na^+, Cl^-, and K^+. This provides the basis for the diagnostic "sweat test," which measures Na^+ and Cl^- in sweat collected by stimulating the glands by pilocarpine iontophoresis. A sweat chloride concentration of 50 to 60 mEq/liter is borderline, but one above 60 mEq/liter is clearly abnormal. It is particularly important to know that an adequate amount of sweat (> 50 mg) has been collected, as well as the patient's age, since sweat chloride normally increases with age.

The abnormal sweat losses are of clinical significance in heat-stressed patients, particularly infants and may lead to severe hyponatremic dehydration. Often, it provides an early diagnostic clue when the mother notes that her child's skin tastes "salty."

Hypochloremic metabolic alkalosis and hypokalemia may result from abnormal sweat and stool losses of electrolytes, vigorous diuretic therapy, or renal tubular dysfunction from antibiotic therapy (carbenicillin, gentamicin). In patients with severe obstructive airway disease, chloride depletion and the resulting inability to reduce serum bicarbonate may lead to alkalosis, depression of respiratory drive, and an inability to improve carbon dioxide retention. The syndrome of inappropriate antidiuretic hormone secretion may be present in older patients.

Males with CF are generally sterile, and obstructive pathologic changes are found in the vas deferens and epididymis; testes are normal. In females, the character of the cervical mucus is abnormal, but many affected females have borne children successfully. There is often a delay in menarche and development of secondary sexual characteristics due to the chronic lung disease.

Early diagnosis, institution of physical therapy and nutrition counseling, vigorous antibiotic therapy, and careful follow-up are important aspects of the comprehensive regional CF treatment programs. These programs have undoubtedly improved the outlook for patients with cystic fibrosis, although many of the modes of therapy remain empirical and without well-controlled studies of efficacy. Specifically, mist tent therapy, bronchial lavage, intermittent positive pressure breathing, continuous "suppressive" antibiotic therapy, aerosol therapy, postural drainage, and breathing exercises have been advocated in this disease without clear evidence of their benefit. In the absence of a specific known defect to which therapy can be directed, empirical therapy will probably remain a major part of the treatment programs.

History

1. Andersen, D. Cystic fibrosis of pancreas and its relation to celiac disease: Clinical and pathological study. *Am. J. Dis. Child.* 56:344, 1938.
   A classic paper separating the clinical picture in infants with CF (particularly the frequency of pulmonary infections) from that in infants with the "celiac syndrome" and a normal pancreas.
2. diSant' Agnese, P., et al. Abnormal electrolyte composition of sweat in cystic fibrosis of pancreas: Clinical significance and relationship to disease. *Pediatrics* 12:549, 1953.

A description of the development of the diagnostic sweat test. (Levels of electrolytes in sweat have been stated to have no relationship to the severity or expression of disease, but there is a subgroup of patients with lower sweat electrolyte content and milder disease: J. Pediatr. *100:357, 1982, and JAMA 239:2676, 1978.)*

Reviews

3. Taussig, L. (ed.). *Cystic Fibrosis.* New York: Thieme-Stratton, 1984.
   Includes many current reviews of both clinical and research aspects of CF; an excellent first source.
4. Wood, R. E., Boat, T. F., and Doershuk C. F. Cystic fibrosis. *Am. Rev. Respir. Dis.* 113:833 1976.
   A complete and readable review, with an extensive bibliography (503 references).

The Clinical Spectrum

5. Shwachman, H., Redman, A., and Khaw, K. Studies in cystic fibrosis: Report of 130 patients diagnosed under three months of age over a 20 year period. *Pediatrics* 46:335, 1970.
   A review of one group's extensive clinical experience.
6. Shwachman, H., Kulezycki, L., and Khaw, K. Studies in cystic fibrosis: A report on sixty-five patients over 17 years of age. *Pediatrics* 36:689, 1965.
   The disease is not limited to infants, as once thought. (Also see reference 29.)

Pathophysiology

7. diSant' Agnese, P., and Davis, P. Research in cystic fibrosis. *N. Engl. J. Med.* 295:481, 1976.
   A comprehensive survey of the research literature on the basic defect in cystic fibrosis (202 references).
8. Talamo, R., Rosenstein, B., and Berninger, R. Cystic Fibrosis. In J. Stanbury et al. (eds.), *The Metabolic Basis of Inherited Disease.* New York: McGraw-Hill, 1983.
   An update of the many biochemical abnormalities described in CF as well as excellent clinical summary (533 references). (Elegant studies in isolated sweat glands demonstrated abnormal permeability to chloride as the basis for poor reabsorption of NaCl in sweat: Nature *301:421, 1983.)*
9. Wheeler, W., et al. Progression of cystic fibrosis lung disease as a function of serum immunoglobulin G levels. *J. Pediatr.* 104:695, 1984.
   Of patients under 10 years of age, 22 percent had low IgG levels. Low levels correlated with better pulmonary function; supports host inflammatory response as important in lung tissue damage in CF. (Low IgG levels in 22 percent of patients under 10 years of age. N. Engl. J. Med. *302;245, 1980.*

Sweat Test

10. Evaluation of testing for cystic fibrosis. *J. Pediatr.* 88:711, 1976.
    Discusses assays for various "factors" in CF, heterozygote testing, screening tests for CF, and the methodology of the sweat test; by a National Academy of Science committee (102 references).
11. MacLean, W. C., Jr., and Tripp, R. W. Cystic fibrosis with edema and falsely negative sweat test. *J. Pediatr.* 83:86, 1973.
    An important caveat.
12. Rosenstein, B., et al. Cystic fibrosis: Problems encountered with sweat testing. *JAMA* 240:87, 1978.
    Both false-positives and -negatives may occur, particularly when methods other than pilocarpine iontophoresis are used.

Gastrointestinal Disease

13. Park, R., and Grand, R. Gastrointestinal manifestations of cystic fibrosis. *Gastroenterology* 81:1143, 1981.
    An excellent clinical review.
14. Lapey, A., et al. Steatorrhea and azotorrhea and their relation to growth and nutrition in adolescents and young adults with cystic fibrosis. *J. Pediatr.* 84:328, 1974.

Growth failure correlates more closely with severity of pulmonary disease than with pancreatic insufficiency. (Improving nutritional status by supplemental parenteral nutrition may result in improved pulmonary status and growth: J. Pediatr. *97:351, 1980; improvement is brief, however:* J. Pediatr. *104:700, 1984.)*

15. Stern, R., et al. Symptomatic hepatic disease in cystic fibrosis: Incidence, course, and outcome of portal systemic shunting. *Gastroenterology* 70:645, 1976.
    The incidence of clinical hepatic disease was 2.2 percent; favorable results were obtained in five patients who underwent portal systemic shunting following gastrointestinal bleeding.

16. Holsclaw, D., Romans, C., and Shwachman, H. Intussusception in patients with cystic fibrosis. *Pediatrics* 48:51, 1971.
    The incidence is approximately 1 percent, and it may be the presenting complaint in an undiagnosed patient. It also may be recurrent, and a trial of reduction with barium enema is warranted. (Rectal prolapse is also an early gastrointestinal complication, affecting 18 percent of children with CF; even a single episode of prolapse is an indication for a sweat test: Gastroenterology *82:707, 1982.)*

17. Mullins, F., Talamo, R., and diSant' Agnese, P. Late intestinal complications of cystic fibrosis. *JAMA* 192:721, 1965.
    So-called meconium ileus equivalent presenting with fecal masses, ileocolic intussusception, volvulus, and fecal impaction in older patients; CF patients who have previously been operated on and have adhesions are at increased risk for serious complications.

Upper Respiratory Tract Disease

18. Taylor B., Evans, J., and Hope, G. Upper respiratory tract in cystic fibrosis: Ear-nose-throat survey of 50 children. *Arch. Dis. Child* 49:133, 1974.
    The universality of sinus disease is documented; nasal polyps are common, occur at a younger age than atopic patients, and are different histologically. (Also see Am. J. Dis. Child. *136:1067, 1982.)*

Lower Respiratory Tract Disease

19. Mellins, R. The site of airway obstruction in cystic fibrosis. *Pediatrics* 44:315, 1969.
    The earliest changes in the small airways produce abnormal distribution of ventilation, progressing to involvement of the larger airways and increased airway resistance—first during forced maneuvers (such as FEV_1) and finally during quiet breathing. (There is a mean decline in FEV_1 of approximately 8 percent per year, but this varies markedly: Am. Rev. Resp. Dis. *114:1085, 1976.)*

20. Stern, R., et al. Treatment and prognosis of massive hemoptysis in patients with cystic fibrosis. *Am. Rev. Respir. Dis.* 117:825, 1977.
    Usually associated with severe disease.

21. McLaughlin, F., et al. Pneumothorax in cystic fibrosis: Management and outcome. *J. Pediatr.* 100:863, 1982.
    Lower recurrence rates for quinacrine sclerosis (12.5%) and parietal pleurectomy (0%).

Cor Pulmonale

22. Stern, R., et al. Heart failure in cystic fibrosis. *Am. J. Dis. Child.* 134:267, 1980.
    Mean survival was only 8 months despite vigorous medical therapy. (For a review of the pathogenesis of cor pulmonale, see Pediatrics *70:728, 1982.)*

Treatment

23. Orenstein, D., et al. The effect of early diagnosis and treatment in cystic fibrosis *Am. J. Dis. Child.* 131:973, 1977.
    Supports the concept that early treatment (such as chest physiotherapy: J. Pediatr. *103:358, 1983.) can improve outcome.*

24. Marks, M. The pathogenesis and treatment of pulmonary infections in patients with cystic fibrosis. *J. Pediatr.* 98:173, 1981.
    *Overview of current use of antibiotic therapy. (Anti-*Pseudomonas *therapy results in improved clinical and lung function:* J. Pediatr. *99:307, 1981; resistant strains are a significant developing problem, however:* J. Pediatr. *104:206, 1984.)*

25. Stokes, D., et al. Sleep hypoxemia in young adults with cystic fibrosis. *Am J. Dis. Child.* 134:741, 1980.
    Hypoxemia worsens at night in some patients with CF; this supports the use of nocturnal oxygen therapy. (Also see Am. Rev. Resp. Dis. 129:712, 1984.)
26. Davis, P., and diSant' Agnese, P. Assisted ventilation for patients with cystic fibrosis. *JAMA* 239:1851, 1978.
    In general, indications are limited to patients with good lung function having an acute reversible exacerbation or elective pulmonary surgery.
27. Boyle, I., et al. Emotional adjustments of adolescents and young adults with cystic fibrosis. *J. Pediatr.* 88:318, 1976.
    To the difficulties of helping patient and family to cope with a chronic, disabling illness are added the problems of adolescent independence, vocational training, marriage and family planning.

Prognosis
28. Stern, R., et al. Course of cystic fibrosis in 95 patients. *J. Pediatr.* 89:406, 1976.
    Of 45 patients diagnosed prior to extensive irreversible pulmonary involvement, only 1 had died over a mean follow-up of 14 years.
29. diSant' Agnese, P., and Davis, P. Cystic fibrosis in adults. *Am. J. Med.* 66:121, 1979.
    Median survival has increased to 21 years by 1978, and there has also been increased recognition of individuals with CF with mild involvement presenting in adulthood.

VI. GASTROINTESTINAL DISORDERS

62. BILIARY ATRESIA AND NEONATAL HEPATITIS
Robert D. White

Both biliary atresia and neonatal hepatitis, in the light of current knowledge, appear to be misnamed. Complete atresia of the bile ducts is not a universal finding in "biliary atresia," and neonatal hepatitis is rarely confined to the first month of life. Nor is the distinction between the two as clear as once thought: biliary obstruction is present to some degree in many patients with neonatal hepatitis, and cellular inflammation is often found in biliary atresia. Both entities present as chronic cholestatic jaundice in the first weeks of life. Current thinking is that a given insult or pathogen may produce self-limited disease (neonatal hepatitis) in some infants and progressive, ultimately fatal disease (biliary atresia) in others. Trisomy 18 and alpha-1-antitrypsin deficiency, for example, are associated with both neonatal hepatitis and biliary atresia. Other causes of neonatal hepatitis include viral infections (hepatitis B, rubella, and cytomegalovirus) and chemical agents (intravenous alimentation solutions). Most cases of both diseases must still be considered "idiopathic," but additional viral, chemical, and genetic pathogens have been proposed, and several are being actively investigated. Each disease has an incidence of slightly less than 1 in 10,000 births.

Infants with biliary atresia or neonatal hepatitis are typically healthy at birth, presenting with mixed hyperbilirubinemia after the first week of life. Their livers are enlarged and firm, and their spleens are usually palpable as well. The urine is dark yellow, and in children in whom biliary obstruction is significant, the stools are acholic. The clinical presentation of hepatitis secondary to chronic intrauterine infection is usually somewhat different, in that symptoms are generally present at birth (see Congenital Infections, Chap. 43).

Differentiation between biliary atresia and neonatal hepatitis is extremely difficult when symptoms first become apparent. In a few patients, there is a history of a previous sibling with neonatal hepatitis or a maternal history of rubella, toxoplasmosis, or syphilis infection during pregnancy. Screening tests for known causes of hepatitis may also be helpful in some cases. Liver function tests are of little value for distinguishing neonatal hepatitis from biliary atresia, except for the rose bengal excretion test. Infants with biliary atresia excrete less than 10 percent of an administered dose of rose bengal sodium I 131 into the bile over a 72-hour period, while 90 percent of infants with neonatal hepatitis excrete more than 10 percent of the administered dose; in borderline cases, administration of cholestyramine or phenobarbital to augment rose bengal excretion may be useful. The test is valuable but difficult to perform; the stool must not be contaminated by urine for 72 hours, and this is often difficult to ensure in a young infant. Levels of 5'-nucleotidase, alpha fetoprotein, and lipoprotein-X differ significantly in infants with neonatal hepatitis and those with biliary atresia, but the limited availability of tests for these levels and the overlap between diseases reduce their usefulness. Percutaneous needle biopsy of the liver is helpful in the diagnosis, as are ultrasonography, technetium scanning, and duodenal and serum bile acid assays. Exploratory laparotomy with operative cholangiography is still necessary to confirm the diagnosis when bile duct obstruction is suspected, however, or when this diagnosis cannot be excluded using less invasive means by 8 to 12 weeks of age.

Until recently, biliary atresia was universally fatal—almost by definition, since recovery was considered evidence that neonatal hepatitis was actually the correct diagnosis. Intrigued by indications that this was a dynamic process, and by postmortem studies that demonstrated patent intrahepatic bile ducts in some infants, Kasai proposed that bile flow could be reestablished in certain cases by removal of the obstructed extrahepatic biliary structures and anastomosis of patent ducts in the porta hepatis to the small intestine. The operation that bears his name was enthusiastically received but is feasible only for 60 percent of infants; 15 to 20 percent of infants have intrahepatic atresia of the bile ducts, and a similar percentage have such severe intrahepatic and extrahepatic obstruction that no ducts of sufficient caliber for anastomosis can be found. The documentation of several cases in which patent ductal tissue undetected during the first procedure was later found and successfully anastomosed has prompted some authors to recommend a "second-look" operation in infants initially believed to have inoperable disease; liver transplantation has also become an alternative for this group.

Even when patent bile ducts are found and anastomosed to the intestine, however, relief of symptoms is uncommon. In approximately one-fourth, bile excretion does not resume. One-half of the remainder experience one or more episodes of ascending cholangitis, due to the proximity of the intestinal flora to the liver. In many, ductal stricture and hepatic cirrhosis follow cholangitis and are ultimately fatal. Overall, approximately 40 to 50 percent of infants with extrahepatic biliary obstruction regain normal liver function following surgery; this "cure" rate appears to be improving as new surgical modifications reduce the incidence of postoperative complications and as the importance of early intervention becomes increasingly appreciated. These infants require considerable supportive care for hepatic insufficiency until their liver disease resolves.

Infants with neonatal hepatitis should receive supportive care; malabsorption, hypoproteinemia, rickets, and their sequelae are common, but can usually be managed successfully. Of affected infants, 50 percent recover fully, and another 20 to 30 percent survive with residual liver disease.

Reviews

1. Bill, A., and Kasai, M. (eds.). Biliary atresia and choledochal cyst. *Prog. Pediatr. Surg.* 6:1, 1974.
   The entire volume is devoted to biliary atresia and neonatal hepatitis.
2. Andres, J., Mathis, R., and Walker, W. Liver disease in infants. *J. Pediatr.* 90:686, 864, 1977.
   An excellent two-part review of basic physiology and the clinical presentation of liver disease in infancy.
3. Thaler, M., and Gellis, S. Studies in neonatal hepatitis and biliary atresia. *Am. J. Dis. Child.* 116:257, 1968.
   This four-part study made a quantum leap in understanding of these disorders.
4. Danks, D., et al. Studies of the aetiology of neonatal hepatitis and biliary atresia. *Arch. Dis. Child.* 52:360, 1977.
   Much more so than the title indicates, this is an extensive study of the natural histories of these disorders. For a similar study of equal and complementary value, see Mowat et al., Arch. Dis. Child. 51:763, 1976.
5. Gartner, L. Cholestasis of the newborn. *Pediatr. Rev.* 5:163, 1983.
   For other recent reviews, see Curr. Probl. Pediatr. 12(12), 1982, and Clin. Pediatr. (Phila.) 22:30, 1983.

Differential Diagnosis

6. Hays, D., et al. Diagnosis of biliary atresia: Relative accuracy of percutaneous liver biopsy, open liver biopsy, and operative cholangiography. *J. Pediatr.* 71:598, 1967.
   A careful study to document the accuracy of these techniques was hampered by the inability to distinguish biliary atresia from neonatal hepatitis, even at autopsy in some cases.
7. Javitt, N., et al. Serum bile acid patterns in neonatal hepatitis and extrahepatic biliary atresia. *J. Pediatr.* 90:736, 1977.
   This study, along with those by Andres et al. on alpha$_1$ fetoprotein (J. Pediatr. 91:217, 1977) and by Campbell and Williams on lipoprotein-X (Ann. Surg. 184:89, 1976), proposes a new test to discriminate neonatal hepatitis from biliary atresia by noninvasive means; none of the studies had more than 25 infants in either category.
8. Manolaki, A., et al. The prelaparotomy diagnosis of extrahepatic biliary atresia. *Arch. Dis. Child.* 58:591, 1983.
   Large series utilizing current diagnostic techniques.

Biliary Atresia

9. Altman, R. Biliary atresia. *Pediatrics* 68:896, 1981.
   Brief summary, oriented toward surgical considerations.
10. Hays, D., and Snyder, W. Life-span in untreated biliary atresia. *Surgery* 54:373, 1963.
    Mean survival was 19 months.
11. Kasai, M., et al. Surgical treatment of biliary atresia. *J. Pediatr. Surg.* 3:665, 1968.
    Kasai describes his landmark surgical series.

12. Weber, T., and Grosfeld, J. Contemporary management of biliary atresia. *Surg. Clin. North Am.* 61:1079, 1981.
    Review with recent mortality/morbidity figures.
13. Lilly, J. Biliary atresia and liver transplantation. *Pediatrics* 74:159, 1984.
    Adds a bureaucratic perspective to the medical report on liver transplantation on p. 140 of the same issue.
14. Lottsfeldt, F., et al. Cholestyramine therapy in intrahepatic biliary atresia. *N. Engl. J. Med.* 269:186, 1963.
    Cholestyramine may provide symptomatic relief by lowering the serum level of bile acids.
15. Daum, F., et al. 25-Hydroxycholecalciferol in the management of rickets associated with extrahepatic biliary atresia. *J. Pediatr.* 88:1041, 1976.
    Rickets is a common but preventable complication of biliary atresia. (Also see J. Pediatr. *94:870, 1979.)*
16. Abramson, S., et al. The infant with possible biliary atresia: Evaluation by ultrasound and nuclear medicine. *Pediatr. Radiol.* 12:1, 1982.
    Ultrasound evidence of normal gallbladder size makes biliary atresia unlikely.

Neonatal Hepatitis

17. Danks, D., et al. Prognosis of babies with neonatal hepatitis. *Arch. Dis. Child.* 52:368, 1977.
    The course of neonatal hepatitis depends in large part on the etiology; e.g., cytomegalovirus-induced disease has a good prognosis, but hepatitis due to the other TORCHES agents (see Congenital Infections, Chap. 43) is often fatal.
18. Watkins, J., Katz, A., and Grand, R. Neonatal hepatitis: A diagnostic approach. *Adv. Pediatr.* 24:399, 1977.
    Nearly 50 pages long (242 references) and followed by an article on hepatitis B infection in infants (p. 455).
19. Schweitzer, I., et al. Viral hepatitis B in neonates and infants. *Am. J. Med.* 55:762, 1973.
    Neonatal infection with the serum hepatitis virus follows two distinct courses: most infants have chronic, subclinical hepatitis and antigenemia, while acute icteric diseases develop in a few, followed by rapid healing and loss of antigenemia.
20. Talamo, R. Basic and clinical aspects of the alpha$_1$-antitrypsin. *Pediatrics* 56:91, 1975.
    An excellent review of this disorder, the importance of which has only recently been appreciated.

63. HEPATITIS
Kenneth B. Roberts

There are many viruses capable of causing hepatitis. In the newborn, congenital infection with the TORCH agents or acquired infection with herpes simplex virus or an enterovirus (Coxsackie, ECHO) can result in a systemic disease process of which hepatitis is a significant component. Older children infected with cytomegalovirus may develop hepatitis, with hepatomegaly and splenomegaly; jaundice, however, is uncommon, enzyme increases are usually modest, and chronic hepatitis is very rare. Subclinical hepatitis is frequent in infectious mononucleosis caused by the Epstein-Barr virus; rarely, acute hepatic failure ensues that clinically may mimic Reye syndrome.

The viruses that cause the majority of cases of hepatitis are those responsible for the diseases designated hepatitis A, hepatitis B, and non-A, non-B hepatitis. Hepatitis A, previously called infectious hepatitis, is usually an acute illness with an incubation period of 14 to 40 days. Hepatitis B, formally called serum hepatitis, is more often insidious in onset, and the incubation period is longer (50–100 days). Although it was once felt that hepatitis A was spread only by fecal-oral means and hepatitis B only by parenteral exposure, it is now clear that these are but the usual routes of infection. Like hepatitis B, non-A, non-B hepatitis is usually transmitted by parenteral exposure, but sporadic cases have been identified.

The timing of various manifestations is usually described in relation to the onset of jaundice. It should be noted, however, that jaundice is much less common in infants and young children than in adults. Anorexia, fever, and malaise may be the major—or only—clinical manifestations; these are also less severe in younger patients. The first detectable abnormality at all ages is bilirubinuria. Urobilinogen appears in the urine later and then disappears at the height of hyperbilirubinemia; its reappearance heralds recovery. Conjugated bilirubin may be increased before the total bilirubin is abnormal. Serum aminotransferase (transaminase) concentrations rise to maximal values about the time jaundice appears. Since aminotransferase levels return toward normal even if the patient becomes clinically worse, they cannot be used to predict the course; elevations that persist for 6 months or more do not preclude complete recovery.

In the preicteric stage, the white blood cell count is often low, and the erythrocyte sedimentation rate is increased. As the illness progresses and hyperbilirubinemia approaches its peak, the sedimentation rate and leukocyte count return to normal. Atypical lymphocytes, suggestive of infectious mononucleosis, may constitute 5 to 25 percent of the white blood cells.

Although hepatitis B is often more severe than hepatitis A (mortality as high as 12% has been reported), it is usually impossible to distinguish the two diseases clinically. Differentiation is based on a history of known exposure and serologic testing. In patients with hepatitis A an IgM antibody against the virus can be demonstrated at the time of presentation with clinical disease; this antibody is generally present for approximately 1 month after onset of illness and is followed by an IgG anti*body* to the virus that may persist for years. Patients with hepatitis B do not have anti*body* to the virus at the time of clinical presentation; rather, the anti*gen* is demonstrable: HBsAg (hepatitis B surface antigen). The presence of various components of the hepatitis B virus or antibody responses to them provides further information, such as timing of the infection and degree of infectiousness: e.g., presence of HBsAb implies immunity; HBeAg is a marker of high infectivity.

Discovery of hepatitis B surface antigen made possible the delineation of several clinical syndromes associated with hepatitis B. As many as 10 to 20 percent of patients have a prodromal illness resembling serum sickness, with rash, urticaria, polyarthralgia, and circulating immune complexes. Some patients have an illness resembling polyarteritis nodosa and others a glomerulonephritis with nodular deposits of hepatitis B surface antigen, immunoglobulins, and complement in the glomerular basement membrane. A small number of patients develop a papular acrodermatitis. The risk of developing hepatocellular carcinoma is increased in individuals infected with hepatitis B virus.

The ability to identify cases of hepatitis A and hepatitis B serologically has led to the recognition of a group of patients with hepatitis from an unspecified cause or causes given the designation *non-A, non-B hepatitis*. This is a major form of posttransfusional hepatitis, and affected patients have a high risk for developing chronic hepatitis; they may also develop bone marrow suppression during or following their episode of hepatitis. At present there is no specific assay available to screen for non-A, non-B hepatitis. It has been demonstrated, however, that eliminating as blood donors individuals with serum alanine aminotransferase (ALT) elevations reduces the incidence of posttransfusional hepatitis.

Bed rest and a low-fat diet have traditionally been prescribed for patients with acute hepatitis; controlled studies have failed to demonstrate any benefit from either. The patient with severe involvement (reflected by a prolonged prothrombin time) should be hospitalized. The administration of corticosteroids is to be discouraged, since the improvement in laboratory values that may occur is only a "biochemical whitewash": the rate of relapse is doubled, and that of chronic hepatitis tripled, with the use of corticosteroids, and they increase mortality in patients with fulminant disease.

Less than 1 percent of adult patients and even fewer children have a fulminant course with death in the first month. Complete recovery occurs in 80 to 90 percent, although in 10 to 12 percent it takes several months. Those in the latter group have normal liver architecture on biopsy, and their disease is classified as chronic persistent hepatitis. Chronic active hepatitis develops in 3 to 5 percent of patients, with alterations in the architectural structure of the liver and, commonly, progression to cirrhosis. (Two forms of chronic active hepatitis may be distinguished, one associated with hepatitis B in adult males, and a second, not associated with hepatitis B, occurring as a progressive auto-immunelike disorder in young females.)

Efforts to prevent the spread of hepatitis are hampered by the heartiness of the viruses. Hepatitis A virus, which is excreted in the stool from 2 weeks before the onset of clinical illness to 1 week after, is resistant to most common means of disinfection, and whole blood contaminated with hepatitis B virus cannot be sterilized with present techniques.

Human immune serum globulin (HISG), administered shortly after exposure to hepatitis A, reduces the development of overt hepatitis, but does not appear to prevent subclinical infection. Prophylaxis with HISG is also appropriate for travelers to areas in which hepatitis A is prevalent and sanitation facilities are inadequate. Hepatitis B immune globulin (HBIG) contains a high titer of antibody to hepatitis B surface antigen. Nevertheless, two injections are required for adequate protection: one within the first week after exposure, and a second, 1 month later. Preexposure prevention of hepatitis B is now possible with inactivated hepatitis B vaccine. Candidates for this vaccine are individuals at high risk of encountering hepatitis B virus, such as patients who receive multiple transfusions (because of hemodialysis, hemophilia, thalassemia, etc.), individuals who reside in institutions for the mentally retarded, immigrants or refugees from areas of high HBV endemicity, household contacts of HBV carriers (especially newborns and infants), health care workers (medical, dental, and laboratory) who come in contact with blood, users of illicit parenteral drugs, and homosexually active males.

At present it is not clear how to manage carriers of hepatitis B surface antigen, particularly if they are pregnant (hepatitis B can be devastating to infants) or are health professionals. Approximately 15 percent of dentists and physicians have serologic evidence of encounter with hepatitis B virus.

Reviews

1. Krugman, S., and Katz, S. Viral Hepatitis. In S. Krugman (ed.), *Infectious Diseases of Children* (7th ed.). St. Louis: Mosby, 1980. P. 90.
   Who better to read concerning hepatitis in children than Krugman?
2. Sherlock, S. (ed.). Virus hepatitis. *Clin. Gastroenterol.* 9(1), 1980.
   Contains 12 chapters, 228 pages, on various aspects, including a specific chapter on infants and children.

Clinical Disease

3. FitzGerald, J., Angelides, A., and Wyllie, R. The hepatitis spectrum. *Curr. Probl. Pediatr.* 11(11), 1981.
   Considers the various forms of hepatitis A and B: acute, subacute, fulminant, chronic, benign, and chronic aggressive.
4. Chilton, L. Viral hepatitis in school-aged children. *Pediatr. Rev.* 4:105, 1982.
   Practical aspects of hepatitis A, B, and non-A, non-B well summarized.
5. Wewalka, F. Clinical course of viral hepatitis. *Clin. Gastroenterol.* 3:355, 1974.
   The clinical aspects are discussed (21 pages, 77 references).
6. Gocke, D. Extrahepatic manifestations of viral hepatitis. *Am. J. Med. Sci.* 270:49, 1975.
   Serum-sickness-like prodrome, polyarteritis nodosa, and glomerulonephritis.
7. Kleinknecht, C., et al. Membranous glomerulonephritis and hepatitis B surface antigen in children. *J. Pediatr.* 95:946, 1979.
   HBsAg more frequently associated with membranous nephropathy than with other forms of kidney diseases.
8. Rubenstein, D., Esterly, N., and Fretzin, D. The Gianotti-Crosti syndrome. *Pediatrics* 61:433, 1978.
   Infantile papular acrodermatitis associated with hepatitis B (and other agents as well: J. Pediatr. 101:216, 1982). Color picture: Am. J. Dis. Child. 136:161, 1982.

Management

9. Silverberg, M., et al. An evaluation of rest and low-fat diets in the management of acute infectious hepatitis. *J. Pediatr.* 74:260, 1969.

"Supervised ad lib diets and activity regimen" do not hurt children with hepatitis *(also see* N. Engl. J. Med. *281:1393, 1969).*

10. Gregory, P., et al. Steroid therapy in severe viral hepatitis. *N. Engl. J. Med.* 294:681, 1976.
    Biochemical improvement at the expense of a more complicated course in patients with severe disease (when treatment is hardest to resist!); double-blind, randomized trial. (See the editorial and letter to the editor in the same issue; also see Am. J. Med. *47:82, 93, 1969.)*

Chronic Active Hepatitis

11. Redeker, A. Treatment of chronic active hepatitis. *N. Engl. J. Med.* 304:420, 1981.
    An editorial review, subtitled "good news and bad news," emphasizing definition of various forms of chronic hepatitis.

Prevention/Control

12. Favero, M., et al. Guidelines for the care of patients hospitalized with viral hepatitis. *Ann. Intern. Med.* 91:872, 1979.
    Emphasizes blood precautions and questions need for specific enteric isolation in continent patients; specific precautions addressed.

13. Stiehm, E. Use of human immune serum globulins. *Pediatr. Rev.* 4:135, 1982.
    Includes indications, dosages, and schedule of administration for HISG and HBIG. Official CDC recommendations published in Ann. Intern. Med. *96:193, 1982, and in* Clin. Pediatr. *(Phila.) 21:313, 1982. Updated:* Ann. Intern. Med. *101:351, 1984.*

14. Chin, J. Prevention of chronic hepatitis B virus infection from mothers to infants in the United States. *Pediatrics* 71:289, 1983.
    How to use serologic tests, HBIG, and hepatitis B vaccine.

15. Hadler, S., et al. Hepatitis A in day-care centers: A community-wide assessment. *N. Eng. J. Med.* 302:1222, 1980.
    The key figures were infants less than 2 years of age.

16. Centers for Disease Control. Inactivated hepatitis B virus vaccine. *Ann. Intern. Med.* 97:379, 1982.
    The "official" recommendations regarding the vaccine, indications for its use, and prevaccination serologic screening. (Krugman's view: JAMA 247:2012, 1982; safety reaffirmed: JAMA 249:745, 1983.)

17. Szmuness, W., et al. Hepatitis B vaccine: Demonstration of efficacy in a controlled clinical trial in a high-risk population in the United States. *N. Engl. J. Med.* 303:833, 1980.
    Safe and effective; implications discussed in an editorial on page 874.

18. Mulley, A., Silverstein, M., and Dienstag, J. Indications for use of hepatitis B vaccine, based on cost-effectiveness analysis. *N. Engl. J. Med.* 307:644, 1982.
    A discussion of the relative merits of vaccinating everyone, screening everyone and vaccinating those without evidence of immunity, and neither vaccinating nor screening but passively immunizing those with known exposure.

Non-A, Non-B Hepatitis

19. Robinson, W. The enigma of non-A, non-B hepatitis. *J. Infect. Dis.* 145:387, 1982.
    Currently the most frequent cause of posttransfusion hepatitis. (Also see Ann. Intern. Med. *92:539, 1980.)*

Occupational Hazard

20. Smith, J., et al. Comparative risk of hepatitis B among physicians and dentists. *J. Infect. Dis.* 133:705, 1976.
    The news is not good.

---

64. CHRONIC DIARRHEA AND MALABSORPTION
Margaret E. Mohrmann

The child with abnormal stools presents one of the more common diagnostic problems with which the pediatrician is faced. The initial evaluation of such a patient should determine whether or not an abnormality indeed exists. Because there is a wide range of normal stool patterns in childhood, defining diarrhea solely as frequent, loose stools may be misleading. For example, that definition aptly describes the normal stool pattern of a breast-fed infant; conversely, a child with significant fat malabsorption (steatorrhea) may pass only one or two firm stools daily. A diagnosis of diarrhea must take into account both the patient's usual stool pattern and the nature (color, consistency) of the stools passed. Chronic diarrhea may be defined as diarrhea that persists beyond a period of time, perhaps 2 weeks, that could reasonably be ascribed to an acute episode of gastroenteritis.

Important aspects to consider in the initial interview include the presence or absence of associated symptoms; a recent history of gastroenteritis, or a past history of constipation, diarrhea, or both; and the relationship of the onset of diarrhea to diet or dietary changes. A detailed family history should also be obtained. The physical examination should help define the chronicity and nutritional significance of the disorder, with measurements of height, weight, and head circumference being most revealing in this regard.

Decisions as to the extent of further evaluation of chronic diarrhea are difficult and cannot be approached dogmatically. In general, growth retardation ("failure to thrive") is the single most compelling reason to perform an elaborate workup. The child whose growth continues to follow a normal percentile curve is unlikely to have significant disease.

Among children with persistent diarrhea whose growth is unaffected, the largest fraction are presumed to have recurrent bouts of gastroenteritis. A diagnosis of "chronic nonspecific diarrhea" has been used for children who have intermittent episodes of increased stool frequency and amount, without signs of growth retardation, malnutrition, or dehydration. Most of these patients present at about 1 year of age and have family histories of functional bowel problems. This syndrome probably represents the pediatric equivalent of the "irritable colon" in adults and requires no therapy other than reassurance; over 90 percent of such patients will be free of diarrhea after the age of 3 years. Children with *Giardia lamblia* infestation of the small bowel may continue to grow normally, as may patients with specific food allergies causing diarrhea.

Children with chronic diarrhea but with normal growth need few diagnostic tests when first seen. These should include hemoglobin determination, stool culture, examination of the stool for blood and parasites, urinalysis, and urine culture, since persistent diarrhea may be the only manifestation of urinary tract infection in the very young. If the results of these studies are normal, the patient is probably best managed with observation alone.

In contrast, an infant who is failing to gain weight at an appropriate rate, or an older child with evidence of growth retardation, requires a careful study of bowel function, even if the stool is of normal frequency and consistency. The history and physical examination of the child and the gross appearance of the stool are usually helpful in determining the initial direction of a staged search for evidence of malabsorption of dietary sugar, fat, or protein. Sugar malabsorption causes watery, acid diarrhea that excoriates the buttocks; steatorrhea is usually associated with frothy, bulky stools that need not be increased in frequency; protein malabsorption—or protein-losing enteropathy—is almost always accompanied by some degree of steatorrhea and may present as hypoproteinemic edema.

The most common cause of sugar malabsorption is transient lactase deficiency of the postgastroenteritis period. Lactase is the least abundant and the most superficially located of the mucosal enzymes; it is "the first to go and the last to return," occasionally requiring 3 to 6 months to return to normal levels after an acute episode of diarrhea. Congenital alactasia is a rare cause of sugar malabsorption, distinguishable from secondary lactase deficiency only by mucosal biopsy. Approximately 70 percent of adult blacks, but only 5 to 10 percent of adult Caucasians, have a late-onset "hypolactasia," theoretically due to a gradual loss of only one of the two functional lactases. Other disorders of disaccharide absorption—specifically, sucrase-isomaltase deficiency—are rare. Transient defects of monosaccharide absorption infrequently occur after severe diarrhea. A rare congenital defect in glucose-galactose absorption, necessitating the use of fructose as the only dietary sugar, has also been described.

Screening tests for sugar malabsorption detect either the unabsorbed sugars themselves or the products of their digestion by intestinal bacteria. Clinitest tablets may be used to detect reducing substances (all dietary sugars except sucrose) in the stool. Bacterial fermentation of intraluminal sugar results in the production of hydrogen, which i, freely absorbed into the blood, excreted via the lungs, and can be measured in expired air. The production of hydrogen ions also lowers the pH of the stool, but, because of the wide range of stool pH values in healthy infants, this test is probably more reliable in follow-ing an individual patient than as a screen. Tolerance tests for specific sugars may be performed by giving a standard oral dosage of the sugar in question, followed by serial examinations of blood and stool, and measurements of breath hydrogen content to assess digestion and absorption. Such tests should be conducted under close supervision, since even a test dose may cause significant diarrhea and dehydration in an affected child. In a child with probable postgastroenteritis transient lactase deficiency, tolerance tests are unnecessary; a trial of lactose-free formula is a more reasonable—and therapeutic—approach.

A broad range of disease states may cause steatorrhea, including disorders of bile metabolism, pancreatic enzyme production, and mucosal integrity. Cystic fibrosis is the most common cause of significant steatorrhea in children in the United States and should receive prime consideration in the differential diagnosis of malabsorption even in the absence of respiratory symptoms and growth retardation. In a patient with apparent pancreatic enzyme deficiency but with a normal sweat chloride determination, a diagno-sis of Shwachman syndrome (pancreatic insufficiency and neutropenia) should be enter-tained. The child with steatorrhea caused by gluten sensitivity (celiac disease) presents in the second 6 months of life with growth retardation, abdominal distention, muscle wasting and hypotonia, anorexia, and marked irritability, with an appearance of total misery; the stools are pale, bulky, frothy, and malodorous. Only half the patients with celiac disease have this classic syndrome, however; others may present with vomiting alone or with manifestations of vitamin deficiencies.

Cow milk protein intolerance, found in fewer than 1 percent of the total population when specific milk protein challenge tests are used to confirm the diagnosis, has its onset in the first 6 months of life. Vomiting and diarrhea (steatorrhea) are the most common symptoms, but there is a significant incidence of eczema, asthma, and anaphylaxis; the child's tolerance of milk protein usually returns to normal by 24 to 30 months of age. Abetalipoproteinemia is a rare disease that presents in infancy as steatorrhea and acanthocytosis, followed later in childhood by retinal and neurologic changes.

The examination of a single stool specimen for fat is not as valid a quantitative test for steatorrhea as a 3- or 5-day fecal fat determination. Indirect evidence of fat mal-absorption may be obtained from determinations of serum carotene, calcium, and the prothrombin time, which are indicators of absorption of the fat-soluble vitamins A, D and K. A sweat chloride level should be obtained in every child with malabsorption of fat. Radiologic examination of the gastrointestinal tract with barium may show mucosal edema or other abnormalities. The D-xylose absorption test can be used to evaluate mucosal integrity; although some authors feel that the test adds nothing to clinical findings, others believe it to be useful in deciding which patient should have a mucosal biopsy performed. Criteria for the use of a peroral biopsy of the duodenal or jejunal mucosa vary considerably, with the only definite indications being a strong suspicion of celiac disease (with plans for instituting a gluten-free diet) or a severely growth-retarding or life-threatening diarrhea in a child for whom a diagnosis has not been made by other means.

Protein malabsorption is most commonly seen in syndromes of pancreatic insufficiency and is accompanied by steatorrhea. (Only rarely, as in the case of enterokinase deficiency, is protein malabsorption an isolated finding.) Intestinal lymphangiectasia is a protein-losing enteropathy characterized by hypoproteinemia, hypogammaglobuline-mia, steatorrhea, and lymphopenia; it may be a primary disorder, with generalized dilatation of lymphatics, or occur as a result of constrictive pericarditis. Many patients who have mucosal damage and malabsorption as a result of sensitivity to cow milk protein will exhibit protein loss, hypoproteinemia, and edema. Similarly, any disease causing severe mucosal injury may result in a clinically significant loss of protein, reflected by decreased serum levels of protein, albumin, and gamma globulin. Intestinal protein loss can be substantiated by demonstrating exudation of radioactively labeled albumin, for example, into the gut lumen.

In addition to specific syndromes of sugar, fat, or protein malabsorption, there are numerous disorders that cause generalized mucosal damage and chronic diarrhea, including drug effects, acrodermatitis enteropathica, familial chloride diarrhea, inflammatory bowel disease, and severe iron deficiency. Persistent diarrhea is a major manifestation of many immunodeficiency states, especially selective IgA deficiency, severe combined immunodeficiency, and the "variable immune deficiency" of adults. Although the cause of the diarrhea remains obscure, many of the immuno-deficiency-related malabsorptive disorders are associated with infestation by *Giardia lamblia*, a protozoan parasite diagnosed most readily by demonstration of the trophozoite in duodenal aspirates or mucosal biopsies (only infrequently are *Giardia* cysts identified in the stool).

It has become clear that clinical disorders of bowel function often cannot be absolutely categorized into specific derangements of digestion, or absorption, or both; e.g., most children with significant steatorrhea have evidence of secondary disaccharidase deficiency. However, close attention to the patient's growth, nutritional status, and stool pattern can result in an appropriate and efficient plan of diagnosis and management.

Reviews and Management

1. Ament, M. Malabsorption syndromes in infancy and childhood. *J. Pediatr.* 81:685, 867, 1972.
   A comprehensive review of gastrointestinal physiology, tests of function, and causes of malabsorption. The disease is classified on the basis of age at presentation and type of stools. (A more recent and briefer review by the same author is in Pediatr. Ann. *11:125, 1982.)*

2. Lo, C., and Walker, W. Chronic protracted diarrhea of infancy: A nutritional disease. *Pediatrics* 72:786, 1983.
   An excellent, extensively referenced paper, which, after reviewing etiologies and diagnostic studies, gives appropriate emphasis to the important role of malnutrition in perpetuating the diarrhea (a concept presented previously in Pediatrics *41:712, 1968).*

3. Fitzgerald, J., and Clark, J. Chronic diarrhea. *Pediatr. Clin. North Am.* 29:221, 1982.
   A discussion of mechanisms of disease and a logical approach to evaluation; possible diagnoses are organized by the nature of the stool (watery, fatty, or bloody).

4. Sunshine, P., Sinatra, F., and Mitchell, C. Intractable diarrhoea of infancy. *Clin. Gastroenterol.* 6:445, 1977.
   Excellent overview concentrating on possible causes and diagnostic measures. (This issue of Clin. Gastroenterol. *is a symposium on pediatric gastroenterology and includes several helpful articles.)*

5. Lloyd-Still, J. Chronic diarrhea of childhood and the misuse of elimination diets. *J. Pediatr.* 95:10, 1979.
   The author cites a relatively high incidence of iatrogenic malnutrition and speculates that the empiric use of gluten-free diets is masking the true incidence of celiac disease in the United States.

6. MacLean, W., et al. Nutritional management of chronic diarrhea and malnutrition: Primary reliance on oral feeding. *J. Pediatr.* 97:316, 1980.
   The article emphasizes the efficacy and advantages of the enteral route for nutritional repletion and discusses the common errors of reasoning and implementation that interfere with the appropriate use of oral feedings. (The return of some intestinal function is faster in children given oral feedings than in those receiving intravenous alimentation only: J. Pediatr. *87:695, 1975.)*

Chronic Nonspecific Diarrhea

7. Davidson, M., and Wasserman, R. The irritable colon of childhood (chronic nonspecific diarrhea syndrome). *J. Pediatr.* 69:1027, 1966.
   An excellent study of 186 patients, with a discussion of clinical manifestations and typical course; recommends the use of a full diet, not because it is curative but because a restricted diet is unnecessary and may prolong the diarrhea. (For a more recent review, see Pediatr. Rev. *3:153, 1981.)*

8. Cohen, S., et al. Chronic nonspecific diarrhea: Dietary relationships. *Pediatrics* 64:402, 1979.
   Most patients with the disorder had less than adequate fat intakes; increasing dietary fat to recommended levels resulted in resolution of the diarrhea in almost all. (A high

daily fluid intake is implicated as the cause of chronic diarrhea in some children: J. Pediatr. *102:836, 1983.)*

Sugar Malabsorption

9. Lebenthal, E. Small intestinal disaccharidase deficiencies. *Pediatr. Clin. North Am.* 22:757, 1975.

A brief review of classification, presentation, and diagnosis; for a good overview of pathophysiology, see Arch. Dis. Child. *42:341, 1967.*

10. Antonowicz, I., et al. Congenital sucrase-isomaltase deficiency. *Pediatrics* 49:847, 1972.

A study of 10 children with this disorder, the most common congenital form of carbohydrate intolerance. (Also see J. Pediatr. *103:491, 1983; includes a good discussion of differential diagnosis.)*

11. Soeparto, P., et al. Role of chemical examination of the stool in diagnosis of sugar malabsorption in children. *Arch. Dis. Child.* 47:56, 1972.

The use of Clinitest tablets as a screen for reducing substances and paper chromatography to detect the type of sugar; pH is generally unreliable as a screen, although it may be useful in following an individual patient.

12. Barr, R., et al. Breath tests in pediatric gastrointestinal disorders: New diagnostic opportunities. *Pediatrics* 62:393, 1978.

An enthusiastic review of the tests' diagnostic accuracy and utility in children. (For a study of the sensitivity of the breath hydrogen test, see J. Pediatr. *97:609, 1980; for the usefulness in following the recovery of bowel function in infants with acquired carbohydrate malabsorption, see* J. Pediatr. *102:371, 1983.)*

Fat Malabsorption: Pancreatic Insufficiency

13. Shwachman, H. Gastrointestinal manifestations of cystic fibrosis. *Pediatr. Clin. North Am.* 22:787, 1975.

Emphasis on the spectrum; note that pancreatic dysfunction may be minimal or absent in true cystic fibrosis. (For more on pancreatic function, normal and abnormal, see Adv. Pediatr. *25:223, 1978.)*

14. Shwachman, H., et al. The syndrome of pancreatic insufficiency and bone marrow dysfunction. *J. Pediatr.* 65:645, 1964.

Original description (five cases) of Shwachman syndrome, with a comprehensive listing of diagnostic features.

Fat Malabsorption: Celiac Disease

15. Lebenthal, E., and Branski, D. Childhood celiac disease: A reappraisal. *J. Pediatr.* 98:681, 1981.

A helpful comprehensive review that stresses the need for small bowel biopsies for diagnosis.

16. Young, W., and Pringle, E. 110 children with celiac disease, 1950–1969. *Arch. Dis. Child.* 46:421, 1971.

A misdiagnosis rate of 8 to 10 percent without biopsy; importance of "subclinical" relapses in teenagers who go off the diet and who may have growth retardation and/or iron- or folate-deficiency anemia without gastrointestinal symptoms.

Fat Malabsorption: Other Causes

17. Lebenthal, E. Cow's milk protein allergy. *Pediatr. Clin. North Am.* 22:827, 1975.

A practical, reasonable discussion of the known facts and remaining questions (15 pages, 52 references). (Also see Adv. Pediatr. *25:1, 1978, and* Pediatrics *60:477, 1977.)*

18. Kuitunen, P., et al. Malabsorption syndrome with cow's milk intolerance. *Arch. Dis. Child.* 50:351, 1975.

Emphasizes the need for a cow milk protein challenge, since mucosal changes are often indistinguishable from those in other malabsorption syndromes; the mucosa was still significantly abnormal in many at 1 year of age when clinical sensitivity had cleared. (Also see commentary, p. 347.)

19. Kornzweig, A. Bassen-Kornzweig syndrome: Present status. *J. Med. Genet.* 7:271, 1970.

A five-page review of the abetalipoproteinemia syndrome; if betalipoprotein is present at 10 to 20 percent of normal levels, there will be no symptoms or pathologic changes.

Fat Malabsorption: Diagnostic Studies

20. Tully, T., and Feinberg, S. A roentgenographic classification of diffuse diseases of the small intestine presenting with malabsorption. *Am. J. Roentgenol.* 121:283, 1974.
Four diagnostic categories, based on the presence or absence of small bowel dilatation and on the appearance of mucosal folds.

21. Buts, J., et al. One-hour blood xylose test: A reliable index of small bowel function. *J. Pediatr.* 92:729, 1978.
Test found reliable in study of 435 children; companion article (p. 725 of same issue) reports high false-negative and false-positive rates in 33 children and refutes usefulness of test, as does a similar study reported in J. Pediatr. *99:245, 1981.*

22. Townley, R., and Barnes, G. Intestinal biopsy in childhood. *Arch. Dis. Child.* 48:480, 1973.
The study included 1172 children, 1247 biopsies; the youngest patient was 3 weeks old, most were outpatients, 34 percent had mucosal abnormalities, and there was only one complication.

Protein Malabsorption

23. Waldmann, T. Protein-losing enteropathy. *Gastroenterology* 50:422, 1966.
A lengthy review emphasizing diagnostic techniques and the broad spectrum of etiologies (see also references 13, 14, 17, and 18).

Miscellaneous Causes of Malabsorption

24. Faloon, W. Drug production of intestinal malabsorption. *N.Y. State J. Med.* 70:2189, 1970.
A four-page article on varying degrees of drug effects on absorption, ranging from steatorrhea caused by calcium carbonate to mucosal flattening by methotrexate.

25. Neldner, K., and Hambidge, K. Zinc therapy of acrodermatitis enteropathica. *N. Engl. J. Med.* 292:879, 1975.
A case report with a discussion of possible defects in zinc metabolism.

26. Ament, M. Inflammatory disease of the colon: Ulcerative colitis and Crohn's colitis. *J. Pediatr.* 86:322, 1975.
A thorough, classic review article (11 pages, 97 references). (For a recent update, see N. Engl. J. Med. *306:775, 837, 1982.)*

27. Oski, F. The nonhematologic manifestations of iron deficiency. *Am. J. Dis. Child.* 133:315, 1979.
A review that includes a brief section on the spectrum of clinical and histologic abnormalities of the gastrointestinal tract that may be found in iron deficiency. (For an older, but more detailed review, see Pediatrics *33:83, 1964.)*

Immunodeficiency States

28. Ament, M. Immunodeficiency syndromes and gastrointestinal disease. *Pediatr. Clin. North Am.* 22:807, 1975.
An overview of types of gastrointestinal lesions and absorptive defects associated with various immunodeficiency states. Giardia *infestation is commonly linked to malabsorption in the immune-incompetent person; bacterial overgrowth in the small intestine has not been shown to cause malabsorption.*

29. Wolfe, M. Giardiasis. *Pediatr. Clin. North Am.* 26:295, 1979.
A review of clinical manifestations, diagnostic methods, and treatment.

30. Dubois, R., et al. Disaccharidase deficiency in children with immunologic deficits. *J. Pediatr.* 76:377, 1970.
Emphasizes the importance of secretory IgA for normal gastrointestinal function; sugar intolerance was related to the loss of mucosal integrity.

65. ULCERATIVE COLITIS
Kenneth B. Roberts

Until about a decade ago, all children with inflammatory disease of the colon were considered to have ulcerative colitis (UC). With the identification of Crohn disease of the colon as an entity, it is clear that some of the older reviews on ulcerative colitis in children included patients with Crohn. Ulcerative colitis can usually be distinguished from Crohn disease: involvement characteristically begins in the rectum and extends proximally without "skip areas." The perianal area is unaffected, and inflammation limited to the mucosa. In Crohn disease (see Chap. 66), involvement is patchy, perianal ulcers and fistulas are common, and inflammation involves all layers of the intestinal wall (transmural). Although no single measure successfully distinguishes between UC and Crohn colitis, the results of clinical evaluation (including proctoscopy and radiographic and histologic studies) strongly suggest one or the other diagnosis in about 80 percent of patients with inflammatory bowel disease. Entities other than Crohn disease from which ulcerative colitis must be distinguished are the so-called irritable colon of childhood, bacterial and amebic dysenteries, malignancy, the hemolytic-uremic syndrome, and collagen vascular diseases.

Children constitute about 15 percent of the patients with ulcerative colitis. The disease is rare in infants under the age of 1 year, and its frequency increases progressively throughout childhood. The female preponderance in adult-onset ulcerative colitis is not seen in the pediatric age group, and, in some series, boys outnumber girls 2 : 1. Ulcerative colitis is more common in Jews than non-Jews and tends to cluster in families.

The most common presenting complaint is diarrhea, often mucoid and bloody. Tenesmus and abdominal pain are common and palpation of the abdomen often produces tenderness. Impaired growth and maturation may be apparent, but is usually less striking than in Crohn disease. Extraintestinal manifestations, such as arthritis, dermatitis, liver disease, and fever, are common and may antedate gastrointestinal symptoms. Rectal fistulas do not occur, and perianal disease is rare.

Proctoscopy reveals diffuse involvement of the rectum, with vascular congestion, multiple small ulcerations, diffuse fine granularity and friability, purulent exudate, and occasionally, inflammatory polyps. Once the disease is well established, rectal narrowing may be noted, with mucosal dullness reflecting loss of the normal vascular pattern.

A barium enema demonstrates an abnormal rectum with disease extending proximally, including a "backwash ileitis" in 20 to 30 percent of patients: the notable x-ray features are decreased distensibility of the rectum and contraction and shortening of the colon, with diffuse, symmetric serration of margins. On postevaluation films, the mucosa appears coarsened and irregular. Widening of the presacral space and loss of the normal haustral pattern are commonly seen but do not differentiate ulcerative colitis from Crohn disease.

Biopsy specimens reveal acute and chronic inflammation limited to the mucosa. Loss of mucus from the epithelial cells is characteristic of active disease and is followed by atrophy of the glands in severe cases. Specimens obtained at proctocolectomy show not only the superficial inflammatory changes, but crypt abscesses, hemorrhage, and ulcerations as well.

Approximately 10 percent of children with UC have what is defined as mild disease, that is, fewer than four bowel movements per day and no constitutional signs. Moderately severe disease, consisting of diarrhea with abdominal cramps and fever, is uncommon in children; progression to severe disease is the rule. Severe disease consists of diarrhea with more than six bowel movements per day, anemia, fever, tachycardia, weight loss, and an incidence of toxic megacolon of 2 to 5 percent.

Toxic megacolon is a massive dilatation of the colon involving all layers, including the muscularis. Although it is usually a complication of well-established severe disease, it may be the presenting feature of ulcerative colitis. The mortality associated with toxic megacolon remains high (on the order of 25%), despite vigorous medical management including intravenous fluids, corticosteroids, antibiotics, constant nasogastric suction, and prohibition of oral intake. Emergency colectomy is purported to reduce mortality to 5 percent, but is not the universally accepted approach to management. Other indications for surgery include perforation, massive hemorrhage, worsening in the first several hours despite "resuscitative" medical management, lack of clinical improvement by 48 to 72 hours, or failure of the megacolon to recede by 12 to 14 days.

The other colonic complication of ulcerative colitis is cancer, which occurs at a rate of 20 percent per decade after the first 10 years of the disease; thus, colonic cancer develops in 50 percent of patients with ulcerative colitis after 35 years of disease. At present, there is no way to ensure early detection of cancer.

As noted, extracolonic manifestations are common and include growth retardation that is not improved by administration of growth hormone. Growth occurs if disease can be controlled *and* calorie intake is adequate; a growth spurt frequently occurs after colectomy. Arthritis of either a rheumatoid type or an ankylosing spondylitis type develops in 20 percent of patients. The rheumatoid type of arthritis is peripheral, associated with mucocutaneous lesions, and benign; it may precede the gastrointestinal symptoms. Its course is unrelated to the severity of the diarrheal disease; it will remit following colectomy. The ankylosing spondylitis type of arthritis is unassociated with mucocutaneous lesions and is progressive. It also proceeds unrelated to the severity of the diarrheal disease but does not necessarily respond to colectomy and may prove to be a severe, disabling feature of the illness. A high percentage of these children have histocompatibility antigen HLA-W27. Mucocutaneous lesions include erythema nodosum, pyoderma gangrenosum, and oral ulcers. Hepatic involvement is characterized by periportal lymphocytic inflammation, which may progress to ductal proliferation, portal and periportal fibrosis, liver necrosis, and cirrhosis. The hepatitis may improve following colectomy—although this is not yet clear—but once cirrhosis is present, the damage is irreversible. Although the significance is unclear, multiple immunologic abnormalities have been noted, including high antibody titers to both epithelial cells and cross-reacting enterobacterial antigens. Circulating lymphocytes may be cytotoxic for colonic epithelial cells, and patients may have abnormal immunoglobulin patterns, anergy to dinitrochlorobenzene (DNCB), and circulating antigen-antibody complexes.

Systemic corticosteroids are of benefit for acute severe disease, and, as part of an in-hospital regimen, hydrocortisone enemas may have a salutary effect on localized proctocolitis. Once remission is obtained, sulfasalazine (Azulfidine) is administered as oral maintenance therapy. The drug is absorbed in the upper gastrointestinal tract and excreted into the bile; it is split into its components, sulfapyridine and 5-aminosalicylate, by mucosal bacteria. The sulfapyridine is absorbed, but the salicylate stays in the colon. The drug was developed because of the belief that the disease might have infectious and inflammatory components; it now appears that the salicylate is the active agent and that the sulfapyridine acts merely as a carrier, delivering the salicylate to the mucosa of the colon.

Immunosuppressive agents have been studied in UC and do not appear to be useful. Emergency colectomy is indicated for massive bleeding, perforation, and perhaps, as previously noted, for toxic megacolon. Elective protocolectomy is performed to prevent cancer and to provide relief from debilitation. Colectomy has beneficial effects on the peripheral arthritis, skin disease, growth impairment, and clubbing of the fingers and may halt progressive liver dysfunction; it prevents cancer and cures the gastrointestinal disease ("no colon, no colitis"). Colectomy does not halt the progression of ankylosing spondylitis and, although it does help certain features, creates the problems of coping with an ileostomy. As more experience is gained in children with the ileoanal anastomosis or "pull through" procedure, such adjustment problems may be lessened.

Reviews

1. Ament, M. Inflammatory disease of the colon: Ulcerative colitis and Crohn's colitis. *J. Pediatr.* 86:322, 1975.
   An excellent place to start.
2. Kelts, D., and Grand, R. Inflammatory bowel disease in children and adolescents. *Curr. Probl. Pediatr.* 10(5), 1980.
   A 40-page review, 102 references; for other extensive reviews see Adv. Pediatr. *26:311, 1979, or* Clin. Gastroenterol. *9(2), 1980.*
3. Schachter, H., and Kirsner, J. Definitions of inflammatory bowel disease of unknown etiology. *Gastroenterology* 68:591, 1975.

Clinical, proctoscopic, radiographic, and pathologic characteristics of known inflammatory bowel diseases, with a plea for standard nomenclature.

4. Kirsner, J., and Shorter, R. Recent developments in "non-specific" inflammatory bowel disease. *N. Engl. J. Med.* 306:775,837, 1982.
   An extensive two-part overview of multiple aspects (391 references).

Series

5. Goel, K., and Shanks, R. Long-term prognosis of children with ulcerative colitis. *Arch. Dis. Child.* 48:337, 1973.
   A study of 25 children, with extracolonic manifestation in 76 percent; the course was of the "chronic intermittent" type in 76 percent and was limited to a single attack in 16 percent.

6. Jalan, K., et al. An experience of ulcerative colitis: II. Short term outcome. *Gastroenterology* 59:589, 1970.
   Mortality in severe cases was 26.4 percent, with hypoalbuminemia, hypokalemia, and elevated alkaline phosphatase signaling a poor prognosis; 399 patients.

7. Jalan, K., et al. An experience of ulcerative colitis: III. Long term outcome. *Gastroenterology* 59:598, 1970.
   A relapse rate of 27 percent per year irrespective of severity; mortality in those moderately ill during the first attack was 2.4 percent per year.

8. Ein, S., Lynch, M., and Stephens, C. Ulcerative colitis in children under one year: A twenty-year review *J. Pediatr. Surg.* 6:264, 1971.
   Rare, but it does occur in infants under 1 year (these authors saw eight cases in 20 years). The course was not chronic: the children either improved or rapidly became worse.

Intestinal Complications

9. Norland, C., and Kirsner, J. Toxic dilatation of colon (toxic megacolon): Etiology, treatment and prognosis in 42 patients. *Medicine* (Baltimore) 48:229, 1969.
   In 70 percent, symptoms subsided with medical management, but only eight patients did not require an operation. (The average hospital stay was 83 days.)

10. Binder, S., Patterson, J., and Glotzer, D. Toxic megacolon in ulcerative colitis. *Gastroenterology* 66:909, 1974.
    Advocates of early operation feel that their mortality of 5.6 percent is less than the reported 23.1 percent because of their aggressive posture toward performing colectomy (also see Surg. Clin. North Am. 56:95, 1976).

11. Devroede, G., et al. Cancer risk and life expectancy of children with ulcerative colitis *N. Engl. J. Med.* 285:17, 1971.
    The classic analysis of 601 children that determined the cancer risk to be 20 percent per decade after the first 10 years.

12. Sachar, D., and Greenstein, A. Cancer in ulcerative colitis: Good and bad news. *Ann. Intern. Med.* 95:642, 1981.
    A brief editorial review of present knowledge concerning incidence, risk factors, and prevention.

Extracolonic Aspects

13. Greenstein, A., Janowitz, H., and Sachar, D. The extra-intestinal complications of Crohn's disease and ulcerative colitis: A study of 700 patients. *Medicine* (Baltimore) 55:401, 1976.
    Colitis-related complications are joint, skin, mouth, and eye disease.

14. Berger, M., Gribetz, D., and Korelitz, B. Growth retardation in children with ulcerative colitis: The effect of medical and surgical therapy. *Pediatrics* 55:459, 1975.
    Low-dose steroids are shown to regard growth significantly; high-dose steroids may help growth by controlling disease but are less effective in doing so than is colectomy and have the potential to retard ultimate growth.

15. Kane, W., Miller, K., and Sharp, H. Inflammatory bowel disease presenting as liver disease during childhood. *J. Pediatr.* 97:775, 1980.
    A report of four cases, with the recommendation that the workup of a patient with liver disease of unknown etiology includes tests on inflammatory bowel disease. (Colectomy

may halt progression of liver disease if performed prior to the development of cirrhosis: Mayo Clin. Proc. *47:36, 1972.)*

16. Lindsley, C., and Schaller, J. Arthritis associated with inflammatory bowel disease in children. *J Pediatr.* 84:16, 1974.
    Arthritis of two types occurred in 21 percent of patients with UC: peripheral (a few large joints, benign) and central (ankylosing spondylitis, progressive); mucocutaneous lesions were present with the former but not with the latter. There was no obvious relationship between these extracolonic manifestations and the severity of ulcerative colitis.

17. Thayer, W. Are the inflammatory bowel diseases immune complex disease? *Gastroenterology* 70:136, 1976.
    An editorial with 25 references (also see reference 4 for a detailed, well-referenced discussion).

Therapy

18. Peppercorn, M. Sulfasalazine. *Ann. Intern. Med.* 101:377, 1984.
    A review of a drug commonly used for UC: studies, pharmacology, and reactions.

19. Khan, A., Piris, J., and Truelove, S. An experiment to determine the active therapeutic moiety in sulphasalazine. *Lancet* 2:892, 1977.
    Salicylate wins—and wins again: N. Engl. J. Med. *303:1499, 1980. (Prospects for a "next generation" of sulfasalazinelike drugs:* Gastroenterology *83:1138, 1982.)*

66. CROHN DISEASE
Kenneth B. Roberts

Crohn disease is an inflammatory disorder of unknown etiology affecting all levels of the intestinal tract. It is half as common in children as ulcerative colitis (UC) and is distinguished from UC by transmural involvement (i.e., involvement not limited to the mucosa) and the tendency to form granulomas, fistulas, and abscesses; perianal disease and a patchy distribution of affected areas are characteristic. Although it was once believed that Crohn disease was confined to the small intestine (regional ileitis), it is now apparent that the colon is involved in one-half the children with Crohn disease.

The demographic characteristics of Crohn disease are similar to those of UC: the disease runs in families, and the incidence in Jews is approximately 6 times that in non-Jews; the disorder is particularly uncommon in blacks, American Indians, and Spanish-Americans. The sexes are affected equally. Crohn disease is uncommon in infants, but when it occurs, it is usually severe, with intestinal obstruction a prominent feature. The disease is most common among adolescents and young adults, but careful histories often reveal signs or symptoms that predate the diagnosis by many months or years.

The clinical presentation of Crohn disease is usually much less dramatic than that of UC: crampy abdominal pain and mucoid, bloody diarrhea are unusual. When abdominal pain and diarrhea are present, they are usually overshadowed by fever and growth retardation or by joint complaints. (The exception to this generalization is acute Crohn disease of the ileum, which may mimic appendicitis sufficiently to require laparotomy to establish the correct diagnosis.)

Approximately 5 percent of children with Crohn disease present with predominant perianal manifestations: perianal fistula, abscess, or hypertrophy and edema of rectal tags. Rectal strictures are not uncommon in this situation.

Joint disease is of two types, as in UC (see Chap. 65), but is less common than in UC. Eye manifestations include episcleritis, uveitis, and iridocyclitis. Skin lesions, aphthous ulcers, and clubbing also occur. Renal stones and gallstones are common in adult patients with Crohn disease, but the incidence in children is unknown. Local complications of intestinal disease include fistulas, abscesses, fibrosis, and obstruction; the ureters may be irritated by direct extension of the inflammation from the gastrointestinal tract, resulting in a functional or anatomic obstruction and hydronephrosis.

There is no laboratory test diagnostic of Crohn disease. Anemia and elevation of the erythrocyte sedimentation rate are usually present. At proctoscopic examination particular attention should be paid to the perianal area. A barium enema is suggestive of Crohn colitis when "skip areas" are identified, ulcers are greater than 2 mm in depth, and fistulas or abscesses are visualized. In the small bowel, findings are wide separation of adjacent loops, suggesting thickening of the bowel wall, replacement of normal mucosal pattern by a "cobblestone" appearance, narrowing and rigidity of segments of bowel with pseudodiverticula, and trapping of barium in fissures. Histologically, inflammation is not limited to the mucosa but is transmural; noncaseating granulomas are present in 30 to 50 percent of patients.

Conservative medical management consists of (1) anti-inflammatory agents such as sulfasalazine (Azulfidine) for colonic involvement and steroids; (2) bowel management with hydrophilic colloids and antimotility agents as needed; and (3) psychologic support. Recently, there has been greater enthusiasm for intensive corticosteroid therapy at the onset of treatment to gain control over the disease and reverse growth failure. Although the corticosteroids themselves have adverse effects on linear growth, such effects are quantitatively less severe for many patients than is uncontrolled Crohn disease. Parenteral nutrition may be required in some children and adolescents.

Intestinal perforation or obstruction, massive hemorrhage, or toxic megacolon are certain indications for operative intervention, but these complications are infrequent, and the place of surgery in the management of patients with Crohn disease is uncertain. Indications that have been proposed include fistulas, strictures, rectal bleeding, perianal disease, growth failure, and small-bowel carcinoma. (Carcinoma is more common in patients with Crohn disease than in the general population, but nevertheless is still infrequent.) Surgery is not curative in Crohn disease, as in ulcerative colitis, and a recurrence is virtually ensured. It is estimated that 80 percent of patients with Crohn disease come to operation at some time; the correct timing of procedures is usually a difficult decision for the physician, surgeon, and patient.

Disease confined to the small bowel is said to be associated with a better prognosis, but colonic disease offers the hope of cure by colectomy. At present, Crohn disease is a chronic, often debilitating, and sometimes mutilating inflammatory disorder of unknown cause, for which adequate treatment is lacking. Management is geared to control of disease activity while maximizing growth. Requirements for medication are often high, and associated morbidity is significant. Psychologic support is of critical importance.

History

1. Crohn, B., Ginzburg, L., and Oppenheimer, G. Regional ileitis: A pathological and clinical entity. *JAMA* 251:73, 1984.
   The 1932 classic description is reprinted, with an editorial commentary (p. 80). (A two-page reminiscence by Crohn introduces a 270-page symposium: Clin. Gastroenterol. *1:263, 1972.)*
2. Janowitz, H. Crohn disease: 50 years later. *N. Engl. J. Med.* 304:1600, 1981.
   An editorial to an article on the role of initial location of disease in recurrence and reoperation rates (p. 1586), briefly reviewing areas of progress since the 1932 report.

Reviews

3. Gryboski, J. Crohn disease in children. *Pediatr. Rev.* 2:239, 1981.
   An excellent general review of incidence, etiology, diagnosis, clinical course, complications, and therapy.
4. Singleton, J. (ed.). The national cooperative Crohn disease study. *Gastroenterology* 77:827, 1979.
   A series of 12 articles (more than 100 pages) on more than 1000 patients with Crohn disease, with attention to clinical course, effect of various drugs, factors determining recurrences after surgery, complications, and more.
5. Kirsner, J., and Shorter, R. Recent developments in "non-specific" inflammatory bowel disease. *N. Engl. J. Med.* 306:775,837, 1982.
   An extensive two-part overview (391 references).

Diagnosis

6. Miller, R., and Larsen, E. Regional enteritis in early infancy. *Am. J. Dis. Child.* 122:301, 1971.
   Rare; severe.

7. Burbige, E., Huang, S., and Bayless, T. Clinical manifestations of Crohn's disease in children and adolescents. *Pediatrics* 55:866, 1975.
   Extraintestinal manifestations and delays in diagnosis are stressed.
8. Dyer, N., and Dawson, A. Diagnosis of Crohn's disease: A continuing source of error. *Br. Med. J.* 1:735, 1970.
   A correct diagnosis is rarely made early.

Colonic Disease
9. Ament, M. Inflammatory disease of the colon: Ulcerative colitis and Crohn's colitis. *J. Pediatr.* 86:322, 1975.
   A good place to start your reading on the subject.
10. Schacter, H., and Kirsner, J. Definitions of inflammatory bowel disease of unknown etiology. *Gastroenterology* 68:591, 1975.
    Crohn disease is characterized and distinguished from other inflammatory bowel diseases.
    Also see Ulcerative Colitis (Chap. 65).

Complications
11. Greenstein, A., Janowitz, H., and Sachar, D. The extra-intestinal complications of Crohn's disease and ulcerative colitis: A study of 700 patients. *Medicine* (Baltimore) 55:401, 1976.
    Complications related to small bowel disease included malabsorption, gallstones, kidney stones, hydronephrosis, and hydroureter; colitis-related complications were joint, skin, mouth, and eye disease.
12. Rosenthal, S., et al. Growth failure and inflammatory bowel disease: Approach to treatment of a complicated adolescent problem. *Pediatrics* 72:481, 1983.
    A review of pathogenesis, evaluation, and various forms of treatment.
13. Lindsley, C., and Schaller, J. Arthritis associated with inflammatory bowel disease in children. *J. Pediatr.* 84:16, 1974.
    Clinical correlations of various complications.
14. Weedon, D., et al. Crohn's disease and cancer. *N. Eng. J. Med.* 289:1099, 1973.
    The incidence was 20 times greater than in control children.

Management
15. Whittington, P., Barnes, H., and Bayless, T. Medical management of Crohn's disease in adolescence. *Gastroenterology* 72:1338, 1977.
    Advocates aggressive use of steroids to get disease under control.
16. Motil, K., et al. The effect of disease, drug, and diet on whole body protein metabolism in adolescents with Crohn disease and growth failure. *J. Pediatr.* 101:345, 1982.
    Caloric insufficiency, rather than inflammation or steroid therapy, is primarily responsible for growth failure (confirmation in the form of improved growth with increased calories: Gastroenterology *80:10, 1981). (Also see reference 12.)*
17. Sleisenger, M. How should we treat Crohn disease. *N. Engl. J. Med.* 302:1024, 1980.
    *An editorial attempt to resolve conflicting reports of the benefit of immunosuppressives in Crohn disease (*N. Engl. J. Med. *302:981, 1980, versus the national cooperative Crohn disease study).*
18. Kirsner, J. Current medical and surgical opinions on important therapeutic issues in inflammatory bowel disease. *Am. J. Surg.* 140:391, 1980.
    A survey of gastroenterologists and surgeons regarding issues such as indications for surgery, surgical approaches, and postoperative problems; "opinions . . . were more concordant than might have been anticipated."
19. Fonkalsrud, E., et al. Surgical management of Crohn's disease in children. *Am. J. Surg.* 138:15, 1979.
    A summary of 50 patients, representing 57 percent of the children followed for Crohn disease during the 12-year period. (Another series: J. Pediatr. Surg. *16:449, 1981.)*
20. Homer, D., Grand, R., and Colodny, A. Growth, course, and prognosis after surgery for Crohn's disease in children and adolescents. *Pediatrics* 59:717, 1977.
    Linear growth improved following surgery only in children who were prepubertal and who had no early recurrence of disease activity.

Prognosis

21. Gryboski, J., and Spiro, H. Prognosis in children with Crohn's disease. *Gastroenterology* 74:807, 1978.

Children with ileocolitis had the highest number of extracolonic manifestations and operations and required steroid therapy the longest; those whose gastrointestinal disease was limited to the small intestine (duodenum excluded) had fewer extraintestinal problems and had better therapeutic responses.

VII. RENAL, FLUID, AND ELECTROLYTE DISORDERS

57. HYPERNATREMIC DEHYDRATION
Kenneth B. Roberts

One-fourth of children hospitalized because of diarrhea and dehydration have sodium concentrations above 150 mEq/dl. Mortality in these children is 4 to 5 times that associated with hypotonic dehydration, and survivors may suffer permanent sequelae. Hyperosmolarity per se is not the only problem; it is the inability of sodium to enter cells and consequent shifts in body water that are hazardous. In addition, other metabolic derangements accompany the elevation of serum sodium—some iatrogenically induced—which may further compromise the child.

A hypernatremic state may come about because of loss of water in excess of solute, failure to replace water loss, administration of excess solute, or combinations of these events. Loss of water in excess of solute can occur from the gastrointestinal tract with diarrhea or vomiting, from the kidney as in diabetes insipidus, from the skin with environmental stress or fever, from the lungs during hyperventilation or fever, and from iatrogenic causes such as overvigorous dialysis. Failure to replace water loss is particularly likely in infants who are unable to indicate thirst, but it may occur at any age if fluid intake is interfered with by nausea, vomiting, stupor, coma, inability to swallow, or an inappropriate lack of thirst. Administration of excess solute (salt poisoning) results from errors in mixing infant formula or from the administration of highly concentrated tube feedings and causes a syndrome even more devastating than hypertonic dehydration. Hypertonic dehydration occurs most commonly in infants with diarrhea, who may be at risk from all of these mechanisms: the loss of hypotonic diarrheal fluid; the inability to respond to thirst; excessive sweating secondary to fever; loss of fluid through the lungs from hyperventilation induced by both fever and acidosis; the limited capacity of the kidney to concentrate urine (particularly if the infant is very young); and the possibility of being offered a high-solute-load formula such as boiled skim milk.

Clinical recognition of hypernatremia is often difficult because the usual signs of severe dehydration, which are those of circulatory insufficiency, are deceptively mild. The intravascular volume is supported by the water-drawing force of the excess osmols, so that skin turgor may not be poor even with a 10 percent weight loss. The skin is classically described as "doughy," but it is not always so; more reliable findings are dry tongue and mucous membranes. The infant is usually lethargic and apathetic when left alone, but exceeding irritable when aroused; convulsions may occur but are more commonly associated with the treatment phase if the hypernatremia is corrected too rapidly. Increased muscular tone and reflexes may be present, and nuchal rigidity may be pronounced; usually, the number of cells in the cerebrospinal fluid is not increased, but an elevation of the protein concentration is common. In the presence of hypernatremia and hypokalemia, mild hypocalcemia occurs, rarely, to the point of tetany. Hyperglycemia is common and blood glucose concentration can reach high levels (> 600 mg/dl). Hyperventilation may be present because of acidosis and fever. The combination of hyperglycemia, hyperventilation, acidosis, and dehydration, particularly when ketonuria is also present, may suggest the diagnosis of diabetic ketoacidosis; a determination of serum sodium readily establishes the correct diagnosis.

The major risk in hypernatremic dehydration is intracranial hemorrhage. As extracellular sodium increases, water leaves the cell to equalize osmolarity, and the extracellular space is preserved at the expense of the intracellular space, which shrinks. A peculiar finding of experimental studies in which hyperosmolar solutions are infused is that more osmols are measured than can be accounted for; the excess are termed *idiogenic osmols*. It is hypothesized that certain intracellular substances that are usually osmotically inactive (such as proteins, phosphates, or sulfates) can become more osmotically active to protect the intracellular compartment. The substances may be harmful to the working of the cell, however, and might account for the ease of inducing cerebral edema by the too-rapid infusion of hypotonic fluids during the treatment phase. As these idiogenic osmols become unable to keep up with the rising hypernatremia, the brain "shrinks" away from the skull, damaging bridging veins and causing subdural hemorrhages; intracerebral hemorrhages also occur but are less common. The electroencephalogram shows anterior slowing and posterior low-voltage fast activity, with occasional spike and slow-wave complexes.

The kidneys are also a target organ for damage in hypernatremic dehydration. Acute tubular necrosis may develop: the histologic correlate is vacuolation of the convoluted tubules and extreme changes in the collecting ducts, with separation of the epithelium from the basement membrane.

The goals of treatment are slow rehydration, both to support the circulation and to replenish the intracellular volume; too rapid rehydration, particularly with electrolyte-free solutions, can lead to intracranial bleeding and seizures. The slow, steady method of replacement proposed by Finberg has proved safe and effective. If renal failure has supervened or if salt poisoning is a prominent feature, peritoneal dialysis may be required.

Reviews

1. Finberg, L. Treatment of dehydration in infancy. *Pediatr. Rev.* 3:113, 1981.
   Hypernatremic dehydration is reviewed along with other forms of dehydration.
2. Gruskin, A., et al. Serum sodium abnormalities in children. *Pediatr. Clin. North Am.* 29:907, 1982.
   Hypernatremic dehydration considered as well as other hypernatremic states; an extensive treatise on sodium physiology (38 pages, 94 references).

Epidemiology

3. Paneth, N. Hypernatremic dehydration of infancy. *Am. J. Dis. Child.* 134:785, 1980.
   A scholarly review of the epidemiology.
4. Rowland, T., et al. Malnutrition and hypernatremic dehydration in breast-fed infants. *JAMA* 247:1016, 1982.
   Occurs gradually without parental awareness.

Series

5. Bruck, E., et al. Pathogenesis and pathophysiology of hypertonic dehydration with diarrhea. *Am. J. Dis. Child.* 115:122, 1968.
   A good description of the illness in 59 infants.

Brain

6. Finberg, L., Luttrell, C., and Redd, H. Pathogenesis of lesions in the nervous system in hypernatremic states. *Pediatrics* 23:46, 1959.
   Produced central nervous system hemorrhage and clinical neurologic abnormalities in kittens by injecting salt; discusses idiogenic osmols.
7. Hogan, G., et al. Electrophysiologic response of the rabbit brain to chronic hypernatremic dehydration and rehydration. *Pediatrics* 50:769, 1972.
   Produced electroencephalographic abnormalities by injecting salt; seizures were related to rapid rehydration and were not seen in animals who slowly rehydrated themselves ad lib.

Acidosis

8. Hill, L., et al. Role of tissue hypoxia and defective renal acid excretion in the development of acidosis in infantile diarrhea. *Pediatrics* 47:246, 1971.
   Not usually major factors; when they are, there is almost always an underlying metabolic acidosis.
9. Winters, R., et al. The mechanisms of acidosis produced by hyperosmotic infusions. *J. Clin. Invest.* 43:647, 1964.
   Dilution of extracellular HCO_3^- by water transferred from the intracellular space.
10. Sotos, J., et al. Studies in experimental hypertonicity. *Pediatrics* 30:180, 1962.
    Transfer of intracellular H^+.

Hyperglycemia

11. Arieff, A., et al. Studies on mechanisms of cerebral edema in diabetic comas. *J. Clin. Invest.* 52:571, 1973.
    If blood sugar is lowered rapidly, water shifts (and cerebral edema) may occur.

Hypocalcemia

12. Finberg, L. Experimental studies of the mechanisms producing hypocalcemia in

hypernatremic states. *J. Clin. Invest.* 36:434, 1957.
Occurs when Na is high and K is low.

Prognosis

13. Macaulay, D., and Watson, M. Hypernatremia in infants as a cause of brain damage. *Arch. Dis. Child.* 42:485, 1967.
"Backwardness and maladjustment" were related to the neurologic status at the time of the illness, but not to the degree of hypernatremia.

Treatment

14. Bruck, E., et al. Therapy of infants with hypertonic dehydration due to diarrhea. *Am. J. Dis. Child.* 115:281, 1968.
A controlled study demonstrating a greater frequency of seizures with 10% dextrose in water than with electrolyte solutions.
15. Miller, N., and Finberg, L. Peritoneal dialysis for salt poisoning. *N. Engl. J. Med.* 263:1347, 1960.
For salt poisoning (not hypernatremic dehydration).
Also see reference 1.

68. HEMATURIA AND PROTEINURIA

Margaret E. Mohrmann

Hematuria in the context of acute nephritis (see Chap. 69) and proteinuria associated with the nephrotic syndrome (see Chap. 71) present few diagnostic problems for the pediatrician. Asymptomatic isolated hematuria or proteinuria, on the other hand, is often perplexing to the physician. The problem is not an uncommon one: approximately 5 percent of school-aged children have hematuria or proteinuria at some time.

Hematuria is defined as three or more red blood cells (RBCs) per high-power field (hpf), found in two centrifuged specimens of freshly voided urine. It is important to show that the hematuria is persistent since transient hematuria is found in some people after vigorous exercise, after minor trauma, with fever, or in a lordotic posture. The ortho-toluidine test strip (Hemastix) is very sensitive (trace = 1–3 RBC/hpf) but is also positive in the presence of free hemoglobin, myoglobin, or certain peroxidase-producing bacteria. False-negative results, generally due to the presence of ascorbic acid, are rare.

Gross hematuria usually indicates either acute glomerulonephritis or a nonglomerular cause of bleeding (e.g., cystitis, renal stones); the benign types of hematuria may present with visible blood in the urine during relatively minor infections, especially of the upper respiratory tract. It is quite unusual for a patient with any type of chronic glomerulonephritis to experience episodes of gross hematuria. Visible glomerular bleeding is brown (smoky, tea- or Coca Cola–colored), while bleeding from other sites is usually bright red and may include clots. Certain drugs (e.g., rifampin, phenolphthalein) and other substances (e.g., pigment in beets) may cause urine to *appear* bloody; the dipstick test easily differentiates this discoloration from true hematuria.

The causes of hematuria are numerous but the list can be shortened considerably by specifying hematuria that is asymptomatic and isolated (i.e., without proteinuria). For example, although the lower urinary tract can be a source of hematuria (due to cystitis, renal stones, a urethral foreign body, or a bleeding diathesis) such bleeding is rarely asymptomatic.

Common causes of extraglomerular renal hematuria include major trauma; hydronephrosis, in which bleeding frequently follows minor trauma and is often visible; and hemoglobinopathies, especially sickle cell trait and hemoglobin SC disease. Polycystic disease of the kidneys may also present with hematuria, but usually proteinuria and, less often, hypertension are also present. Up to 25 percent of children with Wilms tumor have hematuria but this is seldom the sole manifestation of disease. Hemangioma of the kidney and renal tuberculosis are rare causes of hematuria in children.

Glomerular hematuria, suggested by the presence of RBC casts in the urinary sediment, may be due to acute or chronic nephritis or to a benign hematuria syndrome. The nephritis of Henoch-Schönlein syndrome (Chap. 91) can occur weeks after resolution of the more characteristic symptoms. Chronic nephritides that commonly present with hematuria are hereditary nephritis (Alport syndrome) and membranoproliferative glomerulonephritis, both of which usually also cause simultaneous proteinuria. Systemic lupus erythematosus rarely presents as nephritis alone.

It is unclear whether Berger disease (IgA mesangial nephropathy) should be considered a form of chronic nephritis or one of the benign hematuria syndromes. The disease is characterized by persistent or intermittent microscopic hematuria with episodes of gross hematuria during mild infections; immunofluorescent staining of renal biopsy material reveals mesangial deposition of IgA and IgG. The prognosis is excellent although hematuria will persist; the small number of patients who have progressed to renal failure have been noted to have persistent proteinuria as well as hematuria.

Most children with asymptomatic isolated hematuria have one of the benign hematuria syndromes, which may be clinically indistinguishable from Berger disease. Familial hematuria (autosomal dominant inheritance) is not associated with proteinuria or impaired renal function, in contradistinction to hereditary nephritis. Benign (idiopathic persistent, benign recurrent) hematuria may be a normal variant.

Evaluation of a child with hematuria begins with a thorough history, including: family history of renal disease, hematuria, hearing loss, hemoglobinopathies, or bleeding disorders; drug use (e.g., anticoagulants, aspirin, sulfonamides); trauma; abdominal or suprapubic pain; and recent illnesses. If the hematuria has been visible, description of an episode (color, when the blood appeared in the urinary stream, associated symptoms) is helpful. Physical examination is directed toward detecting evidence of acute nephritis (hypertension, edema) or chronic renal disease (pallor, growth failure), abdominal mass or tenderness, rash, joint abnormalities, or congenital anomalies.

Laboratory evaluation of all children with persistent hematuria must include examination of freshly voided urine for RBC casts and protein. Any amount of protein (more than an occasional "trace") in the presence of microscopic hematuria is abnormal; in the case of gross hematuria, protein excretion over 500 mg/sq m/day is significant. Other studies to be obtained on all patients are urine culture, complete blood count, serum electrolytes, urea nitrogen and creatinine, complement, and serologic tests for evidence of streptococcal infection. Hemoglobin electrophoresis should be performed in black children with hematuria.

Although most authorities consider intravenous pyelography an essential part of the workup, the test is normal in all but a few patients. Cystoscopy is rarely helpful in evaluating microscopic hematuria and only infrequently reveals the cause of asymptomatic gross hematuria in children; bladder tumors are rare in children and usually present with symptoms of voiding dysfunction rather than with hematuria.

The child with a normal evaluation to this point may be considered to have either benign hematuria or Berger disease and should be followed at 6- to 12-month intervals for any clinical changes. Renal biopsy should be considered in the presence of persistent (longer than 8 weeks) hypocomplementemia and/or hypertension, significant proteinuria, or abnormal renal function in a patient without an acute nephritis syndrome whose pyelogram is unrevealing. Biopsy seldom reveals a treatable disease but may provide a diagnosis and, thus, a more accurate prognosis.

Hematuria is usually more frightening to both patients and physicians, but proteinuria is more likely to indicate serious renal disease. Even so, the majority of children with asymptomatic isolated proteinuria have a benign variation of normal renal function.

The initial diagnosis of proteinuria is made on the basis of a positive dipstick test: a strip impregnated with tribromophenol blue (Albustix) changes color in the presence of a protein concentration of 30 mg/dl or greater. Results may be falsely negative if the urine is very dilute or falsely positive if it is alkaline. The true definition of proteinuria requires a timed urine collection, traditionally a 24-hour collection: in children protein excretion greater than 100 mg/sq m/day is abnormal.

The list of etiologies of asymptomatic isolated proteinuria is far shorter than that for hematuria. Membranous and membranoproliferative glomerulonephritis may present with isolated proteinuria but are more likely to cause simultaneous hematuria and/or the nephrotic syndrome. Chronic pyelonephritis and renal hypoplasia infrequently cause proteinuria alone.

Most children under the age of 6 years with asymptomatic isolated proteinuria have either benign persistent proteinuria or subclinical (early) minimal-change nephrotic syndrome. Older children often have orthostatic proteinuria, a normal variant in which the first morning urine is protein-free but subsequent urines, excreted after the child is upright and active, contain variable amounts of protein (less than 1 gm/sq m/day).

Initial evaluation of a child with proteinuria includes many of the historical points noted in the discussion of hematuria, plus questions about episodes of edema, urinary tract infection, and exposure to heavy metals. During the physical examination, one should note the presence or absence of hypertension, edema, and growth failure.

Once the presence of persistent proteinuria has been established by a positive screening test on three or more separate occasions, further evaluation should include careful analysis of freshly voided urine for blood and casts, urine culture, and a 24-hour urine collection. If the excretion of protein is less than 100 mg/sq m/day and all else is normal, there is no need to continue the workup. Patients with abnormal protein excretion require measurement of serum electrolytes, urea nitrogen and creatinine, and testing for orthostatic proteinuria by comparison of a first morning specimen with urine excreted later in the day. Serum protein electrophoresis, cholesterol, and complement may also be obtained at this stage.

Children who are over the age of 6 years, exhibit orthostatic excretion of protein, have normal renal function and serum protein concentration, and whose protein excretion is less than 1 gm/sq m/day require no further evaluation but should be followed for any change. Those with nephrotic syndrome should be evaluated accordingly (see Chap. 71). In all other patients, renal ultrasonography or intravenous pyelography should be performed to rule out renal hypoplasia, polycystic disease, and chronic pyelonephritis. Electrophoresis of urinary protein may be helpful; selective excretion (i.e., predominantly albumin) usually indicates mild glomerular disease, such as minimal change nephrotic syndrome, while nonselective proteinuria implies either severe glomerular disease ("leakage" of large-molecular-weight globulins) or tubular disease (failure to resorb small-molecular-weight globulins). Relative indications for renal biopsy include: nephrotic syndrome in children less than 1 year or greater than 8 years old, hematuria, abnormal renal function, hypocomplementemia, and tubular proteinuria.

A child with persistent hematuria *plus* proteinuria, who does not fit the symptom complex or laboratory characteristics of acute nephritis or minimal-change nephrotic syndrome, almost always has serious renal disease, usually chronic glomerulonephritis, and requires intravenous pyelography or ultrasonography followed, in most instances, by renal biopsy.

Reviews

1. West, C. Asymptomatic hematuria and proteinuria in children: Causes and appropriate diagnostic studies. *J. Pediatr.* 89:173, 1976.
   Excellent discussion, especially of practical differential diagnosis; recommendations concerning workup need to be tempered by information in reference 2 to be truly "appropriate."

2. Dodge, W., et al. Proteinuria and hematuria in school children: Epidemiology and early natural history. *J. Pediatr.* 88:327, 1976.
   Largest series (12,000 children) for prevalence figures; conclusions include fruitlessness both of screening programs and of complex evaluations of isolated hematuria and proteinuria in absence of other abnormalities. (For a review of the cost effectiveness of screening children for proteinuria and hematuria by this author, see Am. J. Dis. Child. 131:1274, 1977.)

3. James, J. Proteinuria and hematuria in children: Diagnosis and assessment. *Pediatr. Clin. North Am.* 23:807, 1976.
   Succinct and thorough.

4. Alyea, E., and Parish, H. Renal response to exercise: Urinary findings. *JAMA* 167:807, 1958.
   Well-done study showing incidences of 70 to 100 percent proteinuria, 50 to 80 percent hematuria, and 60 to 80 percent cylindruria after various types of vigorous athletic activity; all abnormalities cleared within 24 hours after exercise.

Hematuria

5. Northway, J. Hematuria in children. *J. Pediatr.* 78:381, 1971.
   Remains the most complete review.
6. Lieberman, E. Workup of the Child with Hematuria. In E. Lieberman (ed.), *Clinical Pediatric Nephrology.* Philadelphia: Lippincott, 1976.
   Presents in outline form an exhaustive review of important points to be sought in history and physical examination, plus interpretation of laboratory findings.
7. Kaplan, M. Hematuria in childhood. *Pediatr. Rev.* 5:99, 1983.
   A general review, including a flow diagram approach to diagnosis.
8. Vehaskari, V., et al. Microscopic hematuria in school children: Epidemiology and clinicopathologic evaluation. *J. Pediatr.* 95:676. 1979.
   Study of almost 9000 children; findings agree with reference 2; conclusion that renal biopsy is seldom warranted.
9. Wyatt, R., et al. Hematuria in childhood: Significance and management. *J. Urol* 117:366, 1977.
   Cogent arguments against cystoscopy and biopsy as part of the workup; emphasizes benign nature of isolated hematuria.
10. Sears, D. The morbidity of sickle cell trait. *Am. J. Med.* 64:1021, 1978.
    Brief discussion of hematuria with literature review.
11. Rodicio, J. Idiopathic IgA nephropathy. *Kidney Int.* 25:717 1984.
    A complete review, with 134 references. (Also see Kidney Int. 22:643, 1982, and Annu. Rev. Med. 28:37, 1977.)
12. McConville, J., et al. Familial and non-familial benign hematuria. *J. Pediatr.* 69:207, 1966.
    Descriptions of 10 children with familial and 7 with nonfamilial hematuria; distinguishes familial hematuria from Alport nephritis.
13. Stapelton, F., et al. Hypercalciuria in children with hematuria. *N. Engl. J. Med.* 310:1345, 1984.
    Nearly 30 percent of children with unexplained hematuria had hypercalciuria as the likely cause.
14. Schoeneman, M., et al. Idiopathic persistent microscopic hematuria in children: Prognostic features. *N. Y. State J. Med.* 79:1714, 1979.
    Retrospective study that associates proteinuria of more than 1 gm/day and/or biopsy findings of interstitial fibrosis and foam cells with a poor prognosis; these findings, when present, appeared within 12 months of onset of hematuria in the majority.

Proteinuria

15. Ettenger, R. Workup of the Child with Proteinuria. In E. Lieberman (ed.), *Clinical Pediatric Nephrology.* Philadelphia: Lippincott, 1976.
    Organization and thoroughness similar to that of reference 6.
16. Feld, L., Schoeneman, M., and Kaskel, F. Evaluation of the child with asymptomatic proteinuria. *Pediatr. Rev.* 5:248, 1984.
    Includes a good discussion of protein handling by the kidney.
17. Ward, M. The office determination of proteinuria in adolescents. *Pediatr. Ann.* 7:97, 1978.
    Well-organized approach with helpful charts.
18. Houser, M. Assessment of proteinuria using random urine samples. *J. Pediatr.* 104:845, 1984.
    Random urine samples for protein-creatinine ratio were as reliable and less burdensome than 12- or 24-hour timed urine collections.
19. McLaine, P., and Drummond, K. Benign persistent asymptomatic proteinuria in childhood. *Pediatrics* 46:548, 1970.
    Follow-up of six patients; emphasize "benign."
20. Rytand, D, and Spreiter, S. Prognosis in postural (orthostatic) proteinuria. *N. Engl. J. Med.* 305:618, 1981.
    The long-term prognosis in this condition is favorable. (Also see the companion editorial, p. 639.)

69. ACUTE POSTSTREPTOCOCCAL GLOMERULONEPHRITIS
Kenneth B. Roberts

Acute poststreptococcal glomerulonephritis is a nonsuppurative sequela of group A beta-hemolytic streptococcal infection. Unlike rheumatic fever, glomerulonephritis may follow streptococcal infection either of the pharynx or of the skin (see Chap. 105), but only certain strains of streptococci are nephritogenic. The pathogenesis is not precisely understood; the theory in current favor is that circulating immune complexes are deposited in the kidney.

The most common clinical feature of glomerulonephritis is edema, frequently of the eyelids and face; often, the edema is recognized by the family but not by the physician except in retrospect after diuresis. Hypertension is the next most common sign and is due primarily to the increase in vascular volume; it may be symptomatic, with headache and vomiting, but more often, like the edema, is not apparent until recovery, when a lower blood pressure is recorded. Hypertensive encephalopathy occurs in less than 5 percent of the patients; papilledema is rare, and residua are uncommon. Circulatory congestion, the result of fluid and electrolyte retention, is manifested clinically as "congestive heart failure" and radiographically by cardiomegaly and increased pulmonary vascular markings; myocardial function and cardiac output are normal (or above normal). The affected child appears pale because of the edema and hemodilution; mild anemia, with unchanged red cell mass, is due to the increased intravascular fluid. Any of these clinical findings may be absent in biopsy-proved glomerulonephritis.

During the acute phase of glomerulonephritis, the patient excretes a reduced amount of urine with high specific gravity. A variable degree of proteinuria is noted in individual voidings, but the 24-hour quantity is usually not massive, and the nephrotic syndrome is rare. Gross hematuria occurs in over one-third of the patients (up to 70% of hospitalized patients) and gives the urine its smoky, rusty, tea-, or Coca-Cola–colored appearance. The gross hematuria usually disappears after a few days but may continue for up to 2 weeks; microscopic hematuria persists long after the gross hematuria has cleared. Red cell casts are seen more frequently in acid than in alkaline urine and are most easily found at the edge of the coverslip during microscopic examination of freshly voided urine. Hyaline and granular casts are usually present, but do not have the same significance.

Serum complement is decreased, apparently due to decreased synthesis and to increased breakdown as a result of reaction with immune complexes; levels are usually normal by 6 weeks. The sedimentation rate is almost always increased, but neither the magnitude of the increase nor the return to normal correlates well with the severity of the disease. Cholesterol is initially elevated in 40 percent of patients and returns to normal within 3 to 4 weeks. Serum albumin may also be abnormal, but the slight decrease is usually due to hemodilution rather than to proteinuria. During the acute stage, the concentrations of creatinine and urea nitrogen in the serum are increased, and creatinine clearance is reduced.

Renal biopsy is rarely necessary; the characteristic findings are hypercellular glomeruli, compressed capillary lumens, and infiltration by leukocytes and macrophages. Immunofluorescence techniques demonstrate the foci of complement and immunoglobulin on the epithelial side of the basement membrane.

Poststreptococcal glomerulonephritis may be subclinical, as demonstrated both by complement levels and by biopsy in the siblings of children with clinical acute glomerulonephritis. In addition, many children have mild proteinuria and microscopic hematuria during acute streptococcal infections. Although this is usually ascribed to the "toxic phase" of febrile illness, it may also occur with impetigo, in the absence of constitutional symptoms. Hematuria that is not associated with proteinuria or persists after the toxic period is cause for concern and periodic follow-up. Subclinical poststreptococcal glomerulonephritis is a possibility in such situations, but it is also possible that the streptococcal infection is coincidental, superimposed on previously unrecognized renal disease.

Treatment of poststreptococcal glomerulonephritis is supportive and consists of fluid and vigorous salt restriction during the oliguric or anuric phase and control of circulatory congestion and hypertension. Many pediatricians also prescribe penicillin to eradicate any persistent streptococci.

Although recurrences have been noted, they are uncommon. The number of nephritogenic strains of streptococci in the community is usually limited, and type-specific immunity protects against reinfection. Penicillin prophylaxis, as would be prescribed after acute rheumatic fever, is therefore not warranted.

The prognosis for children with acute poststreptococcal glomerulonephritis is considered to be uniformly good. However, other glomerulonephritides that are not so benign may mimic acute poststreptococcal disease; these include other postinfection nephritides, familial nephritis (Alport syndrome), membranoproliferative glomerulonephritis, and the nephritides of Henoch-Schönlein syndrome, systemic lupus erythematosus, polyarteritis nodosa, bacterial endocarditis, and toxins.

Reviews

1. McCrory, W. Glomerulonephritis. *Pediatr. Rev.* 5:19, 1983.
   A readable overview of clinical and laboratory features, differential diagnosis, and treatment.
2. Jordan, S., and Lemire, J. Acute glomerulonephritis: Diagnosis and treatment. *Pediatr. Clin. North Am.* 29:857, 1982.
   Includes a general discussion (classification and pathogenesis) of immune complex-mediated glomerulonephritis.
3. Nissenson, A., et al. Poststreptococcal acute glomerulonephritis: Fact and controversy. *Ann. Intern. Med.* 91:76, 1979.
   An overview of the "straightforward" areas and discussion of the controversies in pathogenesis and prognosis as well. (More on these controversial areas: Paediatrician 8:307, 1979.)

Diagnosis

4. Ingelfinger, J., Davis, A., and Grupe, W. Frequency and etiology of gross hematuria in a general pediatric setting. *Pediatrics* 59:557, 1977.
   Gross hematuria was common in acute glomerulonephritis, but the converse was not true: only 4 percent of children with gross hematuria had acute glomerulonephritis.
5. Madaio, M., and Harrington, J. The diagnosis of acute glomerulonephritis. *N. Engl. J. Med.* 309:1299, 1983.
   A step-by-step approach, starting with determination of serum complement.
6. Kirkpatrick, J., and Fleisher, D. The roentgen diagnosis of the chest in acute glomerulonephritis in children. *J. Pediatr.* 64:492, 1964.
   Abnormalities (cardiomegaly, evidence of circulatory congestion) in 86 percent.
7. Vardi, P., et al. The heart in acute glomerulonephritis: An echocardiographic study. *Pediatrics* 63:782, 1979.
   Confirms data obtained prior to echocardiography: the signs of heart failure are not due to myocardial damage but to fluid overload (so digoxin is of no value: J. Pediatr. 69:1054, 1966).
8. Dunn, M. Acute glomerulonephritis with normal results from urinalyses. *JAMA* 201:113, 1967.
   Includes a review of reported cases up to 1967.
9. Habib, R., and Loriat, C. Acute Glomerulonephritis or the Syndrome of "Postinfectious Glomerulonephritis of Acute Onset." In P. Royer et al. (eds.), *Pediatric Nephrology.* Philadelphia: Saunders, 1974.
   Emphasizes that disorders can mimic acute glomerulonephritis clinically in the "acute" stage but have different histologic features, course, and prognosis.
10. Gubler, M., et al. Alport's syndrome: A report of 58 cases and a review of the literature. *Am. J. Med.* 70:493, 1981.
    Something to think about in differential diagnosis.

Subclinical Infection

11. Derrick, C., Reeves, M., and Dillon, H. Complement in overt and asymptomatic nephritis after skin infection. *J. Clin. Invest.* 49:1178, 1970.
    The siblings of index cases dropped their complement: some also developed hematuria.
12. Dodge, W., Spargo, B., and Travis, L. Occurrence of acute glomerulonephritis in sibling contacts of children with sporadic acute glomerulonephritis. *Pediatrics* 40:1028, 1967.

In one-fourth to one-half of index case families, a sibling had biopsy changes of glomerulonephritis.

13. Rodriquez-Iturbe, D., Rubio, L., and Garcia, R. Attack rate of poststreptococcal nephritis in families. *Lancet* 1:401, 1981.
    Secondary attack rate in siblings approached 40 percent; the ratio of subclinical to clinical cases was 4:1.

14. Sagel, I., et al. Occurrence and nature of glomerular lesions after group A streptococcal infections in children. *Ann. Intern. Med.* 79:492, 1973.
    Among 248 children with streptococcal infection, there were 15 with abnormal urine, 19 with decreased complement, and 20 with both; all were asymptomatic and in all the biopsy findings were suggestive of acute glomerulonephritis.

Prevention

15. Wannamaker, L. Differences between streptococcal infections of the throat and of the skin. *N. Engl. J. Med.* 282:23,78, 1970.
    Infection in either site may lead to acute glomerulonephritis if the strain is nephritogenic.

16. Weinstein, L., and LeFrock, J. Does antimicrobial therapy of streptococcal pharyngitis or pyoderma alter the risk of glomerulonephritis? *J. Infect. Dis.* 124:229, 1971.
    A review of the evidence leaves the question unanswered.
    Also see Streptococcal Infections, Chapter 105.

Treatment

17. Repetto, H., et al. The renal functional response to furosemide in children with acute glomerulonephritis. *J. Pediatr.* 80:660, 1972.
    It worked.

18. Powell, H., et al. Plasma renin activity in acute poststreptococcal glomerulonephritis and the haemolytic-uraemic syndrome. *Arch. Dis. Child.* 49:802, 1974.
    Acute glomerulonephritis is a low-renin state (useful information when contemplating treatment of hypertension).

Natural History and Prognosis

19. Dodge, W., et al. Post-streptococcal glomerulonephritis: A prospective study in children. *N. Engl. J. Med.* 286:273, 1972.
    Younger children with better initial biopsies do well in short-term follow-up.

20. Lewy, J., et al. Clinicopathologic correlations in acute poststreptococcal glomerulonephritis: A correlation between renal functions, morphologic damage and clinical course of 46 children with acute poststreptococcal glomerulonephritis. *Medicine* (Baltimore) 50:453, 1971.
    Cellular and protein excretion do not reliably identify patients with severe changes on biopsy. Poor prognostic signs are: severely depressed creatinine clearance, marked azotemia, obliterated glomerular capillaries, and epithelial cell proliferation (48 pages, many photomicrographs, 71 references).

21. Roy, S., Wall, H., and Etteldorf, J. Second attacks of acute glomerulonephritis, *J. Pediatr.* 75:758, 1969.
    Uncommon, but they occur; the biopsies appeared no worse the second time around.

22. Potter, E., et al. Twelve to seventeen-year follow-up patients with poststreptococcal acute glomerulonephritis in Trinidad. *N. Engl. J. Med.* 307:725, 1982.
    The prognosis appears to be good after endemic or epidemic APSGN.

70. HEMOLYTIC-UREMIC SYNDROME
Kenneth B. Roberts

Hemolytic-uremic syndrome (HUS) is an entity of unknown origin that primarily affects infants and young children. Although uncommon, it is one of the most frequent causes of acute renal failure in infants without underlying structural renal disease. Precise incidence figures are unavailable, and the epidemiology is confused by conflicting reports from widely separated centers. In the two large series from this hemisphere, affected children in California were older than those in Argentina, suffered a more severe prodrome but a shorter period of oliguria or anuria, and proved to have a better prognosis. Despite these differences, the syndrome is distinctive: a prodrome followed by the triad of thrombocytopenia, hemolytic anemia, and acute renal failure.

Virtually all patients have a prodromal illness, but the type of illness seems to depend on the patient's age. Infants usually have diarrhea that may be bloody and can mimic ulcerative colitis or shigellosis; it should be noted that ulcerative colitis is exceedingly rare in this age group. Older children may begin with symptoms of an upper respiratory tract infection. In both age groups, vomiting often becomes pronounced shortly before the acute phase of illness. At this time, anemia and pallor rapidly become prominent; the hematocrit can fall by 50 percent in 48 hours. Fever, abdominal pain, vomiting, and failure to void are frequent accompanying complaints. On examination, small ecchymoses and purpura may be noted, along with petechiae; central nervous system signs (drowsiness, convulsions, or coma) are also present. One-half the patients have organomegaly, one-half have hypertension, and one-third are edematous.

The most striking laboratory features are elevation of serum creatinine and urea nitrogen, and hematologic abnormalities. Platelets are acutely decreased (below 50,000/cu mm) in one-half the patients; megakaryocytes are present in the marrow, and the thrombocytopenia usually resolves within a few weeks. The anemia may be marked with fragmented forms, burr cells, and other evidences of hemolysis readily apparent on peripheral blood smear; the Coombs test is negative.

Most patients at this stage are oliguric if not frankly anuric. Serum complement is normal. Renal biopsy reveals fibrin thrombi and cortical necrosis.

Hemolytic-uremic syndrome is highly suggestive of thrombotic thrombocytopenic purpura (TTP) in adults; the classic features of TTP include the three in childhood HUS, plus fever and variable neurologic manifestations. TTP in adults carries a worse prognosis than does HUS in children; it is possible that the two disorders are age-related manifestations of the same disease, with the cause unknown. Suggestions of an immune dysfunction, a postinfectious reaction, or a toxic reaction to environmental pollutants have been proposed but remain unproved.

Vigorous supportive care is the essence of therapy. Heparin has been tried, although without apparent benefit. Recent reports express skepticism about the benefit of drugs designed to interfere with platelet function, such as aspirin and dipyridamole, as well as the use of drugs such as streptokinase to dissolve thrombi. Of importance are rigorous attention to fluid balance, control of hypertension, transfusions as needed, and early institution of peritoneal dialysis.

Acute mortality in HUS has been reported as high as 25 percent, but recent estimates are closer to 5 percent. It is not clear whether the change is due to an alteration in the disease, diagnosis of milder cases, or earlier use of dialysis. Central nervous system signs, such as convulsions or coma, are associated with decreased survival rates, more closely resembling those in adult TTP.

Hypertension, present in 25 percent of patients in the acute phase, is present in less than 10 percent of patients 1 month after the illness. The incidence of hypertension then increases, however, and after 5 years is 45 percent, probably as a reflection of chronic renal damage.

Chronic renal failure is the major sequela of HUS. It occurs in approximately 30 percent of patients, two-thirds of whom demonstrate an initial improvement. Of patients who are oliguric for less than 1 week, 62 percent recover totally by 6 to 12 months, and an additional 14 percent recover, but more slowly. The remaining 24 percent improve, but then renal function deteriorates. The figures are similar for patients oliguric for between 1 and 3 weeks, except that more patients are in the slow-recovery group. Patients who are oliguric for more than 3 weeks have the worst prognosis: one-third progress directly to chronic renal failure, and renal function deteriorates in an additional 18 percent after an initial inprovement.

Reviews
1. Fong, J., deChadarevian, J., and Kaplan, B. Hemolytic-uremic syndrome: Current concepts and management. *Pediatr. Clin. North Am.* 29:835, 1982.
   An extensive review (21 pages, 161 references).

2. Musgrave, J. The hemolytic-uremic syndrome: A clinical review. *Clin. Pediatr.* (Phila.) 17:218, 1978.
An overview.

Series

3. Gianantonio, C., et al. The hemolytic-uremic syndrome. *J. Pediatr.* 64:478, 1964.
The large Argentina experience is described (58 patients at the time of the review). (Also see references 8 and 17.)

4. Tune, B., et al. The hemolytic-uremic syndrome in California: A review of 28 nonheparinized cases with a long-term follow-up. *J. Pediatr.* 82:304, 1973.
A California series of 27; differs in many respects from the Argentina experience.

5. Dolislager, D., and Tune, B. The hemolytic-uremic syndrome: Spectrum of severity and significance of prodrome. *Am. J. Dis. Child.* 132:55, 1978.
An update of the experience in California (reference 4), with a discussion of geographic differences.

Coagulopathy

6. Avalos, J., et al. Coagulation studies in the hemolytic-uremic syndrome. *J. Pediatr.* 76:538, 1970.
Low platelets were a constant finding, but the pattern of coagulation test abnormalities was not uniform. The contention that disseminated intravascular coagulation is the central common event is not supported.

7. Katz, J., et al. Platelet, erythrocyte, and fibrinogen kinetics in the hemolytic-uremic syndrome of infancy. *J. Pediatr.* 83:739, 1973.
By the time of clinical presentation, a renal lesion seems already to be established without "further" intravascular coagulation.

8. Gianantonio, C., et al. The hemolytic-uremic syndrome. *Nephron* 11:174, 1973.
The pathologic findings suggest disseminated intravascular coagulation. The clinical findings in 678 patients are reported.

9. Katz, J., et al. Coagulation findings in the hemolytic-uremic syndrome of infancy: Similarity to hyperacute renal allograft rejection. *J. Pediatr.* 78:426, 1971.
Likened more to rejection than to disseminated intravascular coagulation. Platelets were decreased, fibrin split products were present, but clotting factors were not reduced.

Selected Aspects

10. Goldstein, M., et al. Hemolytic-uremic syndrome. *Nephron* 23:263, 1979.
Points out similarities and differences between adults and children with the disease.

11. Kaplan, B., Chesney, R., and Drummon, K. Hemolytic uremic syndrome in families. *N. Engl. J. Med.* 292:1090, 1975.
Family members with the disease concurrently had a better prognosis than when an interval of more than 1 year separated cases; speculation about environmental and genetic factors.

12. Drummond, K. Hemolytic uremic syndrome—then and now. *N. Engl. J. Med.* 312;116, 1985.
An editorial update of recent data regarding pathogenesis, clinicopathologic correlations, and classification.

13. Ray, C., et al. Enteroviruses associated with the hemolytic uremic syndrome. *Pediatrics* 46:378, 1970.
Various infectious agents have been incriminated as "triggers" (Shigella, J. Pediatr. 84:312, 1974, and N. Engl. J. Med. 298:927, 1978; Coxsackie B virus, J. Infect. Dis. 127:698, 1973; and so forth).

14. Whittington, P., Friedman, A., and Chesney, R. Gastrointestinal disease in the hemolytic-uremic syndrome. *Gastroenterology* 76:728, 1979.
Gastrointestinal involvement is common and may appear to be the primary disease. (Warn your surgeon: J. Pediatr. Surg. 13:597, 1978.)

Therapy

15. Kaplan, B., et al. An analysis of the results of therapy in 67 cases of the hemolytic-uremic syndrome. *J. Pediatr.* 78:420, 1971.

Peritoneal dialysis was of apparent value; heparin was of no benefit. Confirmed: Am J. Dis. Child. *132:59, 1978.*

16. Gomperts, E., and Lieberman, E. Hemolytic-uremic syndrome. *J. Pediatr.* 97:419 1980.

    An editorial accompanying an article on aspirin and dipyridamole therapy (p. 473, stating the problems in evaluating various proposed forms of therapy.

Prognosis

17. Gianantonio, C., et al. The hemolytic-uremic syndrome. *J. Pediatr.* 72:757, 1968.

    Prognosis (with respect to chronic renal disease) was apparently related to the duration of acute oliguria; findings at 3 or 6 months can be misleading.

18. Janssen, F., et al. Short and long-term prognosis of the hemolytic-uremic syndrome *Arch. Fr. Pediatr.* 31:59, 1974. (Reported in S. Gellis, *Year Book of Pediatrics* Chicago: Year Book, 1975. P. 252.)

    Mortality was 15 percent; concentrating ability was last abnormality to improve Hematologic findings were normal in 3 months, renal in 1 year. After 1 year, azotemia persisted in 10 percent, abnormal sediment in 21 percent, hypertension in 5 percent

19. Upadhyaya, K., et al. The importance of non-renal involvement in hemolytic-uremic syndrome. *Pediatrics* 65:115, 1980.

    Extent and severity of nonrenal involvement important in outcome. (More on CNS involvement: Am. J. Dis. Child. *134:869, 1980.)*

71. NEPHROTIC SYNDROME
Richard A. Cohn

The nephrotic syndrome (NS) consists of heavy proteinuria (in excess of 1 gm/sq m/day), hypoalbuminemia (less than 2.5 gm/dl), edema, and hypercholesterolemia (greater than 250 mg/dl). The prime abnormality is an alteration in the structural or functional integrity (or both) of the glomerular filter, which ordinarily permits less than 0.03 percent of plasma albumin to reach the tubules. A small increase in permeability, while still restricting over 99 percent of plasma albumin, can overwhelm the resorptive capacity of the tubules and result in heavy proteinuria. The features of NS are either a direct consequence of protein loss or a result of compensatory mechanisms.

Edema (periorbital, peripheral, scrotal, or abdominal) is the usual presenting complaint and may be massive. The pathogenesis is related to (1) decreased plasma oncotic pressure and transudation of water into the extravascular compartment, and (2) decreased effective plasma volume, causing enhanced salt and water resorption in distal nephron sites via secondary hyperaldosteronism and secretion of antidiuretic hormone.

The incidence of NS is estimated at 2 cases per 100,000 children/year. In contrast to adults with NS, children with NS usually have primary renal disease rather than systemic disorders such as systemic lupus erythematosus (SLE) or diabetes mellitus. Recent renal biopsy studies have permitted the characterization and differentiation of several primary renal disorders leading to NS in children.

By far the most common cause of NS in children is *minimal change nephrotic syndrome* (MCNS). More than 75 percent of children with NS and more than 90 percent of those 1 to 6 years of age have this form. The term *minimal change* refers to the paucity of abnormalities seen by light microscopy; terms formerly used include *nil lesion* and *lipoid nephrosis*. It is this disorder that determines the overall epidemiology of NS in childhood: the majority of affected patients are symptomatic by age 6, and boys predominate 2 : 1.

Blood pressure is elevated transiently in 20 percent of children with MCNS. Gross hematuria is extremely rare, but microscopic hematuria occurs in 25 percent of patients when proteinuria is present. Histologically, the glomeruli are normal or minimally abnormal by light microscopy; no immunoglobulin and complement components are seen by fluorescence microscopy. Alterations of epithelial podocytes are detected by electron microscopy.

Treatment consists of medication to reduce proteinuria, salt restriction to control edema, and measures to prevent and treat complications. Proteinuria remits in more than 90 percent of children with MCNS within 4 weeks of initiating prednisone therapy (often within 7–10 days). Two-thirds of those whose NS responds to prednisone will have a relapsing course, however, usually for several years; most children ultimately achieve prolonged or permanent remissions, particularly by early adolescence. In some children, the NS becomes resistant to steroids after earlier responses or requires intoxicating doses to maintain remissions; for these patients, immunosuppressive medication (cyclophosphamide, nitrogen mustard, or chlorambucil) has been used, but there is concern about the undesirable associated effects, particularly sterility and the threat of malignancy.

Dietary sodium should be restricted, but fluid restriction is not helpful and may be dangerous in these children since their intravascular volumes may already be low. Moreover, children with MCNS are predisposed to vascular thromboses, particularly when taking steroids. Patients with respiratory embarrassment, skin breakdown, or massive edema may benefit from an intravenous infusion of concentrated albumin followed by furosemide.

The most common serious complication of MCNS is bacterial infection (e.g., cellulitis, peritonitis, pneumonia, sepsis), especially at sites of edema. Contributing factors include hypoimmunoglobulinemia and reduced opsonic activity from loss of properdin factor B in the urine, and other immunologic abnormalities caused by both the disease and the treatment. Children should receive pneumococcal vaccine, and appropriate precautions should be taken when steroids are being administered such as avoidance of live viral vaccines and administration of varicella-zoster immune globulin (VZIG) following exposure to chickenpox if the dose of prednisone is high and the child is not already immune. Bacterial infection should be treated early and aggressively; *Streptococcus pneumoniae* and *Escherichia coli* are the most frequent organisms.

The prognosis for children with MCNS is excellent. Renal function remains normal in those who respond to medication, whether relapses are frequent or not.

Of children with NS, 10 percent (or nearly one-half of those who do not have minimal-change disease) have *focal segmental glomerular sclerosis*. As in minimal-change disease, most are males, have apparent disease by age 8, and are normocomplementemic; hypertension and hematuria are more common than in MCNS. Histologic examination reveals a portion of glomeruli with a segment of hyalinosis, devoid of nuclei and adherent to Bowman's capsule; capillary lumens are obliterated. The remaining tufts in an involved glomerulus are normal. Juxtamedullary glomeruli are often affected earliest, but progression to generalized involvement occurs commonly. IgM, C3, C4, and often properdin can be demonstrated by immunofluorescence in sclerosing segments; collapse of capillary loops and sclerosis are evident on electron microscopy. The relationship of this lesion to "minimal change" is unsettled; some feel that sclerosis may develop over time in a child with MCNS; others feel that the sclerotic lesion is present at the onset, but, since it is focal in nature, it may be missed on early biopsies, particularly if juxtamedullary glomeruli are not sampled.

In 20 percent of patients with focal segmental glomerular sclerosis, the NS responds to steroids and to cytotoxic drugs. Relapses may be frequent, but a complete remission is often achieved; in some, progression to end-stage renal disease (ESRD) occurs, despite the initial response. In 80 percent of patients, however, the NS does not respond initially to either steroid therapy or cytotoxic drugs. The nephrotic state is persistent, and hypertension and renal insufficiency develop, often within 2 years of diagnosis. Renal transplantation is generally successful, although NS, with focal sclerosis, may recur.

Approximately 7 percent of children with NS have *membranoproliferative* (mesangiocapillary) *glomerulonephritis*. These patients are usually older children who present with NS or an acute nephritis syndrome (gross hematuria, edema, hypertension) or both; they may present with asymptomatic hematuria and proteinuria. Reduced renal function, hypertension, and hypocomplementemia are common. The characteristic histologic appearance is mesangial proliferation and expansion around capillary walls. The glomeruli are enlarged and lobular, with either subendothelial or intramembranous deposits apparent on electron microscopy. Immunoglobulins and complement are found on capillary loops in a peripheral-lobular distribution by fluorescence microscopy.

Prednisone and immunosuppressive agents do not induce remissions in this form of NS and may cause severe toxicity, particularly hypertensive encephalopathy. Most of the patients have a slowly progressive course over many years, often into ESRD. Occasionally, renal function stabilizes with persistent proteinuria; complete remissions do occur but are unusual. The lesions may recur after renal transplantation.

Mesangial proliferative glomerulonephritis is present in 5 percent of children with NS. There usually is an initial remission with steroids, but frequent relapses and steroid dependency are common; in some children, steroids are ineffective from the outset. The response to cyclophosphamide or chlorambucil is highly variable, ranging from none to long-term remission. IgM is often seen in the mesangium by fluorescence microscopy, and mesangial electron-dense deposits are present on electron microscopy.

Membranous glomerulopathy (extramembranous glomerulonephritis, membranous glomerulonephritis) is present in less than 5 percent of children with NS. Neither sex predominates, and age distribution is scattered. Hematuria and hypertension may or may not be present; renal function and complement levels are generally normal at the time of presentation. Histologic findings include uniformly thickened capillary walls in all glomeruli, lack of proliferative changes in glomeruli, and typical spikes along the basement membrane on silver stain. Electron microscopy reveals deposits on the epithelial side of the thickened glomerular basement membrane. Uniform granular deposits of IgG, C3, and often C4 are seen on the outer aspect of the basement membrane by immunofluorescence.

Although therapy in children with membranous glomerulopathy is generally ineffective, one-third to one-half have spontaneous clinical improvement over months or years; an equal number continue to have proteinuria but maintain normal renal function. Approximately 10 percent, primarily older children, continue in a nephrotic state and progress slowly to ESRD.

Congenital NS is a rare familial disorder transmitted in an autosomal recessive pattern, with a higher frequency in families of Finnish ancestry. These patients have severe proteinuria from birth, have disproportionately more ascites and less peripheral edema than other patients with NS, and generally fail to thrive. Response to steroid therapy is uncommon, and large doses of diuretics are required. Many advocate prophylactic antibiotic therapy, since overwhelming sepsis is not uncommon in this group. Renal function may remain normal for years, but most of these patients ultimately develop ESRD. The nephrotic state does not recur after renal transplantation, lending support to evidence that abnormal biochemical structure of the glomerular capillary is the basic underlying defect. Antenatal diagnosis is now possible, since elevated levels of alpha fetoprotein are present in the amniotic fluid, with concomitantly high levels in maternal blood.

How does one approach a given patient once NS has been diagnosed? Should a renal biopsy be performed initially, or should steroid therapy be started? Most authorities agree that children younger than age 8 who are normotensive, do not have hematuria, and have normal renal function can be given a trial of steroid therapy, with a renal biopsy to be done later if the NS is unresponsive. Biopsy prior to using prednisone should be considered in patients less likely to have MCNS: older children (especially girls) and those with hypocomplementemia, significantly reduced renal function, or a concomitant acute nephritis syndrome. If treatment is prescribed without histologic diagnosis, these patients in particular must be monitored closely to reduce potential morbidity from steroid therapy.

Reviews

1. Barnett, H., et al. The Nephrotic Syndrome. In C. Edelmann, Jr. (ed.), *Pediatric Kidney Disease*. Boston: Little, Brown, 1978.
   Comprehensive overview with excellent chapters on all pathologic entities that cause NS.

2. International Study of Kidney Disease in Children. Nephrotic syndrome in children: Prediction of histopathology from clinical and laboratory characteristics at time of diagnosis. *Kidney Int.* 13:159, 1978.
   Details of 521 unselected patients.

3. Rance, C., Arbus, G., and Balfe, J. Management of the nephrotic syndrome in children. *Pediatr. Clin. North Am.* 23:735, 1976.
   A review of the clinical presentation, pathologic varieties, and therapy (94 references).

4. Grupe, W. Primary nephrotic syndrome in childhood. *Adv. Pediatr.* 26:163, 1979.
   Long (39 pages, 131 references) but worth reading; the section on drug therapy is

particularly good and includes an important critique of what steroids may and may not do for NS and of the relative merits of cyclophosphamide and chlorambucil.

5. Oliver, W., and Kelsch, R. Nephrotic syndrome due to primary nephropathies. *Pediatr. Rev.* 2:311, 1981.
   Brief but complete.

Pathology and Pathogenesis

6. White, R., Glasgow, E., and Mills, R. Clinicopathological study of nephrotic syndrome in childhood. *Lancet* 1:1353, 1970.
   Details of glomerular morphology and the clinical course are given.

7. Brenner, B., Hostetter, T., and Humes, H. Molecular basis of proteinuria of glomerular origin. *N. Engl. J. Med.* 298:826, 1978.
   An excellent, readable summary of glomerular permeability.

8. Michael, A., McLean, R., and Roy, L. Immunological aspects of the nephrotic syndrome. *Kidney Int.* 3:105, 1973.
   A review of pathogenesis, complement function, and morphology. (Also see Lancet *2:556, 1974, for the hypothesis that relapses are related to lymphocyte changes.)*

Complications

9. International Study of Kidney Disease in Children. Minimal change nephrotic syndrome in children: Deaths during the first 5 to 15 years' observation. *Pediatrics* 73:497, 1984.
   A review of long-term problems. The pattern of response to steroids appears to be of prognostic significance.

10. Wilfert, C., and Katz, S. Etiology of bacterial sepsis in nephrotic children. *Pediatrics* 42:840, 1968.
    A short review of sites and agents causing infections; for studies of immunologic competence in children with NS, see J. Infect. Dis. *140:1, 1979.*

11. Speck. W., Dresdale, S., and McMillan, R. Primary peritonitis and the nephrotic syndrome. *Am. J. Surg.* 127:267, 1974.
    A short review of 39 episodes of peritonitis in 22 patients. (Also see Am. J. Dis. Child. *136:732, 1982.)*

12. Kendall, A., Lohmann, R., and Dossetor, J. Nephrotic syndrome: A hypercoagulable state. *Arch. Intern. Med.* 127:1021, 1971.
    Coagulation tests and thromboembolic complications in 35 patients are described.

Minimal Change Nephrotic Syndrome

13. International Study of Kidney Disease in Children. The primary nephrotic syndrome in children: Identification of patients with minimal change nephrotic syndromes from initial response to prednisone. *J. Pediatr.* 98:561, 1981.
    Ninety-two percent of responders and 25 percent of nonresponders had MCNS; additional criteria are needed to justify biopsy in nonresponders.

14. Siegel, N., et al. Long-term follow-up of children with steroid-responsive nephrotic syndrome. *J. Pediatr.* 81:251, 1972.
    Of 61 patients, 51 had a relapsing course that became evident in first 2 years after diagnosis; relapses continued to be steroid-responsive.

15. International Study of Kidney Disease in Children. Nephrotic syndrome in children: A randomized trial comparing two prednisone regimens in steroid-responsive patients who relapse early. *J. Pediatr.* 29:239, 1979.
    Longer course of steroids increased the duration of remission but after 6 months there was no difference between the 2 groups. (For a lengthy general review of steroid uses and effects, see Ann. Intern. Med. *84:304, 1976.)*

16. Siegel, N., et al. Steroid-dependent nephrotic syndrome in children: Histopathology and relapses after cyclophosphamide treatment. *Kidney Int.* 19:454, 1981.
    Much greater likelihood of long-term remission after cyclophosphamide in MCNS than in focal sclerosis or mesangial proliferative NS. (Also see J. Pediatr. *92:304, 1978, and* Pediatrics *57:948, 1976. For a review of cyclophosphamide, see* Ann. Intern. Med. *80:531, 1974; for discussion of gonadal dysfunction, see* J. Pediatr. *84:831, 1974; and 91:385, 1977.)*

17. Williams, S., et al. Long-term evaluation of chlorambucil plus prednisone in the

idiopathic nephrotic syndrome of childhood. *N. Engl. J. Med.* 302:929, 1980.
Short-term, low-dose therapy with chlorambucil effects remissions in most patients. (For more on the toxicity of chlorambucil, see J. Pediatr. 92:299, 1978, and 97:653, 1980.)

Focal Segmental Glomerular Sclerosis

18. Case Records of the Massachusetts General Hospital. Recurrent focal glomerulonephritis. *N. Engl. J. Med.* 294:1108, 1976.
    Clinicopathologic discussion (8 pages, 45 references).
19. Nash, M., et al. The significance of focal sclerotic lesions of glomeruli in children. *J. Pediatr.* 88:806, 1976.
    The clinical course in 27 children is described. (For the association of renal tubular abnormalities with focal sclerosis and poor prognosis, see J. Pediatr. 97:918, 1980.)
20. Habib, R. Focal glomerular sclerosis. *Kidney Int.* 4:355, 1973.
    An excellent summary.
21. Hoyer, J., et al. Recurrence of idiopathic nephrotic syndrome after renal transplantation. *Lancet* 2:343, 1972.
    The title is the message. (For a comprehensive review, see Transplantation 32:512, 1981.)

Other Causes of Nephrotic Syndrome

22. West, C., and McAdams, A. The chronic glomerulonephritides of childhood. *J. Pediatr.* 93:1, 167, 1978.
    Excellent, well-referenced, brief discussions of several disorders (two-part review).
23. Kim, Y., and Michael, A. Idiopathic membranoproliferative glomerulonephritis. *Annu. Rev. Med.* 31:273, 1980.
    Thorough and current (76 references); clearly distinguishes types I and II. (For the largest series in children, see Clin. Nephrol. 1:194, 1973; for an uncontrolled study suggesting improved survival with alternate-day prednisone therapy, see Clin. Nephrol. 13:117, 1980.)
24. Brown, E., et al. The clinical course of mesangial proliferative glomerulonephritis. *Medicine* (Baltimore) 58:295, 1978.
    Review of 44 patients (14 with NS).
25. Habib, R., et al. Extramembranous glomerulonephritis in children. *J. Pediatr.* 82:754, 1973.
    The course in 50 children is described. (For results of an alternate-day prednisone trial in adults with this disorder, see N. Engl. J. Med. 301:1301, 1979.)
26. Kleinknecht, C., et al. Membranous glomerulonephritis with extra-renal disorders in children. *Medicine* (Baltimore) 58:219, 1979.
    Review of this entity associated with SLE, hepatitis, syphilis, etc. in children. (Membranous glomerulopathy may be the only manifestation of SLE in some children: J. Pediatr. 88:394, 1976.)
27. Kaplan, B., Bureau, M., and Drummond, K. The nephrotic syndrome in the first year of life. *J. Pediatr.* 85:615, 1974.
    Classification of infantile nephrotic syndrome is presented. (For more on the clinical and laboratory features of congenital nephrotic syndrome, see Nephron 11:101, 1973; for value of alpha fetoprotein in prenatal diagnosis, see Lancet 2:123, 1976.)

72. URINARY TRACT INFECTION

Richard A. Cohn

Infection within the urinary tract is the most common condition confronting the pediatric nephrologist. Significant bacteriuria occurs in approximately 1 percent of neonates, predominantly males and premature infants, and 2 to 3 percent of preschool children, mostly females; 5 percent of girls have significant bacteriuria at some point during their school years.

Clinical manifestations of urinary tract infection (UTI) vary with the age of the patient. Signs in the neonatal period may be nonspecific and include weight loss, failure to thrive, unexplained jaundice, diarrhea, and central nervous system abnormalities (hypotonia, hypothermia, absent reflexes, irregular respirations). Sepsis is commonly associated with UTI in this age group, and concomitant maternal infection occurs in one-half the affected newborns. Children between 1 month and 2 years of age may present with unexplained fevers, failure to thrive, colic (especially before and during voiding), dribbling, vomiting, and abdominal distention. Children over age 2 generally have symptoms referable to the urinary tract: fever, dysuria, urgency, frequency, lower abdominal pain, flank tenderness, and enuresis.

It is essential that the diagnosis of urinary tract infection be established properly. Bacteriuria is significant when culture of a clean-catch urine demonstrates more than 100,000 organisms of a single species per milliliter. Diagnostic accuracy approaches 95 percent if, prior to treatment, a second clean-catch urine confirms the findings of the first. In most proved UTIs, in fact, there are more than 1 million organisms/ml, whereas contaminated specimens contain less than 10,000 per ml. If the colony count is between 10,000 and 100,000, another sample should be obtained and cultured. A single suprapubic aspirate or a meticulously clean, catheterized specimen showing any growth in culture indicates true infection. False-negative results can occur with high urine volumes of low osmolality, prior antibiotic therapy, extreme urinary acidity, or obstruction of the infected kidney or ureter. Specimens should be refrigerated until plated to avoid bacterial multiplication in vitro, since the duplication time of enteric organisms is less than 30 minutes at room temperature.

Leukocytes and unstained bacteria seen on light microscopy are unreliable indicators of UTI. The presence of bacteria on gram-stained smears of fresh, *un*centrifuged urine correlates well with colony counts in excess of 100,000 per ml, but microscopy cannot substitute for culture as the diagnostic procedure.

Once UTI has been properly diagnosed, the child merits special attention. Physical examination should include a search for hypertension, funduscopic changes, abdominal masses, vertebral anomalies, and neurologic disturbances associated with the neurogenic bladder. In males particularly, observation of the urinary stream should be made: a weak stream despite straining suggests the possibility of posterior urethral valves. Laboratory studies should include assessment of renal function.

A major structural abnormality of the urinary tract may underlie a UTI, and radiologic evaluation is therefore indicated after an initial infection. (Many defer radiography in girls over 3 years of age with cystitis until after a recurrence.) Intravenous pyelography and voiding cystourethrography can detect obstruction, parenchymal renal disease, vesicoureteral reflux, stones, vertebral anomalies, and other abnormalities. Voiding cystourethrography should be performed after sterilization of the urine. Urologic consultation is indicated when significant pathologic changes are found on physical and radiologic examination. Most neonates with UTI have anatomically normal urinary tracts, but young females beyond the neonatal period have a 15 percent incidence of major upper urinary tract disease; reflux is detected in 30 percent; in males the incidence of abnormalities is higher. In addition to anatomic changes, other factors that are often associated with UTI in children include constipation, the use of crude soap or bubble bath, and foreign bodies in the vagina and urethra; in adolescent girls, as in adult women, intercourse may predispose to cystitis, and pregnancy to cystitis and pyelonephritis.

Differentiation of lower from upper tract infection may be of prognostic and therapeutic importance: cystitis is rarely associated with upper tract damage. Unfortunately, symptoms in children are less reliable than in adults in localizing the site of infection. Various direct and indirect techniques that may help identify the locus of infection include ureteral culturing, bladder washout, specific serum antibody levels to pathogens, urinary lactic dehydrogenase isoenzyme fractionation, urinary concentrating ability, and fluorescent-antibody coating of organisms. A radionuclide renal scan (using technetium glucoheptonate) may be the most sensitive way of diagnosing pyelonephritis.

Escherichia coli is the pathogen in approximately 75 percent of childhood UTIs, *Klebsiella, Proteus* (especially *P. mirabilis*), *Pseudomonas, Streptococcus* (especially *S. fecalis*), and *Staphylococcus* species account for most others, particularly in patients who have had prior antibiotic therapy or an operation or who have altered host resistance.

Uncomplicated first infections generally are treated for 10 to 14 days with a sulfonamide or ampicillin although recent studies indicate a single dose of antibiotic is effective in some patients with uncomplicated cystitis. Pyelonephritis is treated for a minimum of 2 to 3 weeks. Patients with anatomic abnormalities or frequent recurrences may benefit from long-term, low-dose suppressive therapy; nitrofurantoin or the combination of tri-methoprim and sulfamethoxazole in a single daily dose appears successful in suppressing infection. Antibiotic treatment of recurrent or complicated infections is based on the sensitivity of the responsible organisms.

Management includes careful follow-up of the patient, with repeat urine cultures at regular intervals, even in asymptomatic patients, since recurrences occur in up to 80 percent. Disease in children with anatomically normal urinary tracts rarely progresses to chronic pyelonephritis and renal insufficiency if recurrences of UTI are appropriately managed. Recent studies of patients with renal transplants show a very low incidence of pyelonephritis as the cause of renal failure, and patients in whom pyelonephritis is the cause of end-stage renal disease usually have a major underlying structural abnormality of the urinary tract (e.g., dysplasia, obstructive uropathy). Histopathologically, chronic interstitial nephritis, which includes pyelonephritis, may be caused by other factors in the absence of infection, such as analgesic abuse, nephrocalcinosis, drugs (thiazides, penicillins, cephalosporins, and others), toxins (lead, cadmium, mercury), irradiation, hyperuricemia, and diabetes mellitus.

Specific abnormalities of the urinary tract, especially when complicated by UTI, can cause progressive renal damage, particularly obstruction and reflux. Underlying ob-struction anywhere along the urinary tract, from collecting ducts to urethral meatus, predisposes to stasis, infection, and scarring. Not uncommonly, symptoms of infection bring the child to the physician and, on further testing, the obstruction is revealed. Underlying neurologic incompetence occurs in patients with myelodysplasia, diabetes mellitus, spinal cord tumors, and other central nervous system diseases; intermittent catheterization or diversion of the urinary tract may be required to halt progressive renal damage in these patients.

Reflux (retrograde flow of urine from bladder to ureter) is caused by incompetence of the ureterovesical junction. The normal ureter tunnels obliquely through the submucosa of the bladder wall and inserts on the trigone. The muscular tone of the bladder, coupled with the angled ureteral tunnel, normally prevents retrograde flow. Congenital abnor-malities of the submucosal ureter, ureteral orifice, or bladder wall predispose to reflux. Cystitis, with resulting mucosal edema, can itself cause reflux in an otherwise normal system, but minor reflux into the lower ureter is of little concern and generally resolves with control of infection and growth of the patient. Reflux of infected urine into the kidney, however, especially if the ureter is dilated, can cause severe damage and may not respond to medical management. Antireflux surgery is indicated for (1) recurrent infec-tions despite continuous antibiotic therapy; (2) failure of renal growth on sequential radiographic studies; (3) the development or progression of renal scarring despite ade-quate medical management; or (4) persistent, high-grade reflux that does not subside over 1–2 years of follow-up, particularly in a young child. Long-term follow-up and study of all patients with urologic, neurologic, and reflux problems is mandatory if chronic renal failure on an infectious basis is to be avoided.

Screening programs for the detection of bacteriuria in asymptomatic children were popular a decade ago. These programs were directed at early detection of UTI, reduction of morbidity, and selection of children with structural abnormalities at risk for chronic renal disease. It is not clear that such programs were efficient or effective in detecting the children at risk, and widespread application to school-age populations appears now to be unjustified. Appropriate clinical suspicion of symptomatic patients, accurate diag-nosis, and effective treatment remain the mainstays for preventing the morbidity and complications of UTIs in children.

Reviews

1. Stephens, F. Urologic aspects of recurrent urinary tract infection in children. *J. Pediatr.* 80:725, 1972.
   A superb paper on UTIs, reflux, dysplasia, and surgery (11 pages, 56 references).
2. Kunin, C. *Detection, Prevention and Management of Urinary Tract Infections* (3rd ed.). Philadelphia: Lea & Febiger, 1979.

Everything you always wanted to know about UTIs in a 320-page monograph.
3. Mathieu, H. Urinary Infection. In P. Royer et al. (eds.), *Pediatric Nephrology.* Philadelphia: Saunders, 1974.
   Discusses the major topics under the subject of UTI.
4. Travis, L., et al. Urinary tract infections in children. *Curr. Probl. Pediatr.* 4(3), 1974.
   A self-instructional manual on UTIs with examination and answers provided (55 pages, 69 references). (For a brief overview of the subject, see Pediatrics *60:508, 1977.)*

Epidemiology and Natural History

5. Kunin, C. Epidemiology and natural history of urinary tract infection in school age children. *Pediatr. Clin. North Am.* 18:509, 1971.
   A complete review of concepts, methods, epidemiology, and therapeutic considerations.
6. Roberts, K., et al. Urinary tract infections in infants with unexplained fever: A collaborative study. *J. Pediatr.* 103:864, 1983.
   Urine cultures advised in girls 0–2 years of age with unexplained fever, but not in boys.
7. Dodge, W. Cost effectiveness of renal screening. *Am. J. Dis. Child.* 131:1274, 1977.
   A critical review of the natural history of asymptomatic bacteriuria, with good references; this article is a gem.
8. Kunin, C., et al. Detection of UTI in 3-to-5-year-old girls by mothers using a nitrite indicator strip. *Pediatrics* 57:829, 1976.
   A representative screening program.
9. Randolph, M., Morris, K., and Gould, E. The first UTI in the female infant. *J. Pediatr.* 86:342, 1975.
   Follow-up of 800 baby girls and their UTIs for 10 years.
10. Cardiff-Oxford Bacteriuria Study Group. Sequelae of covert bacteriuria in school girls. *Lancet* 1:889, 1978.
    A prospective, controlled study that argues against bacteriuria screening programs for girls age 5 years and older. (For a confirmatory study, see J. Pediatr. *92:194, 1978.)*

Diagnosis

11. Pryles, C., and Lustik, B. Laboratory diagnosis of UTI. *Pediatr. Clin. North Am.* 18:233, 1971.
    An excellent summary of diagnostic laboratory tests.
12. Thomas, V., Shelokov, A., and Forland, M. Antibody coated bacteria in the urine and the site of urinary tract infection. *N. Engl. J. Med.* 290:588, 1974.
    A description of simple reliable methods of differentiating upper from lower tract infections. (For a study in children showing poor correlation, see J. Pediatr. *92:188, 1978.)*
13. Smellie, J., et al. Clinical and radiological features of UTI in childhood. *Br. Med. J.* 2:1222, 1964.
    A tabulation of clinical and x-ray findings in 200 children with UTI.

Reflux

14. Aperia, A., Brogerger, O., and Ericsson, N. Effect of vesicoureteral reflux on renal function in children with recurrent urinary tract infection. *Kidney Int.* 9:418, 1976.
    Severe reflux was associated with diminished renal function.
15. Shah, K., Robins, D., and White, R. Renal scarring and vesicoureteric reflux. *Arch. Dis. Child.* 53:210, 1978.
    The younger infants appear to be at greatest risk of marked reflux, with consequent renal damage.
16. Belman, A. The clinical significance of vesicoureteral reflux. *Pediatr. Clin. North Am.* 23:707, 1976.
    Mild reflux tends to improve.
17. Girdany, B., and Price, S. Vesicoureteral reflux and renal scarring. *J. Pediatr.* 86:998, 1975.
    A short summary of controversies regarding reflux.

Therapy

18. Bergstrom, T., et al. Studies of urinary tract infections in infancy and childhood: Short or long-term treatment in girls with first or second-time urinary tract infections uncomplicated by obstructive urological abnormalities. *Acta Paediatr. Scand.* 57:186, 1968.

In terms of 1-year cure rate, 10 days was as good as 2 months.

19. Savage, D., et al. Controlled trial of therapy in covert bacteriuria of childhood. *Lancet* 1:358, 1975.

Questions the benefit of treatment in the absence of symptoms; also see J. Pediatr. 92:194, 1978, and Lancet 1:889, 1978.

20. Shapiro, E., and Wald, E. Single-dose amoxicillin treatment of urinary tract infections. *J. Pediatr.* 99:989, 1981.

Also see Pediatrics 67:796, 1981, Br. Med. J. 1:1175, 1979, and J. Pediatr. 102:623, 1983.

---

73. CHRONIC RENAL FAILURE
Richard A. Cohn

Chronic renal failure (CRF) is a permanent, generally progressive reduction in renal function. Four major categories encompass the major definable causes in children, each representing approximately 20 to 25 percent of the total. The most common cause in older children and adolescents is *glomerulonephritis*. Both primary renal diseases (e.g., hemolytic-uremic syndrome, focal glomerular sclerosis, and membranoproliferative nephritis) and systemic disorders (e.g., Henoch-Schönlein syndrome, systemic lupus erythematosus, and vasculitis) may cause CRF. Acute poststreptococcal glomerulonephritis in children rarely progresses to CRF. *Hereditary nephropathies* include medullary cystic disease, hereditary nephritis with sensorineural deafness (Alport syndrome), cystinosis, oxalosis, and congenital nephrotic syndrome. *Renal hypoplasia-dysplasia* causes renal insufficiency early in infancy and may present as failure to thrive, often with rickets and acidosis. Patients with *obstructive* or *reflux nephropathy* commonly present with hypertension or recurrent infections of the urinary tract. Urinary tract infections, in the absence of anatomic or functional abnormalities, rarely cause CRF.

Most children with creatinine clearance values in excess of 30 ml/minute/1.73 sq m are asymptomatic, although growth may be impaired; below this level of renal function, anorexia, pallor, polyuria, weakness, fatigue, and, in adolescents, delayed puberty may be noted. With clearances below 15 ml/minute/1.73 sq m, medical intervention is usually necessary to correct metabolic disturbances; below 5 ml/minute/1.73 sq m, dialysis and transplantation are generally required, and the condition is termed *end-stage renal disease (ESRD)*.

The uremic syndrome (uremia) refers to the group of clinical signs and symptoms that are due both to the reduction in functioning renal mass and to compensatory mechanisms elicited in response to the altered physiology. A normocytic normochromic *anemia* accompanies advanced CRF, caused by deficient production of renal erythropoietic factors, increased hemolysis of extracorpuscular origin, and a bleeding tendency. *Bleeding* is in part due to inhibition of normal platelet function by toxins, notably guanidinosuccinic acid, and may result in cutaneous and gastric hemorrhage. *Hypertension,* commonly a feature in the glomerulopathies, is related to salt and water retention and occasionally to excessive renin release. In patients with obstructive nephropathy, hypoplasia-dysplasia, and medullary cystic disease, hypertension may not be present even in the late stages of CRF because of salt wasting. *Acidosis* results from urinary bicarbonate wasting, diminished tubular production of bicarbonate and other buffers, and impaired excretion of dietary acid. *Neurologic disturbances* include changes in mental status, peripheral neuropathies, and seizures that may precipitate the need for, and are often relieved by, dialysis. *Ophthalmologic changes* include blindness, nystagmus, the "red-eye syndrome," and band keratopathy, the latter two resulting from calcium deposition. *Gastrointestinal manifestations* are nausea, vomiting, ulceration and bleeding, hiccups, and pancreatitis.

The most constant *immune change* is diminished T lymphocyte function. *Dermatologic phenomena* include pruritus, dry skin, easy bruisability, and terminally, uremic "frost." A degree of *glucose intolerance* may be seen, due to diminished peripheral sensitivity to insulin; *hypertriglyceridemia* may contribute to accelerated atherosclerosis. *Cardiac complications* include congestive heart failure and pericarditis.

Osteodystrophy and *disordered calcium metabolism* result from diminished synthesis of 1,25-dihydroxycholecalciferol (1,25–vitamin D_3) by the failing kidney and from phosphorus retention in proportion to the fall in glomerular filtration rate. Inadequate 1,25–vitamin D_3 results in diminished intestinal calcium absorption, which leads to hypocalcemia and stimulates parathyroid hormone (PTH) release and calcium mobilization from bone. Skeletal resistance to PTH develops in uremia with 1,25–vitamin D_3 deficiency. Lack of 1,25–vitamin D_3 is in part responsible for the rachitic changes seen in prepubertal children. Hyperphosphatemia additionally aggravates this sequence by directly suppressing 1,25–vitamin D_3 synthesis, which causes reciprocal depression of serum calcium levels and further increases PTH production. Therapy must be directed at both reducing intestinal phosphate absorption (by lowering dietary intake and using phosphate-binding drugs) and administering potent synthetic vitamin D preparations (e.g., dihydrotachysterol, 25–hydroxy-vitamin D_3, or 1,25–dihydroxy-vitamin D_3).

Alterations in *salt and water metabolism* allow for urinary excretion of up to one-third of filtered sodium and water, in contrast to the less than 1 percent normally excreted. Natriuretic factors have been postulated, but not proved, to play a role in this regulation. *Hyperkalemia* rarely occurs until the very late stages except in the event of acidosis, infection, excess dietary intake of potassium, or inappropriate use of spironolactone.

Uremic toxins, including nitrogenous wastes (e.g., urea, ammonia, guanidines), magnesium, fluoride, cadmium, and possibly middle-sized molecules of unknown composition, natriuretic factors, PTH, and other hormones contribute to the nausea, anorexia, and lack of well-being in patients with CRF. Dietary therapy directed toward reducing nonessential amino acid intake, the use of ketoanalogues, and high caloric loads aid in symptomatic improvement.

Anticipation of the potential metabolic problems that may arise, with their correction whenever possible, is important in reducing morbidity from ESRD. Institution of early dialysis and transplantation may further prevent unnecessary complications from developing when it becomes clear that a patient's kidneys are becoming serious liabilities.

Because of the refinements in pediatric dialysis and transplantation over the last decade, ESRD in children is no longer an inevitably fatal condition. Both peritoneal and hemodialysis are now technically feasible for long periods, even in infants. Dialysis is as successful in children as it is in adults, but in contrast to its use in adults, dialysis should be viewed as a temporary procedure in children, preparatory to transplantation or until recovery from acute renal failure (ARF).

The decision to initiate dialysis in children with ARF or ESRD is dependent on many variables and must be individualized with each patient. In ARF, determinants include the levels of serum potassium, calcium, phosphorus, uric acid, urea, creatinine, and bicarbonate; the degree of fluid overload; and the likelihood of rapid or spontaneous recovery. In ESRD, in addition to these factors, the availability of a transplant donor, distance of the dialysis center from the patient's home, and the effect on other family members are considered. Most important in both situations is the overall quality of life and the likelihood of significant change on dialysis. For example, initiating dialysis can be delayed in a patient with ESRD despite a serum creatinine of 10 mg/dl if symptoms are tolerable and stable, but should be started earlier in children experiencing serious uremic complications or with complete failure to thrive despite optimal medical management. One must remember that the normal levels of serum creatinine in infants and small children are lower than in older children and adults; the former may require dialysis and transplantation when the serum creatinine approaches 5 to 6 mg/dl.

Hemodialysis requires access to the circulation via external cannulas or internal arteriovenous fistulas, systemic anticoagulation, sophisticated mechanical equipment, and highly trained personnel. In units where these are available and in regular use for children, hemodialysis, as compared with peritoneal dialysis, is the more efficient and preferred technique because of the high clearance rates, shorter treatment periods, and greater precision in the chemical control of the patient. Dialyzers and tubing can be tailored to the size and needs of even premature infants. Treatments generally are given for 4 to 6 hours 3 times weekly, with frequent monitoring of vital signs, weight, coagulation values, hematocrit, and dialyzer function. In centers in which the staff has extensive experience with dialysis, morbidity from the procedure is extremely low.

Peritoneal dialysis can be performed in a child of any size and is preferable in patients in whom cardiovascular function is seriously compromised, who cannot tolerate anticoagulation, or in whom vascular access is unavailable or difficult. The clearance of electrolytes, metabolites, and toxins is lower than with hemodialysis, and thus 24 hours are required to achieve results comparable to 4 hours of hemodialysis. Therapy can be instituted on pediatric wards with regular nursing personnel.

Continuous ambulatory peritoneal dialysis (CAPD) has recently been adapted to pediatric patients and permits home dialysis by the parent or patient. Through a permanent, silastic peritoneal catheter, four exchanges are performed daily, each "dialysis" lasting 4 to 8 hours. Commercially available dialysis solutions are available in bags ranging from 250 to 2000 ml. By being dialyzed "continuously," patients on CAPD avoid the large swings in blood pressure, body chemistry, and fluid status experienced when on hemodialysis. Most patients feel better on CAPD, in part due to improvements in diet, fluid intake, medications needed, and avoidance of hemodialysis needles and psychologic dependence on the machine. Peritonitis and parental "fatigue" are factors that may limit usefulness in certain patients. CAPD appears to be most useful in patients not likely to undergo imminent transplantation or who live great distances for hemodialysis centers.

Children on dialysis generally have poor growth and poor nutrition; remain anemic, weak, and tired; and are psychologically debilitated by their total dependence. When deterioration of function has progressed to ESRD, transplantation is, at present, the best long-term therapeutic choice. Once accepted into a transplantation program, the child undergoes a thorough pretransplantation evaluation, including HLA-A, B, and DR typing, voiding cystourethrogram, serologic and psychologic testing, completion of immunizations, and a dental evaluation. If urinary tract infection, hypertension, reflux, or nephrotic syndrome has complicated the clinical course, nephrectomy is often performed prior to transplantation. A relative with the closest HLA match (HLA-identical sibling or HLA partially matched parent or sibling) is the most preferable donor to minimize the time on dialysis and provide a kidney with the greatest likelihood of long-term function. Almost 80 percent of kidneys transplanted into children function well 5 years later.

After transplantation, prednisone and azathioprine are usually administered as "maintenance" therapy; in some centers, antilymphocyte globulin and irradiation to the graft at the time of transplantation are also given. Despite immunosuppressive treatment, acute rejection episodes may occur and are usually treated by temporarily increasing corticosteroid therapy. Other complications that may arise include infections, growth retardation, cataracts, aseptic necrosis of bone, pancreatitis, diabetes mellitus, gastrointestinal bleeding, and hypertension, all of which are, in part, related to steroid therapy. Infections that occur may be bacterial (especially in splenectomized hosts), viral (particularly herpesviruses—zoster, simplex, and cytomegalovirus), or fungal (*Candida, Nocardia, Aspergillus*). Immunosuppression predisposes to an increased incidence of malignancy, notably of the skin and lymphoid organs. Psychologic problems arise even when graft function is excellent. Finally, recurrence of the original renal disease in the transplanted kidney has been noted, particularly in membranoproliferative glomerulonephritis, idiopathic nephrotic syndrome with focal glomerular sclerosis, IgA nephropathy, and primary hyperoxaluria.

Renal transplantation has emerged from the experimental phase and is an acceptable and improving mode of therapy for children with ESRD.

General Reviews

1. Weiss, R., and Edelmann, C. End-stage renal disease. *Pediatr. Rev.* 5:295, 1984.
   A readable, general review of ESRD in children: recognition, evaluation, complications, and management.
2. Merrill, J., and Hampers, C. Uremia. *N. Engl. J. Med.* 282:953, 1014, 1970.
   A systematic two-part review of the metabolic changes, signs, and symptoms in renal failure (16 pages, 150 references).
3. Broyer, M. Chronic Renal Failure. In P. Royer et al. (eds.), *Pediatric Nephrology.* Philadelphia: Saunders, 1974.
   A series of nearly 300 children (also available in Nephron 11:209, 1973).

4. Avner, E., et al. Mortality of chronic hemodialysis and renal transplantation in pediatric end-stage renal disease. *Pediatrics* 67:412, 1981.
   Mortality was low for children dialyzed or transplanted and was comparable to rates in adults.

Hematologic Aspects
5. Fried, W. Hematologic complications of chronic renal failure. *Med. Clin. North Am.* 62:1363, 1978.
   Reviews the causes of complications such as anemia and bleeding. (Also see Nephron 25:106, 1980.)
6. Janson, P., et al. Treatment of the bleeding tendency in uremia with cryoprecipitate. *N. Engl. J. Med.* 303:1318, 1980.
   Cryoprecipitate shortens the bleeding time, reducing the risk of bleeding, particularly in surgical patients who are uremic.

Metabolic Aspects
7. Relman, A. The acidosis of renal disease. *Am. J. Med.* 44:706, 1968.
   A review of the pathogenesis of acidosis in chronic renal failure.
8. Lewy, J., and New, M. Growth in children with renal failure. *Am. J. Med.* 58:65, 1975.
   A brief review of factors retarding growth.
9. DeFronzo, R., et al. Carbohydrate metabolism in uremia: A review. *Medicine* (Baltimore) 52:469, 1973.
   Uremia and glucose intolerance are discussed (9 pages, 126 references).

Neurologic Disorders
10. Raskin, N., and Fishman, R. Neurologic disorders in renal failure. *N. Engl. J. Med.* 294:143, 1976.
    A detailed two-part review of the effects of uremia on the nervous system (11 pages, 140 references).

Immunologic Function
11. Goldblum, S., and Reed, W. Host defenses and immunologic alterations associated with chronic hemodialysis. *Ann. Intern. Med.* 93:597, 1980.
    Comprehensive review of the subject. (Also see Arch. Intern. Med. 136:682, 1976, and Nephron 14:195, 1975.)

Hyperlipidemia
12. Pennisi, A., et al. Hyperlipidemia in pediatric hemodialysis and renal transplant patients. *Am. J. Dis. Child.* 130:957, 1976.
    Hyperlipidemia correlated with premature coronary artery disease.

Osteodystrophy
13. Massry, S., and Ritz, E. The pathogenesis of secondary hyperparathyroidism of renal failure. *Arch. Intern. Med.* 138:853, 1978.
    Also see Am. J. Med. 58:48, 1975.
14. Coburn, J., Hartenbower, D., and Brickman, A. Advances in vitamin D metabolism as they pertain to chronic renal disease. *Am. J. Clin. Nutr.* 29:1283, 1976.
    A detailed review of vitamin D alterations and therapy in chronic renal disease (13 pages, 111 references).

Therapy
15. Bennett, W. Drug therapy in renal failure *Ann. Intern. Med.* 93:62, 286, 1980.
    Comprehensive, including virtually every important medication and its use in patients with ESRD (2 parts, 1000 references).
16. Gilchrest, B., et al. Relief of uremic pruritus with ultraviolet phototherapy. *N. Engl. J. Med.* 297:136, 1977.
    Study demonstrating that UV light is a safe, inexpensive, and effective treatment for uremic pruritus.

17. Chesney, R., et al. Increased growth after long-term oral 1,25-vitamin D in childhood osteodystrophy. *N. Engl. J. Med.* 298:238, 1978.
    Also see Pediatrics *68:559, 1981, and* Arch. Intern. Med. *140:1030, 1980.*
18. Brickman, A., et al. Action of 1,25-vitamin D$_3$, a potent, kidney-produced metabolite of vitamin D$_3$ in uremic man. *N. Engl. J. Med.* 287:891, 1972.
    The benefit of active vitamin D therapy in patients with ESRD is discussed.

Dialysis

19. Mauer, S., and Lynch, R. Hemodialysis techniques for infants and children. *Pediatr. Clin. North Am.* 23:843, 1976.
    A general review of important considerations involved in hemodialysis in children.
20. Manis, T., and Friedman, E. Dialytic therapy for irreversible uremia. *N. Engl. J. Med.* 301:1260, 1321, 1979.
    Basic hemodialysis principles and complications.
21. Baum, M., et al. Continuous ambulatory peritoneal dialysis in children. *N. Engl. J. Med.* 307:1537, 1982.
    An excellent comparison of hemodialysis versus CAPD in kids.
    (For a review of a large clinical experience of CAPD in adults, see Ann. Intern. Med. *92:609, 1980.)*

Transplantation

22. Mauer, S., and Howard, R. Renal Transplantation in Children. In C. Edelmann, Jr. (ed.), *Pediatric Kidney Disease.* Boston: Little, Brown, 1978.
    A comprehensive, detailed chapter on all aspects of transplantation in children (162 references).
23. Herrin, J. Pediatric renal transplantation. *Kidney Int.* 18:519, 1980.
    Excellent review and discussion (10 pages, 44 references).
24. Guttmann, R. Renal transplantation. *N. Engl. J. Med.* 301:975, 1038, 1979.
    A two-part review. (For an update of current developments, see Ann. Intern. Med. *100:246, 1984.)*
25. Fine, R., et al. Long-term results of renal transplantation in children. *Pediatrics* 61:641, 1978.
    Assessment of patient and graft survival, growth, psychosocial adaptation, and rehabilitation in 69 children. (For a discussion of renal retransplantation, see J. Pediatr. *95:244, 1979.)*
26. Hodson, E., et al. Renal transplantation in children ages 1 to 5 years. *Pediatrics* 61:458, 1978.
    Results in children less than 5 years of age comparable to those in older children.
27. Moel, D., and Butt, K. Renal transplantation in children less than 2 years of age. *J. Pediatr.* 99:535, 1981.
    Poor graft survival in infants that received cadaveric kidney transplants.
28. Korsch, B., et al. Kidney transplantation in children: Psychological follow-up study on child and family. *J. Pediatr.* 83:399, 1973.
    A study of 35 patients and controls, revealing overall rehabilitation of most patients within 1 year of operation but persisting psychologic problems in many (which may be manifested as noncompliance: Pediatrics *61:872, 1978).*
29. Merion, R., et al. Cyclosporine: Five years' experience in cadaveric renal transplantation. *N. Engl. J. Med.* 310:148, 1984.
    Graft and patient survival rates were higher with cyclosporine than with conventional immunosuppressive agents, and the need for corticosteroids was reduced. (Also see Ann. Intern. Med. *101:667, 1984, and* J. Pediatr. *106:45, 1985.)*

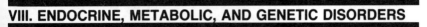

VIII. ENDOCRINE, METABOLIC, AND GENETIC DISORDERS

74. CONGENITAL ADRENAL HYPERPLASIA

John T. Hayford, Jr., and Margaret E. Mohrmann

Congenital adrenal hyperplasia (CAH) refers to a group of genetic disorders involving the metabolism of cholesterol to active steroid compounds such as cortisol. The biochemical and somatic consequences result from both an insufficiency of normal adrenal hormones and an excess of intermediate metabolites. The clinical expression is variable and depends on the metabolic pathways affected, the genetic sex of the patient, the severity of the block, and the degree to which the adrenals can respond to maximal ACTH stimulation.

Three general classes of hormone are produced in the adrenals: glucocorticoids, mineralocorticoids, and sex steroid hormones. Although each class has its own specific substrates, some enzymes act in more than one pathway; a single enzyme deficiency can therefore disrupt the production of more than one hormone. (The detailed metabolism of cholesterol to active steroids will not be reviewed here; diagrams useful for visualizing the results of blocks at various steps are available in the referenced reviews and in most comprehensive textbooks.)

In 95 percent of cases of CAH, the cause is deficiency of 21-hydroxylase, an enzyme that participates in both the mineralocorticoid and glucocorticoid pathways; 30 percent of patients have clinical salt losing. The decrease in cortisol synthesis induces excess ACTH secretion, leading to partial or complete compensation of cortisol production, but at the expense of excessive substrate diversion into the androgenic steroid pathway. Increased production of testosterone precursors causes virilization in virtually all patients, both directly and through peripheral conversion of the precursors to testosterone. As discussed on page 97, androgenic stimulation in intrauterine life leads to masculinization of the external genital organs irrespective of genetic sex. Males with CAH have increased pigmentation, especially of the areolae and scrotum, an enlarged penis, and a thin scrotum; however, these changes are subtle and are rarely detected before adrenal crisis develops. Affected females often present with ambiguous genitalia, ranging from clitoromegaly, or slight labial fusion, or both, to a phenocopy of a bilaterally cryptorchid male.

More advanced degrees of virilization are in general associated with more severe metabolic blockade and salt loss; the less severe 21-hydroxylase defects without salt losing usually cause less severe somatic changes. Females without salt losing usually have some degree of virilization, resulting in early diagnosis, but a mild 21-hydroxylase deficiency in a male may not be recognized until later childhood, when he is noted to have precocious phallic enlargement and sexual hair growth, accelerated somatic growth, increased pigmentation, and, on occasion, salt craving. A major clue in males that differentiates CAH from true sexual precocity is the lack of testicular enlargement to account for the secondary sexual characteristics.

Infants with the salt-losing variety of CAH (66 percent of the total) are usually asymptomatic during the first week of life; a mild elevation of serum potassium may be the only clue to what is to come. During the second week, lethargy, poor weight gain, vomiting, and dehydration occur. Pyloric stenosis commonly is suspected at this time, but hyperkalemia and hyponatremia suggest the true cause; recognition and treatment at this stage are lifesaving.

The diagnosis is confirmed by documentation of increased production of steroid precursors. Testosterone and its precursors are measured in the urine as 17-ketosteroids; these levels are normally elevated in neonates, and values must therefore be interpreted with caution. Measurement of 17-hydroxycorticosteroids is not useful, since levels of these hormones are often normal as a result of the excessive ACTH secretion. The most specific biochemical marker is elevation of 17-hydroxyprogesterone (17-OHP), the steroid substrate in the glucocorticoid pathway normally hydroxylated by the deficient enzyme. This hormone may now be measured by a microfilter paper radioimmunoassay, raising the possibility of newborn screening for 21-hydroxylase deficiency. The major urinary metabolite of 17-OHP, pregnanetriol, is also elevated and can be a diagnostic marker; however, delay in its elevation during the first weeks of life has been reported.

In addition to the preceding, diagnosis in the older child requires a demonstration that the androgenic steroids are elevated because of ACTH stimulation and not because of an active adrenal tumor. This is proved by a reduction of 17-ketosteroid or pregnanetriol excretion, or both, in response to ACTH-suppressing doses of dexamethasone.

The discovery of close linkage between the autosomal recessive gene for the defect in 21-hydroxylase and the human leukocyte antigen (HLA) system has resulted in an accurate means of identifying heterozygous carriers of the gene in families with an affected child. Prenatal diagnosis of this enzyme block may be possible by demonstration of elevated levels of 17-OHP and Δ4-androstenedione in amniotic fluid.

Treatment of the neonate in adrenal crisis is directed at correction of the dehydration and salt loss. Vigorous electrolyte and fluid therapy, combined with exogenous mineralocorticoid replacement (desoxycorticosterone acetate, DOCA), is the mainstay of therapy. Glucocorticoid therapy can safely be delayed until completion of the diagnostic tests that have been outlined. On confirmation of the diagnosis, glucocorticoid at 3 to 4 times the replacement dose is required for approximately 1 week to ensure rapid suppression of ACTH release.

Long-term management requires physiologic replacement of glucocorticoids. No advantage of one hormone preparation over another has been demonstrated conclusively. Careful titration of the dose is extremely important to ensure optimal growth, especially in the first year of life, when inadequate therapy can lead to a reduction in ultimate height. The dosage of replacement therapy must be increased during infections, during and after surgical procedures, and following trauma.

The goals and measures of adequate glucocorticoid replacement therapy are (1) normal hormone levels and (2) normal growth and skeletal maturation. Serum levels of 17-OHP and Δ4-androstenedione are probably the best indicators of metabolic control. There are no biochemical assays which assess excessive glucocorticoid replacement, an obvious potential complication of therapy.

Mineralocorticoid replacement is required for those with a salt-losing tendency. Adequacy of replacement is assessed by periodic monitoring of electrolyte concentrations and blood pressure; salt craving is a symptom of inadequate therapy. Even in those patients without clinical salt-losing, some deficiency of mineralocorticoid usually exists and replacement often makes hormonal control easier to maintain.

Gender assignment in patients with 21-hydroxylase defects should always be in agreement with genetic sex, since these patients have the potential for normal sexual function. Surgical intervention is often required in the female and should be a multistage effort completed within the first 2 years of life for optimal psychosexual development.

The overall prognosis for somatic, sexual, and psychosocial growth and development is excellent with careful management.

Other forms of CAH collectively account for only 5 percent of cases. 11-Hydroxylase deficiency is similar in its manifestations and treatment to 21-hydroxylase deficiency, except that hypertension is prominent, due to mineralocorticoid excess; the blood pressure usually returns to normal with adequate glucocorticoid replacement.

Nonvirilizing CAH is rare. Some forms are incompatible with life (cholesterol desmolase deficiency) or may lead to death in the neonatal period before the nature of the problem is recognized (3-hydroxysteroid dehydrogenase deficiency). 17-Hydroxylase deficiency results in inadequate glucocorticoid and sex steroid hormones and excessive mineralocorticoids. Because there is no androgenic steroid activity, the external genital phenotype is female. Patients usually are detected because of hypertension, sexual infantilism, or both.

Reviews

1. Wilkins, L. The diagnosis of the adrenogenital syndrome and its treatment with cortisone. *J. Pediatr.* 41:860, 1952.
   A classic review by one of the physicians instrumental in unraveling the biochemical defects in CAH.

2. Bongiovanni, A., and Root, A. The adrenogenital syndrome. *N. Engl. J. Med.* 268:1283, 1342, 1391, 1963.
   Another classic review, with a complete discussion of pathophysiology and clinical findings (161 references).

3. Bongiovanni, A. Disorders of the Adrenal Cortex. In S. Kaplan (ed.), *Clinical Pediatric and Adolescent Endocrinology.* Philadelphia: Saunders, 1982.
   An up-to-date textbook review.

4. Bacon, G., et al. *A Practical Approach to Pediatric Endocrinology* (2nd ed.). Chicago: Year Book, 1982.
   The 22-page section on CAH (part of the chapter entitled Abnormal Adrenal Function) is especially good for its clear presentation of steps in diagnosis and management.
5. Hughes, I. Congenital and acquired disorders of the adrenal cortex. *Clin. Endocrinol. Metab.* 11:89, 1982.
   Lucid, well-referenced section on CAH, presenting a thorough, timely review.
6. New, M., and Levine, L. New developments in congenital adrenal hyperplasia. *Pediatr. Ann.* 10:346, 1981.
   An update of an earlier, excellent review (Pediatr. Ann. 3(8):27, 1974). (For much greater detail and an extensive bibliography, see Rec. Prog. Horm. Res. 37:105, 1981.)

Diagnosis

7. Qazi, H., and Thompson, M. Genital changes in congenital virilizing adrenal hyperplasia. *J. Pediatr.* 80:653, 1972.
   An analysis of the severity of virilization in females with 21-hydroxylase deficiency.
8. Tyler, F., and West, C. Laboratory evaluation of disorders of the adrenal cortex. *Am. J. Med.* 53:664, 1972.
   Discussions of the various adrenal function tests and interpretations. (Also see reference 4.)
9. Fife, D., and Rappaport, E. Prevalence of salt-losing among congenital adrenal hyperplasia patients. *Clin. Endocrinol.* (Oxf.) 18:259, 1983.
   Of patients with 21-hydroxylase deficiency, 66 percent are salt losers; this figure is higher than previous estimates of 30 to 50 percent, perhaps because of better detection or longer survival of patients.
10. Hughes, I., and Winter, J. The application of a serum 17-hydroxyprogesterone radioimmunoassay to the diagnosis and management of congenital adrenal hyperplasia. *J. Pediatr.* 88:766, 1976.
    The best test to date for the diagnosis of the 21-hydroxylase deficiency.
11. Dupont, B., et al. Close genetic linkage between HLA and congenital adrenal hyperplasia (21-hydroxylase deficiency). *Lancet* 2:1309, 1977.
    Study showing segregation of the CAH trait with HLA; the gene appears to be closest to the HLA-B locus.
12. Lorenzen, F., et al. Hormonal phenotype and HLA genotype in families of patients with congenital adrenal hyperplasia (21-hydroxylase deficiency). *Pediatr. Res.* 13:1356, 1979.
    A mild enzymatic deficiency (abnormal elevation of 17-OHP after ACTH stimulation) confirms the validity of HLA identification of heterozygous siblings of affected children.
13. Krensky, A., et al. Identification of heterozygote carriers of congenital adrenal hyperplasia by radioimmunoassay of serum 17-hydroxyprogesterone. *J. Pediatr.* 90:930, 1977.
    Also see page 924 of the same issue.
14. Marcus, E., et al. Prenatal diagnosis of congenital adrenal hyperplasia. *Am. J. Med. Genet.* 4:201, 1979.
    A case report of an accurate diagnosis based on amniotic fluid levels of 17-OHP. (Also see J. Pediatr. 86:310, 1975.)
15. Emans, S., et al. Detection of late-onset 21-hydroxylase deficiency congenital adrenal hyperplasia in adolescents. *Pediatrics* 72:690, 1983.
    An "attenuated" form of CAH should be considered in the differential diagnosis of hirsutism in an adolescent female.

Management

16. Brook, C., et al. Experience with long-term therapy in congenital adrenal hyperplasia. *J. Pediatr.* 85:12, 1974.
    An analysis of results in 93 treated children.
17. Riddick, D., and Hammand, C. Long-term steroid therapy in patients with adrenogenital syndrome. *Obstet. Gynecol.* 45:15, 1975.
    A comprehensive clinical review (26 patients).

18. Winter, J. Current approaches to the treatment of congenital adrenal hyperplasia. *J. Pediatr.* 97:81, 1980.
    An editorial review.
19. Cavallo, A., et al. The use of plasma androstenedione in monitoring therapy of patients with congenital adrenal hyperplasia. *J. Pediatr.* 95:33, 1979.
    A reliable test that is usually easier to obtain than the 24-hour urine collection needed for measurement of 17-ketosteroids.
20. Barrett, T., and Gonzales, E. Reconstruction of the female external genitalia. *Urol. Clin. North Am.* 7:455, 1980.
    Discussion of reduction clitoroplasty and vaginoplasty in 23 patients.

Prognosis
21. Rappaport, R., et al. Linear growth rate, bone maturation and growth hormone secretion in prepubertal children with congenital adrenal hyperplasia. *Acta Paediatr. Scand.* 62:513, 1973.
    An analysis of the factors influencing ultimate height, noting the hazards of excessive as well as inadequate replacement therapy. (Also see J. Pediatr. 97:93, 1980.)
22. Klingensmith, G., et al. Glucocorticoid treatment of girls with congenital adrenal hyperplasia: Effects on height, sexual maturation and fertility. *J. Pediatr.* 90:996, 1977.
    Attention to compliance and the adequacy of the dose; height was normal, but menarche was delayed.

75. THYROID DISORDERS
John T. Hayford, Jr., and Margaret E. Mohrmann

Disorders of thyroid function in childhood frequently confront the pediatrician with a diagnostic dilemma. The initial symptoms are often subtle or misleading, and the same disorder may present in markedly different ways at different ages.

Neonatal hypothyroidism occurs in 1 in 4000 live births, a figure determined by mass screening of newborns. Thyroid hypofunction is due to partial or complete failure of thyroid gland development in at least 85 percent of cases and only rarely is a result of thyrotropin (TSH) deficiency. The clinical identification of the newborn with hypothyroidism is often difficult. Only occasionally does an infant present with features of the classic symptom complex, such as large tongue, hoarse cry, umbilical hernia, hypotonia, poor peripheral circulation (mottling, cold hands and feet), or lethargy (which may be interpreted by the parents as the sign of a "good baby"). Retrospective analysis of findings in infants whose disease was diagnosed after the neonatal period has identified other, more subtle clues: a gestation longer than 42 weeks; feeding difficulties; delayed passage of stools; prolonged, unexplained hyperbilirubinemia; large fontanelles (especially posterior); and respiratory distress in an infant weighing over 2.5 kg.

The appropriate initial laboratory test is a thyroxine (T4) level; one must be aware that normal T4 values in the newborn are higher than in older children and adults. The finding of a low or borderline T4 for age necessitates measurement of the TSH level, which normally approximates adult values after the first 72 hours of life. An elevated TSH confirms the diagnosis of primary hypothyroidism; a normal TSH level in the face of a low T4 requires study of the hypothalamic-pituitary axis.

Lifetime thyroid hormone replacement therapy should be started as soon as the diagnosis of hypothyroidism is made; dosage adjustments are based on the TSH level. When laboratory findings are equivocal, and clinical suspicion of thyroid insufficiency persists, replacement therapy should be instituted for a minimum of 2 years to ensure normal thyroxine-dependent brain maturation before reevaluating the need for therapy. Three-fourths of children whose treatment is started before the age of 3 months and is maintained without significant interruption have at least average intellectual development; of those treated after 3 months of age or inadequately treated, only a small number attain normal intelligence levels, although their somatic growth may be normal. It is postulated that children who have mental deficiencies despite early and adequate replacement therapy suffered irreversible cerebral damage from thyroid deficiency in utero; methods of diagnosing and treating intrauterine hypothyroidism are being studied.

Goiter in the newborn may be associated with decreased, normal, or increased thyroid function and may be large enough to require partial excision to relieve respiratory embarrassment. Defective hormonogenesis due to enzyme deficiency, rarely evident in the neonatal period, results in compensatory hypertrophy of the gland and either a hypothyroid or a euthyroid state; thyroid replacement is necessary to reduce the goiter. Thyroid-suppressing thioamides (propylthiouracil, methimazole) or iodide salts (e.g., potassium iodide for the treatment of asthma), when taken by the mother during pregnancy, may cause a euthyroid goiter in the infant; the goiter resolves gradually without treatment.

Hyperthyroidism, unusual in the newborn, is most often associated with maternal Graves disease. When transient, as in the majority of cases, it is thought to be caused by transplacental passage of a thyroid-stimulating immunoglobulin. An affected infant not only has a goiter, but also has signs of increased thyroid hormone activity, such as tachycardia, irritability, excess movement, weight loss, and, occasionally, proptosis. The disease can usually be controlled by short-term thioamide therapy or potassium iodide or both, but beta-adrenergic blockade with propranolol is occasionally necessary for the relief of severe symptoms such as congestive heart failure. A small percentage of infants with neonatal Graves disease continue to need thyroid suppression for an indeterminate length of time. These children are thought to have familial hyperthyroidism, unrelated to maternal thyroid stimulators.

Thyroid dysfunction is much more common in the child and adolescent than in the neonate and has a striking predilection for females. Goiter due to congenital defects in thyroid hormonogenesis and thyroid failure secondary to hypothalamic or pituitary insufficiency characteristically present in this age group, but chronic lymphocytic thyroiditis (CLT, Hashimoto thyroiditis) accounts for the majority of hypothyroid children. The pathogenesis of CLT is unclear; however, lymphocytic infiltration seen on histologic sections of thyroid, association with failure of other endocrine organs, and elevated antithyroid antibodies suggest an autoimmune etiology.

The euthyroid child with CLT usually presents with an asymptomatic goiter—a firm, pebbly or nodular, nontender gland. When T4 is normal, an elevated TSH level will help to differentiate thyroiditis from simple goiter. The most common presenting complaint of the hypothyroid child with CLT is short stature; the bone age is retarded, as are the body proportions. The classic symptoms of thyroid hypofunction (e.g., lethargy, cold intolerance, constipation), if present, are often minimized or ignored by the patient and family and must be questioned for carefully. Physical examination may reveal immature facies with an undeveloped nasal bridge, skin and hair abnormalities, edema, and slow relaxation of the deep tendon reflexes. Laboratory diagnosis is based on a decreased T4 and an elevated TSH, often accompanied by increased titers of antithyroid antibodies. Thyroid imaging and radioactive iodine uptake studies are unnecessary and the results may be misleading. The child with thyroiditis, whether euthyroid or hypothyroid, requires thyroid hormone replacement therapy to reduce the goiter or to relieve the thyroid deficiency.

Hyperthyroidism in childhood and adolescence is usually due to Graves disease, although some children with CLT are hyperthyroid initially. All but a few affected children present with thyroid enlargement, and most have symptoms and signs of excessive thyroid activity, such as tremors, emotional lability, weight loss, and tachycardia. Physical examination reveals a diffusely enlarged, soft, boggy thyroid gland without nodules; other physical findings suggest increased metabolic activity. The ophthalmopathy characteristic of adult Graves disease is considerably less common in hyperthyroid children. The clinical diagnosis is confirmed by the finding of increased concentrations of circulating thyroid hormones, with elevation of T3 (by radioimmunoassay) often being the most sensitive test; suppression tests may be used to demonstrate the gland's autonomy.

Hyperthyroidism is treated initially with thioamide blockade; partial thyroidectomy may be necessary if medical management is unsuccessful. The use of radionuclide ablation of the thyroid in children is controversial and probably should be avoided until more is known about the genetic and carcinogenic implications of such therapy. Thyroid storm, rare in childhood, may require beta-adrenergic blockade with propranolol. Most children with hyperthyroidism no longer require therapy after about 3 years of thio-amide suppression. Patients must be carefully observed for the hypothyroidism that may develop after thyroidectomy, with oversuppression by thioamides, or in the natural progression of CLT.

Thyroid nodules in children are more likely to be carcinomatous (incidence, 40–50%) than are similar masses in adults; adenomas and colloid cysts account for the majority of benign nodules. Involvement of the lymph nodes, esophagus, or recurrent laryngeal nerves increases the likelihood of malignancy, but the absence of lymphadenopathy or of associated symptoms in no way rules out the possibility of thyroid carcinoma. Open biopsy is essential for evaluation of all single or multiple thyroid masses in children and adolescents and should not be delayed by other diagnostic maneuvers, such as thyroid imaging or thyroxine suppression tests. Benign lesions may be treated by simple excision; carcinoma requires extensive resection of all involved areas. Because malignant tumor remnants are frequently sensitive to TSH, high-dose thyroxine replacement should be used in the postoperative period; radiotherapy may also be indicated.

Reviews

1. Ingbar, S., and Woeber, K. The Thyroid Gland. In R. Williams (ed.), *Textbook of Endocrinology* (6th ed.). Philadelphia: Saunders, 1981.
   An authoritative review of thyroid physiology and disease.
2. Kaplan, S. (ed.). *Clinical Pediatric and Adolescent Endocrinology*. Philadelphia: Saunders, 1982.
   Contains five clear, concise, well-referenced chapters on all aspects of normal and abnormal thyroid function in the young.
3. Reiter, E., et al. Childhood thyromegaly: Recent developments. *J. Pediatr.* 99:507, 1981.
   A thorough review of infiltrative and neoplastic processes manifested as goiter. (For a detailed discussion of the immunopathogenesis of childhood goiters, see Pediatr. Rev. 5:259, 1984.)

Thyroid Function Tests

4. Yao, Y. A current view of thyroid function tests. *Hosp. Pract.* 16(9):149, 1981.
   Uneven text but many helpful tables and diagnostic flow diagrams.
5. Fisher, D. Advances in the laboratory diagnosis of thyroid disease. *J. Pediatr.* 82:1, 187, 1973.
   A very readable two-part guide to the use and interpretation of the tests.
6. Erenberg, A., et al. Total and free thyroid hormone concentrations in the neonatal period. *Pediatrics* 53:211, 1974.
   An analysis of the lability of thyroid function in the newborn period. (For normative data in preterm infants, see J. Pediatr. 92:963, 1978, and Am. J. Dis. Child. 131:842, 1977.)

Neonatal Hypothyroidism

7. Fisher, D., and Klein, A. Thyroid development and disorders of thyroid function in the newborn. *N. Engl. J. Med.* 304:702, 1981.
   A well-written, detailed treatise; many of the transient and subtle abnormalities described have been recognized only since the advent of widespread screening of newborns.
8. Committee on Genetics, American Academy of Pediatrics. Screening for congenital metabolic disorders in the newborn infant: Congenital deficiency of thyroid hormone and hyperphenylalaninemia. *Pediatrics* 60:389, 1977.
   Contains basic recommendations for newborn screening. (For an update, see Pediatrics 69:104, 1982; for a brief progress report on international screening results, see J. Pediatr. 102:653, 1983; and for a discussion of problems to be aware of in a screening program, see Pediatrics 70:16, 1982.)
9. Fisher, D. Hypothyroidism in childhood. *Pediatr. Rev.* 2:67, 1980.
   Congenital and acquired hypofunction reviewed. (For a similar, but less detailed, review, see Pediatr. Clin. North Am. 26:33, 1979.)
10. Smith, D., et al. Congenital hypothyroidism: Signs and symptoms in the newborn period. *J. Pediatr.* 87:958, 1975.

A retrospective analysis of the clinical findings in 15 patients.
11. Committee on Drugs, American Academy of Pediatrics. Treatment of congenital hypothyroidism. *Pediatrics* 62:413, 1978.
    This remains the clearest, most accessible paper on the subject.
12 Smith, D., Blizzard, R., and Wilkins, L. The mental prognosis in hypothyroidism of infancy and childhood. *Pediatrics* 19:1011, 1957.
    A study of 128 children, 79 of whom had signs of disease before 6 months of age; prognosis was related to the time of onset of therapy and to osseous evidence of intrauterine thyroid deficiency. (A 25-year follow-up of 10 of these patients showed continued intellectual growth in adulthood: J. Pediatr. 93:432, 1978.)
13. Klein, A., Meltzer, S., and Kenny, F. Improved prognosis in congenital hypothyroidism treated before age three months. *J. Pediatr.* 81:912, 1972.
    In 31 patients, the IQ was over 85 in 78 percent of those treated before 3 months of age, but in only 14 percent of those treated after 3 months.
14. MacFaul, R., et al. Neurological abnormalities in patients treated for hypothyroidism from early life. *Arch. Dis. Child.* 53:611, 1978.
    Despite normal IQ scores, many patients (77% in this series) have evidence of abnormal brain function, such as learning and behavior disorders, the incidence of which is unrelated to the time of institution of therapy. (Preliminary studies of hypothyroid infants detected by mass screening seem to show similar results: J. Pediatr. 102:19, 1983.)

Neonatal Hyperthyroidism

15. Hollingsworth, D., Mabry, C., and Eckerd, J. Hereditary aspects of Graves' disease in infancy and childhood. *J. Pediatr.* 81:446, 1972.
    Contains seven case reports; evidence suggests autosomal recessive inheritance, with predominant expression in females.
16. Hollingsworth, D., and Mabry, C. Congenital Graves' disease. *Am. J. Dis. Child.* 130:148, 1976.
    Four case reports, with a long-term follow-up, as well as a cogent argument against long-acting thyroid stimulator as the cause in all cases. (See the commentary on p. 133 of the same issue.)
17. Daneman, D., and Howard, N. Neonatal thyrotoxicosis: Intellectual impairment and craniosynostosis in later years. *J. Pediatr.* 97:257, 1980.
    Problems arose despite early and adequate therapy, raising the possibility of intrauterine damage.

Childhood Hypothyroidism

18. Fisher, D., and Beall, G. Hashimoto's thyroiditis. *Pharmacol. Ther.* (B) 1:445, 1976.
    An excellent, comprehensive review of pathophysiology, clinical spectrum, and therapy (90 references). (Also see reference 22.)
19. Rallison, M., et al. Occurrence and natural history of chronic lymphocytic thyroiditis in childhood. *J. Pediatr.* 86:675, 1975.
    The incidence among over 5000 adolescents was 1.2 percent; spontaneous cure occurred in many.
20. Monteleone, J., et al. Differentiation of chronic lymphocytic thyroiditis and simple goiter in pediatrics. *J. Pediatr.* 83:381, 1973.
    The diagnosis of CLT by immunofluorescent antibody studies is discussed.
21. Hung, W., et al. Clinical, laboratory, and histologic observations in euthyroid children and adolescents with goiters. *J. Pediatr.* 82:10, 1973.
    Criteria for diagnosing CLT without biopsy are considered. (For data on congenital goiter, see J. Pediatr. 86:753, 1975.)

Childhood Hyperthyroidism

22. Lee, W. Thyroiditis, hyperthyroidism, and tumors. *Pediatr. Clin. North Am.* 26:53, 1979.
    A succinct discussion of childhood Graves disease.
23. Barnes, H., and Blizzard, R. Antithyroid drug therapy for toxic diffuse goiter (Graves' disease): Thirty years' experience in children and adolescents. *J. Pediatr.* 91:313, 1977.

A study of 104 patients; good results were obtained with a combination of thioamide and L-thyroxine; the 1-hour perchlorate discharge test was used to determine the dosage schedule. (Also see Pediatrics *54:565, 1974.)*

24. Collen, R., et al. Remission rates of children and adolescents with thyrotoxicosis treated with antithyroid drugs. Pediatrics 65:550, 1980.
    Remissions occurred in one-half the patients within 5 years of diagnosis.

25. Buckingham, G., et al. Hyperthyroidism in children: A reevaluation of treatment. Am. J. Dis. Child. 135:112, 1981.
    Comparison of medical and surgical therapy in 107 patients; a related editorial (p. 109) supports use of radioactive iodine therapy, a position opposed in N. Engl. J. Med. *303:217, 1980. Review of drugs:* N. Engl. J. Med. *311:1353, 1984.*

Thyroid Masses

26. Bachrach, L., et al. Use of ultrasound in childhood thyroid disorders. J. Pediatr. 103:547, 1983.
    A sensitive noninvasive technique that is especially useful in the evaluation of focal lesions.

27. Kirkland, R., et al. Solitary thyroid nodules in 30 children and report of a child with a thyroid abscess. Pediatrics 51:85, 1973.
    Carcinoma was present in 12 of 30 patients; 4 of the 12 had had neck irradiation previously; biopsy of all nodules is recommended. (Also see reference 22.)

28. Hopwood, N., et al. Functioning thyroid masses in childhood and adolescence. J. Pediatr. 89:710, 1976.
    Recommends surgical removal of autonomously functioning nodules because of the cancer risk and for relief of hyperthyroid symptoms.

76. HYPOGLYCEMIA

John T. Hayford, Jr., and Margaret E. Mohrmann

Hypoglycemia is not a disease per se, but a consequence of many different disorders of metabolism, all of which result in inadequate concentrations of intracellular glucose by one or more of three mechanisms: (1) inadequate substrate availability; (2) disordered endogenous glucose storage, synthesis, or both; and (3) accelerated glucose utilization. Most of the symptoms and signs of hypoglycemia (tachycardia, sweating, pallor), especially when it is acute, are those of epinephrine response to the fall in blood sugar. The central nervous system is particularly sensitive to reductions in glucose concentration, as reflected by disordered cerebral function; additional clinical manifestations are usually aspects of the particular primary disease.

The concentration of blood glucose defined as hypoglycemia is age-dependent. Neonatal hypoglycemia is commonly defined as blood glucose less than 20 mg/dl in a preterm infant and less than 30 mg/dl in a full-term infant. Blood glucose less than 40 mg/dl after the first week of age is abnormal. These concentrations represent statistical definitions of the lower limit of normal; the true relationship between blood glucose concentration and compromise of glucose-dependent metabolic processes has not been adequately defined. Nevertheless, maintenance of blood glucose above these concentrations is the minimal criterion of the adequacy of any therapeutic regimen.

Hypoglycemia is most common in the neonatal period, occurring in 2 to 5 infants per 1000 full-term infants of normal birth weight; both gestational and postnatal complications increase the risk of hypoglycemia in the newborn. Neonatal hypoglycemia can be separated into categories for etiologic and prognostic consideration. Early "transitional" hypoglycemia occurs in a heterogeneous population of neonates and is often associated with maternal diabetes, severe erythroblastosis, intrapartum fetal distress, or postpartum asphyxia. Excessive insulin production is thought to cause hypoglycemia in infants of diabetic mothers and in those with severe erythroblastosis, but the pathophysiology of the failure in glucose homeostasis in infants with transitional hypoglycemia is unknown. Hypoglycemia usually occurs within the first 12 hours of life, is frequently asymptomatic, resolves rapidly, and seldom recurs. Early, frequent feeding (or parenteral glucose if necessary) is the therapy of choice until the problem resolves. Diagnosis, suggested by the perinatal history, is confirmed by the brief clinical course; additional evaluation of glucose metabolism is not indicated.

"Transient" hypoglycemia is a disturbance of neonatal glucose homeostasis that differs from transitional hypoglycemia in several ways. A history of maternal toxemia in the antenatal period is often found in infants with transient hypoglycemia, whereas intrapartum and/or postpartum distress is less common. Intrauterine growth retardation, in which head circumference may be normal, but height—and particularly weight—are disproportionately small, occurs in nearly 75 percent of these hypoglycemic infants. In contrast to transitional hypoglycemia, hypoglycemia in these infants has a more delayed onset, is frequently symptomatic, and tends to persist beyond the first day of life. The diagnosis is usually based on an appropriate history and physical examination, the exclusion of secondary causes of hypoglycemia, and the clinical course. Extensive workups for syndromes of insulin excess, hepatic enzyme defects, and disorders of amino acid metabolism can be deferred, unless the physical findings or clinical course renders the diagnosis of transient hypoglycemia untenable; for example, if large doses of intravenous glucose (over 12 mg/kg/hour) are needed to maintain blood glucose above 40 mg/dl or if improvement is not seen by the second week of life, the diagnosis should be reconsidered.

Significant depression of blood glucose associated with congenital or acquired abnormalities of the cardiovascular or central nervous system, sepsis, hypocalcemia, or severe asphyxia is classified as "secondary" hypoglycemia. Abrupt cessation of parenteral glucose administration is a common cause of secondary hypoglycemia, due to delay in the suppression of insulin secretion after discontinuation of the glucose.

In contrast with hypoglycemia that is limited to the first days of life, hypoglycemia that recurs or persists beyond the second week of life is more commonly associated with a specific defect in hormone, carbohydrate, or amino acid metabolism. Insulin excess is the major endocrine cause of hypoglycemia. On histologic examination, the pancreas shows variable degrees of beta-cell hyperplasia or neoplasia; insulin secretion can range from an excessive insulin secretory response to total autonomy. Hypopituitarism (either isolated growth hormone or multiple pituitary tropic hormone deficiency) may be a cause of hypoglycemia in the neonatal period, but more commonly presents in early childhood. Primary deficiency of adrenal or thyroid hormones may also be associated with hypoglycemia, usually mild. Some types of glycogen storage disease and certain disorders of amino acid metabolism are characterized by persistent hypoglycemia. Diagnosis requires the measurement of substrates and enzyme activities to pinpoint the defect. Glucose levels obtained during a fast and at specific times after feeding may suggest either excessive glucose utilization (e.g., insulin excess) or inadequate glucose production (e.g., glycogenosis type I—von Gierke disease) and thereby allow the workup to be more specific and selective.

Hypoglycemia is much less common in children than in infants and usually involves a more limited differential diagnosis. The two major causes of hypoglycemia in childhood are ketotic hypoglycemia and insulin excess. Ketotic hypoglycemia is usually seen in underweight males, between the ages of 2 and 7 years who have a history of low birth weight. Symptomatic hypoglycemia occurs after a prolonged fast (e.g., in the morning after a light supper and a long sleep) or during periods of anorexia from mild illnesses. This disorder probably represents an exaggeration of the normal age-dependent response to starvation, as most preschool children can be shown to become hypoglycemic and ketonemic with fasting, a fact that has important implications for the practice of preoperative fasting in this age group. Frequent feedings and avoidance of fasting are effective treatment and are generally needed only until late childhood, since the disorder is "outgrown" by that time. Syndromes of excessive insulin secretion are documented by incomplete or absent suppression of circulating insulin concentrations during hypoglycemia and by an increased insulin secretory response to provocative testing. In older children, islet cell adenoma is the predominant cause of hyperinsulinism. Treatment is directed at suppression of insulin secretion with sympathomimetic drugs, or diazoxide, or both; subtotal pancreatectomy or surgical removal of an insulin-producing tumor may be necessary. Hypoglycemia in the young child may also be caused by an endocrine or hepatic enzyme deficiency or by the ingestion of substances such as salicylate, alcohol, or oral hypoglycemic agents (e.g., tolbutamide).

Reviews

1. Cornblath, M., and Schwartz, R. *Disorders of Carbohydrate Metabolism in Infancy* (2nd ed.). Philadelphia: Saunders, 1976.
   An excellent reference for problems with hypoglycemia, with an extensive discussion of and bibliography for most disorders.
2. Cornblath, M. Hypoglycemia in infancy and childhood. *Pediatr. Ann.* 10:356, 1981.
   An excellent, concise review with many helpful practical points about evaluation and treatment.
3. Senior, B., and Wolfsdorf, J. Hypoglycemia in children. *Pediatr. Clin. North Am.* 26:171, 1979.
   A good summary of physiology and differential diagnosis.
4. Aynsley-Green, A. Hypoglycemia in infants and children. *Clin. Endocrinol. Metab.* 11:159, 1982.
   Detailed, thorough, and well referenced.
5. Pagliara, A., et al. Hypoglycemia in infancy and childhood. *J. Pediatr.* 82:365, 558, 1973.
   A two-part review article discussing the physiology of normal and disordered carbohydrate metabolism.

Neonatal Hypoglycemia

6. Lubchenco, L., and Bard, H. Incidence of hypoglycemia in newborn infants classified by birth weight and gestational age. *Pediatrics* 47:831, 1971.
   An important paper relating birth weight and gestational age to the risk of hypoglycemia.
7. Milner, R. Neonatal hypoglycemia, 1979. *J. Perinat. Med.* 7:185, 1979.
   A concise, thorough review emphasizing pathophysiology and a logical plan of evaluation and therapy.
8. de Leeuw, R., and de Vries, I. Hypoglycemia in small for dates newborn infants. *Pediatrics* 58:18, 1976.
   "Transitional" hypoglycemia in 24 percent; a relative lack of metabolizable lipids is postulated.

Syndromes of Insulin Excess

9. Yakovac, W., et al. Beta cell nesidioblastosis in idiopathic hypoglycemia of infancy. *J. Pediatr.* 79:226, 1971.
   A clinical and pathologic description of an increasingly recognized cause of persistent neonatal hypoglycemia.
10. Stanley, C., and Baker, L. Hyperinsulinism in infancy: Diagnosis by demonstration of abnormal response to fasting hypoglycemia. *Pediatrics* 57:702, 1976.
    A report of biochemical observations that aid in the differentiation of hyperinsulinemic hypoglycemia from other hypoglycemic syndromes.
11. Baker, L., et al. Diazoxide treatment of idiopathic hypoglycemia of infancy. *J. Pediatr.* 71:494, 1967.
    Initial observation on a clinically important modality of therapy.
12. Thomas, C., et al. Neonatal and infantile hypoglycemia due to insulin excess. *Ann. Surg.* 185:505, 1977.
    Case reports and review of the literature on surgical intervention.

Ketotic Hypoglycemia

13. Colle, E., and Ulstrom, R. Ketotic hypoglycemia. *J. Pediatr.* 64:632, 1964.
    A good clinical description.
14. Habbick, B., et al. Diagnosis of ketotic hypoglycemia of childhood. *Arch. Dis. Child.* 46:295, 1971.
    A report of the authors' experience with 20 cases, emphasizing diagnostic criteria.
15. Haymond, M., et al. Ketotic hypoglycemia: An amino acid substrate-limited disorder. *J. Clin. Endocrinol. Metabol.* 38:521, 1974.
    Documents low levels of alanine and postulates a lack of gluconeogenetic substrate as the cause of ketotic hypoglycemia. (See reference 3 for a refutation based on evidence that alanine is primarily derived from glucose and that its demonstrated deficiency is due to—not a cause of—hypoglycemia.)

16. Chaussain, J., et al. Glycemic response to 24-hour fast in normal children and children with ketotic hypoglycemia. *J. Pediatr.* 82:438, 1973, and 85:776, 1974.
   Inadequate gluconeogenesis causes a drop in blood glucose in all fasting children, but the drop is more significant in those with ketotic hypoglycemia.
17. Dahlquist, G., et al. Ketotic hypoglycemia of childhood: A clinical trial of several unifying etiologic hypotheses. *Acta Paediatr. Scand.* 68:649, 1979.
   Concludes that ketotic hypoglycemia represents part of the spectrum of normal development of adaptation to starvation.

77. DIABETES MELLITUS
John T. Hayford, Jr., and Margaret E. Mohrmann

"Juvenile" diabetes mellitus (in current terminology, insulin-dependent diabetes mellitus, IDDM) is a chronic metabolic disease resulting from a lack of insulin and characterized by hyperglycemia, a tendency to ketoacidosis, and the development of vascular complications. It is unusual in infants; the incidence of new cases is highest around age 11 and appears to have been increasing during the past several decades; the current prevalence is approximately 1 per 1000 children.

Recent studies of the actions of glucagon and somatostatin have demonstrated significant abnormalities, but have also affirmed the primacy of insulin deficiency in the pathophysiology of IDDM. Juvenile diabetes mellitus is distinguished from adult diabetes mellitus (which occasionally has its onset in childhood) by the absolute lack of insulin in the former and the resistance to the effects of normal to increased amounts of insulin in the latter. Those who lack insulin are generally thin; those with insulin resistance tend to be obese, and in some cases their disease may be controlled by diet alone.

The cause of diabetes mellitus is unknown. Familial clustering is well recognized, but the genetic details of the "predisposition" to DM remain obscure. A greater percentage of children with IDDM than of unaffected children have histocompability antigens (HLA) B8 and B15 and diseases thought to be of autoimmune origin (e.g., chronic lymphocytic thyroiditis). Viral infections have been shown experimentally to cause diabetes mellitus in animals, and there are some epidemiologic data suggesting an increased incidence of IDDM in humans following Coxsackie virus and mumps infections. It is possible that in certain children with genetic predisposition, viruses (or other environmental agents) trigger an anti-beta-cell (autoimmune) response that results in IDDM.

Without adequate insulin, children with IDDM generally have a normal to increased appetite (polyphagia), but, because carbohydrate calories are "wasted" in the urine, these children lose (or do not gain) weight. Increased intake of fluids (polydipsia) is caused by the glucose-induced osmotic diuresis (polyuria). A clear history of polyuria and polydipsia, with or without polyphagia, and the finding of hyperglycemia and glucosuria are sufficient for the diagnosis of IDDM. A glucose tolerance test is necessary for diagnosis only in the rare child with adult-type, insulin-resistant DM. Often the diagnosis is not made until ketosis and acidosis develop; at that point, the history and the presence of hyperglycemia and large amounts of ketones in the urine and blood serve to differentiate diabetic ketoacidosis from such disorders as salicylate intoxication and Reye syndrome.

Once the diagnosis is established and the child is in reasonable metabolic balance (see Diabetic Ketoacidosis, Chap. 7), the child and family require education, but it must be recognized that the emotional impact of the diagnosis makes learning an inefficient process. The fear of injections, the specter of a restricted life, and the apparent complexity of the relationship of insulin needs, exercise, and diet are all concerns that require attention. Child and parents must be assured that experienced, sympathetic assistance is readily available.

The goals of therapy are to achieve good control of hyperglycemia and to prevent complications. There continues to be much controversy over the definition and optimal degree of "control," the means of achieving it, and the most accurate method of assessing it. Since current evidence appears to incriminate hyperglycemia (with or without ketoacidosis) as the cause of vascular complications of diabetes, the American Diabetes Association advocates tight control (i.e., keeping the blood glucose concentration as close to normal as possible) through dietary management and frequent injections of insulin: this recommendation is accepted by an increasing number of physicians who care for children with diabetes. However, no regimen based on intermittent injections of insulin can accomplish minute-to-minute adjustments in response to fluctuating needs (as the normal pancreas does); mechanical devices that are able to make such adjustments and provide a more physiologic insulin response have numerous disadvantages. Since long term continuous monitoring of blood glucose is not practical, it is difficult to assess the exact degree of control in an individual patient. Serial determinations of urine glucose concentrations, while satisfactory to detect trends and gauge caloric losses, do not accurately reflect rapid variations in blood glucose. Home blood glucose monitoring is a more direct method of assessment but also has the disadvantage of measuring only a single point on an everchanging curve. The glycosylated hemoglobin level is probably a good indicator of the degree of control over time and may therefore be important for studies correlating control with the rate of complications, but it is not useful for day-to-day adjustments of insulin dose. Since attempts to normalize blood glucose concentrations run the risk of producing hypoglycemia, some clinicians who treat children with IDDM prefer to accept some degree of hyperglycemia (and glucosuria) to protect against central nervous system damage from hypoglycemia. Thus, although "tight control" is desirable it may be more a theoretical than a practically achievable goal at present. Normal growth and development, without episodes of hypoglycemia or ketoacidosis, remain the minimal criteria of acceptable management.

The basic elements of any diabetes regimen are insulin, diet, exercise, and psychologic support. The type of insulin and the frequency of injections vary among centers that care for a large number of children with IDDM; most recommend one or two daily injections of NPH or Lente insulin with or without added regular (CZI) or Semilente insulin. There are numerous studies in progress on the use of a portable pump to deliver a continuous subcutaneous infusion of insulin; the role of such a device in the management of IDDM remains unclear. Research continues on islet cell transplantation.

An acceptable degree of dietary control may be accomplished by instructing the child and his family to keep the child's caloric intake relatively constant from day to day and to avoid high-carbohydrate foods. Some pediatricians prefer the somewhat stricter "exchange" diet system, and a few continue to recommend a stringent "weighed" diet.

The supportive aspects of care cannot be overemphasized. The child with diabetes must not only tolerate (and administer to himself or herself) insulin injections but must also assume a degree of responsibility unknown to his or her peers (e.g., major exercise and dietary changes must be planned). The inescapable burdens of urine and/or blood testing, dietary restrictions, injections, and protective parents combine to produce overt depression at some time in almost all children with diabetes; this is especially true in adolescents, whose depression is often expressed as rebellion. Supportive medical guidance, continuing detailed education, open communication, and opportunities to enjoy activities with other children with IDDM (such as in summer camps) help the child maintain a good self-image. The psychologic health of the child with diabetes ultimately depends in large part on the realization that he or she can control the disease and need not be controlled by it.

The physical complications of IDDM are of three types: (1) acute metabolic decompensation (diabetic ketoacidosis, Chap. 7), (2) disturbances of growth and development, and (3) chronic vascular disorders. The vascular disease that occurs in diabetes affects virtually every organ but is most evident in the eyes, kidneys, and nervous system. Retinopathy, renal failure, and peripheral neuropathy are seldom symptomatic in children, but are responsible for considerable morbidity in young adults with IDDM.

Reviews

1. Sperling, M. Diabetes Mellitus. In S. Kaplan (ed.), *Clinical Pediatric and Adolescent Endocrinology*. Philadelphia: Saunders, 1982.
   A well-balanced current textbook review; a good summary of much of the information in this chapter is found in Pediatr. Clin. North Am. 26:149, 1979.
2. Castells, S. (ed.). Symposium on juvenile diabetes. *Pediatr. Clin. North Am.* 31(3), 1984.

A collection of 15 articles on various issues, including pathogenesis, complications, and selected aspects of management. (For another "Symposium on childhood diabetes," see Pediatr. Ann. 12(9), 1983.)

3. Ehrlich, R. Diabetes mellitus in childhood. *Clin. Endocrinol. Metab.* 11:195, 1982.
   An excellent review of basic knowledge and recent advances.
4. Rosenbloom, A., Kohrman, A., and Sperling, M. Classification and diagnosis of diabetes mellitus in children and adolescents. *J. Pediatr.* 99:320, 1981.
   Important definitions and diagnostic criteria from the National Diabetes Data Group.

Etiology and Epidemiology

5. Cahill, G., and McDevitt, H. Insulin-dependent diabetes mellitus: The initial lesion. *N. Engl. J. Med.* 304:1454, 1981.
   A comprehensive review of research data, with emphasis on the heterogeneity of the disease and the role of viral induction of autoimmune beta cell destruction.
6. Zonana, J., and Rimoin, D. Current concepts in genetics: Inheritance of diabetes mellitus. *N. Engl. J. Med.* 295:603, 1976.
   A review of the data. (A recent report suggests recessive inheritance with 50 percent penetrance: N. Engl. J. Med. 297:1036, 1977; greater heterogeneity suggested: Diabetes 27:599, 1978.)
7. Gamble, D. Relation of antecedent illness to development of diabetes in children. *Br. Med. J.* 281:99, 1980.
   A survey of 1663 children with new onset IDDM showed a significantly greater incidence of mumps in the 6 months prior to the onset of diabetes. (Also see reference 5.)
8. Fleeger, F., et al. Age, sex, and season of onset of juvenile diabetes in different geographic areas. *Pediatrics* 63:374, 1979.
   Notes fall and winter onset and an increasing incidence of IDDM. (Also see J. Pediatr. 91:706, 1977.)

Pathophysiology

9. Vaisrub, S. The primacy of insulin. *JAMA* 236:1274, 1976.
   A brief editorial summarizes the studies suggesting significant roles for glucagon and somatostatin and the studies confirming the "primacy" of insulin; only a few references are included, but they are the key ones.
10. Fajans, S., et al. The various faces of diabetes in the young: Changing concepts. *Arch. Intern. Med.* 136:194, 1976.
    An excellent essay contrasting classic juvenile-onset diabetes and maturity-onset diabetes in children with respect to metabolic abnormalities, natural history, and inheritance. (Also see reference 1.)

Control: The Controversy

11. Cahill, G., Etzwiler, D., and Freinkel, N. "Control" and diabetes. *N. Engl. J. Med.* 294:1004, 1976 (or *Diabetes* 25:237, 1976).
    On the basis of studies linking vascular disease to poor control (referenced), the American Diabetes Association urges that control be tighter.
12. Malone, J., et al. Good diabetic control: A study in mass delusion. *J. Pediatr.* 88:943, 1976.
    Demonstrates the practical problem in defining "control"; an editorial on page 1074 of the same issue outlines realistic, but minimal goals of management.

Control: Assessment

13. Malone, J., et al. The role of urine sugar in diabetic management. *Am. J. Dis. Child.* 130:1324, 1976.
    Good for assessing trends but not for hour-to-hour decisions. (For a discussion of the usefulness of 24-hour fractional urine glucose determinations, see Pediatrics 53:257, 1974.)
14. Javanovic, L., and Peterson, C. The clinical utility of glycosylated hemoglobin. *Am. J. Med.* 70:331, 1981.
    A review of the studies to date; the value of the test is further confirmed in N. Engl. J. Med. 310:341, 1984.

Control: Monitoring and Management

15. Tamborlane, W., and Sherwin, R. Diabetes control and complications: New strategies and insights. *J. Pediatr.* 102:805, 1983.
Lucid, balanced view of information to date. (Also see Pediatrics *74:1079, 1984.)*

16. Brouhard, B. Control and monitoring for the child with insulin-dependent diabetes mellitus. *Am. J. Dis. Child.* 137:787, 1983.
An excellent, well-referenced review containing much practical information.

17. Langdon, D., James, F., and Sperling, M. Comparison of single- and split-dose insulin regimens with 24-hour monitoring. *J. Pediatr.* 99:854, 1981.
No advantage was consistently demonstrable for a two-dose regimen; similar results reported in Br. Med. J. *291:414, 1980.*

18. Gaffner, M., et al. Self-monitoring of blood glucose levels and intensified insulin therapy: Acceptability and efficacy in childhood diabetes. *JAMA* 249:2913, 1983.
It can be done.

19. Schiffrin, A., et al. Feasibility of strict diabetes control in insulin-dependent diabetic adolescents. *J. Pediatr.* 103:522, 1983.
Better control of blood glucose levels was achieved with continuous subcutaneous infusions than with frequent injections of insulin; in the same issue, an editorial (p. 573) by a psychologist and parent of a diabetic child suggests more subtle benefits of good control.

20. Wilson, D. Excessive insulin therapy: Biochemical effects and clinical repercussions. *Ann. Intern. Med.* 98:219, 1983.
A review of the subtle clinical manifestations, including the Somogyi phenomenon, and pathophysiologic bases of chronic hyperinsulinism. (For a review of the problems in identifying the Somogyi effect in children, see J. Pediatr. *84:672, 1974.)*

21. White, N., et al. Identification of type I diabetic patients at increased risk of hypoglycemia during intensive therapy. *N. Engl. J. Med.* 308:485, 1983.
Use of a brief intravenous infusion of insulin to identify those with inadequate counterregulatory hormone responses; a study of counterregulatory responses, reported in N. Engl. J. Med. *307:1106, 1982, was unable to distinguish those patients who are at higher risk of hypoglycemia.*

22. Schmitt, B. An argument for the unmeasured diet in juvenile diabetes mellitus. *Clin. Pediatr.* 14:68, 1975.
A review of various dietary regimens in use; recommends "unmeasured" diet (different from "free" diet). (For the classic demonstration that an "unmeasured" regimen is not harmful, see Diabetes *14:239, 1965.)*

Control: Results

23. Rudolf, M., et al. Effect of intensive insulin treatment on linear growth in the young diabetic patient. *J. Pediatr.* 101:333, 1982.
Normalization of blood glucose levels resulted in a near doubling of growth rate, confirming findings reported in N. Engl. J. Med. *305:303, 1981.*

24. White, N., et al. Reversal of neuropathic and gastrointestinal complications related to diabetes mellitus in adolescents with improved metabolic control. *J. Pediatr.* 99:41, 1981.
More evidence in support of "good control."

Insulin Delivery Research

25. Golden, M., et al. Use of a glucose-controlled insulin infusion system in children and adolescents with insulin-dependent diabetes. *Pediatrics* 70:36, 1982.
Short-term use of the system (requires hospitalization) is helpful in understanding the patient's unique insulin needs and in educating the patient and family about factors that influence blood glucose levels.

26. Rizza, R., et al. Control of blood sugar in insulin-dependent diabetes: Comparison of an artificial endocrine pancreas, continuous subcutaneous insulin infusion, and intensified conventional insulin therapy. *N. Engl. J. Med.* 303:1313, 1980.
Comparable "good" control with all three; the choice of treatment method should be tailored to the individual patient.

27. Metas, A., Sutherland, D., and Najarian, J. Current studies of islet and pancreatic transplantation in diabetes. *Diabetes* 25:785, 1976.

More recent research (in animals) is presented in Am. J. Med. *70:589, 1981.*

Psychologic Aspects

28. Greydanus, D., and Hofmann, A. Psychological factors in diabetes mellitus: A review of the literature with emphasis on adolescence. *Am. J. Dis. Child.* 133:1061, 1979.
    Balanced and well-referenced; also see Clin. Pediatr. (Phila.) *16:1151, 1977.*
29. Ahnsjö, S., et al. Personality changes and social adjustments during the first three years of diabetes in children. *Acta Paediatr. Scand.* 170:321, 1981.
    No significant differences between children with diabetes and a control group; the authors conclude that the medical regimen (considered to be one of "strict control") did not result in demonstrable psychologic abnormalities.
30. Johnson, S., et al. Cognitive and behavioral knowledge about insulin-dependent diabetes among children and parents. *Pediatrics* 69:708, 1982.
    Their knowledge is frighteningly poor. (Schoolteachers of children with IDDM also know little about the disease: Arch. Dis. Child. *58:692, 1983.)*

Prognosis

31. Lestradet, H. Long-term study of mortality and vascular complications in juvenile-onset (type I) diabetes. *Diabetes* 30:175, 1981.
    A statistical survey of a large number of patients with IDDM, all managed by the same protocol and followed for up to 26 years, at which time 85 percent had retinopathy. A 40-year follow-up of 73 patients, reported in Diabetes *24:559, 1975, shows a similar prevalence of retinopathy and a high rate of nephropathy. (For a review of recent advances in diabetic retinopathy, see* Am. J. Med. *70:595, 1981.)*
32. Rosenbloom, A., et al. Limited joint mobility in childhood diabetes mellitus indicates increased risk for microvascular disease. *N. Engl. J. Med.* 305:191, 1981.
    This finding may identify a group of patients who would more clearly benefit from tight control; further information on these patients is reported in J. Pediatr. *101:874, 1982.*

---

78. METABOLIC ERRORS
Robert D. White

Many congenital enzyme deficiencies that cause disability or death in children have been discovered. These enzyme defects are usually inherited in autosomal recessive fashion and are collectively described as the "inborn errors of metabolism." The number and rarity of these disorders prohibit individual discussion of each here; instead, they will be grouped as disorders of amino acid metabolism, disorders of carbohydrate metabolism, and lysosomal storage disorders.

The extraordinary complexity of protein metabolism is reflected in the many *inborn errors of amino acid synthesis and degradation* that have been described. These disorders produce increased blood and tissue levels of various amino acids and, in the case of urea cycle defects, of ammonia as well. The degree of deficiency of an enzyme and the toxicity of its accumulated substrate are major determinants of the time of onset, type, and severity of symptoms. Ammonia, for example, is highly toxic; therefore, urea cycle defects usually cause severe illness (with lethargy, vomiting, and metabolic acidosis) shortly after the initiation of feedings and are often fatal in the neonatal period. Accumulation of the branched-chain amino acids, caused by an enzyme deficiency in the degradation pathway of these substances, produces a disease (commonly known as maple syrup urine disease because of the characteristic odor of the urine) that has similar clinical features. Phenylketonuria (PKU) and many other aminoacidopathies, on the other hand, typically produce no symptoms in the neonatal period, but instead present with feeding difficulties, developmental delay, or hepatic disease later in infancy or childhood.

At present, PKU and maple syrup urine disease are detected in most neonatal screening programs, prior to the onset of their symptoms. Newborn screening for these disorders has been undertaken because (1) they are treatable, and (2) they are sufficiently common causes of serious morbidity (if untreated) to warrant the expense of a mandatory screening program. Diagnosis of the other inborn errors of amino acid metabolism demands a high clinical index of suspicion, since the early signs of disease, as noted earlier, are nonspecific; only occasionally are specific clues found, such as a peculiar body or urine odor, or a history of a previous sibling who died in infancy of an unexplained illness. Consequently, blood ammonia levels and blood and urine amino acid concentrations should be determined in any neonate with persistent, unexplained vomiting or metabolic acidosis, and in infants with unexplained feeding difficulties, failure to thrive, developmental delay, or hepatomegaly.

Treatment of an acutely ill neonate suspected of having an inborn error of amino acid metabolism frequently cannot await definitive diagnosis; all protein intake should be discontinued in such patients, and exchange transfusion or peritoneal dialysis should also be considered if acidosis or lethargy are life-threatening. Long-term control of symptoms can frequently be accomplished by a special diet.

Phenylketonuria is the most common and extensively studied of the aminoacidopathies. Classic PKU is caused by an absence of phenylalanine hydroxylase, the enzyme that converts phenylalanine to tyrosine. Phenylalanine accumulation is usually insidious in early infancy; signs, when they occur, include irritability, vomiting, an eczematoid rash, and a musty odor. Profound mental retardation usually becomes apparent later in infancy. Most affected children have blond hair and blue eyes (probably due to reduced synthesis of tyrosine and melanin), and some have cerebral palsy, seizures, or behavior problems. The defect is inherited as an autosomal recessive disorder; it occurs in 5 to 7 children per 100,000 live births in the United States; but is considerably more common in Ireland, Great Britain, Germany, and Poland and less common in Sweden and Finland.

Newborn screening tests are capable of detecting infants with even mild elevations of phenylalanine in the blood; of this group, however, only 5 percent prove to have PKU, while an additional 1 to 2 percent have a similar but somewhat milder metabolic disorder. The remainder are normal infants with transient, benign elevation of phenylalanine levels. The sensitivity of screening is somewhat dependent on the infant's age and protein intake at the time the sample is taken; 5 to 10 percent of patients with PKU will have normal phenylalanine levels if screening is done before 4 days of age. Retesting at the first well-baby visit is therefore recommended for all infants initially screened in the first 3 days of life.

The therapy of PKU entails strict adherence to a diet that contains only minimal amounts of phenylalanine; the most satisfactory results have been obtained when this is instituted before the infant is 3 to 4 weeks of age. Intellectual development is normal for most children treated in this manner. Unresolved questions include the safety of terminating the special diet after several years and the prognosis for infants born to women with diet-controlled PKU.

Disorders of carbohydrate metabolism include the glycogen storage diseases, galactosemia, and fructose intolerance. Seven glycogen storage diseases have been identified; each results from a specific enzyme deficiency in glycogen synthesis or breakdown. In some (types I, III, IV, and VI), carbohydrate intermediates accumulate in and damage primarily the liver, while the others affect skeletal muscle (types V and VII) or skeletal and cardiac muscle (type II) most prominently. This group of disorders should be considered in an infant or child with unexplained hepatomegaly, muscle weakness, or hypoglycemia.

Galactosemia results from a hereditary deficiency of galactose-1-phosphate uridyl transferase, which catalyzes the conversion of galactose-1-phosphate to glucose; its incidence is approximately 2 to 3 cases per 100,000 live births. In this disorder, galactose and galactose-1-phosphate accumulate in the lens, liver, brain, and kidney. Thus, shortly after birth, intake of lactose (a disaccharide composed of galactose and glucose) leads to a severe illness characterized by hepatomegaly, jaundice, irritability, vomiting, cataracts, and hypoglycemia. Rapid diagnosis is possible through demonstration of galactose in the urine (positive Clinitest, negative glucose oxidase test; also found in fructose intolerance), but the results of this test may be negative if vomiting has already prompted removal of lactose from the diet. A more specific diagnosis is possible by assay of the enzyme activity in the patient's red blood cells. Treatment consists of a galactose-free diet; this produces a dramatic resolution of symptoms and permits normal physical growth.

Hereditary fructose intolerance usually produces a severe neonatal illness that resembles galactosemia in most respects, except that cataracts and brain damage are not commonly found.

Lysosomal storage disease comprises over 25 disorders (encompassing the sphingolipidoses, mucolipidoses, and mucopolysaccharidoses). This group of disorders is even more heterogeneous than the previous two; the only common abnormality is deficiency of a lysosomal enzyme, which results in accumulation of the unmetabolized substrate within the lysosomes. Cellular damage eventually occurs, especially in organs in which metabolism of the substrate is normally high. Reticuloendothelial system involvement is most common, resulting in hepatomegaly; central nervous system damage is also frequent and characteristically produces progressive neurologic impairment after a period of normal development. Even within a single disease entity, however, the severity of symptoms often varies markedly from one patient to another. Diagnosis requires specialized laboratory tests, and in most cases specific therapy is not available.

Tay-Sachs disease (G_{M2} gangliosidosis) is the most common of the sphingolipidoses; it is caused by a deficiency of hexosaminidase A and results in accumulation of G_{M2} ganglioside within the gray matter of the brain. Affected infants are normal for 3 to 6 months, then begin to regress; muscular weakness progresses to paralysis, and blindness develops over the next 12 to 18 months. Death commonly occurs at 3 to 5 years of age, even with excellent supportive care.

Certain features of Tay-Sachs disease have made it a "preventable" disorder: (1) Heterozygotes (carriers) of the Tay-Sachs gene can be detected; (2) affected fetuses can be identified during early gestation. In addition, the "target population" is relatively small and well defined, since this disorder is much more common in Jewish persons of Ashkenazi (eastern European) descent than in the general population. These characteristics make it *possible* to prevent Tay-Sachs disease; prevention is also *desirable*, since this disorder is always fatal by early childhood. Consequently, a screening program has been undertaken in which adults of Jewish descent are screened (voluntarily) to determine whether or not they are carriers of the Tay-Sachs gene. If a couple in which both partners are heterozygous then decide to have a child, aminocentesis is performed in the second trimester of pregnancy to determine the activity of hexosaminidase A in fetal cells; the gestation of affected fetuses can be terminated by therapeutic abortion. This program has been well received and successful in reducing the incidence of Tay-Sachs disease and, as such, serves as a model program for prevention of some types of serious genetic disease.

General

1. Ampola, M. (ed.). Symposium on early detection and management of inborn errors. *Clin. Perinatol.* 3(1), 1976.
   Excellent articles reviewing the field. For a symposium on genetic disorders, see Pediatr. Clin. North Am. *25(3), 1978.*

2. Stanbury, J., et al. (eds.). *The Metabolic Basis of Inherited Disease* (5th ed.). New York: McGraw-Hill, 1983.
   Extensive reviews.

3. O'Brien, D., and Goodman, S. The critically ill child: Acute metabolic disease in infancy and early childhood. *Pediatrics* 46:620, 1970.
   A plan for the initial workup in an infant in whom an inborn error of metabolism is suspected. For a more recent review focusing on the sick neonate, see Pediatr. Clin. North Am. *25:431, 1978.*

4. Danks, D. Management of newborn babies in whom serious metabolic illness is anticipated. *Arch. Dis. Child.* 49:576, 1974.
   A plan of care for neonates when a previous sibling may have died from an inborn error of metabolism.

5. Burton, B., and Nadler, H. Clinical diagnosis of the inborn errors of metabolism in the neonatal period. *Pediatrics* 61:398, 1978.
   A practical approach based on the presenting symptom.

6. Mace, J., et al. The child with an unusual odor. *Clin. Pediatr.* (Phila.) 15:57, 1976.
   Most have inborn errors of metabolism, although ingestion of pine oil is a close second!

7. Morrow, G. Nutritional management of infants with inborn metabolic errors. *Clin. Perinatol.* 2:361, 1975.
Approach to management; specific therapy is considered only briefly.

Prenatal Screening

8. Milunsky, A. Prenatal diagnosis of genetic disorders. *N. Engl. J. Med.* 295:377, 1976.
A short review; a longer discussion appeared in volume 283 of the same journal (pp. 1370, 1441, 1498).
9. Holtzman, N. Genetic screening: For better or for worse? *Pediatrics* 59:131, 1977.
Ethical considerations. For a similar discussion by a multidisciplinary group, see N. Engl. J. Med. *286:1129, 1972.*
10. Massachusetts Department of Public Health. Cost-benefit analysis of newborn screening for metabolic disorders *N. Engl. J. Med.* 291:1414, 1974.
Impressive savings in terms of dollars and morbidity are documented from screening programs.
11. Simpson, L. (ed.). Antenatal diagnosis of genetic disorders. *Clin. Obstet. Gynecol.* 24:1005, 1981.
Several articles on various facets, including legal and ethical considerations.

Disorders of Amino Acid Metabolism

12. Scriver, C., and Rosenberg, L. *Amino Acid Metabolism and Its Disorders.* Philadelphia: Saunders, 1973.
A thorough review of specific disorders. A similar compendium appears in Clin. Endocrinol. Metab. *3(1), 1974.*
13. Hsia, Y. Inherited hyperammonemic syndromes. *Gastroenterology* 67:347, 1974.
A long review, with 172 references.
14. Frimpter, G. Aminoacidurias due to inherited disorders of metabolism. *N. Engl. J. Med.* 289:835, 895, 1973.
Briefly surveys several disorders characterized by aminoaciduria.
15. Holliday, M., et al. Special diets for infants with inborn errors of amino acid metabolism. *Pediatrics* 57:783, 1976.
The products available for the management of PKU and certain other aminoacidopathies are discussed. (For management of some urea cycle defects, see Pediatrics *68:290, 1981.)*
16. Scriver, C., et al. Screening for congenital metabolic disorders in the newborn infant: Congenital deficiency of thyroid hormone and hyperphenylalaninemia. *Pediatrics* 60:389, 1977.
Guidelines, ethical considerations, and unresolved problems. (For an update of unresolved problems, see Pediatrics *69:104, 1982.)*
17. Holtzman, N., Welcher, D., and Mellits, E. Termination of restricted diet in children with phenylketonuria: A randomized controlled study. *N. Engl. J. Med.* 293:1121, 1975.
The results of this small trial suggest that a special diet is unnecessary after early childhood. (Also see J. Pediatr. *94:534, 1979.)*
18. Naylor, E., and Guthrie, R. Newborn screening for maple syrup urine disease (branched-chain ketoaciduria). *Pediatrics* 61:262, 1978.
Reviews current experience with screening and management.
19. Donn, S., and Banagale, R. Neonatal hyperammonemia. *Pediatr. Rev.* 5:203, 1984.
Provides another chance to learn the urea cycle, this time with some meaningful clinical correlation. (Also see Pediatrics *68:271, 1981.)*

Disorders of Carbohydrate Metabolism

20. Cornblath, M., and Schwartz, R. *Disorders of Carbohydrate Metabolism in Infancy* (2nd ed.). Philadelphia: Saunders, 1976.
An extensive review of each disorder.
21. Moses, S., and Gutman, A. Inborn errors of glycogen metabolism. *Adv. Pediatr.* 19:95, 1972.
Easy reading, despite the complexity of the diseases under discussion.
22. Levy, H., and Hammersen, G. Newborn screening for galactosemia and other galactose metabolic defects. *J. Pediatr.* 92:871, 1978.

Most infants detected by screening were not suspected on clinical grounds to have galactosemia.

Lysosomal Storage Diseases

23. Kolodny, E. Lysosomal storage diseases. *N. Engl. J. Med.* 294:1217, 1976.
    A brief overview.
24. McKusick, V., et al. The genetic mucopolysaccharidoses. *Medicine* (Baltimore) 44:445, 1965.
    A scholarly review that suffers little from its age.
25. Legum, C., Schorr, S., and Berman, E. The genetic mucopolysaccharidoses and mucolipidoses: Review and comment. *Adv. Pediatr.* 22:305, 1975.
    A good introductory discussion of these disorders.
26. Malone, M. The cerebral lipidoses. *Pediatr. Clin. North Am.* 23:303, 1976.
    Treatment is limited, but diagnosis is important in terms of preventing the birth of affected siblings.
27. Kaback, M., and O'Brien, J. Tay-Sachs: Prototype for prevention of genetic disease. *Hosp. Pract.* 8(3):107, 1973.
    The historical and ethical aspects of Tay-Sachs research and screening are discussed.

79. MALFORMATION SYNDROMES

Robert D. White

There are literally thousands of syndromes of human malformation. Most are extremely rare; the practicing pediatrician may encounter only 10 or 20 in a lifetime. Identification of congenital syndromes is clinically important for several reasons. Some defects are incompatible with life, while others produce lifelong illness or disability. Many syndromes are associated with mental retardation, often severe or profound. In addition, nearly all malformations impose a psychologic burden on both child and parents. Management of such diverse problems must obviously be highly individualized, but in every case, a pediatrician or family practitioner should accept the responsibility for providing general medical care and for coordinating contact with specialists. Parents also need a clear description of their child's syndrome and its implications, with counseling and support provided over months or years. Probably the families most neglected in this respect are those whose child dies shortly after birth.

Congenital malformations are the leading cause of neonatal death in full-term infants. Some are caused by an excess or deficiency of chromosomal material. Others are single-gene defects that may be located on the autosomes or the sex chromosomes and may be dominant, recessive, or with variable penetrance. Still others are described as multifactorial, which means that a complex interplay of multiple gene defects, or environmental factors, or both is believed responsible for the pattern of malformations. Finally, there is a large group of malformations caused by teratogens. Thalidomide is probably the most (in)famous of these, and alcohol and hydantoins the most common (of those currently identified). Many more teratogens have been implicated in fetal malformations, including: other drugs taken by the mother, such as warfarin, aminopterin, and aspirin; irradiation; infection (e.g., rubella); and maternal disease (diabetes mellitus). The precise mechanisms by which these environmental or genetic factors cause malformations are still poorly understood. Some may inhibit DNA synthesis (rubella, aminopterin), while others may alter the chemical and hormonal milieu during a critical period of morphogenesis, but these are still largely unproved hypotheses.

Identification of a syndrome of malformations in a specific child begins with delineation of all detectable anomalies. This entails a thorough physical examination, even when several anomalies are immediately apparent. Life-threatening malformations of the heart, urinary tract, and gastrointestinal system are not always obvious, and extremely useful clues may be obtained from findings as subtle as nipple spacing, ear structure, or dermatoglyphics. Many important syndromes, in fact, consist entirely of abnormalities subtle enough to have been overlooked on multiple examinations. A carefully taken history is also imperative, with the family pedigree and information on maternal exposure to drugs, irradiation, or infection of paramount importance. Based on the data obtained from the history and physical examination, identification of the patient's syndrome is usually possible, using one or more of the several reference books available for this purpose. It must be remembered that many malformation complexes have not yet been formally described, and that it is rare for an individual patient to display all the classic features of a particular syndrome. Laboratory tests and radiography may be extremely useful as confirmatory evidence when a tentative diagnosis has been made and are occasionally helpful when the patient's malformation complex does not appear to "fit" a known syndrome. Chromosomal analysis is indicated when several major malformations are present; other tests of occasional value include tissue biopsy and viral titers.

Down syndrome is one of the common syndromes with which pediatricians must be familiar; its overall incidence is 1 per 625 live births. Down syndrome is characterized by a constellation of dysmorphic features and mental retardation and is due to an excess of chromosomal material. Affected patients usually have three number 21 chromosomes instead of the usual two; all somatic cells therefore contain 47 chromosomes. Maternal age appears to be an important factor in the incidence of this syndrome; the disorder is uncommon (1 in 1500 live births) in neonates of 15- to 30-year-old women but the incidence increases with very low or high maternal age, reaching 1 in 50 live births when conception occurs beyond the age of 45 years. It is believed that trisomy results from nondisjunction of the number 21 chromosome during meiosis.

A small proportion (3–4%) of children with the classic features of Down syndrome have 46 chromosomes. Although the chromosome number is normal, an excess of genetic material still exists; special staining ("banding") of the chromosomes demonstrates that a third 21 chromosome is translocated, attached centromere to centromere to another chromosome, usually number 15 or 22. Translocation of chromosome 21 may also be present in one of the child's parents (who has a normal amount of genetic material but only 45 chromosomes, since two normal chromosomes have fused into one). In this instance, 50 percent of this parent's gametes will contain the translocation chromosome and a normal chromosome 21; when the abnormal gamete combines with a normal gamete, the resulting conceptus will have Down syndrome. Maternal age obviously has little bearing on the incidence of this variant.

A second variant of classic Down syndrome is the mosaic form. In these children, only certain cells contain the extra chromosome, perhaps because nondisjunction does not occur until after cellular division begins in the embryo. The clinical spectrum is extremely variable, depending on the number and location of defective cells; some patients may even have a normal appearance and normal intelligence.

Clinical diagnosis of Down syndrome relies on the recognition of a typical constellation of physical signs. No single anomaly is present in every case, but the appearance of children with Down syndrome is nevertheless remarkably constant. They have a flat facial profile, somewhat primitive ear structure, blunting of the inner eye angle or frank epicanthal folds, muscular hypotonia with joint laxity, and simian creases. A typical radiographic finding in infants with Down syndrome is flaring of the iliac wings. Some "characteristic" features, such as a rounded head, upward-slanting palpebral fissures, Brushfield spots on the iris, protruding tongue, and stubby hands and fingers are not always readily apparent in newborns. Other components of this syndrome are present in only a minority of patients, but because of their importance should be sought in every child believed to have Down syndrome; these include congenital heart defects in 40 percent (principally, septal defects), intestinal stenosis or atresia, and leukemia or leukemoid reactions.

Developmental delay is usually apparent by 6 to 10 months of age; IQs are between 40 and 60 in most children and are above this level in only rare cases, many of which are in children with mosaicism. Preliminary reports suggest that early, intensive "schooling" may improve the outlook to some degree.

Definitive diagnosis is accomplished by chromosomal analysis. Chromosomal analysis should also be performed in the parents, since one may be a mosaic or a translocation carrier.

The management of a child with Down syndrome begins with support and counseling of the parents by discussing the cause, manifestations, and prognosis and answering their questions. Parents may suppress the expression of grief and guilt during early interviews, especially if the physician is unfamiliar to them; the impact of the diagnosis must be recognized and counseling done patiently, usually with considerable repetition. Formal genetic counseling should be deferred, at least until chromosomal analysis is complete. Parents of children with Down syndrome have formed groups in many areas to provide a valuable source of continuing support.

Books

1. Smith, D. *Recognizable Patterns of Human Malformation* (3rd ed.). Philadelphia: Saunders, 1982.
   The single most useful reference, with an especially helpful section that lists syndromes associated with any given malformation.
2. Smith, D. *Recognizable Patterns of Human Deformation*. Philadelphia: Saunders, 1981.
   Those disorders that are due to physical limitation in utero.
3. McKusick, V. *Mendelian Inheritance in Man: Catalogue of Autosomal Dominant, Autosomal Recessive, and X-Linked Phenotypes* (6th ed.). Baltimore: Johns Hopkins University Press, 1983.
   This massive compendium includes every syndrome transmitted in mendelian (single-gene) fashion known at the time of publication.
4. Shepard, T. *Catalog of Teratogenic Agents* (4th ed.). Baltimore: Johns Hopkins University Press, 1983.
   Could a drug taken during pregnancy be responsible for a malformation? This is the place to start.
5. Warkany, J. *Congenital Malformations*. Chicago: Year Book, 1971.
   Many syndromes not included in reference 1 are discussed.

General

6. Smith, D. An approach to clinical dysmorphology. *J. Pediatr.* 91:690, 1977.
   An introduction to the study of syndromes. Discussed in greater depth in an earlier article by the same author (J. Pediatr. 69:1150, 1966).
7. Kalter, H., and Warkany, J. Congenital malformations. *N. Engl. J. Med.* 308:424, 491, 1983.
   Complements a previous review in the same journal, 295:204, 1976.
8. Kaback, M. (ed.). Symposium on medical genetics. *Pediatr. Clin. North Am.* 25(3), 1978.
   Includes several articles on malformation syndromes (craniofacial, neural tube, connective tissue, and skeletal).
9. Warkany, J. Prevention of congenital malformations. *Curr. Probl. Pediatr.* 13(7), 1983.
   Until recently, a monograph on this subject would not have been possible, but the same civilization that has found preventive measures has also discovered that many malformations are caused by its own creations: drugs, environmental toxins, and irradiation.
10. Jones, K. (ed.). The developmental pathogenesis of structural defects. *Semin. Perinatol* 7:237, 1983.
    The issue is devoted to known embryologic alterations and their sequelae
11. Feingold, M., and Bossert, W. Normal values for selected physical parameters: An aid to syndrome delineation. *Birth Defects* 10(13), 1974.
    Are the ears really low set? Is there hypertelorism? This monograph tells how to measure and provides normal values. Available from National Foundation—March of Dimes.
12. Juberg, R. . . . but the family history was negative. *J. Pediatr.* 91:693, 1977.
    Outlines several reasons why a patient with a genetically determined disorder might present with a negative family history.
13. Drotar, D., et al. The adaptation of parents to the birth of an infant with a congenital malformation: A hypothetical model. *Pediatrics* 56:710, 1975.

Parental reaction to the birth of a malformed child proceeds through predictable stages. Constructive intervention is based on the parents' needs during each stage.

14. Wilson, M. Genetic counseling. *Curr. Probl. Pediatr.* 5(7), 1975.
    Includes recurrence risks for many syndromes and recommended guidelines for counseling. For an update on recurrence rates, see Pediatr. Rev. *6:141, 1984.*

Down Syndrome

15. Rex, A., and Preus, M. A diagnostic index for Down syndrome. *J. Pediatr.* 100:903, 1982.
    High confidence level using phenotypic findings.
16. Gayton, W., and Walker, L. Down syndrome: Informing the parents. *Am. J. Dis. Child.* 127:510, 1974.
    Parents want to be told early, while they are together, and they want continued support.
17. Smith, D., and Wilson, A. *The Child with Down's Syndrome.* Philadelphia: Saunders, 1973.
    Ideal for parents and good reading for physicians as well. Covers the scientific background and questions parents ask.
18. Aronson, M., and Fallstrom, K. Immediate and long-term effects of developmental training in children with Down's syndrome. *Dev. Med. Child Neurol.* 19:489, 1977.
    Intensive preschool training for 18 months yielded impressive gains, but the difference between experimental and control groups had largely disappeared 12 months later.

Other Syndromes Related to Excess or Deficiency of Chromosomal Material

19. Gerald, P. Sex chromosome disorders. *N. Engl. J. Med.* 294:706, 1976.
    A brief summary of Klinefelter (XXY), Turner (XO), and other syndromes characterized by abnormal numbers of sex chromosomes.
20. Taylor, A. Patau's, Edwards' and cri du chat syndromes: A tabulated summary of current findings. *Dev. Med. Child Neurol.* 9:78, 1967.
    A review of the literature on these syndromes, also known as trisomy 13, trisomy 18, and deletion of the short arm of 5, respectively.

Syndromes Related to Maternal Drug Intake During Pregnancy

21. Clarren, S., and Smith, D. The fetal alcohol syndrome. *N. Engl. J. Med.* 298:1063, 1978.
    Perhaps the most common teratogenic cause of mental deficiency.
22. Hanson, J., et al. Risks to the offspring of women treated with hydantoin anticonvulsants, with emphasis on the fetal hydantoin syndrome. *J. Pediatr.* 89:662, 1976.
    Of infants exposed to hydantoins in utero, the characteristic syndrome of malformations and growth and developmental delay develop in 10 percent; another 30 percent have features that are suggestive but not diagnostic.
23. Smith, D. Fetal drug syndromes: Effects of ethanol and hydantoins. *Pediatr. Rev.* 1:165, 1979.
    By the individual who did most to elucidate these conditions.

Other Common Syndromes

24. Nora, J., et al. The Ulrich-Noonan syndrome (Turner phenotype). *Am. J. Dis. Child.* 127:48, 1974.
    Usually known as Noonan syndrome or male Turner syndrome.
25. Jones, K., and Smith, D. The Williams elfin facies syndrome. *J. Pediatr.* 86:718, 1975.
    Hypercalcemia and supravalvar aortic stenosis were originally considered inherent features of this syndrome, but they are actually uncommon, and the characteristic facies is consistent.
26. Ptacek, L., et al. The Cornelia de Lange syndrome. *J. Pediatr.* 63:1000, 1963.
    A survey; again, facial features are the most useful diagnostic clue.

27. Hall, B., and Smith, D. Prader-Willi syndrome. *J. Pediatr.* 81:286, 1972.
    Classic diagnostic tetrad consists of hypotonia, obesity, mental retardation, and hypogonadism.
28. Townes, P. Fragile-X syndrome. *Am. J. Dis. Child.* 136:389, 1982.
    A common genetic cause of mental retardation, perhaps second in frequency only to Down syndrome.

IX. NEUROMUSCULAR DISORDERS

80. SEIZURE DISORDERS

William R. Leahy, Jr., and Kenneth B. Roberts

A seizure is an "abnormal, sudden, excessive electrical discharge of neurons (gray matter) which propagates down the neuronal processes (white matter) to affect an end organ in a clinically measurable fashion." Such events may be subtle or dramatic and affect 5 percent of children at one time or another during childhood. Most children who experience a seizure do not have epilepsy, however; the term should be reserved for the disorder affecting only 0.5 to 1.0 percent of children, in which seizures are recurrent, paroxysmal, and unprovoked by metabolic derangements such as hypoglycemia.

The most frequent precipitant to seizures in children who do not have epilepsy is fever, and approximately 3 percent of children between the ages of 3 months and 5 years have a "febrile seizure," unassociated with CNS infection or other explainable cause. The event usually occurs early in a febrile illness, during the initial rapid rise in body temperature. The child loses consciousness and has generalized tonic-clonic movements; although the convulsion is frightening to behold and appears to the parents to last a long time, the duration is characteristically on the order of several minutes.

Of children who have one febrile seizure and do not receive prophylactic anticonvulsant therapy, approximately 30 to 40 percent have another; the recurrence does not constitute epilepsy. Risk factors for developing epilepsy include a family history of epilepsy; evidence of neurologic damage or impaired development prior to the febrile seizure; and an "atypical" febrile seizure, such as one that is focal or prolonged beyond 20 to 30 minutes. If none of the risk factors is present, the risk of subsequent epilepsy is 2 to 3 percent; if two or three factors are present, the risk is 13 percent.

Daily therapy with phenobarbital or valproic acid (Depakene) is effective in preventing recurrences, but routine use of these drugs is discouraged by many authors because of the toxicity and side effects that occur in a large number of treated children; moreover, there is no evidence that prophylactic therapy has an effect on the ultimate prognosis.

Nonfebrile seizures are classified into different types on the basis of clinical manifestations and the electroencephalogram (EEG). Knowledge of the various types is important (1) when eliciting a history to determine that an episode was in fact a seizure, (2) when selecting therapy, and (3) when counseling about the prognosis.

The International League Against Epilepsy has proposed classifying seizures into two main groups depending on how much of the brain is affected at the onset of the seizure: partial seizures begin in a localized focus; generalized seizures involve both hemispheres simultaneously. (For completeness, there is a third group: "unclassified.") Partial seizures are further subdivided into three types: simple partial, in which consciousness is preserved; complex partial, in which consciousness is impaired (formerly called psychomotor or temporal lobe); and partial seizures, which spread to become generalized. Generalized seizures are subdivided into six types: absence (formerly petit mal), tonic-clonic (formerly grand mal), tonic or clonic, myoclonic, atonic, and infantile spasms.

In simple partial seizures, the symptoms produced depend on the area of the brain affected and may be motor, sensory, autonomic, or psychic. Anticonvulsants used include phenobarbital, phenytoin (Dilantin), carbamazepine (Tegretol), and primidone (Mysoline).

Complex partial seizures consist of altered behavior for which the patient is amnesic but during which some interaction with the environment may occur. Manifestations fall into three categories: subjective experiences, automatisms, and postural changes. An aura may usher in the more intense portion of the seizure, during which semipurposeful movements occur. The pattern lasts from several minutes to hours and is followed by postictal depression. Carbamazepine, primidone, phenobarbital, and valproic acid are among the anticonvulsants prescribed to treat this disorder.

Absence seizures are episodes of momentary loss of awareness during which no motor activity other than rolling or blinking of the eyes is noted. The attacks are brief, 5 to 10 seconds in duration, appearing without an aura and with no postictal depression; there may be many attacks per day, sufficient to impair school performance. The child may be accused of "daydreaming" and misbehaving, creating additional pressure for the affected child. The EEG is characteristic, with a spike-wave discharge at a rate of 3 per second. It is thought that such activity originates from the diencephalon or thalamic areas.

Pure absence seizures appear limited to school-age children and adolescents, are amenable to treatment with ethosuximide (Zarontin) and other anticonvulsants, and have an excellent prognosis. Other seizure types may be associated with absence, however.

Tonic-clonic seizures are characterized by stiffness followed by rhythmic shaking of the trunk and extremities. Consciousness is lost, and incontinence is frequent. The convulsive stage is followed by postictal drowsiness and, often, by confusion. Focal neurologic findings, such as weakness (Todd paralysis), if present, are transient.

The anticonvulsants most commonly used for tonic-clonic seizures include phenobarbital, phenytoin, carbamazepine, and valproate.

Mixed convulsions consist of a combination of any of the preceding disorders. These often require the administration of several anticonvulsants simultaneously for control. It is generally preferred to "push" a single drug to efficacy or to toxicity before changing medication or adding a second, however.

Three convulsive disorders, which are less common but distinctive, deserve special attention because of the difficult management and poor prognosis: myoclonic, infantile spasms, and atonic seizures.

Myoclonic convulsions are characterized by a single contraction or repetitive contractions of a single muscle or group of muscles. These seizures are often associated with degenerative, infectious, and progressive diseases of the central nervous system, such as subacute sclerosing panencephalitis (SSPE), and with metabolic disorders, such as uremia and hepatic failure.

Infantile spasms consist of a sudden flexion or extension of the body resembling an exaggerated Moro reflex. These often occur in clusters, affect infants between 3 and 9 months of age, and are associated with an EEG pattern described as hypsarrhythmia.

Although primarily idiopathic, infantile spasms may be symptomatic of an underlying disorder, such as tuberous sclerosis, neurofibromatosis, phenylketonuria, or congenital malformations of the central nervous system. In 90 percent the prognosis for intellectual development is poor. By age 3 the spasms are often replaced by atonic or tonic-clonic seizures.

To control myoclonic attacks and infantile spasms, ACTH or corticosteroids are usually given. The benzodiazepines—diazepam and clonazepam—and valproic acid have also been tried, but the seizures are usually exceedingly refractory to medication.

Atonic spells are sudden momentary loss of posture and tone without aura or postictal depression. These spells, often multiple during the day, occur in children 1 to 7 years old and are often associated with brain damage.

A child who has a seizure deserves a thorough initial evaluation in an attempt to define an underlying cause. A clear description of the ictal event is important. In addition, a detailed account of any acute illness, the child's past medical history, development, and family history should be elicited. The general examination should be thorough, with particular attention to the possibility of acute (e.g., meningitis) or chronic (e.g., tuberous sclerosis) disease and to the neurologic examination. An EEG may assist in better defining the abnormality. Supplementary investigation may include determination of blood sugar, calcium, and electrolytes. More extensive studies (e.g., lumbar puncture, brain scan, computerized axial tomography, angiography) are indicated when the initial evaluation suggests the presence of CNS infection or a mass lesion.

In 70 to 80 percent of children with epilepsy, anticonvulsant medication is effective in controlling seizures. Each anticonvulsant has associated toxicity and side effects, however, such as behavioral difficulties with phenobarbital, hypertrichosis and gingival hyperplasia with phenytoin, and hepatotoxicity with valproic acid. Recent series have demonstrated that most children with epilepsy who, with medication, are seizure-free for 4 years, can successfully have their medication tapered and stopped. If seizures recur, they are most likely in the first year after cessation of therapy. The group at highest risk of recurrence includes those with numerous seizures prior to control and those whose EEG is abnormal prior to termination of anticonvulsant treatment.

Convulsive disorders often have a devastating emotional impact on the child and the family; the emotional "morbidity" may far outweigh the physical danger. Thus, a comprehensive approach must be taken by the clinician caring for the child with a seizure disorder: Support and guidance may be needed in many matters of life-style, such as participation in sports, driving an automobile, and choosing a career. The ultimate goal of management is to minimize disability and maximize developmental potential.

Reviews
1. Delgado-Escueta, A., Treiman, D., and Walsh, G. The treatable epilepsies. *N. Engl. J. Med.* 308:1508, 1576, 1983.
   A recent and comprehensive review of the various forms of epilepsy, including clinical description and therapy.
2. Engel, J., et al. Recent developments in the diagnosis and therapy of epilepsy. *Ann. Intern. Med.* 97:584, 1982.
   A UCLA interdepartmental conference on epilepsy, with emphasis on recent developments in diagnosis and therapy plus a brief discussion of surgery and EEG-biofeedback training.
3. Oppenheimer, E., and Rosman, N. Seizures in childhood: An approach to emergency management. *Pediatr. Clin. North Am.* 26:837, 1979.
   A practical approach to status epilepticus, recurrent seizures, and nonepileptic disorders with recommendations for evaluation and therapy.

Laboratory Evaluation
4. Lewis, D., and Freeman, J. The electroencephalogram in pediatric practice: Its use and abuse. *Pediatrics* 60:324, 1977.
   Electroencephalography is explained.
5. Berman, W., and Johnson, B. The questionable value of routine skull radiography in clinical evaluation of children with recurrent convulsions. *J. Pediatr.* 90:598, 1977.
   A report of 130 cases; skull films provided relevant information in very few.
6. Yang, P., et al. Computed tomography and childhood seizure disorders. *Neurology* 29:1084, 1979.
   Of 256 children, 33 percent had abnormal CT scans; of those whose physical examination and EEG were normal, however, only 5 percent had abnormal scans, and only 2.7 percent of scans were of therapeutic import.

Febrile Seizures
7. NIH Consensus Development Conference on Febrile Seizures. Febrile seizures: Long-term management of children with fever-associated seizures. *Pediatrics* 66:1009, 1980.
   The state of the art regarding evaluation, treatment, and prognosis of febrile seizures. (For further discussion of the controversy regarding treatment, see J. Pediatr. 94:177, 1979, Neurology 29:287, 1979, and Arch. Dis. Child. 56:81, 1981.)
8. Nelson, K., and Ellenberg, J. Predictors of epilepsy in children who have experienced febrile seizures. *N. Engl. J. Med.* 295:1029, 1976.
   Data from the NIH Collaborative Perinatal Project: Risk factors identified include prior neurologic or developmental abnormalities and prolonged seizure. Similar findings from the Mayo Clinic: Neurology 29:297, 1979. (Lack of relationship to complex partial seizures: Am. J. Dis. Child. 137:123, 1983.)
9. Ellenberg, J., and Nelson, K. Febrile convulsions and later intellectual performance. *Arch. Neurol.* 35:17, 1978.
   Additional data from the NIH study; no decrement in IQ or academic performance noted at age 7 in children with a history of febrile seizures compared to siblings.

Partial Seizures
10. Freeman, J., and Vining, E. Focal epileptic seizures. *Pediatr. Rev.* 1:141, 1979.
    A description of various types and an approach to evaluation and treatment. (For another concise review, see N. Engl. J. Med. 309:536, 1983.)
11. Falconer, M., et al. Etiology and pathogenesis of temporal lobe epilepsy. *Arch. Neurol.* 10:233, 1964.
    Classic clinical-pathologic correlations.
12. Aird, R., and Crawther, D. Temporal lobe epilepsy in childhood: Clinical expressions observed in 125 affected children. *Clin. Pediatr.* (Phila.) 9:409, 1970.
    The strength of this review is the number of patients.

Absence Seizures

13. Holowach, J., et al. Petit mal epilepsy. *Pediatrics* 30:893, 1962.
    The clinical course in 88 children is reviewed.
14. Holmes, G. Therapy of petit mal (absence) seizures. *Pediatr. Rev.* 4:150, 1982.
    An excellent, recent review of classification, characteristics, and therapy.
15. Charlton, M., and Yahr, M. Long-term follow-up of patients with petit mal. *Arch. Neurol.* 16:595, 1967.
    Tonic-clonic seizures developed in the majority of 275 patients before age 16.

Infantile Spasms

16. Gibbs, E., et al. Diagnosis and prognosis of hypsarrhythmia and infantile spasms. *Pediatrics* 13:66, 1954.
    A review of 237 cases; seizures decreased with age (50% had no seizures after age 3). (Value of neuroradiology: J. Pediatr. *100:47, 1982.)*
17. Jeavons, P., et al. Long-term prognosis in infantile spasms: A follow-up report of 112 cases. *Dev. Med. Child Neurol.* 12:413, 1970.
    Good prognosis depends on cause rather than on therapy.
18. Singer, W., et al. The effect of ACTH therapy upon infantile spasms. *J. Pediatr.* 96:485, 1980.
    Suggests that early treatment improves prognosis. (ACTH versus prednisone: J. Pediatr. *103:641, 1983, and* Neurology *33:966, 1983.)*

Management

19. Hauser, W., et al. Seizure recurrence after a first unprovoked seizure. *N. Engl. J. Med.* 307:522, 1982.
    Data to consider when deciding whom to treat: overall, 27 percent of those with a first seizure had a recurrence; in those with a history of prior neurologic "insult," the rate was 34 percent, whereas without such a history the rate was 17 percent.
20. Woodbury, D., et al. *Anti-Epileptic Drugs.* New York: Raven, 1982.
    The most comprehensive text on anticonvulsant drugs. For a brief "bottom line" review, see Med. Lett. Drugs Ther. *25:81, 1983; intermediate length:* Pediatr. Clin. North Am. *28:179, 1981, and 23:443, 1976.*
21. Dodson, W., et al. Management of seizure disorders: Selected aspects. *J. Pediatr.* 89:527, 695, 1976.
    A two-part review, including the pharmacology of anticonvulsants, use of the ketogenic diet, and surgical treatment.
22. Emerson, R., et al. Stopping medications in children with epilepsy: Predictors of outcome. *N. Engl. J. Med.* 304:1125, 1981.
    After 4 seizure-free years of therapy, treatment was stopped without further seizures in most children; risk factors for recurrence identified. (Also see N. Engl. J. Med. *306:831, 861, 1982.)*
23. Camfield, C., et al. Side-effects of phenobarbital in toddlers: Behavioral and cognitive aspects. *J. Pediatr.* 95:361, 1979.
    Patients given phenobarbital prophylaxis for febrile seizures compared with untreated patients; no IQ differences but phenobarbital appeared to affect memory and comprehension and to produce behavior changes.
24. American Academy of Pediatrics Committee on Drugs. Anticonvulsants in pregnancy. *Pediatrics* 63:331, 1979.
    The teratogenic effects and potentials of anticonvulsants are discussed.
25. Hodgman, C., et al. Emotional complications of adolescent grand mal epilepsy. *J. Pediatr.* 95:309, 1979.
    An important consideration in management.

81. SPINAL DYSRAPHISM

William R. Leahy, Jr.

Incomplete closure of the neural tube during the fourth week of embryonic life gives rise to spina bifida, an anomaly that may be mild or severe, depending on the extent of the neural elements involved.

Spina bifida occulta, or failure of closure of the posterior vertebral arch, is a mild malformation present in about 10 percent of children, usually in the lumbar area. Often, there is a hairy dimple or dermal sinus in the skin of the lower back, or a conspicuous mass due to an underlying lipoma or teratoma. Urinary incontinence and a mild gait disturbance may evolve as the child grows older. Computerized tomography of the spine with metrizamide instilled in the CSF, is an excellent method of defining the extent of the lesion.

Spina bifida cystica is a term encompassing two types of disorders. The meningocele is a cystic lesion on the back in which the meninges protrude through a bony defect. The spinal cord and rootlets remain uncompromised, so that neither motor or sensory deficits in the legs nor incontinence is noted, and prognosis for full neurologic function is excellent. Meningomyelocele is a more devastating lesion. This disorder occurs primarily in the lumbar or lumbosacral area as a cystic distention of both the meninges and the spinal cord or nerve rootlets through the abnormal opening of the spinal arch. The incidence of this disorder varies from a low of 0.2 per 1000 births in Japan to 4.2 per 1000 births in Ireland.

Impairment directly related to the meningomyelocele includes paralysis and incontinence; in addition, hydrocephalus due to the Arnold-Chiari malformation is usually present (see Chap. 82). Medical and surgical treatment includes the following: providing continued emotional support and counseling; closing the spinal defect early (to both prevent meningitis and limit neurologic deterioration); treating meningitis, if already present; establishing and maintaining a well-functioning, noninfected "shunt" for hydrocephalus; developing a socially acceptable regimen for bowel incontinence; controlling urinary incontinence (with particular attention to infection and deterioration in the renal function); utilizing bracing, physical therapy, and/or orthopedic procedures (to achieve the maximal level of functional ambulation possible and to ameliorate deformities). Since the efforts of many disciplines are required, regional "teams" have been developed to deal with this problem; there remains the need for a generalist to coordinate the activities of the specialists and to ensure communication with the family. With a full-scale effort, the majority of children with meningomyelocele will survive with IQs in the normal range.

Many children, however, despite vigorous care and multiple operative procedures, do not achieve a desirable "quality of life"; such outcomes have prompted consideration of "selective treatment." It has been proposed that children not be treated if they have one or more of the following: gross paralysis of the legs; high lesions; kyphosis or scoliosis; grossly enlarged head at birth; intracerebral birth injury; or other major congenital defects, such as Down syndrome or cardiac malformations. Some groups have attempted to predict which children will have limited intelligence, using an estimate of brain mass or cerebral mantle thickness. Without treatment, death usually occurs in the first 2 years of life from meningitis or progressive hydrocephalus; chronic renal failure is a later cause of death. Of untreated infants, 20 percent survive, however, and a "wait-and-see" position is difficult to endorse, since delayed treatment is not as effective in preserving function as early, vigorous therapy. In this country, there have been no generally accepted criteria for "selection," and the subject itself remains controversial.

Whether or not selective treatment is considered, the initial examination is of great importance in assessing the level of disability. In general, the more neural elements that are involved, and the higher the lesion, the greater the neurologic deficit. A determination should be made regarding the spinal cord level of motor and sensory deficits; the posture of the lower limbs and the nature of the deformity result from muscle imbalance and suggest the level of cord functioning. Attention should also be directed toward signs of hydrocephalus or cranial nerve lesions. Frequent, small-volume dribbling of urine and constant leakage of meconium from a patulous anus are indicators of future problems with continence.

Despite the major advances in the neurosurgical, orthopedic, and urologic management of children with meningomyelocele, treatment remains frustrating and inadequate; clearly, prevention is more desirable. Families with one affected child have a 5 percent chance of a subsequent child having a neural tube defect, and it now appears possible to detect open neural tube defects during the second trimester of pregnancy by measuring alpha fetoprotein in amniotic fluid; elevations may also be present in maternal serum.

Meningomyelocele Reviews

1. Shurtleff, D. Myelodysplasia: Management and treatment. *Curr. Prob. Pediatr.* 10(3), 1980.
   A 98-page, comprehensive review of all aspects (153 references).
2. Golden, G. Neural tube defects. *Pediatr. Rev.* 1:187, 1979.
   A brief overview of multiple aspects, with added discussion in subsequent volume: 2:58, 1980.
3. Fishman, M. Recent clinical advances in the treatment of dysraphic states. *Pediatr. Clin. North Am.* 23:517, 1976.
   The clinical aspects are stressed.

Series

4. Laurence, K. The natural history of spina bifida cystica. *Arch. Dis. Child.* 39:41, 1964.
   Infection is the most common immediate cause of death, followed in frequency by progressive hydrocephalus (407 cases).

Initial Assessment

5. Stark, G., Neonatal assessment of the child with myelomeningocele. *Arch. Dis. Child.* 46:539, 1971.
   Filled with "pearls."

"Selective Treatment"

6. Lorber, J. Results of treatment of myelomeningocele: An analysis of 524 unselected cases with special reference to possible selection for treatment. *Dev. Med. Child Neurol.* 13:279, 1971.
   The classic study suggesting no treatment for children with gross paralysis of the legs, high lesions, kyphosis or scoliosis, grossly enlarged head at birth, intracerebral birth injury, or other major congenital defects (reaffirmed in Arch. Dis. Child. *47:854, 1972). For other reports of "selective treatment," see* N. Engl. J. Med. *291:1005, 1974, and* Pediatrics *72:450, 1983.*
7. Freeman, J. The shortsighted treatment of myelomeningocele: A long-term case report. *Pediatrics* 53:311, 1974.
   But not all children selected for no treatment have early deaths (editorial comment by Lorber, p. 307).

Neurosurgical Aspects

8. John, W., et al. A controlled trial of immediate and delayed closure of spina bifida cystica. *Arch. Dis. Child.* 38:18, 1963.
   Closure of the defect during the first 48 hours of life is associated with improved survival, a lower incidence of sepsis and meningitis, and a shorter hospital stay (40 cases).
   Also see Hydrocephalus, Chapter 82.

Orthopedic Aspects

9. Sharrard, W. The orthopaedic surgery of spina bifida. *Clin. Orthop.* 92:195, 1973.
   Encyclopedic (28 pages).
10. DeSouza, L., and Carroll, N. Ambulation of the braced myelomeningocele patient. *J. Bone Joint Surg.* [A] 58:1112, 1976.
    The outlook for teenagers and young adults.

Bladder and Bowel

11. Klauber, G., et al. Current approaches to evaluation and management of children with myelomeingocele. *Pediatrics* 63:663, 1979.
    A review by the AAP Section on Urology's Action Committee on Myelodysplasia, emphasizing clean intermittent catheterization. (Also see Pediatrics *72:203, 1983.)*

12. Wald, A. Use of biofeedback in treatment of fecal incontinence in patients with meningomyelocele. *Pediatrics* 68:45, 1981.
   Accompanied by a brief editorial review of the various problems associated with spina bifida, p. 136.

Epidemiology
13. Mortimer, E. The puzzling epidemiology of neural tube defects. *Pediatrics* 65:636, 1980.
   Brief editorial review of the epidemiology. (Incidence appears to be declining: Pediatrics *69:511, 1982, and 70:333, 1982.)*

Prognosis
14. Soare, P., and Raimondi, A. Intellectual and perceptual motor characteristics of treated myelomeningocele children. *Am. J. Dis. Child.* 131:199, 1977.
   Among children with treated hydrocephalus, 63 percent had IQs above 80; perceptual-motor skills were impaired.
15. McLone, D., et al. Central nervous system infections as a limiting factor in the intelligence of children with myelomeningocele. *Pediatrics* 70:338, 1982.
   A review of 167 patients, implicating ventriculitis and the recurrence of ventriculitis as major factors in the depression of intellectual performance.
16. Hayden, P., et al. Adolescents with myelodysplasia: Impact of physical disability on emotional maturation. *Pediatrics* 64:53, 1979.
   The greatest impediments to emotional growth included lack of appropriate chores, decreased opportunities for peer interaction, and uncertainties about bowel and bladder continence. (Special counseling needed by adolescents: Clin. Pediatr. [Phila.] *22:331, 1983.)*

Support
17. Colgan, M. The child with spina bifida: Role of the pediatrician. *Am. J. Dis. Child.* 135:854, 1981.
   Provider of medical care, coordinator, and advocate.
18. Leonard, C. Counseling parents of a child with meningomyelocele. *Pediatr. Rev.* 4:317, 1983.
   Based on assessment and current data regarding prognosis.
19. Kolin, I., et al. Studies of the school-age child with meningomyelocele: Social and emotional adaptation. *J. Pediatr.* 78:1013, 1971.
   Evaluation of parents as well as children; the need for communication with the physician is stressed.

Spina Bifida Occulta
20. Anderson, F. Occult spinal dysraphism: A series of 73 cases. *Pediatrics* 55:826, 1975.
   Embryologic and clinical considerations are discussed.

82. HYDROCEPHALUS

William R. Leahy, Jr.

Hydrocephalus occurs in 2 per 1000 live births. It is usually the result of obstruction to the flow of cerebrospinal fluid (CSF), leading to dilatation of the cerebral ventricles and subarachnoid space; the clinical manifestations are those of increased intracranial pressure.

Normally, the CSF is produced by the choroid plexus in the lateral ventricles, flows to the third ventricle and through the aqueduct of Sylvius into the fourth ventricle; from there, CSF enters the cisterns and spinal subarachnoid space. As the fluid bathes the hemispheres, it is absorbed via the arachnoid villi into the cortical venous system.

Obstruction within the ventricular system does not permit CSF free access to the spinal canal, producing so-called noncommunicating hydrocephalus. The most common site of obstruction is between the third and fourth ventricles, with the obstruction caused by stenosis or gliosis of the aqueduct. Varying degrees of narrowing—and obstruction—may occur; the onset of symptoms is usually insidious and may even be delayed until adulthood. A small percentage of cases appear to have a sex-linked pattern of inheritance. Other examples of noncommunicating hydrocephalus are obstructions of the fourth ventricle, the Arnold-Chiari malformation and Dandy-Walker syndrome. The Arnold-Chiari malformation is due to aberrant development of the lower brainstem and cerebellum and usually accompanies meningomyelocele. Dandy-Walker refers to a cyst arising from and obstructing the fourth ventricle.

If the CSF is free to "communicate" with the spinal canal, but absorption over the convexities is deficient, the result is so-called communicating hydrocephalus. The usual cause is scarring due to neonatal anoxia, subarachnoid hemorrhage, or meningitis. Communicating hydrocephalus is half as frequent as noncommunicating hydrocephalus.

A rare cause of hydrocephalus is choroid plexus papilloma, in which overproduction of CSF rather than obstruction is the problem.

The physical signs and symptoms of hydrocephalus vary with the age of the child and the degree of pressure. In infants and young children, the symptoms may be insidious, with failure to thrive, irritability or somnolence, and vomiting. Examination may demonstrate a tense or large anterior fontanelle, distended scalp veins, a divergent strabismus, or spasticity in the lower extremities; often, however, concern is prompted by the observation on repeated examination that the head circumference is increasing too rapidly. Papilledema and other signs of elevated pressure may develop in older children with fused cranial sutures.

As in all children with increased intracranial pressure, diagnostic evaluation for the definition of site and type of pathologic condition should be prompt. Transillumination of the skull may demonstrate evidence of a thin cortical mantle in children with moderate to severe hydrocephalus. Pneumoencephalography has traditionally been the procedure used to delineate the anatomy, but is rapidly being replaced by computerized axial tomography, which is noninvasive, much less dangerous than pneumoencephalography, and can be performed serially to monitor progress once the diagnosis is established and treatment effected.

Several authors have advocated diuretics and hyperosmolar agents to control CSF production or to increase excretion, but this strategy has been of temporary value only, and medical management of hydrocephalus has all but been abandoned. The standard procedure for treatment at present is operative diversion of CSF from a cerebral ventricle to the peritoneum or the right atrium. The major complications of the shunts—infection and nonfunction due to obstruction—are the same whether the diversion is to the peritoneum or the right atrium. Infection, often with organisms of low virulence, usually dismissed as "contaminants," such as *Staphylococcus epidermidis,* can rarely be treated successfully with antibiotics alone; it is necessary to remove the shunt and control CSF pressure with intermittent aspirations of ventricular fluid. Shunts may have to be revised several times during childhood, though occasionally a single procedure will suffice.

It is difficult to define the prognosis for children with hydrocephalus as a group, since outcome is influenced by the presence of associated anomalies. It is clear, however, that to conserve intellectual potential, detection should be early and treatment aggressive. Despite the problems associated with shunts, at present they offer the best opportunity to maximize developmental potential. The clinician must withstand the temptation to consider hydrocephalus synonymous with retardation; often, certain motor functions, such as sitting, may be delayed simply as a consequence of the disproportionately large head. Language development and subsequent tests of intelligence are much more valid indicators of ultimate performance.

Review

1. Bell, W., and McCormick, W. *Increased Intracranial Pressure in Children* (2nd ed.). Philadelphia: Saunders, 1978.

   Chapter 8 is an 83-page tour de force on hydrocephalus; includes more than 400 references.

Aspects of Diagnosis

2. Cheldelin, L., et al. Normal values for transillumination of skull using a new light source. *J. Pediatr.* 87:937, 1975.

Values for the "Chun gun." (Normal values for prematures: J. Pediatr. *91:980, 1977.)*

3. Cernerud, L. The setting sun phenomenon in infancy. *Dev. Med. Child Neurol.* 17:447, 1975.
   A follow-up of 19 infants with this clinical sign; only 8 had hydrocephalus.

4. McCullough, D., et al. Computerized axial tomography in clinical pediatrics. *Pediatrics* 59:173, 1977.
   A review of 725 scans in children with various pathologic entities, including hydrocephalus.

Specific Causes

5. Lorber, J., and Priestley, B. Children with large heads: A practical approach to diagnosis in 557 children, with special reference to 109 children with megalencephaly. *Dev. Med. Child Neurol.* 23:494, 1981.
   The differential diagnosis. (Also see Am. J. Dis. Child. *135:1118, 1981.)*

6. Hart, M. et al. The Dandy-Walker syndrome: A clinicopathological study based on 28 cases. *Neurology* (Minneap.) 22:771, 1972.
   A review of pathology, suggesting that other systemic and central nervous system anomalies may coexist with classic Dandy-Walker syndrome.

7. Kendall, B., and Holland, I. Benign communicating hydrocephalus in children. *Neuroradiology* 21:93, 1981.
   Review of a "benign" and mild form of hydrocephalus increasingly recognized by CT scan; causes and therapy in this controversial entity are discussed.

Experimental Work

8. Hochwald, G. Experimental hydrocephalus: Changes in cerebrospinal fluid dynamics as a function of time. *Arch. Neurol.* 26:120, 1972.
   Alterations of CSF dynamics during the development of acute and chronic hydrocephalus.

9. Rubin, R., et al. The effect of severe hydrocephalus on size and number of brain cells. *Dev. Med. Child Neurol.* 27:117, 1972.
   The white matter is most affected by hydrocephalus; the ventricles may expand without cellular loss.

Shunts

10. Pudenz, R. The surgical treatment of hydrocephalus: An historic review. *Surg. Neurol.* 15:15, 1981.
    A classic; excellent review of shunting procedures.

11. Little, J., Rhoton, A., and Mellinger, J. Comparison of ventriculoperitoneal and ventriculoatrial shunts in hydrocephalic children. *Mayo Clin. Proc.* 47:396, 1972.
    The problems of infection and cardiac decompensation in ventriculoatrial shunts suggest the superiority of the ventriculoperitoneal shunt. (Also see J. Neurosurg. *50:179, 1979.)*

12. Grosfeld, J. Intra-abdominal complications following ventriculoperitoneal shunt procedures. *Pediatrics* 54:791, 1974.
    Superior, but not perfect!

13. Freeman, J., and D'Souza, B. Obstruction of CSF shunts. *Pediatrics* 64:111, 1979.
    Brief and to the point: "Anything that goes wrong with a person with shunted hydrocephalus is due to a shunt problem until proven otherwise."

14. Schoenbaum, J., et al. Infections of CSF shunts: Epidemiology, clinical manifestations and treatment. *J. Infect. Dis.* 131:543, 1975.
    Infection in 27 percent; there is little chance of sterilizing CSF without removal of the shunt. (Infection with H. influenzae *an exception:* J. Pediatr. *97:424, 1980.)*

15. Birnholz, J., and Frigoletto, F. Antenatal treatment of hydrocephalus. *N. Engl. J. Med.* 304:1021, 1981.
    Early report of intrauterine decompression of hydrocephalus.

Prognosis

16. Laurence, K., and Coates, S. The natural history of hydrocephalus: A detailed analysis of 182 unoperated cases. *Arch. Dis. Child.* 37:345, 1962.

A key review for prognosis; 46 percent were noted to have spontaneous arrest of hydrocephalus.

17. Laurence, K. Neurological and intellectual sequelae of hydrocephalus. *Arch. Neurol.* 20:73, 1969.
    A further follow-up on arrested hydrocephalus; 41 percent had IQs over 85, and 22 percent had slowly improved in several respects since the 1962 study.

18. Foltz, E., and Shurtleff, D. Five-year comparative study of hydrocephalus in children with and without operation (113 cases). *J. Neurosurg.* 20:1064, 1963.
    Five-year survival in children who had shunts was 61 percent, but only 22 percent in those who did not have shunts; the IQ was over 75 in 33 percent of the former but in only 5 percent of the latter.

19. Raimondi, A., et al. Intellectual development in shunted hydrocephalic children. *Am. J. Dis. Child.* 127:664, 1974.
    Those with associated myelomeningocele were the brightest; the IQ was unrelated to the number of shunt revisions or "severity" of hydrocephalus prior to surgery, but closely related to the age of initial shunting and shunt function.

83. CEREBRAL PALSY

Eileen P. G. Vining

Cerebral palsy (CP) is defined as a nonprogressive disorder of motion and posture due to brain insults or injury occurring in the period of early brain growth (generally under 3 years of age). The manifestations of a given lesion may change as the nervous system matures, but the insult that caused the lesion is no longer present, and there is no active disease at the time of diagnosis.

Risk factors for cerebral palsy include: (1) low birth weight (associated with diplegia); (2) multiple pregnancy (associated with diplegia); (3) hyperbilirubinemia (associated with extrapyramidal cerebral palsy); (4) neonatal difficulties; and (5) a maternal history of infertility and fetal wastage. Improvements in neonatal intensive care are associated with the survival of more low-birth-weight infants; there does not appear to be a significant increase in the prevalence of cerebral palsy, however. Progress has been made in preventing cerebral palsy, but a current review suggests that many recent cases could have been prevented.

There are also certain developmental observations, often made first by parents, which suggest a possible diagnosis of cerebral palsy. The most frequent is delayed motor development, often with "dissociation" between motor and intellectual developmental milestones. An infant who is strongly right-handed or left-handed before 12 months is at high risk for having hemiplegia. Persistent fisting after 3 months, a paucity of activity, or asymmetry in the use of the extremities warrants suspicions. Toe walking may be a sign of spasticity. Cerebral palsy is also suggested by the presence of drooling, variable muscle tone, grimacing, and retention of primitive reflexes, such as the asymmetric tonic neck reflex, Moro reflex, and positive supporting reaction. Cerebral palsy can be detected clinically by 4 months of age, utilizing expected motor milestones and an assessment of muscle tone.

Other findings that alert the physician to the possibility of spastic cerebral palsy include decreased range of motion, extensor tone in the supine position, clonus, and the presence of pathologic reflexes.

Persistence of primitive reflexes, a poor quality Moro reflex, and reduced or variable muscle tone accompanied by opisthotonic posturing and poor feeding, sucking, or tongue control are hallmarks of extrapyramidal cerebral palsy.

Phelps described the distribution of types of cerebral palsy as being 40 percent spastic, 40 percent athetotic, and 20 percent other forms of extrapyramidal disease; others state that 75 percent of cases are spastic, 15 percent extrapyramidal, and 10 percent mixed. The clinician must remember that a single examination does not establish the classification of the individual patient with cerebral palsy with certainty. The natural history of the disorder demonstrates that certain signs evolve and change with time. Accurate classification is important information for the clinician, since it alerts him to serious abnormalities associated with particular types (e.g., hearing deficits with athe-toid CP) and provides a better basis for counseling.

The spastic limb has persistent and consistent characteristics: (1) muscular hypertonia of the clasp-knife type; (2) extreme hyperreflexia associated with sustained clonus, overflow, and a wide reflexogenic zone; (3) a marked tendency to the development of contractures; and (4) extensor plantar reflex (Babinski's sign). The following topographic patterns of cerebral palsy are defined: (1) hemiplegia involving two limbs on the same side; (2) double hemiplegia involving four limbs, with the upper extremities more af-fected; (3) quadriplegia involving all four limbs, with the lower extremities slightly more affected; and (4) diplegia involving all four limbs, with the lower extremities affected to a markedly greater degree than the upper.

The hallmark of extrapyramidal CP is variability with regard to motion, posture and sleep state of muscle tone, deep tendon reflexes, plantar reflex, and movement disorders. When muscle tone is increased, hypertonicity is "lead-pipe" rather than "clasp-knife" rigidity (i.e., there is a steady increase or decrease of tone during flexion and extension rather than a sense of "give" or "catch," as in spasticity). The child with rigidity is often floppy when asleep. Reflexes may be hyperactive, but rarely is clonus sustained. The plantar reflex is usually flexor (plantar), but involuntary movement may simulate an extensor response. Movement disorders include athetosis, chorea, dystonia, or any com-bination of these.

Comprehensive assessment is necessary for the child with CP because of the multi-plicity of associated handicaps. Mental retardation occurs in 50 to 70 percent of children with CP. Psychologic testing is often difficult because of the motor handicaps of these children and often requires the use of specialized tests and experienced examiners. There appears to be an inverse relationship between intellectual function and the number of extremities involved, with hypotonic children being most adversely affected. The child of normal intelligence with CP is at exceedingly high risk for minimal cerebral dysfunction and the associated learning and behavioral problems. Behavior modification is often useful in changing inappropriate behavior and stimulating more adaptive patterns. Visual problems occur in about 45 percent of children, the most common being stra-bismus. Hearing acuity is diminished in approximately 15 percent, predominantly in children with athetoid CP due to kernicterus. Epilepsy is also common, affecting 66 percent of children with spastic cerebral palsy and 35 percent of children with athetosis.

The therapeutic approach includes careful evaluation of the associated disabilities and the involvement of occupational and physical therapists. The occupational therapist is concerned with the attainment and improvement of upper extremity and self-help skills; the therapist is also instrumental in devising adaptive devices and seating arrangements for these children. Physical therapists deal with lower extremity skills, posture, and locomotion, and assist in the use of braces and crutches that are prescribed by the orthopedic surgeon.

Many medications have been used to ameliorate the motor problems. Diazepam has been widely used, but sedation may be a major problem. Reports exist suggesting benefit from dantrolene, levodopa, and baclofen, but extensive and controlled clinical trials are not available.

Various orthopedic procedures have been employed in the habilitation of these chil-dren, including adductor tenotomies, Achilles tendon releases, and multiple forms of hip surgery. The results are variable and depend on the type of cerebral palsy and post-operative habilitative efforts. Correction of scoliosis, without long-term use of a body brace, is possible using Luque rod instrumentation. Neurosurgical approach to the pa-tient, especially chronic cerebellar stimulation, remains controversial.

Habilitation of children with CP includes placement in appropriate social and edu-cational settings in order to avoid what in the past has been poor integration into society. Between 25 and 45 percent of adults with CP are in competitive employment, although some studies indicate that the social life for adults with CP is limited, with only 10 percent married and one-fourth described as social isolates. It is to be hoped that more appropriate intervention will maximize the potential of each person with CP.

General Reviews
1. Vining, E., et al. Cerebral palsy: A pediatric developmentalist's overview. *Am. J. Dis. Child.* 130:643, 1976.

A brief review: history, definitions, terminology, diagnosis, associated dysfunctions, and habilitation are discussed; a selective bibliography is provided.

2. Capute, A. Developmental disabilities: An overview. *Dent. Clin. North Am.* 18:557, 1974.
A short discussion of mental retardation, CP, and learning disabilities.

3. Molnar, G., and Taft, L. Cerebral Palsy. In J. Wortis (ed.), *Mental Retardation* (vol. 5). New York: Bruner/Mazel, 1973.
An extensive review article (27 pages, 307 references); an excellent source.

4. Crothers, B., and Paine, R. *The Natural History of Cerebral Palsy.* Cambridge, Mass.: Harvard University Press, 1959.
A superb source for description and problems of different types of cerebral palsy.

5. Alberman, E., et al. Cerebral palsy and severe educational subnormality in low-birth weight children: A comparison of births in 1951–53 and 1970–73. *Lancet* 1:606, 1982.
A short review of the impact of improved neonatal care on the prevalence of cerebral palsy.

6. Holm, V. The causes of cerebral palsy: A contemporary perspective. *JAMA* 247:1473, 1982.
An interesting review of etiology and epidemiology, with implications regarding prevention.

7. Molnar, G., Cerebral palsy: Prognosis and how to judge it. *Pediatr. Ann.* 8:596, 1979.
Some good clues to help clinicians counsel and prognosticate.

Diagnosis

8. Illingworth, R. The diagnosis of cerebral palsy in the first year of life. *Dev. Med. Child Neurol.* 8:178, 1966.
A classic; clues to etiology.

9. Ellenberg, J., and Nelson, K. Early recognition of infants at high risk for cerebral palsy: Examination at age four months. *Dev. Med. Child Neurol.* 23:705, 1981.
Collaborative Perinatal Project data regarding predictive power of assessment in first few months.

10. Johnston, R. Motor Function: Normal Development and Cerebral Palsy. In R. Johnston and P. Magrab (eds.), *Developmental Disorders: Assessment, Treatment, Education.* Baltimore: University Park Press, 1976.
The diagrams are exceptionally good.

11. Capute, A. Identifying cerebral palsy in infancy through study of primitive reflex profiles. *Pediatr. Ann.* 8:589, 1979.
Explanation of primitive reflexes, their impact and correlation to function.

12. Holt, K. Medical examination of the child with cerebral palsy. *Pediatr. Ann.* 8:581, 1979.
An excellent developmentalist's approach to the child, especially regarding counseling and routine follow-up.

13. Minear, W. A classification of cerebral palsy. *Pediatrics* 18:841, 1956.
A comprehensive description of classification.

Associated Problems

14. Cruickshank, W. (ed.). *Cerebral Palsy, Its Individual and Community Problems.* Syracuse, N.Y.: Syracuse University Press, 1966.
Very comprehensive with respect to education, vocational guidance, and habilitation.

15. Robinson, R. The frequency of other handicaps in children with cerebral palsy. *Dev. Med. Child Neurol.* 15:305, 1973.
An analysis of associated problems, by type of cerebral palsy.

Treatment

16. Potter, P., and Harryman, S. Physical and occupational therapy for the handicapped child. *Pediatr. Clin. North Am.* 20:159, 1973.
The basic means of intervention; what the therapists do.

17. Scherzer, A., et al. Physical therapy as a determinant of change in the cerebral palsied infant. *Pediatrics* 58:47, 1976.
A good entrée to the debate over therapy; correlates improvement in therapy with increased intelligence prior to therapy.

18. Hoffer, M., et al. New concepts in orthotics for cerebral palsy. *Clin. Orthop.* 102:100, 1974.
    Shows what can be done with bracing, special chairs.
19. Banks, H., and Panagakos, P. The role of the orthopedic surgeon in cerebral palsy. *Pediatr. Clin. North Am.* 14:495, 1967.
    The types of procedures, when useful, and the outcome.
20. Allen, B., and Ferguson, R. L-rod instrumentation for scoliosis in cerebral palsy. *J. Ped. Orthop.* 2:87, 1982.
    A review of previous therapy, with explanation and advantages of this new approach.
21. Penn, R. Chronic cerebellar stimulation for cerebral palsy: A review. *Neurosurgery* 10:116, 1982.
    Excellent review and discussion of the difficulty in evaluating this procedure.

At Home and In Society
22. Blasco, P., et al. Literature for parents of children with cerebral palsy. *Dev. Med. Child Neurol.* 25:642, 1983.
    Literature for parents is reviewed and critiqued. An absolute "must" resource list for pediatricians.
23. Finnie, N. *Handling the Young Cerebral Palsied Child at Home.* New York: Dutton, 1975.
    Good for the physician, necessary for the parent; instructions for carrying, positioning, and feeding.
24. O'Reilly, D. Care of the cerebral palsied: Outcome of the past and needs for the future. *Dev. Med. Child Neurol.* 17:141, 1975.
    A follow-up of 336 patients; data on education, occupation, and employment and suggestions for the future are given.

X. RHEUMATIC DISORDERS

84. JUVENILE RHEUMATOID ARTHRITIS

Margaret E. Mohrmann

The group of disorders known as juvenile rheumatoid arthritis (JRA) might more appropriately be labeled "chronic arthritis of childhood," since the disease seldom bears any resemblance to classic adult rheumatoid arthritis. The distinction between the adult and juvenile types of chronic arthritis was first clearly drawn in 1897 by the pediatrician George Frederic Still, whose original paper remains perhaps the best clinical description of the childhood disease.

There are estimated to be roughly 200,000 children in the United States who have JRA; females predominate almost 3:1. The cause of the disease is unknown, although intriguing connections with infection, immunologic abnormalities, genetic factors, and environmental stress have been described.

In 20 percent of children with JRA, the disease begins as an acute febrile systemic disorder. This subset, often referred to as "Still disease," affects boys as often as girls and may occur at any age, although the median age at onset is 5 years. Antinuclear antibodies (ANA) and rheumatoid factor (RF) are usually absent. Children with this mode of onset have a characteristic intermittent fever with one or two daily temperature spikes and an evanescent salmon-pink rash, which tends to appear at the height of the fever. Hepatosplenomegaly and generalized lymphadenopathy are common. Pericarditis may be present but is seldom clinically significant; myocarditis, on the other hand, although rare, may result in congestive heart failure and death. The characteristic polyarthritis may not be present at the onset of disease, but will usually appear within 6 months; almost one-fourth of these children suffer progressive joint destruction.

Symmetric polyarthritis, involving both large and small joints, is the predominant initial manifestation in 35 to 40 percent of children with JRA; systemic features, when present, are usually limited to mild fever and malaise. Cervical spine involvement may occur and can result in life-threatening atlantoaxial subluxation. The polyarthritis group includes two JRA subsets, a division based on the presence or absence of RF. Two-thirds of children with polyarthritis do not have RF (i.e., are "seronegative") and respond well to treatment; in almost 90 percent the arthritis follows a benign course with eventual complete resolution. Children in the seropositive subset, most of whom also have ANA, have a disease very similar to adult rheumatoid arthritis: more than one-half have severe progressive crippling arthritis, unresponsive to drug therapy. Both subsets occur more often in females; the seronegative group often presents in the preschool years while disease in patients who have RF usually begins in the second decade.

One-fourth of patients with JRA, usually girls, present in the preschool years with asymmetric arthritis affecting only a few large joints (pauci- or oligoarthritis). Sequelae from the typically mild joint disease are rare. Well over one-half the children in this subgroup have ANA; most of those who do develop chronic iridocyclitis, a potential cause of near or total blindness. Iridocyclitis is usually asymptomatic and its course is unrelated to the activity of the joint disease; frequent slit-lamp examinations by an ophthalmologist are necessary to detect ocular involvement and prevent disabling complications.

The fifth subset, affecting 15 percent of children with JRA, is also characterized by a pauciarticular onset but is more common in males and usually appears after the eighth birthday. Knees and ankles are typically involved initially; hips and sacroiliac joints are eventually affected in most. There may be significant involvement of the lumbar spine and many of these children ultimately have disease indistinguishable from ankylosing spondylitis. ANA and RF are absent, but 75 percent of patients in this subset have HLA-B27. Patients may have bouts of acute, symptomatic iridocyclitis, seldom associated with significant sequelae. The prognosis for maintenance of normal gait and posture depends on the severity of spine and pelvic girdle disease and on the adequacy of treatment.

Perhaps as many as 5 to 10 percent of children with chronic arthritis have juvenile psoriatic arthritis. The arthropathy of psoriasis, which may precede the skin manifestations by years, is characterized by a monarticular or pauciarticular onset but an asymmetric polyarticular course. Spondyloarthritis and tenosynovitis involving an entire finger or toe are frequently seen. A family history of psoriasis and the presence of nail pitting may suggest the diagnosis in these patients, many of whom will have significantly disabling chronic joint disease.

The diagnosis of chronic arthritis in children is made on the basis of the history, physical examination, and clinical course; there are no definitive laboratory tests or radiographic procedures, although such tests may be needed to eliminate other diagnoses, such as infectious or neoplastic disease. Diagnosis of chronic arthritis depends on a clear understanding of terms. "Arthritis" means the presence of at least two of the following joint signs: pain, swelling, warmth, erythema, limitation of motion. "Chronic," in this context, implies at least 6 weeks of arthritis; many authorities suggest a time period of 3 months in the absence of extraarticular manifestations. Defining a chronic course is necessary to differentiate JRA from a confusing multitude of transient arthritides (viral, postdysenteric, traumatic). The differential diagnosis must also include: acute rheumatic fever, which may be distinguished by evidence of valvular heart disease and by dramatic relief of joint symptoms with aspirin; septic arthritis, which requires examination and culture of joint fluid for diagnosis; other rheumatic disorders, such as systemic lupus erythematosus, which are often differentiated by characteristic clinical and serologic abnormalities; and the arthritis associated with inflammatory bowel disease.

Optimal treatment of JRA requires an aggressive multidisciplinary effort coordinated by the child's primary physician. Since the major goal of treatment is maintenance of normal joint function, physical therapy is essential, especially considering both the rapidity of development of joint contractures and muscle wasting and the risk of growth retardation in children. The treatment plan should stress regular exercise coupled with adequate rest (not complete bed rest); in general, joint immobilization is contraindicated, although resting splints may be needed to relieve pain and increase range of motion.

Anti-inflammatory agents are used to relieve pain, stiffness, and swelling so joints will function normally and physical therapy may proceed; there is little evidence that any drug used to treat JRA directly affects the process of joint destruction. Aspirin is the drug of choice for all subsets of JRA; at least 90 percent of children will experience significant improvement of symptoms, although the response may come only after several weeks of treatment. Children receiving aspirin therapy are at risk of developing salicylism and appropriate dosing must be ensured by blood salicylate levels. Patients who cannot tolerate the side effects of salicylates and some patients who do not respond to aspirin may be helped by one of the newer nonsteroidal anti-inflammatory drugs (NSAID). Tolmetin is probably as effective as aspirin, may have fewer side effects, and is the only NSAID approved for use in children. Ibuprofen, sulindac, naproxen, and similar agents seem effective and well tolerated but are still being studied in children. Indomethacin, one of the first-line drugs for treatment of adult ankylosing spondylitis, is used in children with the second subset of pauciarticular JRA who do not respond to aspirin.

Children whose articular disease progresses or fails to improve after 6 months of adequate salicylate (or NSAID) and physical therapy are candidates for treatment with gold salts, as are patients who are dependent on steroids for relief of symptoms. Gold is administered in a single weekly intramuscular injection and usually takes 2 to 4 months to effect a clinical response. Patients must be monitored weekly for signs of dermatologic, hematologic, and renal toxicity. One-third of patients experience significant amelioration of disease; one-third do not respond at all; and in one-third the drug is discontinued because of toxic effects. Oral gold preparations are being studied; they appear to be as effective and may be less toxic than parenteral gold. Penicillamine is a potentially useful alternative to gold, although there is little experience with its use in JRA.

Steroids are to be avoided if possible in JRA because of their failure to retard joint destruction and their well-known side effects. The only indications for steroid use are: (1) severe "toxicity", especially life-threatening carditis, in patients with acute systemic disease; (2) iridocyclitis unresponsive to topical therapy; and (3) incapacitating joint symptoms unresponsive to aspirin and gold. Steroids are contraindicated in the presence of spine or hip involvement because of the increased risk of vertebral collapse and femoral head necrosis. Immunosuppressive drugs have been used, with variable results, only in patients with progressive joint destruction who fail to respond to any other form of therapy.

In addition to physical therapy and drug treatment, other aspects of management include orthopedic intervention for release of contractures, synovectomy, or arthroplasty when necessary; annual ophthalmologic examinations for iridocyclitis (children in the high-risk pauciarticular subset should be examined every 3–4 months); and thoughtful psychologic support of the child and family.

Mortality in JRA is estimated at 1 to 5 percent; death is usually due to infection, carditis, or renal failure. In Europe, renal failure due to amyloidosis is the leading cause of death. With appropriate treatment, the overall prognosis for JRA is good: 10 years after diagnosis 50 percent of patients are in complete remission, 20 percent have normal joint function but occasional symptoms of arthritis, and 15 percent are able to work normally despite some joint dysfunction. Optimal use of physical therapy, anti-inflammatory agents, ophthalmologic care, and emotional support can prevent most of the physically and emotionally crippling effects of this disease.

The Classic

1. Still, G. On a form of chronic joint disease in children. *Med. Chir. Trans.* 80:47, 1897.
   Worth reading for superb clinical descriptions as well as for historical interest; conveniently reprinted, with commentary, in Am. J. Dis. Child. *132:192, 1978.*

Reviews

2. Brewer, E., Giannini, E., and Person, D. *Juvenile Rheumatoid Arthritis* (2nd ed.). Philadelphia: Saunders, 1982.
   The most complete source of information.
3. Cassidy, J. *Texbook of Pediatric Rheumatology.* New York: Wiley, 1982.
   The chapter on JRA is well written and thorough (100 pages, 363 references).
4. Schaller, J. Juvenile rheumatoid arthritis. *Pediatr. Rev.* 2:163, 1980.
   Complete but succinct; an excellent place to start.
5. Schaller, J., and Hanson, V. (eds.). Proceedings of the conference on the rheumatic diseases of childhood. *Arthritis Rheum.* 20:145, 1977.
   Book-sized supplement, most of which deals with current knowledge about all aspects of JRA.
6. Ansell, B. Chronic arthritis in childhood. *Ann. Rheum. Dis.* 37:107, 1978.
   Fascinating discussion (the 1977 Heberden Oration) of the heterogeneity of the disease.

Diagnosis and Differential Diagnosis

7. Petty, R., et al. Serologic studies in juvenile rheumatoid arthritis: A review. *Arthritis Rheum.* 20:260, 1977.
   The spectrum of possibilities; earlier but similar information in J. Pediatr. *77:98, 1970.*
8. Espinoza, L., et al. HLA, juvenile rheumatoid arthritis and other disease associations. *Adv. Pediatr.* 26:93, 1979.
   Good general review (141 references).
9. Wedgwood, R., and Schaller, J. The pediatric arthritides. *Hosp. Pract.* 12(6):83, 1977.
   Lucid description of subsets with emphasis on differential diagnosis.
10. Shore, A., and Ansell, B. Juvenile psoriatic arthritis: An analysis of 60 cases. *J. Pediatr.* 100:529, 1982.
    Typical presenting manifestations, clinical course, and diagnostic clues.
11. Schaller, J. The seronegative spondyloarthropathies of childhood. *Clin. Orthop.* 143:76, 1979.
    Differentiates pauciarticular (type II) JRA from other arthritides affecting the spine.
12. Lindsley, C., and Schaller, J. Arthritis associated with inflammatory bowel disease in children. *J. Pediatr.* 84:16, 1974.
    Of patients with IBD-associated joint disease, 75 percent have benign, short-lived peripheral arthritis; the rest have a spondyloarthropathy, which behaves much like ankylosing spondylitis.
13. Sills, E. Errors in diagnosis of juvenile rheumatoid arthritis. *Johns Hopkins Med. J.* 133:88, 1973.
    Reveals the variety of illnesses that can masquerade as JRA.

Joints

14. Miller, J., and Robertson, W. Mechanisms of arthritis in children. *Adv. Pediatr.* 18:151, 1971.
    Helpful basic information.

15. Bywaters, E. Pathological aspects of juvenile chronic polyarthritis. *Arthritis Rheum.* 20:271, 1977.
    The spectrum of joint changes.
16. Beales, J., Keen, J., and Holt, P. The child's perception of the disease and the experience of pain in juvenile chronic arthritis. *J. Rheumatol.* 10:61, 1983.
    The older the child, the more likely he is to have a very unpleasant idea of the internal pathology of his joints and to interpret the sensations emanating from those joints as pain.

Systemic Manifestations

17. Calabro, J., and Marchesano, J. Fever associated with juvenile rheumatoid arthritis. *N. Engl. J. Med.* 276:11, 1967.
    Description of the classic intermittent fever. (For a discussion of JRA presenting in the adult as fever of unknown origin, see Medicine [Baltimore] 52:431, 1973.)
18. Calabro, J., and Marchesano, J. Rash associated with juvenile rheumatoid arthritis. *J. Pediatr.* 72:611, 1968.
    Excellent description (with color pictures) and differentiating points.
19. Bernstein, B., et al. Cardiac involvement in juvenile rheumatoid arthritis. *J. Pediatr.* 85:313, 1974.
    Pericarditis was present in 36 percent of 55 patients, diagnosed by echocardiography; 10 percent had myocarditis. (For additional statistics, see Arthritis Rheum. 20:231, 1977.) *A follow-up study, reported in* Acta Paediatr. Scand. 72:345, 1983, *recommends early use of steroids, regardless of the severity of the symptoms.*

Iridocyclitis

20. Schaller, J., et al. Iridocyclitis in juvenile rheumatoid arthritis. *Pediatrics* 44:92, 1969.
    Information on ocular changes and correlation with other findings. (For further clinical and serologic associations, see Arthritis Rheum. 16:130, 1973, and 17:409, 1974.)
21. Chylack, L., et al. Ocular manifestations of juvenile rheumatoid arthritis. *Am. J. Ophthalmol.* 79:1026, 1975.
    Iridocyclitis found in 17 percent of 210 patients with JRA; this review, including information on treatment and outcome, is summarized in Arthritis Rheum. 20:217, 1977.

Treatment

22. Granberry, W., and Brewer, E. The combined pediatric-orthopedic approach to the management of juvenile rheumatoid arthritis. *Orthop. Clin. North Am.* 9:481, 1978.
    Excellent, detailed coverage of physical therapy and orthopedic contributions to long-term management. (Indications for and success of hip and knee arthroplasty are presented in Clin. Orthop. 182:90, 1984, and Arthritis Rheum. 26:1140, 1983.)
23. Donovan, W. Physical measures in the treatment of juvenile rheumatoid arthritis. *Arthritis Rheum.* 20:553, 1977.
    Includes specific recommendations.
24. Wright, V., and Amos, R. Do drugs change the course of rheumatoid arthritis? *Br. Med. J.* 1:965, 1980.
    Careful assessment of the evidence gives little proof of significant change in the underlying disease.
25. Lindsley, C. Pharmacotherapy of juvenile rheumatoid arthritis. *Pediatr. Clin. North Am.* 28:161, 1981.
    The place to start; thorough and well-referenced. (Another very helpful review is in Drugs 26:530, 1983.)
26. Schaller, J. Chronic salicylate administration in juvenile rheumatoid arthritis: Aspirin "hepatitis" and its clinical significance.*Pediatrics* 62:916, 1978.
    Covers all aspects of salicylate use, not just the reversible transaminase elevations. (For an interesting view of compliance, see Am. J. Dis. Child. 135:434, 1981.)
27. Brewer, E. Nonsteroidal anti-inflammatory agents. *Arthritis Rheum.* 20:513, 1977.
    The most complete review of the drugs in children, giving early data collected by the collaborative study group.

28. Levinson, J., et al. Gold therapy. *Arthritis Rheum.* 20:531, 1977.
    A four-page review of indications for use, toxicity, and efficacy. (For further information and statistics on 63 patients, see Arthritis Rheum. *23:404, 1980; for results of initial studies of orally administered gold, see* J. Pediatr. *102:138, 1983.)*
29. Schaller, J. Corticosteroids in juvenile rheumatoid arthritis. *Arthritis Rheum.* 20:537, 1977.
    Important reading about indications for and dangers of steroids in this disease.

Prognosis
30. Dequeker, J., and Mardjuadi, A. Prognostic factors in juvenile chronic arthritis. *J. Rheumatol.* 9:909, 1982.
    Statistical analysis of 96 patients; poorest functional outcome was seen in those with polyarticular onset and course, in combination with a persistently elevated sedimentation rate and a family history of rheumatic disease.
31. Baum, J., and Gutowska, G. Death in juvenile rheumatoid arthritis. *Arthritis Rheum.* 20:253, 1977.
    Infection, carditis, renal failure. (For a detailed discussion of amyloidosis, see Ann. Rheum. Dis. *27:137, 1968.)*
32. McAnarney, E., et al. Psychological problems of children with chronic juvenile arthritis. *Pediatrics* 53:523, 1974.
    Loss of self-esteem arises from conflict between subtle physical limitations and unrealistic expectations. (However, children with JRA function socially when they become adults much better than would be expected given the degree of disability: J. Pediatr. *100:378, 1982.)*

85. SYSTEMIC LUPUS ERYTHEMATOSUS

Margaret E. Mohrmann

Systemic lupus erythematosus (SLE) is a disorder resulting from the formation of antigen-antibody complexes and the deposition of these complexes in vessel walls and in tissues such as skin, the renal glomerulus, and the choroid plexus in the central nervous system (CNS). The cause of the disease is unknown; theories of pathogenesis usually combine a probable genetic predisposition with a presumed environmental "trigger," such as viral infection, drugs, pregnancy, sunlight, or emotional stress.

Childhood SLE, about one-tenth as common as juvenile rheumatoid arthritis, usually presents in the second decade; the mean age at diagnosis is 12 years and the onset is often temporally associated with menarche. Less than 5 percent of children with SLE will present before the age of 5. The disease has a striking female predominance, although the characteristic adult female-male ratio of 9 : 1 decreases to 4 : 1 in children less than 12 years old.

Over 70 percent of children with SLE present with fever, rash, and arthritis or arthralgia. Another large percentage exhibit weight loss, fatigue, and malaise with or without an arthritis syndrome. Less commonly, the disease at onset is manifested by involvement—primarily or solely—of a single system, occasionally resulting in diagnostic error; examples of such presentations include thrombocytopenic purpura, hemolytic anemia, acute nephritis, nephrotic syndrome, seizures, carditis, pneumonitis, hepatosplenomegaly, recurrent abdominal pain, and sore throat with lymphadenopathy.

Because of the many varied modes of presentation of this disease, the American Rheumatism Association has proposed classification criteria to standardize the diagnosis for research and reporting purposes. The criteria, as revised in 1982, are : (1) malar rash; (2) discoid lesions; (3) photosensitivity; (4) oral or nasopharyngeal ulceration; (5) nonerosive arthritis; (6) the presence of LE cells, antiDNA or antiSm antibody, or a chronic false-positive serologic test for syphilis; (7) persistent protein or cellular casts in the urine; (8) pleuritis or pericarditis; (9) psychosis or convulsions; (10) hemolytic anemia, leukopenia, lymphopenia, or thrombocytopenia; and (11) the presence of antinuclear antibody. The presence, simultaneously or serially, or four or more of these features is highly suggestive of SLE (estimated 96% specificity); however, many patients considered to have SLE have less than four of these manifestations and the proposed standard should not be considered necessary for diagnosis.

Tissue injury and manifestations of disease in SLE are caused by the deposition of immune complexes, the cytotoxic effects of activated components of the complement system, and the action of lysosomal enzymes released by polymorphonuclear leukocytes. The antigens involved in the damaging immune complexes are of nuclear origin and, thus, the major screening laboratory test for the presence of SLE is an assay of antinuclear antibodies (ANA) by indirect fluorescence. The absence of ANA virtually rules out the diagnosis of SLE, but their presence is only suggestive of the disease, since they may be found in several other disease states and occasionally in normal persons. The finding of antibody to native (double-stranded) DNA (anti-dsDNA), on the other hand, is highly specific for SLE; it is probable that most, if not all, of the immune complexes formed in the patient with SLE are dsDNA–anti-dsDNA complexes. The LE cell phenomenon is absent in 30 to 50 percent of children with SLE at the time of diagnosis; the test has largely been replaced by the assays for ANA and anti-dsDNA.

The anti-dsDNA titer is useful not only for diagnosis but also for monitoring the disease, since the quantity of antibody appears to correlate well with disease activity. The participation of activated complement in the process of tissue destruction is reflected in the depressed levels of C3, C4, and CH50 generally found during episodes of active disease, especially nephritis; however, the correlation of disease status with complement level may not be as consistent as with the anti-dsDNA titer.

The goals of therapy are (1) to suppress inflammation, (2) to prevent formation of immune complexes by blocking production of antibodies to DNA, (3) to promote normal growth and development, and (4) to avoid unacceptable side effects of the medications used. Patients with mild disease, primarily manifested as arthritis and fever, often respond well to salicylates alone. Antimalarial agents, such as hydroxychloroquine, are helpful for treatment of skin lesions and mild disease unresponsive to aspirin; the use of this class of drugs is limited by the risk of ocular toxicity. The drug of choice for more severe disease is prednisone; indications for its use include severe "toxicity" (e.g., marked weight loss), active nephritis, carditis, or CNS disease. Rapidly progressive renal disease may respond to intravenous "pulses" of methylprednisolone. "Flares" of fever or joint symptoms that occur while prednisone is being tapered usually respond to aspirin or antimalarials and seldom require an increase in steroid dosage. The toxic effects of prednisone account for many of the complications seen in children with SLE (such as growth retardation, infection, aseptic necrosis of bone). The balance between control of the disease and prevention of steroid toxicity is often difficult to attain; there are no clear guidelines for dosage, timing of doses, and duration of therapy.

Immunosuppressive agents (azathioprine, cyclophosphamide, chlorambucil) are used in those patients with severe disease that is unresponsive to high-dose prednisone or who manifest toxic effects of steroids. In some centers, patients with the most severe type of lupus nephritis (diffuse proliferative glomerulonephritis) are treated with both steroids and cytotoxic agents from the time of diagnosis and have significantly improved survival rates. It is not certain that the increased survival is due to the early use of immunosuppressive therapy, however, since similar rates are now being seen in centers that seldom use these drugs.

In addition to anti-inflammatory drugs, treatment of the child with SLE must include careful attention to diet, rest, exercise, and psychologic support. Patients must be taught to avoid exposure to the sun or to use sun-screening lotions as direct sunlight may precipitate a flare of skin lesions or even of systemic disease activity. Hypertension, due both to nephritis and to steroid therapy, is a common finding and must be meticulously controlled to prevent additional organ damage.

Early reports described SLE in children as a rapidly fatal disorder in more than one-half the patients. It is now apparent that at least 80 percent will survive more than 10 years from diagnosis. The improved prognosis is due not only to wiser use of drugs but also to improved supportive care and increased availability and success of dialysis and renal transplantation. When death occurs, it is usually due to renal failure, CNS disease, or infection. Of the several types of renal lesions seen in patients with SLE, diffuse proliferative glomerulonephritis is the one associated most often with azotemia. CNS disease has protean manifestations and may be difficult to distinguish from steroid-induced neurologic or psychologic abnormalities. Increased susceptibility to infection may be a result of the disease itself, but the major cause is probably the immunosuppressive therapy used; viruses and *Pneumocystis carinii* are the organisms commonly associated with fatalities. Children treated successfully for SLE are at increased risk in adulthood of premature atherosclerotic heart disease (and myocardial infarction) and of malignancies. The former is likely a consequence of lupus vasculitis and prolonged steroid therapy, while the latter is probably a result of immunosuppression.

Two lupuslike syndromes deserve note: "drug-induced lupus" and manifestations of SLE in newborns whose mothers have the disease. Occasionally, a drug (e.g., hydralazine, phenytoin) is the agent that triggers the clinical expression of true SLE. More often, these drugs—and others, such as procainamide and isoniazid (INH)—elicit the development of ANA and mild symptoms of lupus, both of which generally disappear when the drug is discontinued; nephritis and anti-dsDNA are rarely part of this syndrome.

Neonates of mothers with SLE may have serologic abnormalities, occasionally accompanied by discoid lupus and/or hematologic abnormalities. These findings, which are apparently the result of transplacental passage of antibodies, are transient, and the infants should not be considered to have congenital SLE. More serious is an increased incidence of congenital heart block in infants of mothers with SLE.

Reviews

1. Dubois, E. (ed.). *Lupus Erythematosus* (2nd ed.). Los Angeles: University of Southern California Press, 1974.
   Probably the most complete review available, touching on every imaginable facet of the disease (more than 1500 references).
2. Cassidy, J. *Textbook of Pediatric Rheumatology.* New York: Wiley, 1982.
   Contains an excellent, detailed chapter on SLE (69 pages, 214 references).
3. Decker, J., et al. Systemic lupus erythematosus: Contrasts and comparisons. *Ann. Intern. Med.* 82:391, 1975.
   Roundtable discussion of pathogenesis, clinical manifestations, and current research areas; for an update, see Ann. Intern. Med. 91:587, 1979.
4. King, K., et al. The clinical spectrum of systemic lupus erythematosus in childhood. *Arthritis Rheum.* 20:287, 1977.
   Review of 108 patients and their modes of presentation; the review in Pediatr. Clin. North Am. 10:941, 1963, although dated in some areas, remains helpful for clinical descriptions, diagnostic clues, and differential diagnostic features.
5. Tan, E., et al. The 1982 revised criteria for the classification of systemic lupus erythematosus. *Arthritis Rheum.* 25:1271, 1982.
   An attempt to weight the criteria to provide even greater sensitivity and specificity is presented in Arch. Intern. Med. 144:281, 1984.

Lupus Immunology

6. Goldberg, M., et al. Histocompatibility antigens in systemic lupus erythematosus. *Arthritis Rheum.* 19:129, 1976.
   Also see Transplant Rev. 23:3, 1975, for a review of HLA-disease associations.
7. Fernandez-Madrid, F., and Mattioli, M. Antinuclear antibodies (ANA): Immunologic and clinical significance. *Semin. Arthr. Rheum.* 6:83, 1976.
   Review primarily of findings in SLE, with an excellent discussion of clinical relevance. (For a report of a child with SLE and negative assay for ANA, see J. Pediatr. 98:578, 1981.)
8. Cassidy, J. Clinical assessment of immune-complex disease in children with systemic lupus erythematosus. *J. Pediatr.* 89:523, 1976.
   Brief editorial review of available tests and their significance.
9. Lehman, T., et al. The role of antibodies directed against double-stranded DNA in the manifestations of systemic lupus erythematosus in childhood. *J. Pediatr.* 96:657, 1980.
   Study of correlation between anti-dsDNA titers and disease activity. (Complement levels do not correlate consistently with disease activity: J. Pediatr. 89:358, 1976.)

Systemic Manifestations: Nephritis

10. Baldwin, D., et al. The clinical course of the proliferative and membranous forms of lupus nephritis. *Ann. Intern. Med.* 73:929, 1970.

    The classic clinical and histologic classification, continued in Am. J. Med. *62:12, 1977, with addition of mesangial nephritis and recognition of occasional transformation from one type to another. (For a scholarly, detailed review with very specific recommendations for treatment, see* Annu. Rev. Med. *31:463, 1980.)*

11. West, C., and McAdams, A. The chronic glomerulonephritides of childhood. *J. Pediatr.* 93:1, 67, 1978.

    Includes a brief, clear, well-referenced review of lupus nephritis. (For a reminder that the urinary sediment may be normal in a patient with lupus nephritis, see Pediatrics *64:678, 1979.)*

12. Coplon, N., et al. The long-term clinical course of systemic lupus erythematosus in end-stage renal disease. *N. Engl. J. Med.* 308:186, 1983.

    The outcome of dialysis and transplant is not significantly different in patients with SLE compared to those with ESRD from other causes; the nonrenal manifestations of SLE were almost always quiescent during hemodialysis, resulting in discontinuation of immunosuppressive medication in most cases. (Also see editorial comment, p. 218.)

Systemic Manifestations: Central Nervous System

13. Feinglass, E., et al. Neuropsychiatric manifestations of systemic lupus erythematosus. *Medicine* (Baltimore) 55:323, 1976.

    Exhaustive review of 140 patients (15 pages, 76 references).

14. Bennahum, D., and Messner, R. Recent observations on central nervous system lupus erythematosus. *Semin. Arthr. Rheum.* 4:253, 1975.

    Presents the great variety of manifestations and the difficulties involved in diagnosis and treatment. (For a review of neuropathology, see Semin. Arthr. Rheum. *8:212, 1979.)*

Systemic Manifestations: Miscellaneous

15. Budman, D., and Steinberg, A. Hematologic aspects of systemic lupus erythematosus. *Ann. Intern. Med.* 86:220, 1977.

    Detailed attention to the pathogenesis and management of anemia, leukopenia, and thrombocytopenia.

16. Hoffman, B., and Katz, W. The gastrointestinal manifestations of systemic lupus erythematosus: A review of the literature. *Semin. Arthr. Rheum.* 9:237, 1980.

    Especially helpful on differential diagnosis, evaluation and treatment of abdominal pain in patients with SLE.

17. Englund, J., and Lucas, R. Cardiac complications in children with systemic lupus erythematosus. *Pediatrics* 72:724, 1983.

    A succinct review in a grand-rounds format.

Treatment

18. Dubois, E. Antimalarials in the management of discoid and systemic lupus erythematosus. *Semin. Arthr. Rheum.* 8:33, 1978.

    Details of use and toxicity.

19. Fauci, A., Dale, D., and Balow, J. Glucocorticoid therapy: Mechanism of action and clinical considerations. *Ann. Intern. Med.* 84:304, 1976.

    Emphasis on mechanism of immunosuppression. (For a brief, comprehensive discussion of toxic effects, see Am. J. Dis. Child. *132:806, 1978; for recommendations on withdrawal schedules and management of prolonged adrenal suppression, see* Pediatr. Clin. North Am. *26:251, 1979; and for data on the use of pulse methylprednisolone, see* J. Pediatr. *101:137, 1982.)*

20. Fish, A., et al. Systemic lupus erythematosus within the first two decades of life. *Am. J. Med.* 62:99, 1977.

    Strongest argument (73% 10-year survival) for use of azathioprine plus steroids in patients with diffuse proliferative glomerulonephritis.

21. Wagner, L. Immunosuppressive agents in lupus nephritis: A critical analysis. *Medicine* (Baltimore) 55:239, 1976.

    After weighing risks against equivocal efficacy, author takes dim view of the drugs.

22. Shumak, K., and Rock, G. Therapeutic plasma exchange. *N. Engl. J. Med.* 310:762, 1984.
    A helpful review; plasmapheresis has not been proven to be of benefit in SLE, despite occasional anecdotal reports to the contrary (as in Acta Paediatr. Scand. *71:347, 1982).*

Prognosis
23. Meislin, A., and Rothfield, N. Systemic lupus erythematosus in childhood: Analysis of 42 cases with 18 year follow-up. *Pediatrics* 42:37, 1968.
    Ten-year survival was 50 percent in children without nephritis and 20 percent in those with renal disease; much more optimistic figures are to be found in Am. J. Dis. Child. *130:929, 1976. More recent mortality for all ages is reported in* Arthritis Rheum. *24:762, 1981.*
24. Abeles, M., et al. Systemic lupus erythematosus in the younger patient: Survival studies. *J. Rheumatol.* 7:515, 1980.
    Five-year statistics that promise to be at least as good as those reported in reference 20, but without the use of immunosuppressive drugs.

Lupuslike Syndromes
25. Alarcon-Segovia, D. Drug-induced lupus syndromes. *Mayo Clin. Proc.* 44:664, 1969.
    Thorough discussion that emphasizes a genetic-environmental balance determining drug response. (For a more recent appraisal of the relationship between anticonvulsants and SLE, see Arthritis Rheum. *20:308. 1977.)*
26. Schaller, J. Lupus phenomena in the newborn. *Arthritis Rheum.* 20:312, 1977.
    Brief (two pages) but thorough review of noted abnormalities and their significance. (Also see Medicine [Baltimore] *63:362, 1984.)*
27. Scott, J., et al. Connective-tissue disease, antibodies to ribonucleoprotein, and congenital heart block. *N. Engl. J. Med.* 309:209, 1983.
    An important correlation between congenital complete heart block and the presence of anti-Ro(SS-A) in maternal and infant sera (similar information is presented in J. Pediatr. *103:889, 1983). An accompanying editorial (p. 236) is a helpful summary of knowledge to date.*

86. OTHER RHEUMATIC DISORDERS

Margaret E. Mohrmann

Juvenile rheumatoid arthritis and systemic lupus erythematosus represent at least 90 percent of all rheumatic diseases (excluding acute rheumatic fever) in childhood, but there are a few other disorders that deserve mention.

Dermatomyositis and *polymyositis* are distinct manifestations of what is probably a single disease entity. Polymyositis, the more common of the two in adults, is a disease of chronic muscle inflammation; dermatomyositis, at least 10 times more common than polymyositis in children, is the same disease with the addition of a characteristic rash. Females predominate and the usual age of onset in children is 5 to 8 years.

Most children present with insidious muscle weakness, which may be manifested as "clumsiness," difficulty climbing stairs, or, occasionally, an apparent behavior problem in a child who can no longer dress himself or participate in active play. Weakness is generally greater in proximal muscles and in abductors and extensors. Muscles are usually painful and may be swollen or atrophic. Flexion contractures develop rapidly in children and may already be present at the time of diagnosis. Involvement of palatal and respiratory muscles, manifested by a voice change or difficulty swallowing, is ominous; aspiration and respiratory failure may result.

The rash of dermatomyositis typically begins as an erythematous discoloration (with purplish or "heliotrope" hue) of the eyelids; the scaly eruption soon spreads to involve the periorbital and malar areas and the extensor surfaces of the knees, elbows, and digits. There may be underlying brawny edema, especially around the eyes. The skin lesions are but one sign of the diffuse vasculitis typical of dermatomyositis in children; angiopathic changes may also be seen in palatal lesions and in the gastrointestinal tract, where they may result in perforation or hemorrhage.

Dermatomyositis is diagnosed on the basis of the clinical syndrome of muscle pain and weakness coupled with the typical rash, plus elevated levels in the serum of one or more muscle enzymes (creatine phosphokinase, aldolase, SGOT, LDH). The sedimentation rate, although often elevated, may be normal in the presence of active disease. Antinuclear antibodies and rheumatoid factor are usually absent, although low titers may be found transiently. The electromyogram shows a characteristic, though not diagnostic, mixture of myopathic and neuropathic abnormalities. Histologic studies of muscle reveal nonspecific changes; muscle biopsy is seldom necessary for diagnosis. Differential diagnostic considerations include systemic lupus erythematosus, other connective tissue diseases, bacterial and viral myositis, steroid-induced myopathy, Guillain-Barré syndrome, and muscular dystrophy.

Treatment includes daily high-dose steroids (1.5–2.0 mg/kg/day of prednisone) until remission is achieved, as indicated by clinical improvement, usually paralleled by the return of muscle enzymes to normal. Steroids are then tapered and continued at a low dose for 1 to 2 years. Physical therapy is necessary to increase muscle strength and to prevent or ameliorate flexion contractures.

Death from respiratory failure, gastrointestinal perforation and hemorrhage, and infection occurred in 35 to 50 percent of patients prior to the use of steroids; the majority of survivors were crippled. Now, with prednisone and physical therapy, more than 80 percent of patients recover without sequelae and the mortality is less than 10 percent. Although most children are free of disease within 2 years after diagnosis, some will go on to have a chronic or relapsing course for several more years, requiring constant or intermittent prednisone therapy. Almost 50 percent of patients have scattered subcutaneous calcifications, unresponsive to chelation therapy; the calcinosis may be somewhat disabling but usually does not correlate with ultimate prognosis. Of adults with dermatomyositis, 20 percent are found to have an underlying malignancy; this association does not occur in children.

Scleroderma, a very unusual disease in childhood, involves dermal alterations resulting in "hard skin." In children, the disease most often takes the form of localized scleroderma, which may occur either as morphea or as linear scleroderma. Morphea is a well-circumscribed, variably pigmented, shiny patch of initially edematous, then indurated, and ultimately atrophic skin. Although there may be multiple areas in a single patient, their effect is generally cosmetic only. In contrast, the lesions of linear scleroderma are far more extensive, usually involve underlying tissue down to bone, and frequently cross joints, resulting in contractures and limb atrophy. Thus, localized scleroderma, while not life-threatening, can cause marked dysfunction. Progression of the lesions is variable; complete healing is rare. There is no known effective treatment, although physical therapy can be invaluable in maintaining function. Children with scleroderma, especially of the linear type, may present with synovitis; antinuclear antibodies (nonspecific pattern) and rheumatoid factor are often present, and elevated immunoglobulin levels are common. Progressive systemic sclerosis—diffuse scleroderma with visceral involvement—fortunately is rare in children; the mortality is high, with death generally being due to pulmonary or myocardial fibrosis.

The general category of rheumatic disorders also includes syndromes characterized by specific patterns of primary *vasculitis.* The pathologic process is one of inflammation and necrosis of blood vessels, and the nature of the resulting syndrome depends on the size and location of the vessels involved. Primary vasculitis syndromes in children include Henoch-Schönlein syndrome (see Chap. 91); Wegener granulomatosis, with necrotizing lesions of the face, respiratory tract, and kidneys; polyarteritis nodosa, characterized by fever, arthritis, subcutaneous nodules, and severe hypertension; and infantile polyarteritis nodosa, a uniformly fatal disorder that is clinically and pathologically indistinguishable from fatal cases of Kawasaki disease (mucocutaneous lymph node syndrome).

In recent years a new syndrome has been described, known as *mixed connective tissue disease.* This "overlap" syndrome, said to combine features of systemic lupus erythematosus, progressive systemic sclerosis, and polymyositis, is characterized serologically by the presence of antibodies to ribonucleoprotein. Over time, however, most of these patients have a clinical course similar to that seen in one of their "component" diseases, usually systemic sclerosis. It is probably most important to recognize that many patients with rheumatic disorders are not easily classified into a specific disease category and are perhaps better considered to have an undifferentiated connective tissue disease, rather than an entirely new syndrome.

Reviews

1. Cassidy, J. *Textbook of Pediatric Rheumatology*. New York: Wiley, 1982.
   Excellent chapters on dermatomyositis, scleroderma, and systemic vasculitis.
2. Hanson, V. Dermatomyositis, scleroderma and polyarteritis nodosa. *Clin. Rheum. Dis.* 2:445, 1976.
   A good single article covering the more common "other" rheumatic diseases.

Dermatomyositis

3. Schaller, J. Dermatomyositis. *J. Pediatr.* 83:699, 1973.
   Brief (three pages), pithy, thorough editorial review; an excellent and accessible place to begin. (Differential diagnosis: Pediatr. Rev. *6:163, 1984.)*
4. Banker, B., and Victor, M. Dermatomyositis (systemic angiopathy) of childhood. *Medicine* (Baltimore) 45:261, 1966.
   Lengthy but full of good clinical points and pathologic correlations.
5. Bohan, A., and Peter, J. Polymyositis and dermatomyositis. *N. Engl. J. Med.* 292:344, 403, 1975.
   Comprehensive iconoclastic discussion, mostly about adults; seriously questions the efficacy of steroids, a stance challenged in Arthritis Rheum. *20:338, 1977.*
6. Crowe, W., et al. Clinical and pathogenetic implications of histopathology in childhood polydermatomyositis. *Arthritis Rheum.* 25:126, 1982.
   An important, detailed study linking the severity of the vasculopathy, as observed in muscle biopsy material, to the clinical course of the disease.
7. Pachman, L., and Cooke, N. Juvenile dermatomyositis: A clinical immunologic study. *J. Pediatr.* 96:226, 1980.
   Descriptions of 21 patients, emphasizing multisystem involvement and 72 percent incidence of HLA-B8.
8. Sullivan, D., Cassidy, J., and Petty, R. Dermatomyositis in the pediatric patient. *Arthritis Rheum.* 20:327, 1977.
   Fifteen-year study of 41 patients; good prognosis confirms earlier information published by this group in J. Pediatr. *80:555, 1972.*
9. Dubowitz, V. Treatment of dermatomyositis in childhood. *Arch. Dis. Child.* 51:494, 1976.
   Advocates lower doses and shorter duration of prednisone therapy in the belief that overuse of steroids may increase risk of a chronic course.
10. Miller, J. Late progression of dermatomyositis in childhood. *J. Pediatr.* 83:543, 1973.
    Continued physical and psychologic problems more than 5 years after diagnosis; relationship of later course to initial treatment is unclear.
11. Bowyer, S., et al. Childhood dermatomyositis: Factors predicting functional outcome and development of dystrophic calcification. *J. Pediatr.* 103:882, 1983.
    The most important predictor of prognosis is early and adequate steroid therapy. Four patterns of calcinosis are identified (more detailed descriptions are in AJR *142:397, 1984), one of which—a diffuse, lacy, exoskeletonlike pattern—is associated with a severe clinical course. (Natural history with therapy:* J. Pediatr. *105:399, 1984.)*

Scleroderma

12. Kornreich, H., et al. Scleroderma in childhood. *Arthritis Rheum.* 20:343, 1977.
    This article and the following one (p. 351) present a thorough discussion of 63 patients. (For an older series, with excellent clinicopathologic descriptions, see J. Pediatr. *68:243, 1966.)*

13. Kesler, R., et al. Linear scleroderma in children. *Am. J. Dis. Child.* 135:738, 1981.
    Two cases that dramatically point out both the variable progression of the disease and the marked dysfunction that can result.
14. Hochberg, M. The spectrum of systemic sclerosis: Current concepts. *Hosp. Pract.* 16(3):61, 1981.
    Thorough, detailed review of clinical manifestations and etiologic theories.
15. Dabich, L., et al. Scleroderma in the child. *J. Pediatr.* 85:770, 1974.
    Twelve children with progressive systemic sclerosis; specific diagnostic procedures are necessary to document extent of visceral involvement.

Vasculitis

16. Fan, P., et al. A clinical approach to systemic vasculitis. *Semin. Arthr. Rheum.* 9:248, 1980.
    Well-organized, long, thorough review; for a helpful, briefer review, see Hosp. Pract. *17(1):47, 1982.*
17. Fauci, A., et al. The spectrum of vasculitis. *Ann. Intern. Med.* 89:660, 1978.
    Detailed discussion of general pathophysiology and specific disease entities (16 pages, 139 references).
18. Magilavy, D., et al. A syndrome of childhood polyarteritis. *J. Pediatr.* 91:25, 1977.
    Clinical descriptions of 9 patients; 11 others are described in Pediatrics *60:227, 1977.*
19. Landing, B., and Larson, E. Are infantile periarteritis nodosa with coronary artery involvement and fatal mucocutaneous lymph node syndrome the same? Comparison of 20 patients from North America with patients from Hawaii and Japan. *Pediatrics* 59:651, 1977.
    Detailed pathologic study reveals no differences. (For more on Kawasaki disease, see Pediatrics *54:271, 1974;* Pediatr. Rev. *2:107, 1980; and* Am. J. Dis. Child. *134:603, 1980, and 137:211, 1983.)*

"Mixed Connective Tissue Disease"

20. Sharp, G., et al. Mixed connective tissue disease: An apparently distinct rheumatic disease syndrome associated with a specific antibody to an extractable nuclear antigen (ENA). *Am. J. Med.* 52:148, 1972.
    The original paper, describing 25 patients. (For a long-term follow-up of these patients, revealing their tendency to follow the course of a specific rheumatic disorder, see Medicine *[Baltimore] 59:239, 1980.)*
21. Singsen, B., et al. Mixed connective tissue disease in childhood. *J. Pediatr.* 90:893, 1977.
    Descriptions of 14 patients, all with anti-RNP; childhood course contrasted with the syndrome as described in adults. (For a report of four more cases and a review of the literature, see Pediatrics *67:333, 1981.)*
22. LeRoy C., et al. Undifferentiated connective tissue syndromes. *Arthritis Rheum.* 23:341, 1980.
    Well-reasoned plea to avoid designating new syndromes, since it is clear that many patients with overlapping symptoms will ultimately fit other well-established diagnoses.

XI. HEMATOLOGIC DISORDERS

Dennis C. Stokes and Evan Charney

Iron deficiency is the most common nutritional deficiency in children everywhere, and the most common cause of anemia at all ages. The prevalence in childhood varies widely, depending on age, the population studied, and the definition of deficiency employed. Measures of hemoglobin and hematocrit are best defined for 6-month-old to 2-year-old children, in whom iron deficiency is most common; 3 to 24 percent of children in this age group have been found to be iron-deficient by hematocrit screening. If a transferrin saturation of less than 16 percent is used as a measure (the level at which iron becomes a limiting factor in erythropoiesis) 29 to 68 percent of the entire population may be considered iron deficient!

About 95 percent of the iron in the body is contained in the circulating hemoglobin or in storage form as ferritin. Myoglobin iron constitutes 4 percent of total body iron, and various iron-containing enzymes (e.g., cytochromes, catalases), of major metabolic importance, account for less than 1 percent.

The overt problem in severe iron deficiency is anemia. Infrequently, the anemia is profound and causes congestive heart failure; the implications of mild or moderate iron deficiency are more difficult to define. Because of iron's importance as a cofactor, even moderate degrees of deficiency may have physiologic consequences. Mitochondrial changes, decreased myoglobin concentrations, and decreased synthesis of cytochromes and other heme-containing enzymes have all been described, but the long-term effects of these changes and their relationship to the clinical features of iron deficiency require further definition. Until these effects are more clearly defined, the level at which a person is to be considered iron-deficient will remain controversial.

Irritability, anorexia, and lassitude are well-described behavioral changes associated with iron deficiency, and prompt improvements in both developmental scores and behavior have been reported following iron supplementation in iron-deficient children. A mechanism for these changes has been proposed based on deficiency of the iron-containing enzyme monoamine oxidase.

The exact relationship between iron deficiency and increased susceptibility to infection is controversial. Iron is an important growth factor required by many pathogenic organisms, so iron deficiency in the host could therefore theoretically provide resistance to infection; yet some authors have found an increased number of infections in iron deficient children. There is no convincing evidence for a link between iron deficiency and serious defects in immunity or the risk of serious infection, although subtle impairment in T-cell function, reversible with iron therapy, has been documented.

Chronic infection, thalassemia minor, and lead poisoning are confounding diagnoses commonly found in populations at risk for iron deficiency. In chronic inflammation, iron is taken up by the reticuloendothelial system and is not available for red cell synthesis. Consequently, free erythrocyte protoporphyrin levels, reflecting the unavailability of iron for heme synthesis, are mildly elevated, but serum ferritin levels are usually normal. In thalassemia minor, mean corpuscular volume (MCV) and mean corpuscular hemoglobin (MCH) are low, as in iron deficiency, but ferritin and serum iron are normal; targeting and basophilic stippling of the red cells are seen. In significant lead poisoning, free erythrocyte protoporphyrin (EP) is usually markedly elevated.

The "balance sheet" of iron metabolism begins in the intrauterine environment, when the fetus acquires iron across the placenta by an active process that takes place even if the mother is iron-deficient. The bulk of this transplacental iron is acquired in the third trimester of pregnancy; its importance is reflected by the fact that at 1 year of age, almost 50 percent of the infant's hemoglobin iron is derived from this prenatal endowment. A reduction in this iron store, by, for example, premature birth or neonatal blood loss, may be a major cause of later iron deficiency. The newborn's hemoglobin concentration normally averages 15 gm/dl; it progressively falls to 10 to 12 gm/dl over the first 6 to 8 weeks of life, and iron derived from the breakdown of hemoglobin is stored. As the hemoglobin level rises from this physiologic low point, the stored iron is reutilized. Dietary iron will be required sometime between 2 and 6 months of age, depending on the rate of growth and how rapidly the storage iron is depleted. The full-term infant needs to absorb an additional 165 mg of iron from the diet during the first year of life, primarily to supply iron for the doubling in red cell mass that occurs with growth; the premature infant requires substantially more.

Since milk is the principal component of the infant's diet, its influence on iron status is important. Both human and cow milk contain 0.5 to 0.1 mg/liter of iron, but there is a large difference in the percentage absorbed—50 percent from human milk, versus 10 percent from cow milk. This difference in absorption, which is unexplained, helps protect the breast-fed infant from iron deficiency. The intake of whole cow milk may relate to iron deficiency by at least two mechanisms. First, infants who continue to receive the bulk of their nutrition from cow milk may simply exclude richer dietary sources of iron. Second, in up to 50 percent of infants with a large milk intake, chronic gastrointestinal bleeding due to sensitivity to bovine albumin may develop; substituting evaporated milk or commercial formulas for whole cow milk stops the gastrointestinal blood loss.

Absorption of dietary iron varies markedly, depending on the type of food and other dietary factors: ascorbic acid and lactate enhance absorption; phytates (present in many grain products) reduce it. The form of the dietary iron is also important; iron pyrophosphate and iron orthophosphate were formerly used to supplement infant cereals, but subsequent balance studies showed that only 0.9 percent of the iron was absorbed. The iron in meats is largely in the form of heme, the most efficiently absorbed form of iron (utilizing a different mechanism than inorganic iron) and enhances the absorption of iron from vegetable foods. A feedback mechanism exists whereby persons who have iron deficiency, or have increased requirements, will increase their absorption of dietary iron twofold to threefold.

Iron losses throughout life are normally small, mostly from cells shed in the intestine and from the skin (20 μg/kg/day). However, chronic blood loss from the intestinal tract can quickly deplete the borderline iron stores of children, since each milliliter of blood contains 0.5 mg of iron. In adolescence there are increased requirements for iron because of rapid growth; for women, menstrual losses become the primary determinant of iron requirements.

Useful measures of the status of iron stores include the following: (1) red cell indexes, particularly mean corpuscular volume (MCV); (2) free erythrocyte protoporphyrin (EP), a measure of disordered heme synthesis that occurs with depletion of available iron; and (3) serum ferritin. Serum iron and total iron binding to transferrin are also widely available measures; morning specimens should be obtained to avoid possible confusion due to diurnal variations. Serum iron is normal in mild deficiency states. In adults the lack of hemosiderin (macroaggregates of ferritin) in the bone marrow is considered a valuable diagnostic aid; infants and children normally lack hemosiderin in bone marrow, however, since available iron is in use. In fact, its presence may indicate an abnormal state, such as chronic inflammation or hemolysis. The classic iron deficiency anemia smear, with hypochromic, microcytic red cells is seen relatively late in the sequence of iron deficiency, as are the physical signs of anemia, such as pallor and tachycardia.

Serum ferritin, a measure of storage iron, may also be used as an indicator of the body's iron balance. The newborn's level is higher than the mother's level, increases further as hemoglobin concentration declines in the first 2 months of life, and then falls off again as storage iron is mobilized for growth. Infants not receiving any dietary iron may have no measurable ferritin by 6 months of age, and premature infants may deplete their iron stores by 2 months of age. During childhood, levels of ferritin remain low (20 mg/ml), indicating maximal use of daily iron intake and little storage.

Present recommendations to prevent iron deficiency include the following : (1) encouraging mothers to breast-feed their infants; (2) the use of infant formulas or other heat-treated, iron-fortified milk products rather than whole cow milk from 6 to 12 months of age; (3) ensuring adequate dietary or supplemental iron intake by 4 months of age in full-term infants and by 2 months of age in prematures; (4) screening for anemia at 8 to 12 months of age and frequently thereafter for those at particular risk, e.g., premature infants, pregnant teenagers.

Once iron deficiency is detected, the cause must be identified, particularly in age groups in which a deficient intake is unlikely; blood loss, particularly from the gastrointestinal tract, is a prime consideration. Iron deficiency is easily treated with orally administered ferrous salts, best absorbed (and cheapest) as ferrous sulfate (20% elemental iron). Divided daily doses are better tolerated than single doses and produce an increased rate of hemoglobin production. Therapy should be continued for 8 to 12 weeks after hemoglobin concentration is normal, to replenish iron stores. An adequate iron dose should increase the hematocrit by 1 percent per day, with a reticulocyte count rise after 2 or 3 days of treatment.

Failure of suspected iron deficiency to respond to oral iron supplementation should raise questions of (1) incorrect diagnosis, (2) continued occult blood losses, and/or (3) inadequate compliance with the prescribed regimen.

Reviews

1. Dallman, P., Siimes, M., and Stekel, A. Iron deficiency in infancy and childhood. *Am. J. Clin. Nutr.* 33:86, 1980.
   A thorough review covering major issues of iron nutrition by three authorities in the field; 158 references.
2. Smith, N., and Rios, E. Iron metabolism and iron deficiency in infancy and childhood. *Adv. Pediatr.* 21:239, 1974.
   Another comprehensive review.

Iron Metabolism

3. Finch, C., and Huebers, H. Perspectives in iron metabolism. *N. Engl. J. Med.* 306:1520, 1982.
   Reviews iron balance, deficiency, and overload; 118 references.
4. Oski, F. The nonhematologic manifestations of iron deficiency. *Am. J. Dis. Child.* 133:315, 1979.
   Outlines effect of iron deficiency on growth and on a variety of organ systems.
5. Crosby, W. Who needs iron? *N. Engl. J. Med.* 297:543, 1977.
   The problem of defining iron deficiency in the population.
6. Jacobs, A., and Worwood, M. Ferritin in serum: Clinical and biochemical implications. *N. Engl. J. Med.* 292:951, 1975.
   Serum ferritin accurately reflects iron stores; levels are elevated in the anemia of chronic disease, liver disease, iron overload states, and lymphoblastic leukemia.
7. Hillman, R., and Henderson, P. Control of marrow production by the level of iron supply. *J. Clin. Invest.* 48:454, 1969.
   If transferrin saturation is less than 16 percent, the iron supply for hematopoiesis is inadequate.
8. Smith, N. Iron storage in the first five years of life. *Pediatrics* 16:166, 1955.
   A classic article relating body iron stores at different ages to the incidence of iron deficiency anemia.

Incidence and Detection

9. Dallman, P., and Siimes, M. Percentile curves for hemoglobin and red cell volume in infancy and childhood. *J. Pediatr.* 94:26, 1979.
   Normative data on nonindigent white children; those with thalassemia or iron deficiency were excluded.
10. Public Health Service. *Vital and Health Statistics.* Series 11–No. 232, 1982. DHHS Pub. No. (PHS) 83–1682. Washington, D. C.: Government Printing Office, 1982.
    The largest, least selective data base by far, involving 8709 subjects, 3 to 74 years of age, surveyed between 1976–1980: presents hematocrits, concentrations of hemoglobin, serum iron, total iron-binding capacity, and erythrocyte protoporphyrin, plus red cells indices.
11. Dallman, P. New approaches to screening for iron deficiency. *J. Pediatr.* 90:678, 1977.
    The combination of low mean corpuscular volume, low ferritin, and elevated free erythrocyte protoporphyrin is diagnostic, although a therapeutic trial remains the final test. A useful flow chart for the detection of iron deficiency is presented.
12. Driggers, D., et al. Iron deficiency in one year old infants: Comparison of results of a therapeutic trial in infants with anemia or low-normal hemoglobin values. *J. Pediatr.* 98:753, 1981.
    Almost one-half of those with hemoglobin concentrations of 11.0 to 11.4 gm/dl increased their levels by 1 gm/dl after therapeutic trial of Fe: that defines Fe deficiency, authors contend. (Also see J. Pediatr. 98:894, 1981.)
13. Koerper, M., and Dallman, P. Serum iron concentration and transferrin saturation

in the diagnosis of iron deficiency in children: Normal developmental changes. *J. Pediatr.* 91:870, 1977.

Concludes that transferrin saturation less than 16 percent is not adequate to define iron deficiency if the child is not anemic. (Also see pp. 875 and 1027 in the same issue.)

14. Saarinen, U., Siimes, M., and Dallman, P. Iron absorption in infants: High bioavailability of breast milk iron. *J. Pediatr.* 91:36, 1977.

    Infants absorbed 49 percent of labeled iron from human milk, compared to only 10 percent from cow milk. (Iron in human milk may not be sufficient to prevent deficiency after 3 months of age, however: Pediatr. Res. *15:822, 1981.)*

15. Oski, F., and Landaw, S. Inhibition of iron absorption from human milk by baby food. *Am. J. Dis. Child.* 134:459, 1980.

    Addition of supplemental food to diet of breast-fed infants impairs bioavailability of the iron from human milk.

16. Lundstrom, M., Siimes, M., and Dallman, P. At what age does iron supplementation become necessary in low-birth-weight infants? *Pediatrics* 91:878, 1977.

    Three months. (Also see reference 25.)

17. Dallman, P., et al. Hemoglobin concentration in white, black and Oriental children: Is there a need for separate criteria in screening for anemia? *Am. J. Clin. Nutr.* 31:377, 1978.

    The authors say "yes"; blacks average 0.5 gm/dl lower than whites and Orientals. (Also see Am. J. Clin. Nutr. *34:1645, 1981.) Others contend that iron deficiency accounts for most of the difference:* Am. J. Clin. Nutr. *34:2154, 1981.*

Morbidity: Infection

18. Stockman, J. Infections and iron: Too much of a good thing? *Am. J. Dis. Child.* 135:18, 1981.

19. Committee on Nutrition, American Academy of Pediatrics. Relationship between iron status and incidence of infection in infancy. *Pediatrics* 62:246, 1978.

20. Pearson, H., and Robinson, J. The role of iron in host resistance. *Adv. Pediatr.* 23:1, 1976.

    These three discussions are where to start in the extensive literature on iron deficiency and immunity, particularly the last review (119 references).

Morbidity: Behavior and Other Manifestations

21. Pollitt, E., and Leibel, R. Iron deficiency and behavior. *J. Pediatr.* 88:372, 1976.

    A critical review (81 references).

22. Voorhees, M., et al. Iron deficiency anemia and increased urinary norepinephrine excretion. *J. Pediatr.* 86:542, 1975.

    Elevated urinary catecholamine excretion corrected with iron: the behavioral changes of iron deficiency may be related to changes in catecholamine metabolic pathways. (For a more thorough discussion of this issue, see E. Pollitt and R. Leibel, Iron Deficiency: Brain Biochemistry and Behavior. New York: Raven Press, 1982.)

23. Oski, F., and Honig, A. The effects of therapy on the developmental scores of iron deficient infants. *J. Pediatr.* 92:21, 1978.

    Imferon therapy resulted in improved Bayley test scores after 1 week; may reflect better attention span rather than cognitive gains. (Behavior scores improved in iron deficient infants treated with iron orally for 11 days: J. Pediatr. *102:519, 1983.)*

24. Lozoff, B., et al. The effects of short-term oral iron therapy on developmental deficits in iron-deficient anemic infants. *J. Pediatr.* 100:351, 1982.

    In contrast to above reports, 1 week of oral therapy did not reverse the deficits.

Prevention and Treatment

25. Committee on Nutrition, American Academy of Pediatrics. Iron supplementation for infants. *Pediatrics* 58:765, 1976.

    Dosages are 1 mg/kg/day for full-term infants, starting no later than 4 months of age, and 2 mg/kg/day for prematures, starting no later than 2 months of age; upper limit is 15 mg/day.

26. Wilson, J., Lahey, M., and Heiner, D. Studies on iron metabolism: V. Further observations on cow's milk induced gastrointestinal bleeding in infants with iron-deficiency anemia. *J. Pediatr.* 84:335, 1974.

Gastrointestinal losses do not cease when iron deficiency is corrected; reducing milk intake is required.

88. SICKLE CELL DISEASE
Kenneth B. Roberts

Sickle hemoglobin differs from normal hemoglobin by a single amino acid substitution (valine for glutamic acid) in the number 6 position of the beta chain; it can be distinguished from normal hemoglobin by electrophoresis and by its morphologic effect on the red blood cell when exposed to low oxygen tension ("sickling"). Sickle cell disease is caused by the replacement of both normal hemoglobin genes by genes for hemoglobin S (homozygous hemoglobin SS). It is a common inherited disorder in blacks (1 per 600 black newborns) and causes both morbidity and mortality. Combinations of other abnormal hemoglobins with hemoglobin S (such as SC, Sβ-thalassemia, S-persistence of fetal hemoglobin) are distinguished by electrophoresis and often by clinical characteristics: for example, patients with SS do not have a palpable spleen after about age 6, but splenomegaly persists in patients with SC or Sβ-thalassemia; patients with S-persistence of fetal hemoglobin have particularly mild disease, due to the influence of increased amounts of fetal hemoglobin in each cell. When hemoglobin S is paired with normal hemoglobin A, the result is sickle cell trait, found in approximately 10 percent of the American black population. It is important not to confuse sickle cell *trait* with sickle cell *disease*; it is only the latter that is associated with a profound hemolytic anemia, serious illness, and decreased life expectancy.

The clinical course of patients with sickle cell disease is punctuated by the occurrence of episodic events called *crises,* which are of four types: aplastic, hyperhemolytic, sequestration, and vasocclusive (painful) crises. *Aplastic* crises may occur in any type of chronic hemolytic anemia; they are often triggered by infection and last up to 7 to 10 days. Since survival of the red cell in sickle cell disease is 15 to 20 days (rather than the normal 120 days), markedly increased production by the bone marrow is required to maintain even the modest hemoglobin level of 5.5 to 9.5 gm/dl. The consequences of aplastic crises may therefore be profound: hemoglobin may decrease by 50 percent, necessitating transfusions. The delicate balance in sickle cell disease between increased production and premature destruction is also upset in *hyperhemolytic crises.* Again, infection may be the precipitating event, leading to increased icterus, increased reticulocytosis (which distinguishes hyperhemolytic from aplastic crises), and a fall of hemoglobin and hematocrit to two-thirds or less of the usual level. *Sequestration* crises are uncommon but dramatic events in infants and small children with sickle cell disease; the spleen rapidly enlarges and traps most of the circulating red blood cells, leading in some children to shock and death. Recurrent infarctions and fibrosis of the spleen appear to protect against sequestration crises past the age of 5 or 6 years.

By far the most common crises are the *vasocclusive,* or *painful,* type. These are most frequently skeletal or abdominal. Painful symmetric swelling of the hands and feet due to dactylitis (the "hand-foot syndrome") may be the earliest sign of sickle cell disease in an infant. In older children, skeletal pain is more common in the long bones. Children with sickle cell disease have an increased incidence of osteomyelitis (particularly with *Salmonella*), and the differentiation between infarction (vasocclusive crisis) and infection is often difficult. Joint pain and effusion occasionally occur. Avascular necrosis of the hip is also a skeletal complication, but occurs more frequently in children with SC than with SS disease.

Any intraabdominal structure may be affected by ischemic necrosis resulting from compromise of the blood supply by sickled cells. Patients may have recurrent abdominal crises, but in any given episode the distinction between a vasocclusive crisis and an acute (surgical) abdomen, such as from appendicitis, may be difficult.

Sickle cell disease also affects other organ systems, including the nervous system. Cerebrovascular accidents are uncommon in affected infants and children but do occur; a program of regular, repeated transfusions is often instituted after a cerebrovascular accident to prevent recurrence. The lungs are commonly subjected to infarction and infection—again, the differentiation in a given episode may not be possible. Hypoxemia from lower respiratory tract involvement is common and hazardous, since it may promote further sickling. Infarction of renal tissue, particularly in the medullary area, leads to inability to concentrate the urine (hyposthenuria), papillary necrosis, and hematuria; hematuria occurs both in individuals with sickle cell disease and in those with sickle trait and is usually unilateral, the left kidney being more frequently involved. Priapism may occur in children, but is more common toward puberty than earlier. Leg ulcers are not usually a problem until adolescence or early adulthood, but then become a source of continued morbidity.

The greatest threat to life in sickle cell disease is serious overwhelming infection, a common complication in the first 5 years of life. During that time the incidence of meningitis is approximately 5 percent and the incidence of septicemia an additional 4 percent. The pneumococcus is the usual organism, but there is also a marked increase in the incidence of serious *Haemophilus influenzae* infection. The major determinant of inadequate host protection appears to be related to dysfunction of the spleen. Beginning at several months of age, long before anatomic infarction and fibrosis of the spleen have taken place, a state of "functional asplenia" can be demonstrated. During this time, presumably both the antibody-producing and the mechanical-filtering functions of the spleen are compromised. After the age of 5 or 6 years, serious infections become less frequent, possibly because of accumulated antigenic experience, and the hospitalization rate for children with sickle cell disease decreases.

The repeated crises, time lost from school, limited tolerance for strenuous physical activity, and delayed growth and maturation combine to make sickle cell disease not only a physically painful disorder but a potentially emotionally crippling one as well. Children require reassurance that they will not be left to suffer alone and that appropriate analgesia will be prescribed. It is important that children with sickle cell disease not fall behind in school and that opportunities for success be provided.

Although the molecular basis of sickle cell disease was elucidated approximately 4 decades ago, there is still no cure or even satisfactory palliation. Therapy consists primarily of providing analgesia and adequate hydration; in some clinical situations, antibiotics, oxygen, and red blood cell transfusions are also required. Specific agents, such as urea, have been promoted, but without exception the initial enthusiasm has faded, as carefully controlled studies demonstrated their lack of clinical efficacy.

During the 1960s, screening programs were developed to detect persons with sickle trait so that genetic counseling could be provided. It is not clear that the outcome of the programs has been beneficial, however, and such activities have been curtailed. Prenatal determination of sickle cell disease is now available and may be of value in selected families.

Reviews, Series, Natural History

1. Powars, D. Natural history of sickle cell disease—the first ten years. *Semin. Hematol.* 12:267, 1975.
   A retrospective focus on the first decade in over 400 patients.
2. Karayalcin, G., et al. Sickle cell anemia—clinical manifestations in 100 patients and review of the literature. *Am. J. Med. Sci.* 269:51, 1975.
   A retrospective review of 100 patients aged 3 months to 50 years.
3. Davis, J., Vichinsky, E., and Lubin, B. Current treatment of sickle cell disease. *Curr. Probl. Pediatr.* 10(12), 1980.
   An encyclopedic review (64 pages, 178 references)—more than treatment is covered.
4. O'Brien, R., et al. Prospective study of sickle cell anemia in infancy. *J. Pediatr.* 89:205, 1976.
   The clinical course of 12 infants diagnosed in a cord blood screening program.

Crises

5. Pearson, H., and Diamond, L. The critically ill child: Sickle cell disease crises and their management. *Pediatrics* 48:629, 1971.
   A good description of the crises and an approach to management.
6. Jenkins, M., Scott, R., and Baird, R. Studies in sickle cell anemia. XVI. Sudden death

during sickle cell crises in young children. *J. Pediatr.* 56:30, 1960.
Beware the sequestration crisis.

Specific Organ Involvement

7. Bromberg, P. Pulmonary aspects of sickle cell disease. *Arch. Intern. Med.* 133:652, 1974.
   Common problem; secondary to infection, or vascular occlusion, or both.
8. Stevens, M., Padwick, M., and Serjeant, G. Observations on the natural history of dactylitis in homozygous sickle cell disease. *Clin. Pediatr.* (Phila.) 20:311, 1981.
   Dactylitis occurred in 45 percent of 233 infants followed from birth.
9. Keeley, K., and Buchanan, G. Acute infarction of long bones in children with sickle cell anemia. *J. Pediatr.* 101:170, 1982.
   Crisis at least 50 times more common than osteomyelitis; distinction between the two is difficult. (Remember Salmonella as major cause of osteomyelitis in children with sickle cell disease: J. Pediatr. *99:411, 1981.)*
10. Schmidt, J., and Flocks, R. Urologic aspects of sickle cell hemoglobin. *J. Urol.* 106:740, 1971.
    A brief discussion of five genitourinary manifestations (hematuria, papillary necrosis, priapism, pyelonephritis of pregnancy, and hyposthenuria), with emphasis on priapism. (Fertility in males also a problem: Lancet *2:275, 1981.)*
11. Portnoy, B., and Herion, J. Neurological manifestations in sickle cell disease. *Ann. Intern. Med.* 76:643, 1972.
    Neurologic manifestations, two-thirds of which were hemiplegia, were observed in 26 percent.
12. Lindsay, J., Meshel, J., and Patterson, R. The cardiovascular manifestations of sickle cell disease. *Arch. Intern. Med.* 133:643, 1974.
    These were the result of chronic, severe anemia, and vasocclusive events.
13. Sarnaik, S., et al. Incidence of cholelithiasis in sickle cell anemia using the ultrasonic gray-scale technique. *J. Pediatr.* 96:1005, 1980.
    From 12 percent in 2 to 4 year olds to 42 percent in 15 to 18 year olds. (Occurs in patients with SC and Sβ-thalassemia as well as SS hemoglobin: Am. J. Dis. Child. *138:66, 1984; for a series of eight patients with SS disease and gallstones, see* Am. J. Dis. Child. *133:306, 1979.)*

Infection

14. Pearson, H. Sickle cell anemia and severe infections due to encapsulated bacteria. *J. Infect. Dis.* 136:S25, 1977.
    An excellent, concise review of mechanisms and approaches to the problem, with the appropriate references.
15. Overturf, G., Powars, D., and Baraff, L. Bacterial meningitis and septicemia in sickle cell disease. *Am. J. Dis. Child.* 131:784, 1977.
    Confirms the preschool years as the time of highest risk and the pneumococcus as by far the most frequent organism. (The same group reports decreasing major morbidity in pneumococcal disease without prophylaxis or vaccine: JAMA *245:1839, 1981; others confirm benefit of aggressive treatment of febrile youngsters with sickle cell disease: e.g.,* J. Pediatr. *96:199, 1980.)*
16. Rogers, D., Vaidya , S., and Serjeant, G. Early splenomegaly in homozygous sickle cell disease: An indicator of susceptibility to infection. *Lancet* 2:963, 1978.
    *Low fetal hemoglobin levels also a risk factor for early severe disease (*J. Pediatr. *98:37, 1981).*
17. Topley, J., et al. Pneumococcal and other infections in children with sickle cell-hemoglobin C (SC) disease. *J. Pediatr.* 101:176, 1982.
    Serious infection more common in children with SC than with AA hemoglobin, particularly in infancy, and particularly in those infants with early splenomegaly.
18. Buchanan, G., and Glader, B. Leukocyte counts in children with sickle cell disease: Comparative values in the steady state, vaso-occlusive crisis, and bacterial infection. *Am. J. Dis. Child.* 132:396, 1978.

Total leukocyte and PMNs increased during crises and infections; bands increased only in infection.

19. Nottidge, V. Pneumococcal meningitis in sickle cell disease in childhood. *Am. J. Dis. Child.* 137:29, 1983.
    More frequent but not more severe than in children without sickle cell disease.

20. Immunization Practices Advisory Committee, Centers for Disease Control. Pneumococcal polysaccharide vaccine. *Ann. Intern. Med.* 96:203, 1982.
    Unfortunately, children with sickle cell disease do not have a uniformly good antibody response to all the types in the vaccine (J. Pediatr. 100:404, 1982) and failures occur (N. Engl. J. Med. 301:26, 1979). (New "expanded" pneumococcal vaccine: Med. Lett. Drugs Ther. 25:91, 1983.)

Treatment/Prevention

21. Dean, J., and Schechter, A. Sickle-cell anemia: Molecular and cellular bases of therapeutic approaches. *N. Engl. J. Med.* 299:752, 804, 863, 1978.
    Illustrates the molecular basis of sickling; reviews past attempts and future possibilities (three parts, 322 references). (For newer approaches, see J. Clin. Pharmacol. 22:1, 1982, and Blood 62:370, 1983.)

22. Wilimas, J., et al. Efficacy of transfusion therapy for one to two years in patients with sickle cell disease and cerebral vascular accidents. *J. Pediatr.* 96:205, 1980.
    A high recurrence rate after 1 to 2 years of transfusion therapy; with editorial, page 243. (Also see Am. J. Dis. Child. 133:1254, 1979.)

23. Lanzkowsky, P., et al. Partial exchange transfusion in sickle cell anemia. *Am. J. Dis. Child.* 132:1206, 1978.
    For use in serious complications (e.g., "acute lung syndrome") and in preparation for surgery.

24. Whitten, C., and Fischoff, J. Psychosocial effects of sickle cell disease. *Arch. Intern. Med.* 133:681, 1974.
    An excellent essay relevant to supportive management of children with any chronic disease.

Growth and Maturation

25. Jimenez, C., et al. Studies in sickle cell anemia: XXVI. The effects of homozygous sickle cell disease on the onset of menarche, pregnancy, fertility, pubescent changes, and body growth in Negro subjects, *Am. J. Dis. Child.* 111:497, 1966.
    Menarche was delayed, pregnancy complicated, fertility decreased, pubescent changes delayed, and body growth decreased. (Also see N. Engl. J. Med. 311:7, 1984.)

Screening and Sickle Cell Trait

26. Motulsky, A. Frequency of sickling disorders in U.S. blacks. *N. Engl. J. Med.* 288:31, 1973.
    The calculations.

27. Atlas, S. The sickle cell trait and surgical complications. *JAMA* 229:1078, 1974.
    No increased rate of complications was found in a matched-pair patient analysis. (But under certain environmental conditions, individuals with sickle cell trait may be at risk: N. Engl. J. Med. 282:323, 1970.)

28. Rowley, P., and Huntzinger, D. Newborn sickle cell screening: Benefits and burdens realized. *Am. J. Dis. Child.* 137:341, 1983.
    The continuing story of screening program in upstate New York. (For the story from Houston, see Am. J. Dis. Child. 138:44, 1984; for discussion of potential misunderstanding about sickle cell trait following a screening program, see sickle cell "nondisease:" Am. J. Dis. Child. 128:58, 1974.)

29. Boehm, C., et al. Prenatal diagnosis using DNA polymorphisms. *N. Engl. J. Med.* 308:1054, 1983.
    Appears safe and accurate.

89. HEMOPHILIA
Kenneth B. Roberts

The hemophilias are a group of inherited disorders characterized by decreased clotting factor activity, with prolonged and often spontaneous bleeding. Hemophilia A, or classic hemophilia, results from subnormal factor VIII clotting activity. Until recently it was thought that factor VIII was absent, but it is now recognized that material identified antigenically as factor VIII is present although clotting activity is reduced. It is currently believed that factor VIII has three components: factor VIII–related antigen, factor VIII clotting activity, and von Willebrand factor. Patients with classic hemophilia have very low clotting activity (often less than 1%), but normal amounts of antigenic activity. Carriers have normal or low normal activity, disproportionately low for their level of antigenic activity, which is normal. Patients with von Willebrand's disease may have low levels of clotting activity, proportionate to their level of antigenic activity; in addition, because of a deficiency of von Willebrand factor, they also have abnormal platelet function, evidenced by a prolonged bleeding time. Hemophilia B (Christmas disease) results from deficient factor IX activity. Both hemophilias A and B are sex-linked disorders; however, the mutation rate for hemophilia A is said to be upward of 25 percent, one of the highest known in human disease. von Willebrand's disease is autosomally transmitted and thus affects both sexes equally.

For reasons that remain unclear, hemophilia is rarely manifested on the first day of life, even after a difficult delivery. Factor VIII does not cross the placenta, yet only rarely does the newborn with hemophilia experience increased bruising or unusually severe cephalhematomas. Even after circumcision, 75 percent of affected neonates have only mild or no bleeding; a complication from the procedure implies severe disease, defined as less than 1 percent normal activity. The first few months of life are usually a benign period during which the only clinical clues to the diagnosis may be exaggerated bruising from contact with crib slats. When walking—and falling!—begins, excessive bruising and bleeding, particularly of the lip and tongue, are noted. Ecchymoses and soft-tissue bleeding remain common in childhood, but since platelet function and vascular integrity are normal (except in von Willebrand's disease), petechiae are not a feature.

Once the diagnosis of hemophilia is suspected, laboratory confirmation is accomplished in two steps. First, screening tests for coagulation function are made: the platelets are normal in number and the prothrombin time is not prolonged. Bleeding time is usually normal, although recent reports note a number of patients with hemophilia who have prolonged bleeding times for reasons not understood. The earlobe should not be used as a site for this test because bleeding, if prolonged, may be difficult to control. Partial thromboplastin time is prolonged in patients with moderate or severe hemophilia, but is normal in persons with 30 percent or more of normal factor VIII activity. The second step is the identification of the specific factor deficiency. This may be done by correcting the partial thromboplastin time by the addition of specific factors but is best done by specific factor assay. With the advent of cryoprecipitate and specific concentrates, the distinction between hemophilia A and B is of critical therapeutic importance and should be accomplished by an experienced, reliable laboratory.

The most dread complication of hemophilia is intracranial bleeding. It is important to recognize that the clinical signs need not be those of a sudden catastrophe but often reflect slow, persistent oozing; thus, a headache persisting 12 hours or more assumes great significance and should be managed aggressively.

Although soft-tissue hemorrhages usually respond readily to factor replacement therapy, special attention to bleeding involving the floor of the mouth or the neck is mandatory because of the threat of airway compromise. A similar kind of mass effect may compromise neurovascular function in closed spaces such as the forearm; in the retroperitoneum, extensive bleeding can occur with few clinical signs prior to the appearance of evidence that lower extremity function is decreased.

A clinical hallmark of hemophilia is the tendency to spontaneous hemarthroses and the chronic disabling arthropathy that ensues. The knees are most often affected, followed in order by the elbows, ankles, hips, and shoulders. Initially, the joint is tense and tender, and motion is limited. In the subacute stage, the synovium is boggy and thickened, but pain is generally not a feature; osteoporosis is detectable by x-ray examination, but the joint itself appears preserved. If progression continues, the result is a fibrotic, contracted nonfunctional joint. Early treatment of intraarticular bleeding (such as by home treatment programs) decreases the morbidity and retards the development of arthropathy: 10 to 15 percent of patients given optimal early care nevertheless eventually require the services of physical therapists and orthopedic surgeons. The role of acute aspiration of intraarticular blood, installation of chemical agents into the joint (so-called medical synovectomy), operative synovectomy, and total joint replacement is uncertain at present, each major center having its own protocol. Similarly, other therapies for special problems in hemophilia, such as the administration of epsilon-aminocaproic acid for dental bleeding and prednisone for hematuria, are advocated by many groups but are not accepted by all.

The treatment of hemorrhage is based on replacement of missing factor activity to a level required to control bleeding. One unit of activity is defined as the mean level of activity in 1 ml of pooled population plasma; a person may have between 50 and 200 percent activity (i.e., 50–200 units/dl of plasma) and still be "normal." Specific regimens vary from center to center, but all agree on certain basic principles, such as the "normalization" or "supernormalization" of coagulant activity during episodes of life-threatening (e.g., central nervous system) hemorrhage or major surgery. Common bleeding episodes, such as soft-tissue hemorrhages and hemarthroses, may be treated by infusions at home when detected early; home treatment programs are generally regarded as highly successful.

Replacement therapy in children with hemophilia is limited by the development of inhibitors to infused clotting factors. These inhibitors are antibodies of the IgG type and may be present in astronomical titers; they are reported to occur in approximately 10 percent of children with hemophilia. In small children or early in the course of a bleeding event, it may be possible to overwhelm the inhibitor with large amounts of infused factor; eventually, such therapy becomes not only technically unfeasible and taxing on local resources but also futile. "Activated prothrombin complex," although not without problems, may prove useful in such situations.

Analgesia is often required, but agents that interfere with platelet function, such as aspirin, can have devastating effects and should be avoided. There is often dramatic relief of the pain of acute hemarthrosis with prompt factor VIII infusion.

Emotional and psychologic support of both child and family is essential. It is often difficult for an affected child, who feels perfectly well, to accept the limitations on his activities imposed by hemophilia. Because of the inherited nature of the disorder, feelings of guilt may complicate the parents' (particularly the mother's) response. Many centers have established parent groups to permit sharing of problems and methods of coping. Of particular value is a close relationship with a physician who is both supportive and responsive to medical needs.

Reviews and Natural History

1. Buchanan, G. Hemophilia. *Pediatr. Clin. North Am.* 27:309, 1980.
   An excellent, general review.
2. Baehner, R., and Strauss, H. Hemophilia in the first year of life. *N. Engl. J. Med.* 275:524, 1966.
   Serious bleeding is unusual in the neonatal period and first few months of life.
3. Massie, R. *Nicholas and Alexandra.* London: Gollancz, 1968.
   Biography of the last czar and czarina, written by and about the parents of a child with hemophilia; provides insight into the family's suffering.
4. Lewis, J., Spero, J., and Hasiba, U. Death in hemophiliacs, *JAMA* 236:1238, 1976.
   Since the 1930s, the average age at death has increased to 52.

Factor VIII, Diagnosis, and Differential Diagnosis

5. Montgomery, R., and Hathaway, W. Acute bleeding emergencies. *Pediatr. Clin. North Am.* 27:327, 1980.
   Distinguishes hemophilia(s) from other bleeding disorders.
6. Ratnoff, O. Antihemophilic factor (factor VIII). *Ann. Intern. Med.* 88:403, 1978.
   Another review of the structure and function of factor VIII: Blood 58:1, 1981.
7. Klein, H., et al. A co-operative study for the detection of the carrier state of classic hemophilia. *N. Engl. J. Med.* 296:959, 1977.

The use of the ratio of factor VIII antigenic material to coagulant activity is discussed.

8. Firshein, S., et al. Prenatal diagnosis of classic hemophilia. *N. Engl. J. Med.* 300:937, 1979.
   At risk male fetuses with and without hemophilia were correctly identified.

9. Lian, E., and Deykin, D. Diagnosis of von Willebrand's disease. *Am. J. Med.* 60:344, 1976.
   Differentiating hemophilia, von Willebrand's disease, and thrombocytopathy by a combination of the "ratio" test and platelet function tests.

10. Zimmerman, T., Abildgaard, C., and Meyer, D. The factor VIII abnormality in severe von Willebrand's disease. *N. Engl. J. Med.* 301:1307, 1979.
    Severe von Willebrand's disease is a multitude of disorders.

Complications

11. Arnold, W., and Hilgartner, M. Hemophilic arthropathy. *J. Bone Joint Surg.* [A] 59:287 1977.
    A cause of chronic disability that deserves early, vigorous attention (differs from author's previous review: Adv. Pediatr. 21:139, 1974, in its increased emphasis on orthopedic aspects).

12. Blattner, R. Recent developments in the management of hemophilia with particular reference to intracranial bleeding. *J. Pediatr.* 70:449, 1967.
    Beware the prolonged headache.

13. Lancourt, J., Gilbert, M., and Posner, M. Management of bleeding and associated complications of hemophilia in the hand and forearm. *J. Bone Joint Surg.* [A] 59:451, 1977.
    Emphasizes the prevention of contractures.

14. Wolff, L., and Lovrien, E. Management of fractures in hemophilia. *Pediatrics* 70:431, 1982.
    Discusses the medical and orthopedic management of fractures and of pseudotumor (bone destruction from soft-tissue hematoma).

15. Speero, J., et al. The high risk of chronic liver disease in multitransfused juvenile hemophiliac patients. *J. Pediatr.* 94:875, 1979.
    Of 72 patients treated with factor concentrates, 32 had persistently elevated transaminase values, compared with only 1 of 15 treated with cryoprecipitates or fresh-frozen plasma.

16. Desforges, J. AIDS and preventive treatment in hemophilia. *N. Engl. J. Med.* 308:94, 1983.
    An editorial accompanying two reports of impaired cell-mediated immunity in patients with classic hemophilia (pp. 79 and 83).

Selected Aspects of Therapy

17. Honig, G., et al. Administration of single doses of AHF (factor VIII) concentrates in the treatment of hemophilic hemarthroses. *Pediatrics* 43:26, 1969.
    Demonstrates efficacy of a single whopping dose calculated to provide duration of coverage equivalent to that of smaller, more frequent infusions.

18. Smith, P., Keyes, N., and Forman, E. Socioeconomic evaluation of a state-funded comprehensive hemophilia-care program *N. Engl. J. Med.* 306:575, 1982.
    Modern goals include self-treatment, integration of children into school, and satisfying employment of adults.

19. Roberts, H. Hemophiliacs with inhibitors: Therapeutic options. *N. Engl. J. Med.* 305:757, 1981.
    Problems with prothrombin-complex concentrates: Pediatrics 74:290, 1984.

90. IDIOPATHIC THROMBOCYTOPENIC PURPURA
Kenneth B. Roberts

The three cardinal features of idiopathic thrombocytopenic purpura (ITP) in childhood are the following: thrombocytopenia, with a platelet count less than 100,000 per cu mm (usually much less); the presence of normal or increased number of megakaryocytes in the bone marrow; and the absence of other disorders capable of causing thrombocytopenic purpura, such as leukemia or systemic lupus erythematosus (SLE). Some authors also include absence of splenomegaly as a characteristic of ITP, but up to 10 percent of affected children have a palpable spleen tip.

The normal platelet count in the peripheral blood is between 150,000 and 400,000 per cu mm; platelet survival time is 9.9 days, and there is a turnover of 35,000/cu mm/day. In severe ITP the half-life of the platelets may be less than 9 minutes. The problem is one of destruction and reticuloendothelial system removal rather than production; indeed, production is 2 to 8 times normal.

On the basis of age, sex, and outcome, it is clear that ITP is not a single, homogeneous disorder. In younger children (peak age 3–4 years) the sexes are equally affected, and the clinical course is usually benign. In adults and adolescents in their late teens, girls outnumber boys by 2 to 3 : 1, and the course is likely to be protracted and complicated. The initial clinical picture is the same in both groups, however: bruises, petechiae, and purpura are present in virtually all affected children. Gastrointestinal, genitourinary, and mucous membrane bleeding occurs in one-fourth to one-third of patients. The most serious complication is intracranial hemorrhage, which occurs in 1 to 3 percent of children, usually—but not always—in the first month of illness.

Approximately 50 percent of the children with ITP have a history of an infectious illness in the previous 6 weeks, usually an upper respiratory tract infection; chickenpox, rubella, infectious mononucleosis, hepatitis, mumps, measles, and pertussis have also been associated. These children with postinfectious ITP have the shortest, most benign course; 90 percent recover, one-half within 4 to 8 weeks. Mechanisms proposed to explain the development of ITP following viral infection include the trapping of platelets in virus-antibody complexes and the destruction of platelets by virus-stimulated lymphocytes (immunocytes). In up to 85 percent of patients, an IgG antiplatelet antibody can be demonstrated.

The distinction between SLE (see Chap. 85) and ITP may be particularly difficult, and 2 to 3 percent of children felt to have ITP demonstrate evidence of SLE within 10 years of the acute episode. Evidence of SLE develops in approximately one-third of children whose ITP becomes chronic and who require splenectomy.

Treatment with corticosteroids is advocated by many to decrease splenic phagocytosis of platelets, decrease splenic production of antibody against platelets, stabilize small vessels and, possibly, accelerate the spontaneous increase in the platelet count. The routine use of corticosteroids has been questioned, however, because of potential toxicity and a lack of convincing evidence that the incidence of intracranial hemorrhage is reduced. In addition, concern has been expressed that corticosteroids might delay ultimate recovery, or even perpetuate the thrombocytopenia after prolonged administration. Most clinicians presently favor a short course of corticosteroids for their patients with very low platelet counts.

Immunosuppressive agents appear to have no place in acute disease; their role in the management of chronic ITP is uncertain. Platelet transfusions are generally futile, but are administered as an emergency procedure in intracranial hemorrhage, along with splenectomy. Splenectomy is also considered in intractable, chronic ITP if the disease hampers the patient. The role of intravenous gamma globulin is not yet clear.

Mortality during the acute episode is rare, and most patients recover without recognized sequelae. Clinical relapses are unusual and suggest the presence of a disorder such as SLE. "Cure" may be more apparent than real, however; platelet kinetic studies in many patients demonstrate continued peripheral destruction of platelets, although at a rate that can be matched by increased bone marrow production. During intercurrent illness, marrow activity slows, and thrombocytopenia may be manifested. Newborns of mothers with a prior history of ITP may be thrombocytopenic, which presumably is a reflection of persistent maternal antiplatelet IgG. Relapses are unusual and suggest the presence of a disorder such as SLE.

Reviews

1. McClure, P. Idiopathic thrombocytopenic purpura in children: Diagnosis and management. *Pediatrics* 55:68, 1975.
   A brief but thorough review; an excellent place to start.

2. Schulman, I. Idiopathic (immune) thrombocytopenic purpura in children: Pathogenesis and treatment. *Pediatr. Rev.* 5:173, 1983.
   An update, emphasizing newer aspects of therapy and infants born to mothers with ITP.

Series

3. Choi, S., and McClure, P. Idiopathic thrombocytopenic purpura in childhood. *Can. Med. Assoc. J.* 97:562, 1967.
   A review of 239 children with ITP over a 15-year period.
4. Lusher, J., and Zuelzer, W. Idiopathic thrombocytopenic purpura in childhood. *J. Pediatr.* 68:971. 1966.
   Most of this group of 152 children did not have steroid therapy.

Pathogenesis

5. Karpatkin, S., et al. Cumulative experience in the detection of antiplatelet antibody in 234 patients with idiopathic thrombocytopenic purpura, systemic lupus erythematosus and other clinical disorders. *Am. J. Med.* 52:776, 1972.
   Antiplatelet antibody was present in 65 percent of patients with ITP and in 78 percent of those with systemic lupus erythematosus (even though only 4% of latter were thrombocytopenic).
6. Harker, L. Thrombokinetics in idiopathic thrombocytopenic purpura. *Br. J. Haematol.* 19:95, 1970.
   Platelet production increases (2–8 times normal) in proportion to the amount of peripheral destruction.
7. Karpatkin, S., Garg, S., and Siskind, G. Autoimmune thrombocytopenic purpura and the compensated thrombocytolytic state. *Am. J. Med.* 51:1, 1971.
   Combines the observations of references 5 and 6 in an editorial emphasizing that platelet count may be normal during "remissions," despite persistent platelet destruction if marrow can keep up. (Present status of a "platelet Coombs test": N. Engl. J. Med. 309:490, 1983.)
8. McMillan, R., et al. Quantitation of platelet-binding IgG produced in vitro by spleens from patients with idiopathic thrombocytopenic purpura. *N. Engl. J. Med.* 291:812, 1974.
   The spleen not only clears platelets but also is in itself a source of antibody.
9. Shattil, S., and Bennett, J. Platelets and their membranes in hemostasis: Physiology and pathophysiology. *Ann. Intern. Med.* 94:108, 1980.
   In case you want to know more about platelets.

Diagnostic Considerations

10. Lightsey, A. Thrombocytopenia in children. *Pediatr. Clin. North Am.* 27:293, 1980.
    The differential diagnosis.
11. Rabinowitz, Y., and Dameshek, W. Systemic lupus erythematosus after "idiopathic" thrombocytopenic purpura: A review. *Ann. Intern. Med.* 52:1, 1960.
    On recall and review of patients with ITP who underwent splenectomy, SLE was diagnosed or suspected in one-third; need for long-term follow-up is stressed.
12. Radel, E., and Schorr, J. Thrombocytopenic purpura with infectious mononucleosis. *J. Pediatr.* 63:46, 1963.
    Infectious TP in infectious mononucleosis mimicked leukemia.
13. Pui, C., Wilimas, J., and Wang, W. Evans syndrome in childhood. *J. Pediatr.* 97:754, 1980.
    Elaborates on idiopathic thrombocytopenic purpura in combination with autoimmune hemolytic anemia.
14. Miller, B., and Beardsley, D. Autoimmune pancytopenia of childhood associated with multisystem disease manifestations. *J. Pediatr.* 103:877, 1983.
    ITP with neutropenia and anemia; all patients subsequently developed nonhematologic disease manifestations.

Steroids, Intracranial Hemorrhage

15. Woerner, S., Abildgaard, C., and French, B. Intracranial hemorrhage in children with idiopathic thrombocytopenic purpura. *Pediatrics* 67:453, 1981.

A review of the most dreaded complication with an editorial discussion of why we don't know more (p. 570).

16. McClure, P. Idiopathic thrombocytopenic purpura in children: Should corticosteroids be given? And Zuelzer, W., and Lusher, J. Childhood idiopathic thrombocytopenic purpura: To treat or not to treat. *Am. J. Dis. Child.* 131:357, 360, 1977.
Arguments pro and con are given (with Gellis editorial).

17. Weinblatt, M., and Ortega, J. Steroid responsiveness. *Am. J. Dis. Child.* 136:1064, 1982.
Subtitled "A predictor of the outcome of splenectomy in children with chronic immune thrombocytopenic purpura."

Other Treatment

18. Imbach, P., et al. High-dose intravenous gammaglobulin for idiopathic thrombocytopenic purpura in childhood. *Lancet* 1:1228, 1981.
The results in 13 children are reported; 6 of the children had acute ITP, 7 had chronic or intermittent disease.

19. Finch, S., et al. Immunosuppressive therapy of chronic idiopathic thrombocytopenic purpura. *Am. J. Med.* 56:4, 1974.
A report on the treatment of 12 adults with various immunosuppressive drugs, plus a review of the literature and a discussion of problems in interpreting testimonials; concludes that immunosuppressives are a last resort.

20. Ahn, Y., et al. Danazol for the treatment of idiopathic thrombocytopenic purpura. *N. Engl. J. Med.* 308:1396, 1983.
Hormonal therapy was beneficial to some adults with chronic ITP.

Chronic ITP

21. McMillan, R. Chronic idiopathic thrombocytopenic purpura. *N. Engl. J. Med.* 304:1135, 1981.
A thorough review (12 pages, 16 references).

91. HENOCH-SCHÖNLEIN SYNDROME
Kenneth B. Roberts

The diagnostic designations *anaphylactoid purpura* and *Henoch-Schönlein purpura* (HSP) call attention to the purpuric rash, but it has been the association of the rash with visceral manifestations that has fascinated clinicians for over a century. Schönlein (1837) is credited with relating joint findings to the rash; Henoch added the gastrointestinal complaints (1874) and, incidentally, noted renal involvement (1899). As early as 1806, however, Heberden had described the case of a 5-year-old boy with all the cardinal features of HSS: skin, gastrointestinal, renal, and joint involvement and a course marked by recurrences. The diagnosis of HSS remains the province of the clinician with knowledge of the individual features, since there is no pathognomonic laboratory test.

Purpura is considered a sine qua non by most authors, but the lesions first appear as pink, rounded papules, most commonly on the extensor surfaces of the limbs, the buttock, and lower back and only seldom on the face; they may blanch at this stage. Soon they are red and by 24 hours are flat and purpuric. As the lesions clear over 3 to 4 days, the purple color fades to brown and yellow with residual discoloration persisting for up to 10 to 14 days. Petechiae or ecchymoses occur in some patients coincident with the purpura but are by no means universally present; more common is urticaria, which precedes the purpura in one-third of cases. Subcutaneous edema, particularly of the scalp and eyelids, can be a striking feature of HSS, occurring particularly in younger patients; it is frequently painful. This presentation is usually not associated with severe renal involvement and occurs independent of proteinuria and edema elsewhere on the body. Although rash is present in virtually 100 percent of cases (essentially by definition), it is the first sign in only one-half and perhaps need not be purpuric (thus Henoch-Schönlein syndrome).

True arthritis is not a feature of HSS. Periarticular pain and swelling may be noted, most frequently in knees and ankles. Some disability ascribed to "joint pain" is found in most children with HSS (70–80%) and, particularly when combined with an urticarial rash (considered erythema marginatum), may suggest the diagnosis of rheumatic fever. The arthralgia is not of the same intensity as that in acute rheumatic fever, however, and the correct diagnosis can usually be made by careful serial observations and attention to clinical detail.

Abdominal pain is as common a finding as joint pain, but the two do not necessarily appear together. Melena may occur in one-half the patients and is usually associated with pain; the stools are guaiac-positive in another 25 percent. Significant blood loss occurs in from 5 to 15 percent of children with HSS. Vomiting and hematemesis occur with about the same incidence. Between 3 and 6 percent have intussusception; this potentially lethal complication can be difficult indeed to diagnose and is made no easier by the ileoileal location in 50 percent of the reported cases (75% of "usual" intussusceptions in children are ileocolic and therefore easily detected by barium enema). Resection of bowel is commonly required for reduction of intussusception in HSS, reflecting the difficulty in early diagnosis.

Renal manifestations are apparent in about 50 percent of patients with HSS, but, in addition, some children without overt findings show abnormalities on biopsy. Renal involvement is usually detected after the onset of skin and joint complaints; less than one-half of the patients with urinary findings are identified in the first week of illness and "new" abnormalities may appear 4 to 6 weeks after the onset of illness. Hematuria occurs in virtually all children who evidence renal involvement and is more commonly microscopic than gross (1.5:1.0). Children who have only microscopic hematuria have minor focal lesions on biopsy and do not appear to have an impaired prognosis. Nephrotic syndrome and "nephritis syndrome" (i.e., edema, hypertension, azotemia, urinary abnormalities) are likely to be the manifestations of a proliferative glomerulonephritis of greater import.

While skin, joints, gastrointestinal tract, and kidneys may all be involved (as in Heberden's patient), there is a tendency to "subsyndromes," based on the age of the patient. Younger children (around age 2) are more likely to have edema and to be free of the serious gastrointestinal and renal complications, which, in turn, are more likely to be present in patients over age 5.

The laboratory is of assistance only in "ruling out" other diagnostic possibilities. Thrombocytopenia is not seen in this syndrome, and the bone marrow, prothrombin time, partial thromboplastin time, and bleeding time are all normal. Renal failure may be present, as evidenced by azotemia and elevated serum creatinine, but serum complement is not depressed.

Biopsy of the skin reveals perivascular infiltration and is not diagnostic. The renal histologic findings correlate well with the degree of proteinuria and with the minimal change pattern present in mild cases and the diffuse proliferative glomerulonephritis present in severe cases. Again, the changes are not diagnostic. Immunofluorescence reveals IgA in glomeruli, which helps to distinguish HSS from other forms of nephritis such as poststreptococcal glomerulonephritis, once thought to be related to HSS. It now seems clear that the streptococcus does not appear to play a causative role in HSS, nor has any other single infectious agent been implicated. Infections commonly precede HSS, but no relationship has been established.

Allergy has been suggested and emphasized as causative in a multitude of case reports; a lack of understanding of the possible mechanisms is maintained in the designation anaphylactoid.

The course of HSS is marked by relapses and remissions in nearly one-half the patients; the rash seems particularly to recur within the first 6 weeks. The joint findings leave no residua and so are of little concern; similarly, if intussusception or massive hemorrhage does not complicate the acute course, the gastrointestinal manifestations usually resolve completely; some patients will have evidence of small bowel narrowing later on. Of greatest consequence are the urinary abnormalities. These commonly appear after the first week, as noted, and, when heavy proteinuria is present, may reflect an underlying chronic (but not preexisting) proliferative glomerulonephritis. The results of follow-up studies suggest that 25 percent of patients with HSS have chronic urinary findings, but most do well. An assessment at 2 years after the acute episode appears reliable in gauging prognosis, since by that time the ultimate course is more or less apparent, with further deterioration rare and further improvement slow. Follow-up reveals that even in the group with the worst prognosis ("nephritic nephrotics"), 60 percent do well. Over all, 1 to 4 percent progress to end-stage renal disease.

Since the cause is unknown and the course variable, treatment is empirical, symptomatic, and supportive. Antihistamines, still touted by some, have generally been abandoned. Corticosteroids, however, continue to enjoy favor for the treatment of abdominal manifestations in the hope of reducing edema and thus preventing intussusception; data supporting this therapy are not conclusive. Corticosteroids may well be effective in hastening the elimination of the edema seen in the younger children. To date, no therapy for the chronic nephritis of HSS has proved effective.

Memorabilia

1. Marx, K. Henoch purpura revisited. *Am. J. Dis. Child.* 128:74, 1974.
   All the gossip you ever craved about Henoch, followed by a translation of Henoch's address to the Berlin Medical Society in 1874.

Review

2. Silber, D. Henoch-Schoenlein syndrome. *Pediatr. Clin. North Am.* 19:1061, 1972.
   Covers the waterfront (46 references).

Series

3. Allen, D., Diamond, L., and Howell, D. Anaphylactoid purpura in children (Schölein-Henoch syndrome). *Am. J. Dis. Child.* 99:833, 1960.
   The series worth reading (131 patients).

Gastrointestinal

4. Feldt, R., and Stickler, G. Gastrointestinal manifestations of anaphylactoid purpura in children. *Proc. Staff Meet. Mayo Clin.* 37:465, 1962.
   Of nine children with intussusception, five had melena and abdominal pain as the only preoperative manifestations of HSS.

5. Lindenauer, S., and Tank, E. Surgical aspects of Henoch-Schönlein's purpura. *Surgery* 59:982, 1966.
   Reviews 50 intussusceptions from the literature, noting that 24 were ileoileal. Overall mortality was 13 percent in 39 patients who were operated on and 55 percent in the 11 who were not; bowel resection was required in two-thirds of the former.

6. Ching, E., et al. Intussusception in children. *Mayo Clin. Proc.* 45:724, 1970.
   By way of comparison, these 53 children with intussusception not associated with HSS were younger, more likely to have ileocolic intussusception, a lower resection rate (25%), and a better outcome.

7. Glasier, C., et al. Henoch-Schönlein syndrome in children: Gastrointestinal manifestations. *AJR* 136:1081, 1981.
   The x rays may suggest Crohn's disease to your radiologist. (This differential—and others—considered in CPC: N. Engl. J. Med. 302:853, 1980.)

Renal

8. Hurley, R., and Drummond, K. Anaphylactoid purpura nephritis: Clinicopathological correlations. *J. Pediatr.* 81:904, 1972.
   Emphasizes the lack of correlation between the severity of renal and extrarenal manifestations; notes that patients with severe renal disease may present "late" (31 patients).

9. Meadow, S., et al. Schölein-Henoch nephritis. *Q. J. Med.* 41:241, 1972.
   Notes reliability of prognosis at 2-year assessment (88 patients).

10. Koskimies, O., et al. Henoch-Schönlein nephritis: Long-term prognosis of unselected patients. *Arch Dis. Child.* 56:482, 1981.
    Of 141 children with HSS, 28 percent had abnormal urinalysis for more than 1 month, one of whom progressed to renal failure and one to chronic glomerular disease.

Unusual Clinical Presentations

1. Sahn, D., and Schwartz, A. Schönlein-Henoch syndrome: Observations on some atypical clinical presentations. *Pediatrics* 49:614, 1972.
   Includes a child without skin involvement but who presented an otherwise classic picture of HSS.
2. Byrn, J., et al. Unusual manifestations of Henoch-Schönlein syndrome, *Am. J. Dis. Child.* 130:1335, 1976.
   Gastrointestinal manifestations were present for 3 months prior to the appearance of skin lesions.
3. Loh, H.S., and Jalan, O. M. Testicular torsion in Henoch-Schönlein syndrome, *Br. Med. J.* 2:96, 1974.
   A reminder of an infrequent complication.

Pathology and Etiology

4. Giangiacomo, J., and Tsai, C. Dermal and glomerular deposition of IgA in anaphylactoid purpura. *Am. J. Dis. Child.* 131:981, 1977.
   IgA may be involved in pathogenesis. (Link to Berger disease? J. Pediatr. 106:27, 1985.)
5. Ayoub, E., and Hoyer, J. Anaphylactoid purpura: Streptococcal antibody titers, and B_1C-globulin levels. *J. Pediatr.* 75:193, 1969.
   Antibody titers to multiple streptococcal products failed to support the streptococcus as the etiologic agent; complement was normal, too.
6. Ackroyd, J. Allergic purpura, including purpura due to foods, drugs and infections. *Am. J. Med.* 14:605, 1953.
   Often-quoted, lengthy paper that does not document well the view that HSS is a result of allergy to specific agents (despite references to it in that context); gives a good prosaic description of HSS, though.

Steroid Treatment

See references 3 and 4.

XII. NEOPLASTIC DISORDERS

Leukemia is the most common neoplastic disease of childhood, but it is no longer the rapidly fatal disorder it once was: 30 years ago, median survival was 3 to 4 months; today, an initial remission is expected, and the majority of patients are alive 5 years after diagnosis. Long-term "cures" are no longer viewed with astonishment.

The incidence of leukemia is 3 to 4 new cases per 100,000 children per year, with a peak incidence between ages 2 and 6 years. Despite extensive epidemiologic and virologic investigations, no cause for leukemia has been found.

The onset may be insidious or acute. The most common signs and symptoms at the time of diagnosis are fever, pallor, purpura, and/or bone pain. Anemia reflects inadequate production of red blood cells; bleeding is due to inadequate platelet production. Infection is the result both of a reduced number and a decreased effectiveness of white blood cells. Blast cells may or may not appear in the peripheral blood, but it is imperative that the diagnosis of leukemia be established by examination of a specimen of bone marrow. It is usually not difficult to diagnose leukemia from bone marrow aspirates, since in nearly 80 percent a monotonous sheet of lymphoblasts is seen, replacing the normal elements (acute lymphoblastic leukemia, ALL); the bone marrow changes in less common forms of leukemia may be more difficult to diagnose, however.

Therapy has progressed from the use of a single-drug induction-only regimen to the present multistage protocols that attempt to effect "cure" by (1) inducing remission, (2) eliminating cells in "sanctuaries," such as the CNS, and (3) maintaining the remission. Most centers incorporate vincristine and prednisone in induction therapy; these agents are effective (90% induction rate) and cause the least marrow suppression, mucosal ulceration, and nausea among the antileukemic agents. The prednisone may be of additional benefit during the initial period of thrombocytopenia, since it is believed to "stabilize" small blood vessels and thus protect against bleeding. In some centers a third drug is used as well.

Malignant cells in organs such as the central nervous system (CNS) escape the effects of the drugs used to achieve remission. Before attempts were made specifically to eradicate leukemic cells from the CNS at the time of initial diagnosis, signs of CNS leukemia developed in 30 to 70 percent of children who achieved bone marrow remission, and systemic relapse followed shortly thereafter. Specific strategies designed to seek out malignant cells in "protected" sites are commonly called "sanctuary therapy." Sanctuary therapy (currently, craniospinal radiation, intrathecal methotrexate plus cranial radiation, or larger than usual doses of intravenous methotrexate plus intrathecal methotrexate) has dramatically reduced the incidence of CNS leukemia, greatly prolonged remission from active disease, and resulted in apparent cure in more than 50 percent of children with ALL. In recent years, it has become clear that the testes also may act as a sanctuary; late relapses among boys in long-term remission (long enough to be off chemotherapy altogether) have been the result.

Maintenance therapy protocols vary in the number of agents used (2–8) and duration (2–4 years). Relapses may or may not be treated with initial induction therapy; the trend appears to be toward more complicated regimens for each reinduction attempt.

There are metabolic, hematologic, infectious, and psychologic complications, both of the disease and of the therapy. Uric acid nephropathy may result from the deposition of the breakdown products of leukemic cells in the kidneys; alkalinization, hydration, and allopurinol are used to prevent this complication, but peritoneal dialysis may be required once renal failure is present.

Hemorrhage is a severe threat, a result of thrombocytopenia caused by the leukemic process or by the chemotherapy. Platelet concentrate and supportive red cell transfusions may be required.

The major cause of death in leukemia is infection. During active disease, the usual organisms are bacteria (predominantly gram-negative bacilli, such as *Pseudomonas* and *Escherichia coli,* and *Staphylococcus aureus*) and fungi; the risk of serious infection is directly related to the degree of granulocytopenia. Fever in the neutropenic patient must be considered indicative of sepsis; prompt acquisition of specimens for culture and institution of antibiotic therapy are required.

During periods of remission, viruses (especially varicella-zoster and cytomegalovirus) and protozoa are the chief offending organisms of concern. *Pneumocystic carinii,* the cause of a diffuse, interstitial pneumonitis that is fatal in one-third of treated patients, was until recently the most frequent cause of death in patients considered to be in complete remission; trimethoprim-sulfamethoxazole twice daily appears to be effective in preventing this infection.

Much has been learned about the psychologic devastation to the child and family associated with this disease, just as much has been learned about the biology of leukemia, cell kinetics, and multimodal therapy. Although the physician is looked to as a source of optimism and help in conquering the disease, he must be able to recognize, manage and, when appropriate, encourage grief (see Death, Dying, and Mourning, Chap. 18). Although new therapies are being developed and introduced, such as bone marrow transplantation and immunotherapy, enthusiasm for "cure" must not blind members of the health-care team to the need of the child and the family for free communication and a warm supportive relationship.

The prognosis is best for children aged 2 to 6 years with low initial white blood cell counts (less than 10,000 per cu mm). Lymphoblastic leukemia is more responsive to therapy than is nonlymphoblastic, and leukemia caused by lymphocytes with neither B nor T cell markers (null cells) has the most favorable prognosis. T cell leukemia, in contrast, is often rapidly fatal; it accounts for 20 percent of the cases of acute lymphoblastic leukemia and characteristically occurs in older children (in boys 11 times more frequently than in girls), usually in association with an anterior mediastinal mass. As such biologic markers and prognostic factors are delineated, it becomes more apparent that "leukemia" is not a single disease but a group of diseases. Further definition should make possible the selection of more specific therapeutic regimens for each child, to provide maximal effectiveness with a minimum of toxicity.

With the increasing number of long-term survivors, it has become clear that there are late effects. As with the short-term complications, the late effects are related to the treatment as well as to the disease. Three areas of concern are growth and development (physical, intellectual, and sexual), the possibility of a second neoplasm, and psychologic sequelae.

Reviews

1. Sallan, S., Weinstein, H., and Nathan, D. The childhood leukemias. *J. Pediatr.* 99:676, 1981.
   An overview of pathophysiology, cell markers, management, and future trends.
2. Miller, D. Acute lymphoblastic leukemia. *Pediatr. Clin. North Am.* 27:269, 1980.
   An overview with emphasis on prognostic factors. (Acute nonlymphocytic leukemia considered separately in the same volume, p. 345.)
3. Dunn, N., and Maurer, H. The role of the practitioner in the care of children with acute leukemia. *Pediatr. Rev.* 5:81, 1983.
   An excellent overview of what the practitioner needs to know about leukemia (prognosis, treatment, and complications) and the implications of the disease for general pediatric care.

Biologic and Prognostic "Markers"

4. Miller, D. Prognostic factors in childhood leukemia. *J. Pediatr.* 87:672, 1975.
   The best prognosis is in children 2 to 10 years of age, with ALL and white blood cell count < 20,000. (After continuous long-term remission, these factors are no longer predictive, but sex becomes significant: Cancer 48:370, 1981.)
5. Heideman, R., et al. Lymphocytic leukemia in children: Prognostic significance of clinical and laboratory findings at time of diagnosis. *J. Pediatr.* 92:540, 1978.
   One of many reports to point out the poor prognosis associated with T cell leukemia.
6. Douglass, E. The significance of the subclassifications of acute lymphoblastic leukemia. *Adv. Pediatr.* 29:183, 1982.
   A lengthy review of the various markers.

Treatment

7. Frei, E., and Sallan, S. Acute lymphoblastic leukemia: Treatment. *Cancer* 42:828, 1978.
   A review of progress in complete remission induction, CNS prophylaxis, treatment in remission, and related issues such as dose, combinations of drugs, duration of treatment, and treatment failures.

8. Komp, D. Frequency of bone marrow aspirates to monitor acute lymphoblastic leukemia in childhood. *J. Pediatr.* 102:395. 1983.
   Routine, periodic aspirates appear to be unnecessary for clinical care; relapses are usually preceded by clinical clues or abnormalities in peripheral blood.

9. George, S., et al. A reappraisal of the results of stopping therapy in childhood leukemia. *N. Engl. J. Med.* 300:269, 1979.
   Relapse rate was highest in the first year off therapy; there were no relapses among 79 patients who maintained remission for 4 years off therapy. (A follow-up report of long-term survivors from a different group: J. Pediatr. *95:727, 1979.)*

10. Johnson, F., et al. A comparison of marrow transplantation with chemotherapy for children with acute lymphoblastic leukemia in second or subsequent remission. *N. Engl. J. Med.* 305:846, 1981.
    Marrow transplantation appeared superior to conventional chemotherapy. (Brief editorial review of present status of marrow transplantation in children and persistent problems: Pediatrics *72:818, 1983.)*

Complications

11. Holland, P., and Holland, N. Prevention and management of acute hyperuricemia in childhood leukemia. *J. Pediatr.* 72:358, 1968.
    Allopurinol, alkalinzation, and diuresis are discussed.

12. Gaydos, L., Freireich, E., and Mantel, N. The quantitative relation between platelet count and hemorrhage in patients with acute leukemia. *N. Engl. J. Med.* 266:905, 1962.
    The frequency and severity of hemorrhage increased with lower platelet counts without a "threshold point"; all intracranial hemorrhages were associated with < *10,000 platelets/cu mm.*

13. Bodey, G., et al. Quantitative relationships between circulating leukocytes and infection in patients with acute leukemia. *Ann. Intern. Med.* 64:328, 1966.
    The infection rate increased progressively as neutrophils (especially) fell below 1000; it increased further with counts below 500 and further still with counts below 100; duration of neutropenia was also a factor.

14. Pizzo, P. Infectious complications in the child with cancer: I. Pathophysiology of the compromised host and the initial evaluation and management of the febrile cancer patient. II. Management of specific infectious organisms. III. Prevention. *J. Pediatr.* 98:341, 513, 524, 1981.
    A three-part tour de force (altogether, 29 pages, 208 references).

15. Kosmidis, H., et al. Infection in leukemic children: A prospective analysis. *J. Pediatr.* 96:814, 1980.
    Confirms recognized associations: bacterial disease during relapse with granulocytopenia, viral infections during remission. (Also see Am. J. Dis. Child. *122:283, 1971.)*

16. Hughes, W., et al. Successful chemoprophylaxis for *Pneumocystis carinii* pneumonitis. *N. Engl. J. Med.* 297:1419. 1977.
    Trimethoprim-sulfamethoxazole was associated with a lowered incidence not only of Pneumocystis *pneumonia but also of otitis media, upper respiratory tract infection, sinusitis, and cellulitis. (Prevention of chicken pox:* Pediatrics *72:886, 1983.)*

Long-Term Effects

17. Wells, R. The impact of cranial irradiation on the growth of children with acute lymphocytic leukemia. *Am. J. Dis. Child.* 137:37, 1983.
    *Growth is affected; so is neuropsychologic performance (*J. Pediatr. *101:524, 1982), the CT scan (*N. Engl. J. Med. *298:815, 1978), and IQ (*Am. J. Med. *71:47, 1981, and* Lancet *2:1015, 1981).*

18. Wong, K., et al. Clinical and occult testicular leukemia in long-term survivors of acute lymphoblastic leukemia. *J. Pediatr.* 96:569, 1980.
    Another "sanctuary" identified, affecting long-term cure rates in boys. (Testicular irradiation and testosterone insufficiency: N. Engl. J. Med. *309:25, 1983.)*
19. Freeman, A., et al. Comparison of intermediate-dose methotrexate with cranial irradiation for the postinduction treatment of acute lymphocytic leukemia in children. *N. Engl. J. Med.* 303:477, 1983.
    An attempt to get the benefit of CNS prophylaxis and testicular prophylaxis without the toxicity associated with conventional CNS prophylaxis suggests a present inability to have our cake and eat it too.
20. Gilman, P., and Miller, R. Cancer after acute lymphocytic leukemia. *Am. J. Dis. Child.* 135:311, 1981.
    An editorial review of "second cancers" after ALL.

Emotional Support

21. Schulman, J. Coping with major disease: Child, family, pediatrician. *J. Pediatr.* 102:988, 1983.
    Many pearls strung together by the author's easy-to-read writing style. (For a more complete discussion of "The informing interview," see Am. J. Dis. Child. *137:572, 1983.*
22. Mulhern, R., Crisco, J., and Camitta, B. Patterns of communication among pediatric patients with leukemia, parents, and physicians: Prognostic disagreements and misunderstandings. *J. Pediatr.* 99:480, 1981.
    Misunderstandings may result in coping problems; for more on parental discord and divorce associated wih childhood cancer, see Pediatrics *62:184, 1978.*
23. Powazek, M., et al. Emotional reactions of children to isolation in a cancer hospital. *J Pediatr.* 92:834, 1978.
    Anxiety and depression, as you would expect. (Value of isolation questioned: N. Engl. J. Med. *304:448, 1981.)*
24. Cairnes, N., et al. Adaptation of siblings to childhood malignancy. *J. Pediatr.* 95:484, 1979.
    The siblings showed even more distress than the patients.
25. Heffron, W., Bommelaere, R., and Masters, R. Group discussions with the parents of leukemic children. *Pediatrics* 52:831, 1973.
    Such sessions bring out possibly underestimated issues of major trauma such as alopecia.
    Also see Death, Dying, and Mourning, Chapter 18.

93. WILMS TUMOR

Margaret E. Mohrmann

Wilms tumor, so named because of a compilation of cases by Wilms in 1899, is in pathologic terms a nephroblastoma. It is the most common abdominal neoplasm in children, with an incidence of 1 per 125,000 children. The peak incidence is at $3\frac{1}{2}$ years; there is no male or female predominance.

The tumor is most often recognized clinically as an abdominal mass, or increasing abdominal girth or both. Some children complain of abdominal pain or have fever or vomiting; microscopic hematuria is present in 15 to 25 percent. Hypertension and polycythemia are occasionally present, probably due to renin and erythropoietin secretion by the tumor.

Children with certain congenital anomalies have an unusually high incidence of Wilms tumor; sporadic aniridia, hemihypertrophy, and genitourinary malformations are notable examples of such anomalies. A syndrome of male pseudohermaphroditism, glomerulonephritis, and Wilms tumor has been recognized; these children may succumb to the progressive glomerulonephritis despite successful treatment of the tumor.

The evaluation of the young child with an abdominal mass should be accomplished expeditiously. Intravenous pyelography can usually differentiate hydronephrosis, neuroblastoma (see Chap. 94), and Wilms tumor; Wilms is an intrarenal mass that distorts and splays the calyces. Information obtained from the pyelogram may be augmented by abdominal ultrasonography, computerized tomography, or both.

Surgical removal of the tumor is the essential first step in treatment. Prior to nephrectomy, the pyelogram should be reviewed to ensure the presence of a normally functioning contralateral kidney, and a chest roentgenogram should also be examined, since the lungs are a favored site for metastases. Preoperative angiography may be necessary when there is a significant doubt about the diagnosis of neoplasia or about the status of the other kidney.

Intraoperatively, care is taken to clamp the renal pedicle (to avoid spillage of tumor into the peritoneal cavity) and to define the extent of spread within the abdomen by lymph node dissection, examination of the peritoneum and liver, and palpation of the contralateral kidney. In 70 percent of children, the tumor is completely resectable, whether it is confined (stage I) or not confined (stage II) to the kidney. In stage III disease, residual tumor remains in the abdomen (20% of patients). Stage IV, 10 percent of patients, is characterized by hematogenous metastases, most commonly in the lungs and somewhat less frequently in the liver; metastatic lesions may also occur in bone and brain. Bilateral tumors (stage V) occur in 5 to 15 percent of patients; these are thought to represent separate primary lesions rather than metastases and are staged as above for treatment purposes.

Treatment is determined by clinical stage, tumor histology, and, in some instances, protocol randomization. Irradiation, generally used in all but those with stage I disease, is begun within a few days after nephrectomy. Therapy is directed both to the tumor bed and to known sites of involvement, including areas of local spread or contamination within the abdomen and metastatic lesions. Actinomycin D in combination with vincristine in multiple courses is an effective chemotherapeutic regimen and is used for all stages. The addition of adriamycin improves the rate of relapse-free survival in patients with stage II, III, or IV disease.

Intensive therapy of Wilms tumor has, as expected, various complications. In the postoperative period, intestinal obstruction may occur, as a result of surgical insult, radiation, and vincristine-induced ileus. Nonspecific gastrointestinal symptoms—nausea, vomiting, diarrhea—are sequelae of both abdominal irradiation and actinomycin D use. These two modes of therapy also act in concert to produce desquamative dermatitis over the radiation portals; the skin reaction may be severe enough to limit therapy. During the period in which vincristine is given weekly, loss of deep tendon reflexes and paresthesias may occur. Myelosuppression by actinomycin D (especially thrombocytopenia) is usually most pronounced during the initial 2 months of treatment, when chemotherapy and radiotherapy are most intense, but may continue to be a problem during later courses of therapy. Irradiation of pulmonary metastases can result in radiation pneumonitis and decreased pulmonary function, possibly accentuated by the use of actinomycin D, which is a radiomimetic drug. Similarly, the cardiotoxicity of adriamycin may be enhanced by irradiation of the left hemithorax. Other long-term complications of radiation therapy are growth disturbances, scoliosis, and the occurrence of secondary malignancies.

Patients are examined and chest roentgenograms and intravenous pyelograms or computerized tomograms of the chest and abdomen are evaluated frequently during the first years after diagnosis. Since almost 95 percent of relapses occur within 24 months, the 2-year, disease-free survival rate can be considered a reasonably accurate estimate of cure rate.

The major factors affecting survival appear to be tumor histology and clinical stage. "Unfavorable" histology, defined as the presence of anaplasia or sarcomatous changes, is found in only 12 percent of patients but is associated with a 50 to 60 percent mortality, regardless of stage. The mortality in patients with "favorable" histology is 10 percent or less. Considering the factor of clinical stage alone, relapse-free survival is at least 90 percent for patients with stage I disease, almost 80 percent in stages II and III, and 50 percent in stage IV.

As a result of advances in therapy, Wilms tumor now has the most favorable outlook of the common malignant neoplasms in young children. Current research is directed both toward more effective treatment of metastatic and recurrent disease and toward the reduction of therapeutic toxicity in patients with limited disease.

General

1. Lanzkowsky, P. Wilms' Tumor. In P. Lanzkowsky (ed.), *Pediatric Oncology*. New York: McGraw-Hill, 1983.
   A well-written, thorough but concise clinical review, emphasizing diagnosis and a specific treatment protocol.
2. Belasco, J., Chatten, J., and D'Angio, G. Wilms' Tumor. In W. Sutow, D. Fernbach, and T. Vietti (eds.), *Clinical Pediatric Oncology* (3rd ed.). St. Louis: Mosby, 1984.
   Emphasizes histologic characteristics and treatment modalities (332 references).
3. Lemerle, J., et al. Wilms' tumor: Natural history and prognostic factors. *Cancer* 37:2557, 1976.
   A report on 248 patients, excluding 13 with bilateral disease, seen between 1952 and 1967; exhaustive statistics on all aspects of the subject and several prognostic factors are discussed.
4. Baum, E., and Morgan, E. Wilms' tumor. *Pediatr. Ann.* 12:357, 1983.
   Well-balanced current overview of evaluation and therapy.
5. Cohen, M., et al. A rational approach to the radiologic evaluation of children with Wilms' tumor. *Cancer* 50:887, 1982.
   A review of 50 patients in an attempt to reduce unnecessary invasive procedures while ensuring optimal preoperative delineation of tumor extent and postoperative detection of recurrent disease. (Inferior venacavography not as reliable as computerized tomography or ultrasound in detecting intravascular disease: Clin. Pediatr. [Phila.] 21:690, 1982.)

Associated Congenital Anomalies

6. Pendergrass, T. Congenital anomalies in children with Wilms' tumor. *Cancer* 37:403, 1976.
   This article and its predecessor (N. Engl. J. Med. 270:922, 1964) present lists of malformations found in almost 1000 patients.
7. Fraumeni, J., et al. Wilms' tumor and congenital hemihypertrophy. *Pediatrics* 40:886, 1967.
   Five case reports and a literature review, with interesting correlations drawn.
8. Drash, A., et al. A syndrome of pseudohermaphroditism, Wilms' tumor, hypertension, and degenerative renal disease. *J. Pediatr.* 76:585, 1970.
   Two case reports with a detailed discussion; Radiology 141:87, 1981, is a review of nine cases.

Treatment

9. D'Angio, G., et al. The treatment of Wilms' tumor: Results of the National Wilms' Tumor Study. *Cancer* 38:633, 1976.
   Data are presented on 359 randomized patients; actinomycin D and vincristine together are better than either alone; the efficacy of radiation is equivocal in older children and not worth the risk in the very young.
10. D'Angio, G., et al. The treatment of Wilms' tumor: Results of the second National Wilms' Tumor Study. *Cancer* 47:2302, 1981.
    Results in 513 patients: in stage I disease, 6 months of chemotherapy was as effective as 15 months; adriamycin improved survival in stages II–IV, especially when histology was favorable; age by itself did not correlate with survival.
11. Jenkin, R. The treatment of Wilms' tumor. *Pediatr. Clin. North Am.* 23:147, 1976.
    A good review of various regimens for initial therapy and for treatment of metastatic disease.
12. Ehrlich, R., and Goodwin, W. The surgical treatment of nephroblastoma (Wilms' tumor). *Cancer* 32:1145, 1973.
    An interesting and lucid discussion emphasizing the necessity for nephrectomy and for meticulous lymph node dissection. (For a review of difficulties and complications, see Urol. Clin. North Am. 10:399, 407, 1983.)
13. Tefft, M., et al. Postoperative radiation therapy for residual Wilms' tumor. *Cancer* 37:2768, 1976.

Group III patients (70); figures are given to support the use of well-localized radiation fields rather than total abdominal irradiation whenever possible.

14. Cassady, J., et al. Considerations in the radiation therapy of Wilms' tumor. *Cancer* 32:598, 1973.
   An evaluation of prognostic factors in 156 patients; a good discussion of the complications of radiation therapy.

Follow-Up and Outcome
15. Brasch, R., Randel, S., and Gould, R. Follow-up of Wilms tumor: Comparison of CT with other imaging procedures. *AJR* 137:1005, 1981.
   Based on 13 patients, this study concludes that computerized tomography is more accurate and less expensive for detecting and delineating recurrent disease than a combination of "routine" x rays and scans.
16. Beckwith, J., and Palmer, N. Histopathology and prognosis of Wilms tumor: Results from the first National Wilms' Tumor Study. *Cancer* 41:1937, 1978.
   Analysis identifying "favorable" and "unfavorable" histologic patterns; of those patients with anaplastic or sarcomatous changes, 57 percent died, compared to only 7 percent mortality among those with neither finding.
17. Bishop, H., et al. Survival in bilateral Wilms' tumor: Review of 30 National Wilms' Tumor Study cases. *J. Pediatr. Surg.* 12:631, 1977.
   Reports an 87 percent 2-year survival rate; recommendations for management presented.
18. Littman, P., et al. Pulmonary function in survivors of Wilms' tumor. *Cancer* 37:2773, 1976.
   A report on 33 patients, with survival ranging from 4 to 20 years; average vital capacity was 69 percent of normal in the 10 irradiated for lung metastases.
19. Schwartz, A., et al. Leukemia in children with Wilms' tumor. *J. Pediatr.* 87:374, 1975.
   In five patients, leukemia developed 4 to 16 years after the diagnosis of Wilms; all had been treated wih radiation, three received actinomycin D.

94. NEUROBLASTOMA
Margaret E. Mohrmann

The incidence of neuroblastoma, an embryonic tumor of neural crest origin, is second highest among the solid tumors of childhood, exceeded only by tumors of the central nervous system. It is most common in the first years of life; one-third of patients are less than 1 year old and almost one-half are under the age of 2. Approximately 1 in every 200 infants under 3 months of age who come to autopsy for unrelated reasons has adrenal foci of neuroblastoma, often grossly apparent, with areas of calcification and hemorrhage. This is an incidence about 40 times that of clinically evident neuroblastoma, raising the possibility that the majority of infants are able to destroy, or at least control, the malignant focus. Lymphocytic infiltration is often found in histologic preparations of tumor, suggesting active host immune defense as the cause of the unique "spontaneous regression."

The neural crest origin of the tumor explains three notable features: the spectrum of histologic forms, the diverse location of primary foci, and the ability to produce catecholamines. The term *neuroblastoma,* strictly speaking, refers to the most undifferentiated and malignant of the tumors. The term *ganglioneuroma* is applicable when the cell of origin is a mature ganglion cell. *Ganglioneuroblastoma* refers to an intermediate form.

The primary site of the tumor may be any area of neural crest tissue, but in over one-half the patients it is intraabdominal, usually in the adrenal gland; the next most frequent sites are the thoracic and cervical sympathetic ganglia.

Epinephrine, norepinephrine, and dopamine are secreted by 75 percent of neuroblastomas; nonsecreting tumors are usually among those arising from dorsal ganglia.

Since the amines are rapidly catabolized, they infrequently cause symptoms such as hypertension, but their catabolic products (measured in urine as vanillylmandelic acid [VMA], homovanillic acid [HVA], and total metanephrines [TM]) are important diagnostic markers. Moreover, continued or renewed excretion of these amines following treatment implies residual or recurrent disease. Secretion of an enterohormone, vasoactive intestinal peptide, in some patients results in intractable watery diarrhea.

Presenting signs and symptoms vary, depending on the area in which the tumor exerts its mass effect. Abdominal tumors are most often recognized as palpable masses but may cause urinary obstruction. Thoracic tumors may present with bronchial obstruction and respiratory distress. Cervical neuroblastoma can be the cause of unilateral Horner syndrome or brachial palsy. Tumors arising from dorsal ganglia may have "dumbbell" projections through intervertebral foramina and present with symptoms of spinal cord compression. Intracranial tumors, which are rare, present with symptoms characteristic of central nervous system mass lesions.

A unique mode of presentation is that of cerebellar ataxia with or without opsoclonus. The association has been noted often enough to prompt recommendation that the diagnosis of occult thoracic or abdominal neuroblastoma be considered in any child with "idiopathic" cerebellar ataxia or opsoclonus.

Almost two-thirds of patients have metastatic disease at the time of diagnosis; thus, their presenting signs and symptoms are frequently those of disseminated disease (e.g., anorexia and malaise). Neuroblastoma commonly spreads to the liver, skin, bone, and bone marrow, with parenchymal lung metastases a very late and unusual occurrence; spread to the brain is rare. Common signs of specific metastatic foci are hepatosplenomegaly, lymphadenopathy, bone pain, anemia, subcutaneous nodules (especially in infants), proptosis, and periorbital ecchymoses.

Delineation of disease is primarily radiographic. Intravenous pyelography is performed to detect displacement of an intrinsically normal kidney by an adrenal mass; a roentgenogram of the chest may disclose the presence of a posterior mediastinal mass. Metastases to the bone may be seen as lytic lesions in the skull and distal ends of the long bones. Scans of the liver, spleen, and bone may be helpful if indicated by clinical findings. Suspicion of "dumbbell" tumor invasion of the spinal cord is a definite indication for a myelogram.

Bone marrow aspiration may be useful, since over one-half the patients have marrow involvement at the time of diagnosis. Overt changes in the peripheral blood smear imply disseminated disease.

Treatment of neuroblastoma involves multiple modalities and requires a team effort in management. Surgical extirpation is the basic approach in children with well-localized disease and may be the only treatment needed. In patients with metastatic disease, initial removal of the primary tumor does not appear to alter the outcome. Subsequent removal of an initially unresectable tumor reduced in bulk by radiation and chemotherapy may enhance survival.

Irradiation of the tumor bed has not been shown to be beneficial except perhaps in cases where there is gross residual tumor. In metastatic disease, however, radiotherapy is successfully employed as a palliative measure to relieve bone pain or obstructive phenomena. Antineoplastic drugs have been administered, singly and in combinations, often with a good temporary response; toxicity may be considerable, however, and no convincing diminution in mortality can be associated with the introduction of chemotherapy. Cyclophosphamide is probably the most effective agent and has been used in combination with vincristine, dimethyltriazenoimidazole-carboxamide (DTIC), and other agents.

The prognosis is related to the histologic appearance of the tumor (the more mature, the better the prognosis), the age of the child, and the extent of disease at the time of diagnosis. Children under the age of 1 year have a survival rate of 72 percent, compared to 28 percent for those between 1 and 2 years old and to 12 percent for those over 2. Survival rates improve in older children; 50 percent of those with metastases who are over 6 years old at diagnosis survive their disease.

The extent of disease is the basis of the most commonly used staging system. Disease localized to a single organ is stage I (10% of patients), associated with a 2-year survival in 84 percent. Stage II is regional disease confined to one side of the midline; if both sides of the midline are involved, the disease is considered stage III. In stages II and III, each of which represents 10 to 15 percent of patients, survival rates vary greatly, primarily related to the presence or absence of regional lymph node involvement. Well over one-half the children have metastatic disease (stage IV); the 2-year survival rate in this group is only about 5 percent.

A small percentage of affected children, primarily young infants, have a peculiar combination of localized disease (stage I or II) and metastases limited to the liver, skin, and/or bone marrow; bone metastases specifically are absent. These patients constitute a special classification, stage IV-S disease, in which 2-year survival is high (84% as in stage I). Most oncologists recommend that infants less than 1 year old with stage IV-S disease be managed conservatively, since spontaneous regression is possible, and the risks with intensive chemotherapy are great.

The site of the primary tumor is related to the prognosis, but this relationship is not entirely independent of the staging system just described. Thoracic and cervical tumors are associated with a more favorable outcome than tumors in other sites but are also much more likely to present at stage I or II, while abdominal disease is most often stage III or IV when diagnosed.

The key to improving survival in neuroblastoma will probably be understanding the tumor's mechanisms of spontaneous regression, as well as devising methods, perhaps immunologic, of initiating or enhancing that regression.

General

1. Lanzkowsky, P. Neuroblastoma. In P. Lanzkowsky (ed.), *Pediatric Oncology.* New York: McGraw-Hill, 1983.
   Thorough, well-written chapter with detailed emphasis on clinical presentation.
2. Evans, A., et al. Diagnosis and treatment of neuroblastoma. *Pediatr. Clin. North Am.* 23:161, 1976.
   A good brief overview of all aspects (10 pages).
3. Jaffe, N. Neuroblastoma: Review of the literature and an examination of factors contributing to its enigmatic character. *Cancer Treat. Rev.* 3:61, 1976.
   A complete review, with emphasis on regression, maturation, and unusual presentations.
4. Bill, A., and Koop, C. Conference on the biology of neuroblastoma. *J. Pediatr. Surg.* 3:103, 1968.
   A symposium, with brief reports on all aspects of histopathology, behavior, diagnosis, and management of neuroblastoma; more recent studies of the immunology and differentiation of neuroblastoma are reviewed in Dev. Med. Child Neurol. *22:816, 1980.*
5. Bill, A. Studies of the mechanism of regression of human neuroblastoma. *J. Pediatr. Surg.* 3:727, 1968.
   The significant findings are (1) no evidence of a role for "nerve growth factor," and (2) the serum of patients (both cured and with active disease) inhibits in vitro growth of neuroblastoma.

Clinical Manifestations

6. Williams, T., et al. Unusual manifestations of neuroblastoma. *Cancer* 29:475, 1972.
   A case report and review of 165 Mayo Clinic cases.
7. McLatchie, G., and Young, D. Presenting features of thoracic neuroblastoma. *Arch. Dis. Child.* 55:958, 1980.
   A review of seven patients.
8. Punt, J., et al. Neuroblastoma: A review of 21 cases presenting with spinal cord compression. *Cancer* 45:3095, 1980.
   Good clinical discussion; surprisingly high 61 percent survival, probably related in part to the fact that the majority of patients were less than 1 year old at diagnosis.
9. Roberts, K., and Freeman, J. Cerebellar ataxia and "occult neuroblastoma" without opsoclonus. *Pediatrics* 56:464, 1975.
   A case report with a review of 25 cases; emphasis on the observation that 56% of tumors were found on chest roentgenograms, 36% by physical examination, and 8% by abdominal roentgenograms.

Catecholamine Excretion

10. Evans, A., et al. The LaBrosse spot test. *Pediatrics* 47:913, 1971.
    A two-page report giving technical information on the test (how to do it on the ward), with comments about its reliability.
11. Johnsonbaugh, R., and Cahill, R. Screening procedures for neuroblastoma: False-negative results. *Pediatrics* 56:267, 1975.
    Claims that the spot test and test strips are insensitive because of their dependence on the concentration of vanillylmandelic acid in the urine.
12. deGutierrez Moyano, M., et al. Significance of catecholamine excretion in the follow-up of sympathoblastomas. *Cancer* 27:228, 1971.
    Correlation of persistently elevated urinary catecholamine levels with mortality in 31 patients. (For further prognostic correlation, see Cancer 32:898, 1973.)

Staging and Prognosis

13. Evans, A., et al. A proposed staging for children with neuroblastoma. *Cancer* 27:374, 1971.
    The article presenting and explaining the staging system currently in use; includes a good discussion of prognostic factors.
14. Hughes, H., et al. Histologic patterns of neuroblastoma related to prognosis and clinical staging. *Cancer* 34:1706, 1974.
    Proposes a histologic grading system based on the proportion of mature ganglion cells present; correlation of grade, age, stage, and survival (83 cases).
15. Evans, A., et al. Factors influencing survival of children with nonmetastatic neuroblastoma. *Cancer* 38:661, 1976.
    A study of 113 patients showing the predictive value of the staging system. (A similar analysis, reported in Cancer 53:2079, 1984, relates prognosis to stage, histology, and age at diagnosis; treatment had no apparent effect on the outcome of patients with stage IV or IV-S disease.)
16. Hayes, F., et al. Surgicopathologic staging of neuroblastoma: Prognostic significance of regional lymph node metastases. *J. Pediatr.* 102:59, 1983.
    Whether the tumor is resectable or not, 87 percent of patients survive if regional nodes are free of disease; if the nodes are involved, the survival rate is no different from that in stage IV.

Therapy

17. Leikin, S., et al. The impact of chemotherapy on advanced neuroblastoma. *J. Pediatr.* 84:131, 1974.
    A comparison of two vincristine-cyclophosphamide regimens; neither changed survival despite the initial responses.
18. Evans, A. Staging and treatment of neuroblastoma. *Cancer* 45:1799, 1980.
    A brief, helpful review of the data to date, emphasizing the specific utility of radio- and chemotherapy.
19. Mitschke, R., et al. Neuroblastoma: Therapy for infants with good prognosis. *Med. Pediatr. Oncol.* 11:154, 1983.
    Eleven children with stage I, II, III, or IV-S disease, diagnosed in the first year of life, received no or minimal therapy; all survived.
20. Finkelstein, J., et al. Multiagent chemotherapy for children with metastatic neuroblastoma. *Med. Pediatr. Oncol.* 6:179, 1979.
    Survival is not improved by use of cyclophosphamide, DTIC, and vincristine, with or without additional adriamycin; similar to very young infants, children over 6 years of age have a greater chance of surviving stage IV disease.
21. Raaf, J., Cangir, A., and Luna, M. Induction of neuroblastoma maturation by a new chemotherapy protocol. *Med. Pediatr. Oncol.* 10:275, 1982.
    An increase in the percentage of mature ganglion cells in residual tumor after a four-drug regimen supports both the hypothesis that therapy can be directed toward inducing maturation and the concept that "second-look" surgery may be important in understanding and treating this disease.

Stage IV-S

22. Schneider, K., et al. Neonatal neuroblastoma. *Pediatrics* 36:359, 1965.
   Presents four case reports and reviews 40 cases from the literature; emphasizes the high incidence of liver and skin metastases and low incidence of bone involvement in newborns.

23. Evans, A., et al. A review of 17 IV-S neuroblastoma patients at the Children's Hospital of Philadelphia. *Cancer* 45:833, 1980.
   A detailed clinical review recommending no treatment beyond excision of the primary tumor unless metastases are causing significant sequelae.

24. Evans, A., Baum, E., and Chard, R. Do infants with stage IV-S neuroblastoma need treatment? *Arch. Dis. Child.* 56:271, 1981.
   Among 31 conservatively treated infants, there were only four deaths, all of which were due to massive hepatic involvement.

95. HODGKIN DISEASE

Margaret E. Mohrmann

Lymphoma ranks third in frequency among childhood cancers, and Hodgkin disease accounts for about 40 percent of new cases of lymphoma. Among patients under the age of 12 years, there is a male-female ratio of almost 3:1, but in the teens the incidence in girls increases until the equal sex ratio characteristic of the disease in adults is reached. The disease is rare in children less than 2 years of age, and there are only scattered reports of children under 5. There is a peak in incidence between 5 and 8 years of age, followed by a second, larger peak in the mid-teens.

At present, a viral cause is considered most likely, with clustering of cases and geographic variations in incidence lending support to this view. The presumption is that a virus of low virulence causes antigenic changes on the surface of lymphocytes, thereby setting up a chronic immune reaction that eventually leads to neoplastic transformation. The observation that immunosuppressed patients, such as renal transplant recipients, have a much greater (200 times) incidence of lymphoreticular malignancies is explained by the supposition that the virus is more able to wreak its havoc in such an environment.

Of children with Hodgkin disease, 90 percent are first brought to medical attention because of an enlarged, nontender cervical node. Axillary or inguinal node involvement is rarely the initial finding and extranodal presentation is unusual unless the disease is widespread. The diagnosis is made by histologic examination of the node; it is necessary that the entire node be removed and properly processed, since both needle biopsy and frozen section preparation distort nodal architecture. If possible, a node other than a submaxillary or inguinal node should be chosen for biopsy, since these nodes often show the changes of chronic reaction, which make diagnosis more difficult.

The sine qua non for histologic diagnosis is the presence of Reed-Sternberg cells, which are atypical histiocytes with bilobed or multilobed nuclei and large prominent nucleoli ("owl's eyes"). These cells are not completely pathognomonic of Hodgkin disease, since they may be present in other disorders, such as infectious mononucleosis, phenytoin "pseudolymphoma," and, rarely, in rubeola, thymoma, and non-Hodgkin lymphoma. Based primarily on the ratio of Reed-Sternberg cells to lymphocytes, the histologic classification of Hodgkin disease includes four types: (1) nodular sclerosis, the most common, accounting for half the cases; (2) mixed cellularity, accounting for another fourth; (3) lymphocyte predominance, approximately 20 percent; and (4) lymphocyte depletion of either the reticular or diffuse fibrotic type, 5 percent of cases.

Accurate staging of the disease is important for therapeutic and prognostic reasons. If only one lymph node region or one extralymphatic organ is involved, the disease is considered stage I. More extensive disease limited to one side of the diaphragm is stage II. In stage III, both sides of the diaphragm are involved, and stage IV is diffuse, widespread disease, including extralymphatic sites. Approximately 60 percent of children have stage I or II disease when Hodgkin disease is diagnosed; 25 percent have stage III disease; and 15 percent have stage IV disease.

The extent of disease is often difficult to determine clinically; hepatomegaly and splenomegaly are each found on initial physical examination in 10 to 20 percent of patients, but they are not reliable indicators of hepatic or splenic lymphoma. Mediastinal involvement is apparent on a chest roentgenogram in one-half the patients with enlargement of cervical nodes; it is rarely an isolated finding. Examination of the peripheral blood smear is inadequate to detect marrow involvement; a bone marrow biopsy is necessary.

No combination of radionuclide scans, computerized tomography, and lymphangiography has proven to be as satisfactory for delineating the extent of disease as exploratory laparotomy with removal of the spleen, a favored site of involvement in Hodgkin disease. Abdominal exploration changes the stage in almost 40 percent of children, due largely to the opportunity afforded to examine multiple sections of the spleen, to biopsy the liver, and to sample multiple groups of nodes.

Complete staging of the disease includes noting the absence (A) or presence (B) of symptoms: fever, night sweats, and weight loss exceeding 10 percent of normal body weight in the preceding 6 months. Children with Hodgkin disease usually are asymptomatic, and symptoms, when present, are nonspecific (e.g, anorexia and malaise). Fever is present in 25 to 50 percent of children, but the classic Pel-Ebstein relapsing fever pattern is rare; night sweats and pruritus are also infrequent. Overall, the disease is classified "A" in approximately two-thirds of children and "B" in one-third. In all disease stages, children with symptoms have more rapid progression of disease and a lower survival rate than do asymptomatic children.

Stages I and IIA are usually treated with radiotherapy alone. Stages IIB and III (A and B) are treated with total nodal radiotherapy, or chemotherapy, or both. Stage IV disease is generally treated with chemotherapy alone, utilizing so-called MOPP therapy, a combination of nitrogen mustard, vincristine (Oncovin), procarbazine, and prednisone; many other drug combinations are used but none has been consistently better than the MOPP regimen. The optimal combination of radiation and chemotherapy continues to be controversial, especially for those with stage III disease and those with symptoms in any stage.

Hodgkin disease is characterized by a depression of cellular immunity that results in an increased susceptibility to infection, not only by common bacterial organisms but also by fungi, viruses (especially varicella-zoster), and protozoa. Treatment of the disease increases this susceptibility through splenectomy and myelosuppression. Other complications of treatment include growth retardation and skeletal deformities from paraspinal radiation. Nausea and vomiting may prove debilitating, and social problems caused by alopecia may require the full supportive resources of the family and medical team. Abdominal irradiation and the MOPP protocol both cause a high incidence of sterility; mantle irradiation, especially if lymphangiography has preceded it, often results in hypothyroidism.

More than 90 percent of children with well-localized disease (stages I and II) are cured; of patients with stage IV disease, however, only 40 percent of patients can be expected to survive. The outcome of patients with stage III disease (roughly 80% survival overall) probably depends on the extent of intraabdominal spread. Since more than two-thirds of children with Hodgkin disease have the more favorable histologic types (lymphocyte predominance or nodular sclerosis) and about the same proportion have stage I or II disease, the overall prognosis is quite good. Further refinements in radiotherapy and new applications of chemotherapeutic agents should continue to improve the outlook for children with this disease.

General

1. Lanzkowsky, P. Hodgkin's Disease. In P. Lanzkowsky (ed.), *Pediatric Oncology*. New York: McGraw-Hill, 1983.
   A detailed review with excellent sections on clinical manifestations, staging procedures, and therapy.
2. Murphy, S. The Lymphomas, Lymphadenopathy, and Histiocytoses. In D. Nathan and F. Oski (eds.), *Hematology of Infancy and Childhood* (2nd ed.). Philadelphia: Saunders, 1981.
   A well-organized, helpful overview.
3. Tan, C., and Chan, K. Hodgkin's disease. *Pediatr. Ann.* 12:306, 1983.
   A current review of all aspects (Also see Pediatr. Rev. 6:3, 1984.)

4. Aisenberg, A. Malignant lymphoma. *N. Engl. J. Med.* 288:883, 935, 1973.
   A detailed, lucid discussion of the etiology, epidemiology, pathology, and management of lymphoma (122 references), updated in N. Engl. J. Med. 301:1212, 1979.
5. Vianna, N., and Polan, A. Epidemiologic evidence for transmission of Hodgkin's disease. *N. Engl. J. Med.* 289:499, 1973.
   A study of the clustering within schools in New York; discussion of limited implications.
6. Vianna, N., et al. Tonsillectomy and childhood Hodgkin's disease. *Lancet* 2:338, 1980.
   Children who have had their tonsils removed have 3 times the incidence of Hodgkin disease compared to children who still have their tonsils; the significance of this finding and its independence from other risk factors remain unclear and controversial.
7. Norris, D., et al. Hodgkin's disease in childhood. *Cancer* 36:2109, 1975.
   A review of the cases of 116 patients from the Mayo Clinic, 1935–1970, with a complete statistical analysis.
8. Jenkin, R., et al. Hodgkin's disease in children. *Cancer* 35:979, 1975.
   Another retrospective analysis (1958–1973) of 109 cases; the 5-year overall survival improved from 50 to 95 percent over that period.

Diagnostic Evaluation and Staging

9. Hays, D. The staging of Hodgkin's disease in children reviewed. *Cancer* 35:973, 1975.
   Emphasizes techniques and the importance of accurate staging.
10. Sweet, D., Kinnealey, A., and Ultmann, J. Hodgkin's disease: Problems of staging. *Cancer* 42:957, 1978.
    An excellent review of all methods of evaluation; the authors tentatively suggest that the majority of patients can be treated appropriately without surgical staging if extensive clinical studies are performed.
11. Stein, R., et al. Anatomical substages of stage III Hodgkin's disease. *Cancer* 42:429, 1978.
    In adult patients with abdominal involvement limited to the upper abdomen (stage III-1), 5-year disease-free survival was 77 percent compared to 13 percent in those with more extensive abdominal disease (stage III-2); the authors recommend aggressive combined therapy for patients with stage III-2 and radiotherapy alone for those with stage III-1.
12. Muraji, T., et al. Evaluation of the surgical aspects of staging laparotomy for Hodgkin's disease in children. *J. Pediatr. Surg.* 17:843, 1982.
    The results of laparotomy changed the stage in 35 percent of patients; no difference in outcome could be shown between patients with stage III-1 and those with stage III-2 disease.
13. Filler, R., et al. Experience with clinical and operative staging of Hodgkin's disease in children. *J. Pediatr. Surg.* 10:321, 1975.
    A critical evaluation of lymphangiograms in children; details of various aspects of laparotomy are given.
14. Pear, B. Skeletal manifestations of the lymphomas and leukemias. *Semin. Roentgenol.* 9:229, 1974.
    Presents well-illustrated examples of the various osseous lesions.

Therapy

15. Ultmann, J. Current status: The management of lymphoma. *Semin. Hematol.* 7:441, 1970.
    A comprehensive treatment of the subject, with an excellent critique of radiotherapy and various chemotherapeutic agents (15 pages, 99 references).
16. DeVita, V., et al. Combination chemotherapy in the treatment of advanced Hodgkin's disease. *Ann. Intern. Med.* 73:881, 1970.
    The classic study of the MOPP protocol from the National Cancer Institute (43 patients); includes a good discussion of toxicities and of the rationale for combination therapy in general.
17. Tan, C., et al. The changing management of childhood Hodgkin's disease. *Cancer* 35:808, 1975.

A group of 211 children (1929–1974) from Sloan-Kettering; analyzes survivals in "historical groups" and discusses current therapy.

18. Fuller, L., et al. Results of regional radiotherapy in localized Hodgkin's disease in children. *Cancer* 32:640, 1973.

A study of 47 patients in stages I and II only; the 5-year survival rate was 80 percent; variations in radiation, depending on cell type and site of the primary tumor, are explained.

19. Dearth, J., et al. Management of stages I to III Hodgkin disease in children. *J. Pediatr.* 96:829, 1980.

Experience with 37 children concludes that a combination of radiation and chemotherapy is needed for optimal treatment of stages IIB and III.

20. Smith, K., et al. Concurrent chemotherapy and radiation therapy in the treatment of childhood and adolescent Hodgkin's disease. *Cancer* 33:38, 1974.

St. Jude's series of 49 patients, in all stages, all treated with "total therapy"; there were complete remissions in 96 percent (93% of those in stages IIIB and IV); toxicity is said to be justified by the remission rate.

Complications and Outcome

21. Donaldson, S., Glatstein, E., and Vosti, K. Bacterial infections in pediatric Hodgkin's disease: Relationship to radiotherapy, chemotherapy and splenectomy. *Cancer* 41:1949, 1978.

A well-referenced study of the effects of therapeutic intervention on the incidence of bacterial infections in 181 children.

22. Reboul, F., Donaldson, S., and Kaplan, H. Herpes zoster and varicella infections in children with Hodgkin's disease: An analysis of contributing factors. *Cancer* 41:95, 1978.

Infection developed in 35 percent of patients; splenectomy did not affect the incidence, but the combination of radiation and chemotherapy increased the risk to 56 percent. (Also see Acta Paediatr. Scand. 71:269, 1982.)

23. Donaldson, S., and Kaplan, H. Complications of treatment of Hodgkin's disease in children. *Cancer Treat. Rep.* 66:977, 1982.

An excellent review covering the spectrum from postsplenectomy sepsis to growth retardation, sterility, and secondary malignancies.

24. Mauch, P., et al. An evaluation of long-term survival and treatment complications in children with Hodgkin's disease. *Cancer* 51:925, 1983.

Primarily a discussion of radiation therapy with recommendations for limiting complications.

25. Wilimas, J., Thompson, E., and Smith, K. Long-term results of treatment of children and adolescents with Hodgkin's disease. *Cancer* 46:2123, 1980.

A brief report of the experience at St. Jude's with patients in all stages of disease.

96. NON-HODGKIN LYMPHOMA
Margaret E. Mohrmann

As noted in the preceding section, lymphomas collectively rank third in frequency among childhood malignancies. Non-Hodgkin lymphomas (NHL) as a group occur more frequently than do Hodgkin lymphomas by a margin of 3 to 2 and are responsible for 3 times as many deaths. They are 4 times more common in males than in females.

The subclassification of non-Hodgkin lymphomas is based on degree of differentiation, cell type, and nodularity or diffuseness. Well-differentiated and nodular tumors, both associated with better prognoses, are rare in children. One-third to one-half of non-Hodgkin lymphomas affecting children are lymphoblastic tumors, characterized by mediastinal involvement, T cell markers, and frequent leukemic transformation. Undifferentiated lymphomas account for 20 to 40 percent of cases; this category includes

Burkitt lymphomas. Most undifferentiated tumors arise in the abdomen and carry B cell markers.

Burkitt lymphoma was first described in African children in 1958; since then it has become clear that there are marked differences between African Burkitt and American Burkitt tumors. The disease in African children is characterized by primary sites in the jaw (50%) and abdomen (30%), infrequent involvement of the bone marrow, and an infectionlike endemic incidence pattern that suggests the involvement of an arthropodborne virus. On the other hand, children with American Burkitt lymphoma present more often with abdominal disease (usually involving the ovaries or gastrointestinal tract) and have more bone marrow transformation (over 60%) and a sporadic incidence more characteristic of classic neoplasia. Epstein-Barr viral titers are elevated in almost all patients with African Burkitt tumor but in fewer than 30 percent of those with American Burkitt lymphoma.

The staging system for Burkitt tumor is different from that for other lymphomas because of the tumor's unique propensity for facial bone involvement. The system defines stages A and B as tumor involving extraabdominal sites only (A, one; B, two or more), stage C as intraabdominal tumor, and stage D as intraabdominal tumor plus additional sites (other than facial). A fifth stage (AR), designating intraabdominal tumor (stage C) that has been almost completely removed surgically, recognizes the important prognostic value of tumor volume. With aggressive therapy, the survival rate in stages A, B, and AR is usually greater than 80 percent; only 40 percent of children in stages C and D survive. Stage-related prognosis does not differ significantly between African and American Burkitt tumor.

Staging of NHL, other than Burkitt tumors, is both complex and controversial. Earlier systems, based on the staging of Hodgkin disease, were not helpful in predicting outcome or guiding therapy. Systems currently in use classify localized disease as stage I or II, depending on regional lymph node involvement. Stage III includes any mediastinal or paraspinal disease, all extensive intraabdominal disease, and disease involving both sides of the diaphragm. Involvement of the bone marrow, the central nervous system, or both at the time of diagnosis defines stage IV. Intensive chemotherapy regimens result in 80 to 100 percent survival among patients in stages I and II, 75 percent in stage III, and 50 percent in stage IV.

Non-Hodgkin lymphomas are rapidly growing tumors; this is especially true of Burkitt lymphoma, which may have a doubling time of only 24 hours. This observation accounts for two important aspects of therapy: the need for rapid diagnosis and treatment and the frequent occurrence of significant metabolic derangements due to the rapid turnover of tumor cells. Meticulous care is required to treat or prevent problems such as acute renal failure (due to uric acid nephropathy or to urinary tract obstruction by tumor), hypercalcemia, and hyperkalemia, which have caused up to 15 percent of deaths from NHL in some series.

In general, NHL is never treated with radiotherapy alone; however, radiation can play an important role in reducing tumor bulk, especially in life-threatening situations, such as airway obstruction by a mediastinal mass. Multidrug chemotherapy is the sine qua non of successful treatment. All localized disease and diffuse disease that is nonlymphoblastic (including Burkitt lymphoma) respond best to a combination of cyclophosphamide, vincristine, methotrexate, and prednisone. Stage III or IV lymphoblastic lymphoma requires more intensive therapy with a 10-drug regimen, the LSA$_2$-L$_2$ protocol; the toxicity of this treatment is appreciable but may be considered justified in view of the dramatic improvement in disease-free survival associated with its use.

General
1. Shende, A., and Lanzkowsky, P. Non-Hodgkin's Lymphoma. In P. Lanzkowsky (ed.), *Pediatric Oncology.* New York: McGraw-Hill, 1983.
   A current, detailed textbook review.
2. Gardner, R., and Graham-Pole, J. Non-Hodgkin's lymphoma. *Pediatr. Ann.* 12:322, 1983.
   A well-written, thorough, concise review of all aspects of the disease; an excellent place to start.

3. Ziegler, J. Burkitt's lymphoma. *N. Engl. J. Med.* 305:735, 1981.
   A detailed, readable overview of current knowledge, with emphasis on etiology and therapy.
4. Murphy, S. The Lymphomas, Lymphadenopathy, and Histiocytoses. In D. Nathan and F. Oski (eds.), *Hematology of Infancy and Childhood* (2nd ed.). Philadelphia: Saunders, 1981.
   A well-organized review that clearly presents the interrelationships between NHL and the lymphoblastic leukemias.

Staging and Clinical Manifestations

5. Jaffe, N., et al. Role of staging in childhood non-Hodgkin's lymphoma. *Cancer Treat. Rep.* 61:1001, 1977.
   An attempt to identify most useful staging tools by a retrospective analysis of 227 patients.
6. Murphy, S. Classification, staging and end results of treatment of childhood non-Hodgkin's lymphomas: Dissimilarites from lymphomas in adults. *Semin. Oncol.* 7:332, 1980.
   An understandable and concise summary of the enigmas of NHL.
7. Nathwani, B., et al. Non-Hodgkin's lymphoma: A clinicopathologic study comparing two classifications. *Cancer* 41:303, 1978.
   Describes (and manifests) the nature and significance of the classification dilemma.
8. Dorfman, R. Diagnosis of Burkitt's tumor in the United States. *Cancer* 21:563, 1968.
   An interesting discussion of the clinical and pathologic differentiation between childhood Burkitt lymphoma and leukemia, with the conclusion that Burkitt tumor in the United States cannot be clearly distinguished from poorly differentiated lymphocytic lymphoma.
9. Hutter, J., et al. Non-Hodgkin's lymphoma in children: Correlations of CNS disease with initial presentation. *Cancer* 36:2132, 1975.
   In 26 patients, 12 had mediastinal disease; 5 of the 12 had central nervous system disease before leukemic transformation was evident (all died); recommends central nervous system prophylaxis for those with mediastinal involvement, even without marrow disease.
10. Lynch, R., Kjellstrand, C., and Coccia, P. Renal and metabolic complications of childhood non-Hodgkin's lymphoma. *Semin. Oncol.* 4:325, 1977.
    This important paper reviews both complications and the means of prevention.

Therapy

11. Murphy, S. Management of childhood non-Hodgkin's lymphoma. *Cancer Treat. Rep.* 61:1161, 1977.
    A comprehensive review of several treatment regimens and results.
12. Wollner, N., et al. Non-Hodgkin's lymphoma in children. *Cancer* 37:123, 1976.
    A comparison of the LSA₂-L₂ protocol with other therapy; 2-year survival was 11 percent in the nonprotocol group but 76 percent in the LSA₂-L₂ group (45 references). (Also see Pediatr. Clin. North Am. 23:371, 1976.)
13. Wollner, N., Exelby, P., and Lieberman, P. Non-Hodgkin's lymphoma in children: A progress report on the original patients treated with the LSA₂-L₂ protocol. *Cancer* 44:1990, 1979.
    More than 4 years after diagnosis, disease-free survival is 73 percent; important prognostic factors are the amount of tumor, the use of early and aggressive treatment, and the occurrence of complete remission within 2 months of diagnosis.
14. Anderson, J., et al. Childhood non-Hodgkin's lymphoma: The results of a randomized therapeutic trial comparing a 4-drug regimen (COMP) with a 10-drug regimen (LSA₂-L₂). *N. Engl. J. Med.* 308:559, 1983.
    In patients with localized disease both regimens resulted in 84 percent survival, but COMP was less toxic; COMP gave significantly better results in disseminated nonlymphoblastic lymphoma (such as Burkitt) and LSA₂-L₂ was better for wide spread lymphoblastic disease.

97. BRAIN TUMORS
Margaret E. Mohrmann

Brain tumors are the most common solid tumors and the second most common cancer in children. Their incidence is approximately 1 per 50,000 children/year, with the peak incidence occurring in the early school years. Most series show a slight male predominance but no racial predilection.

One-half to two-thirds of childhood intracranial neoplasms are infratentorial in location (compared to 25–30% in adults) and the majority are glial in origin. Classic definitions of "benign" and "malignant" neoplasms have little meaning when discussing tumors of the central nervous system (CNS). More important factors affecting the presentations and prognoses of brain tumors are their location, rapidity of growth, and obstructive (causing increased intracranial pressure) or infiltrative (causing focal neuronal disruption) characteristics.

Infratentorial tumors frequently present with symptoms and signs of increased intracranial pressure due to obstruction of the fourth ventricle. This increase in pressure may be manifested by headache (characteristically present on awakening), vomiting without nausea, an abducens (VI nerve) palsy, or a rapidly enlarging head circumference. In the infant, headache may be represented by irritability and diplopia by blinking, eye rubbing, squinting, or head turning. The tumor may cause traction on structures near the foramen magnum, resulting in nuchal rigidity, wry neck, or a head tilt. Since most posterior fossa tumors involve the cerebellum, signs of neuronal dysfunction usually include disturbances of gait, balance, and motor coordination; nystagmus may also occur.

Supratentorial tumors are more likely to present with focal neurologic abnormalities than with signs of increased intracranial pressure, the evidence of neurologic dysfunction depending on the specific location of the tumor. Frontal lobe lesions may cause mental changes or hemiparesis; temporal lobe tumors often produce seizures. Hypothalamic neoplasms may be manifested by endocrinologic disturbances, such as precocious puberty or diabetes insipidus, or by the "diencephalic syndrome" of marked emaciation and euphoria. A tumor in the area of the pituitary gland, such as a craniopharyngioma, may present with short stature caused by growth hormone deficiency or may result in visual abnormalities due to involvement of the optic chiasm.

The differential diagnosis of intracranial tumors includes other mass lesions, such as brain abscess and subdural hematoma, and other diseases causing neuronal dysfunction, such as encephalitis and lead encephalopathy. The most important diagnostic tool available is contrast-enhanced computed tomography, a technique that has almost eliminated the need for older methods such as pneumoencephalography. In some instances, cerebral angiography may be helpful; myelography is usually necessary in the diagnosis of spinal cord tumors. Plain radiographs of the skull, radionuclide brain scanning, and electroencephalography may play a role in the delineation of tumor in certain patients.

Treatment of brain tumors is primarily surgical, for palliation and, sometimes, for cure. Radiotherapy is frequently used, often with obvious benefit; however, its utility is limited by its immediate effects (cerebral edema, somnolence) and by its potential long-term consequences, including endocrinologic abnormalities and mental retardation. The use of chemotherapy is increasing, although it is still not clear that it improves survival significantly; the blood-brain barrier is probably less an obstacle to the success of chemotherapeutic agents than is the relatively slow growth of most CNS tumors.

Astrocytomas are the most common histologic type of brain tumor in children. They are usually slow-growing, often cystic lesions, the majority of which arise in the cerebellum. When complete surgical removal is not possible, regrowth tends to be slow, and the new mass can often be controlled surgically, resulting in longer survival. Prognosis and potential benefit from irradiation depend on location, malignant grade, amount of residual tumor, and characterization of the tumor as cystic or diffuse.

The most common infratentorial tumor is medulloblastoma, a highly malignant neoplasm that tends to metastasize throughout the cerebrospinal fluid system. Because of its location and rapid growth rate, this tumor is most likely to cause obstruction of the fourth ventricle early in the course of disease and is less likely to be surgically removable. Treatment, therefore, is concerned initially with relief of increased intracranial pressure and thereafter with irradiation of the entire craniospinal axis. The rapid growth rate also makes medulloblastoma unique among CNS tumors in its sensitivity to chemotherapy, although the long-term benefit of such treatment is unclear. Aggressive use of surgery, radiotherapy, and, perhaps, chemotherapy, results in a 25 to 40 percent 10-year survival.

Brainstem gliomas, which usually present with cranial nerve and long tract abnormalities, comprise 10 to 15 percent of childhood CNS tumors. Histologic grading ranges from "benign" astrocytoma to the highly malignant glioblastoma multiforme. These lesions are almost always inoperable and respond poorly to radiation. Five-year survival rates (not disease-free) are 20 to 30 percent.

Although ependymomas may occur on either side of the tentorium, most arise in the fourth ventricle and there produce obstructive hydrocephalus. Complete surgical removal is rarely possible, and the attempt is associated with a high intraoperative mortality. Radiotherapy is often of benefit; prognosis varies markedly with location, histologic grade, and mode of treatment.

Less common primary CNS tumors of childhood include craniopharyngiomas, pinealomas, optic gliomas, meningiomas, and the intracranial lesions associated with neurocutaneous syndromes such as neurofibromatosis (von Recklinghausen disease) and tuberous sclerosis. While CNS involvement in leukemia is common, the brain is rarely a site of metastasis from extracranial solid tumors.

Reviews

1. Vay Eys, J. Malignant Tumors of the Central Nervous System. In W. Sutow, D. Fernbach, and T. Vietti (eds.), *Clinical Pediatric Oncology* (3rd ed.). St. Louis: Mosby, 1984.
   A well-organized and thoroughly referenced review that gives all the important information without being overwhelmingly detailed.
2. Klein, M., and Festa, R. Central Nervous System Malignancies. In P. Lanzkowsky (ed.), *Pediatric Oncology*. New York: McGraw-Hill, 1983.
   This chapter contains much more detail than does reference 1; as a result, it is more difficult to read and to sift for useful information.
3. Walker, R., and Allen, J. Pediatric brain tumors. *Pediatr. Ann.* 12:383, 1983.
   A very good, brief review. (For a similar, although less current, review, see Pediatr. Clin. North Am. *23:131, 1976.)*
4. Yates, A., Becker, L., and Sachs, L. Brain tumors in childhood. *Childs Brain* 5:31, 1979.
   A statistical report on the location and histology of 689 intracranial and spinal cord tumors. (For incidence figures, see Mayo Clin. Proc. *51:51, 1976.)*
5. Gjerris, F. Clinical aspects and long-term prognosis of intracranial tumors in infancy and childhood. *Dev. Med. Child Neurol.* 18:145, 1976.
   Although dated in its information about outcome, this review is an excellent source of data on clinical findings at the time of diagnosis.
6. Raimondi, A., and Tomita, T. Brain tumors during the first year of life. *Childs Brain* 10:193, 1983.
   The important points in this review of 39 patients (representing 11% of children with CNS tumors) are: the majority of tumors were supratentorial; 82 percent of infants had hydrocephalus; the usual presenting signs were bulging fontanelle, increasing head circumference, and delayed development; and the 5-year survival was 22 percent.

Diagnosis

7. Segall, H., et al. Computed tomography in neoplasms of the posterior fossa in children. *Radiol. Clin. North Am.* 20:237, 1982.
   A review of the usefulness of CT and the appearance of various tumors.
8. Handel. S. Computed tomography vs. angiography in the diagnosis of intracranial neoplasms. *Clin. Neurosurg.* 28:502, 1981.
   Although this article does not deal specifically with children, it is helpful in clarifying the sort of information obtainable from each technique and the advantages and disadvantages of each.
9. Miller, J., et al. Combined computed tomographic and radionuclide imaging in the long-term follow-up of children with primary intra-axial intracranial neoplasms. *Radiology* 146:681, 1983.

CT is generally more sensitive than radionuclide imaging but it is difficult to distinguish the effects of radio- and chemotherapy on a tumor from recurrent disease by CT; used together, the two techniques have a 93 percent sensitivity.

Treatment

10. Deutsch, M. Radiotherapy for primary brain tumors in very young children. *Cancer* 50:2785, 1982.
    The incidence of long-term problems is considered low enough to warrant the use of radiotherapy since it appears to improve the chance of cure.
11. Allen, J. Chemotherapy for primary brain tumors. *Pediatr. Ann.* 7:844, 1978.
    A brief description of the theoretical and practical problems with the use of chemotherapy.
12. Danoff, B., et al. Assessment of the long-term effects of primary radiation therapy for brain tumors in children. *Cancer* 49:1580, 1982.
    Follow-up for up to 21 years showed a less than 2 percent incidence of secondary intracranial neoplasms; the occurrence of mental retardation as a sequela was dependent on age at time of diagnosis and tumor location.
13. Kun, L., Mulhern, R., and Crisco, J. Quality of life in children treated for brain tumors. *J. Neurosurg.* 58:1, 1983.
    This study of 30 children shows significant emotional or intellectual abnormalities or both in at least 20 percent; supratentorial location of tumor and total cranial irradiation were associated with a higher risk of impairment.
14. Duffner, P., Cohen, M., and Thomas, P. Late effects of treatment on the intelligence of children with posterior fossa tumors. *Cancer* 51:233, 1983.
    Of 10 children treated with both irradiation and chemotherapy, all had dementia, learning disabilities, or a lowered IQ.

Specific Tumors

15. Raimondi, A., and Tomita, T. Medulloblastoma in childhood. *Childs Brain* 5:310, 1979.
    Five-year survival was 35 percent; repeat attempts at surgical removal did not enhance survival.
16. Littman. P., et al. Pediatric brain stem gliomas. *Cancer* 45:2787, 1980.
    Five-year survival was 30 percent; recommends limited use of surgery, but radiotherapy for all patients.
17. Pierre-Kahn, A., et al. Intracranial ependymomas in childhood. *Childs Brain* 10:145, 1983.
    Five-year survival was 39 percent; recommends variation in radiotherapy depending on location and degree of malignancy.
18. Burr, I., et al. Diencephalic syndrome revisited. *J. Pediatr.* 88:439, 1976.
    A review of 72 patients and discussion of some enigmatic aspects of this syndrome.
19. Thomsett, M., et al. Endocrine and neurologic outcome in childhood craniopharyngioma: Review of effect of treatment in 42 patients. *J. Pediatr.* 97:728, 1980.
    Good analysis of presentation and endocrine status; recommends partial excision plus irradiation if total excision is not possible. (A strong case for aggressive attempts at total excision: Neurosurgery 11:382, 1982.)
20. Merten, D., et al. Meningiomas of childhood and adolescence. *J. Pediatr.* 84:696, 1974.
    A review of 48 cases of an unusual tumor in children.
21. Riccardi, V. Von Recklinghausen neurofibromatosis. *N. Engl. J. Med.* 305:1617, 1981.
    A thorough review; the major morbidity is due to intracranial tumors, most of which first appear in childhood.
22. Monaghan, H., et al. Tuberous sclerosis complex in children. *Am. J. Dis. Child.* 135:912, 1981.
    CNS tumors were found in 4 of 62 children with tuberous sclerosis.

98. MALIGNANT BONE TUMORS

Margaret E. Mohrmann

Neoplasms of bone are uncommon in children, representing slightly less than 5 percent of all childhood cancer. Among adolescents, however, skeletal malignancies are exceeded in frequency only by leukemia, lymphoma, and brain tumors. Osteosarcoma (osteogenic sarcoma) comprises 60 percent and Ewing sarcoma 30 percent of malignant bone tumors in children; the remaining 10 percent include fibrosarcomas, chondrosarcomas, and reticulum cell sarcomas (non-Hodgkin lymphomas of bone).

Osteosarcoma usually occurs in the second decade of life with the peak incidence coinciding with the adolescent growth spurt: 13 to 14 years in females, 14 to 15 years in males. The most common site of origin is the distal femur ("the most rapidly growing end of the most rapidly growing bone"), followed by the proximal tibia and the proximal humerus; almost 50 percent of tumors arise near the knee. The presenting complaint is usually localized pain, which may be accompanied by swelling or warmth; a palpable mass is not an early finding.

The diagnosis is suggested by the radiographic picture of a lytic and sclerotic lesion in the metaphysis of a long bone, but biopsy is required for definitive diagnosis. The serum alkaline phosphatase level is often elevated and may be useful in identification of residual or recurrent disease. Computed tomographic evaluation of the extent of the tumor and angiographic assessment of neurovascular involvement are often used to guide surgical management. Radiographs or computed tomography of the chest is a necessary part of the initial evaluation, since the lungs are usually the first site of metastasis; a skeletal survey or bone scan is indicated to identify other sites of bone disease.

Amputation of the affected limb has long been a mainstay of the treatment of osteosarcoma. However, with clear delineation of disease extent and intensive preoperative chemotherapy, it is now possible, in selected cases, to perform limb-salvage procedures entailing en bloc resection of involved bone and prosthesis implantation. Osteosarcoma is very radioresistant; consequently, radiation therapy is used only for palliation of inoperable lesions. Multidrug chemotherapy regimens usually include adriamycin and high-dose methotrexate with citrovorum factor rescue. The use of such drugs has been associated with an improvement in disease-free survival from less than 20 percent to at least 50 percent; recent studies show 3-year disease-free survival rates of 80 percent. However, it is unclear whether aggressive chemotherapy has improved the cure rate among patients without metastatic disease at the time of diagnosis.

Originally, the presence of pulmonary metastases meant certain death within several months. However, an aggressive approach utilizing chemotherapy and surgical resection has resulted in a significant improvement in length of survival and, sometimes, in cure.

Ewing sarcoma is also found most often in persons between the ages of 10 and 20 years but does not show a peak incidence related to growth rate during that decade. It is rarely seen in blacks. Ewing sarcoma most often arises in the femur but also frequently occurs in flat bones, such as the pelvis, ribs, and sternum. The usual presenting complaints are pain, swelling, and occasionally, fever.

Although the most common x-ray appearance of Ewing sarcoma is that of a lytic lesion in the metaphysis of a long bone, the picture can vary considerably; it is, therefore, not possible to describe a "classic" radiographic appearance of the tumor. Biopsy is necessary for diagnosis, but the other possible diagnoses suggested by the clinical and radiographic findings—osteomyelitis, metastatic neuroblastoma, non-Hodgkin lymphoma, and benign neoplasms—may be difficult to distinguish histologically from Ewing sarcoma. It is often necessary to perform additional tests, such as bone marrow biopsy, to clarify the diagnosis.

High-dose radiation is the primary mode of treatment. Surgical extirpation has been little utilized in the past because of the success of radiotherapy; however, there is now renewed interest in surgical removal as a means both of circumventing severe complications of irradiation (such as cessation of limb growth, bowel and bladder dysfunction, and secondary malignancies) and of improving the usually dismal outcome of patients with pelvic tumors. Effective chemotherapeutic agents include vincristine, actinomycin D, cyclophosphamide, and adriamycin. Intensive combined therapy has improved disease-free survival from less than 20 percent to at least 60 percent in patients with localized disease; those with metastatic disease (20–30% at the time of diagnosis) continue to have a poor prognosis with no more than 10 to 20 percent surviving.

General

1. Jaffe, N. Malignant Bone Tumors. In P. Lanzkowsky (ed.), *Pediatric Oncology*. New York: McGraw-Hill, 1983.
   A thorough and well-organized discussion.
2. Rosen, G. Management of malignant bone tumors in children and adolescents. *Pediatr. Clin. North Am.* 23:183, 1976.
   A detailed review with emphasis on the differential diagnosis of Ewing sarcoma and on chemotherapy.
3. Osborne, R. The differential radiologic diagnosis of bone tumors. *CA* 24:194, 1974.
   An excellent review of basic criteria for evaluating bone lesions and of identifying characteristics of specific tumors.
4. Lukens, J., McLeod, R., and Sim, F. Computed tomographic evaluation of primary osseous malignant neoplasms. *AJR* 139:45, 1982.
   When compared to other imaging techniques (standard radiography, tomography, and radionuclide scanning), CT is not significantly better at identifying the presence of tumor but is clearly the best method of defining the location and extent of disease.
5. deSantos, L., Murray, J., and Ayala, A. The value of percutaneous needle biopsy in the management of primary bone tumors. *Cancer* 43:735, 1979.
   Needle biopsy, in this study, had 93 percent diagnostic accuracy and definite advantages over open biopsy, especially in patients destined for attempts at limb salvage.
6. Eilber, F., et al. Is amputation necessary for sarcomas? A seven-year experience with limb salvage. *Ann. Surg.* 192:431, 1980.
   In 91 percent of 105 patients there were no local recurrences of tumor. (Use of the procedure in children with osteogenic sarcoma: J. Pediatr. Surg. 18:901, 1983.)

Osteosarcoma

7. Rosen, G. Spindle Cell Sarcoma: Osteogenic Sarcoma. In W. Sutow, D. Fernbach, and T. Vietti (eds.), *Clinical Pediatric Oncology* (3rd ed.). St. Louis: Mosby, 1984.
   A well-written, well-referenced encyclopedic review.
8. Tebbi, C., and Freeman, A. Osteogenic sarcoma. *Pediatr. Rev.* 6:55, 1984.
   A current review with a helpful section on the psychologic problems related to having cancer and to amputation. (For another clear, concise review, see Pediatr. Ann. 12:374, 1983.
9. Sutow, W. Multidrug chemotherapy in osteosarcoma. *Clin. Orthop.* 153:67, 1980.
   A brief discussion of the development of current chemotherapeutic protocols and their role in reducing the need for amputation.
10. Goorin, A., Frei, E., and Abelson, H. Adjuvant chemotherapy for osteosarcoma: A decade of experience. *Surg. Clin. North Am.* 61:1379, 1981.
    This review of one center's experience associated improved disease-free survival with increasingly aggressive chemotherapeutic schemes; similar data from other centers are presented on pages 1371 and 1391 of the same issue.

Ewing Sarcoma

11. Nesbit, M., Robison, L., and Dehner, L. Round Cell Sarcoma of Bone. In W. Sutow, D. Fernbach, and T. Vietti (eds.), *Clinical Pediatric Oncology* (3rd ed.). St. Louis: Mosby, 1984.
    Another encyclopedic review, with much emphasis on histologic findings.
12. Tepper, J., et al. Local control of Ewing's sarcoma of bone with radiotherapy and combination chemotherapy. *Cancer* 46:1969, 1980.
    With increasingly intensive therapy, only 7 percent of patients with tumors in the distal extremities had a local recurrence; of those with "central" lesions (pelvis, vertebrae, ribs), 33 percent suffered recurrent disease.

XIII. IMMUNITY AND INFECTIOUS DISEASES

Kenneth B. Roberts

The thorough study of children with apparent immune deficiency, coupled with great strides in basic immunology, has led to major advances in the understanding of host defenses against infection. Knowledge is presently sufficient often to permit tentative identification of a specific immune defect on clinical grounds alone, prior to laboratory confirmation. Yet this area of medicine is still relatively new, and wide gaps in knowledge exist; the delineation of mechanisms and function is incomplete and treatment frustratingly inadequate.

Immunity is conventionally thought of as being of two types, humoral and cellular. In each of these categories there are both nonspecific and specific components. The specific agents of *humoral immunity,* directed toward a particular antigenic target, are antibodies of a specific gamma globulin fraction of plasma. Various classes (IgG, IgM, IgA, IgD, IgE) are recognized, differentiated on the basis of molecular weight, structure, and function. IgG immunoglobulins are relatively small and are actively transported across the placenta; antibodies of this class are associated with protection against infectious agents and are what constitute commercially available human immune serum globulin (HISG) for injection. The infant starts with a full measure of IgG protection acquired transplacentally, but produces little of his own IgG antibodies for several months. Serum levels may drop as low as 200 mg/dl (low normal for an adult is 600 mg/dl). IgM antibodies are larger than IgG, are produced earlier than IgG in infections, and seem to be of particular importance against gram-negative bacteria. They do not cross the placenta and so are normally absent or present in low amounts in cord sera; their presence at birth suggests prenatal infection. IgA is of two types, circulating and secretory. The importance of circulating IgA is unclear; secretory IgA may well have an important role in the local immunity of mucosal surfaces, at least those of the gastrointestinal and respiratory tracts. Like IgM, IgA is normally absent at birth, and its presence implies prenatal infection. The immunoglobulins are produced by plasma cells derived from special lymphocytes designated as *B cells* because of a bursa discovered in chickens that is believed to be the site of the antibody-producing cells (bursa of Fabricius). It is unknown whether or not a bursal equivalent exists in humans and, if so, where it might reside; speculation has focused primarily on Peyer patches of the ileum.

Complement represents the nonspecific arm of humoral immunity. Once stimulated, members of the complement cascade activate each other and in so doing produce chemotactic, opsonic, and other factors that aid in the control of infection. In addition to the classic sequence of complement activation (C1 → C4 → C2 → C3, etc.) an "alternative pathway" (properdin pathway) is recognized in which the first few steps of the classic pathway are bypassed. The results of studies of children with sickle cell disease and of patients with C3b inactivator deficiency suggest that defects in the alternative pathway may have important clinical consequences.

In *cell-mediated immunity,* the antigen-specific functions are carried out by thymus-dependent lymphocytes, the T cells. Activated T cells may serve as memory cells, secrete mediators of cellular immunity called lymphokines, or directly produce specific cytotoxic effects. They play a major role in host defense against viral, fungal, protozoal, and some bacterial pathogens, are responsible for delayed hypersensitivity, and appear to be important in immune surveillance against cancer. Approximately 70 percent of circulating lymphocytes are T cells.

The nonspecific cell-mediated activity is phagocytosis, performed by polymorphonuclear leukocytes, monocytes, and macrophages. Normally, these cells are attracted to the agent to be cleared, ingest the substance, and digest it.

A careful history is of particular importance when the physician suspects that the child may have an undue susceptibility to infection. Concern is often expressed about the number of infections the child has contracted, but a normal child may have 100 infections in the first 10 years, the majority of which are self-limited viral upper respiratory tract infections and gastroenteritis. For the child with recurrent infections localized to a specific area of the body (e.g., urinary tract infections), immune function is less likely to be abnormal than are mechanical factors. Infections associated with immune deficiency are usually not only recurrent but also severe, complicated, or unusual. The pattern of infections often suggests the nature of a possible immune deficiency: a disturbance in B cell function (antibody) should be suspected if a child has recurrent, complicated, or severe pyogenic infections; chronic recurrent *Candida* infection of the scalp, nails, and mucous membranes (mucocutaneous candidiasis), by contrast, would prompt consideration of faulty T cell function. The history and the physical examination are also used to identify known syndromes of which immunodeficiency is a part; an example is the Wiskott-Aldrich syndrome of eczema, thrombocytopenia, and infections, due to defects in both B cell and T cell immunity. Failure to thrive is a notable feature of severe immunodeficiency, and its absence may be reassuring: severe long-standing immunodeficiency is a most unlikely cause of mild recurrent infections in a child with consistent, normal gains in linear growth.

B cell function can be tested by quantitative determination of immunoglobulins and, functionally, by measuring antibody titers to isohemagglutinins (anti-A, anti-B) or to the toxins of diphtheria and tetanus if the child has completed his primary series of immunizations. The presence of lymphoid tissue (e.g., tonsils, lymph nodes) should be sought on physical examination. More sophisticated tests, such as quantitation of peripheral B cells, can be performed when necessary. To assess nonspecific humoral immunity, assays of hemolytic complement function or quantitative assays of C3 and C4 are now widely available; assays of other components of the complement cascade still require the services of research laboratories.

The two screening tests available for assessing T cell immunity are the peripheral lymphocyte count, normally greater than 1200 per cubic millimeter, and skin testing for delayed hypersensitivity. Skin testing in infants may be complicated by lack of exposure to available skin test antigens; in such a situation, immunization with the antigens in diphtheria-pertussis-tetanus vaccine may be given, followed by skin testing with the diphtheria and tetanus components. There are more sophisticated assays of T cell function, such as the response to phytohemagglutinin, which normally activates T-lymphocytes, but these are not available in every laboratory. Except for the absolute count of polymorphonuclear leukocytes in the blood, assessment of nonspecific cell-mediated immunity function is at present available in a limited number of laboratories.

Between one-half and three-fourths of children recognized as immunodeficient have abnormalities of B cell function, and another one-fourth have combined T cell and B cell abnormalities. Only about 5 percent have deficits limited to T cell function, and 1 percent each have complement or phagocytic disorders. In all likelihood, this breakdown reflects the current availability of diagnostic tests rather than the distribution of immune deficits in nature. As knowledge increases, so does the number of clinically identifiable abnormalities.

Advances in treatment have not kept up with increased knowledge of basic immunologic mechanisms. Human immune serum globulin (HISG) is available for children with gamma globulin deficiency, but it provides only IgG and, until recently, required painful monthly intramuscular injections of large quantities to provide protection; a preparation for intravenous infusion is now available. Thymus transplantation is curative in infants with congenital thymic aplasia and is being evaluated in modified form for older children with combined immune deficiency, as is bone marrow transplantation. Supportive therapy requires avoidance of live viral vaccines, such as poliomyelitis vaccine, and prompt recognition and treatment of infection.

Reviews

1. Stiehm, E., and Fulginiti, V. (eds.). *Immunologic Disorders in Infants and Children* (2nd ed.). Philadelphia: Saunders, 1980.

   An excellent chapter on general considerations of immunodeficiency (p. 183), plus many others on specific topics.

2. Miller, M. (ed.). Symposium on the child with recurrent infection. *Pediatr. Clin. North Am.* 24(2), 1977.

   Ten articles review various aspects (150 pages).

3. Jones, J., and Fulginiti, V. Recurrent bacterial infections in children. *Pediatr. Rev.* 1:99, 1979.

   Immune deficiency in perspective; a good place to start for clinical orientation. (For a review with greater emphasis on mechanisms, see N. Engl. J. Med. 310:1237, 1984, for more on laboratory diagnosis, see Pediatr. Clin. North Am. 24:329, 1977.)

4. Rosen, F., Cooper, M., and Wedgewood, R. The primary immunodeficiencies. *N. Engl. J. Med.* 311:235, 300, 1984.
   A thorough 2-part review (19 pages, 260 references).
5. Cooper, M., and Buckley, R. Developmental immunology and the immunodeficiency diseases. *JAMA* 248:2658, 1982.
   Part of a "Primer on Allergic and Immunologic Diseases"; reviews ontogeny of the immune system and gives a brief description of the various immunodeficiency diseases.

Humoral Immunity

6. Bruton, O. Agammaglobulinemia. *Pediatrics* 9:722, 1952.
   The classic description of multiple septic episodes and determination of the underlying cause.
7. Tiller, T., and Buckley, R. Transient hypogammaglobulinemia of infancy: Review of the literature, clinical and immunologic features of 11 new cases, and long-term follow-up. *J. Pediatr.* 92:347, 1978.
   With editorial on page 521 emphasizing the benign nature of transient hypogammaglobulinemia, the lack of need for HISG, and features that distinguish transient from persistent hypogammaglobulinemia.
8. Hausser, C., et al. Common variable hypogammaglobulinemia in children. *Am. J. Dis. Child.* 137:833, 1983.
   The clinical and immunologic observations in 30 patients are reported; the mean age at onset was 5.5 years, at diagnosis 10.5 years.
9. Stiehm, E. Standard and special human immune serum globulins as therapeutic agents. *Pediatrics* 63:301, 1979.
   Same subject, same author, shorter review: Pediatr. Rev. *4:135, 1982.*
10. Tomasi, T. Secretory immunoglobulins. *N. Engl. J. Med.* 287:500, 1972.
    Emphasizes chemical and biologic properties, but with assessment of clinical implications.
11. Winkelstein, J. Opsonins: Their function, identity and clinical significance. *J. Pediatr.* 82:747, 1973.
    As promised in the subtitle.
12. Johnston, R., and Stroud, R. Complement and host defense against infection. *J. Pediatr.* 90:169, 1977.
    A review of the activities of complement and the diseases associated with deficiencies. (Age-related normal values: Am. J. Dis. Child. *135:918, 1981; more on alternative pathway:* N. Engl. J. Med. *303:259, 1980.)*

Cellular Immunity

13. Conley, M., et al. The spectrum of the DiGeorge syndrome. *J. Pediatr.* 94:883, 1979.
    Hypoplasia and malformation or maldescent of the thymus and parathyroid glands (III-IV pharyngeal pouch syndrome); review of 25 patients with emphasis on associated abnormalities and variability. (More on the clinical and immunologic spectrum: J. Clin. Lab. Immunol. *6:1, 1981.)*
14. Winkelstein, J., and Drachman, R. Phagocytosis. *Pediatr. Clin. North Am.* 21:551, 1974.
    Succinct and readable; still useful, even after more than a decade. (For an update on the management of patients with defective phagocyte function, see Rev. Infect. Dis. *6:107, 1984, the thirteenth review in this journal's series on the role of the phagocyte in infection.)*
15. Weetman, R., and Boxer, L. Childhood neutropenia. *Pediatr. Clin. North Am.* 27:361, 1980.
    Followed in the same issue (p. 377) by review of "Neutrophil dysfunction associated with states of chronic and recurrent infection." (For another review of neutropenia in children, including a table of normal values, see Pediatr. Rev. *3:108, 1981.)*
16. Franz, M., Carella, J., and Galant, S. Cutaneous delayed hypersensitivity in a healthy pediatric population: Diagnostic value of diphtheria-tetanus toxoids. *J. Pediatr.* 88:975, 1976.

Expected reaction rates for Candida, *mumps, streptokinase-streptodornase, and DT skin tests suggest superiority of diluted DT as a test for delayed-type hypersensitivity. (Disagreement with the conclusion and the problems of selecting skin test antigens are discussed:* Am. J. Dis. Child. *134:479, 1980.)*

17. Kirkpatrick, C., Rich, R., and Bennett, J. Chronic mucocutaneous candidiasis: Model-building in cellular immunity. *Ann. Intern. Med.* 74:955, 1971.
    A description of the syndrome, associated immune defects, and attempts at correction.

Other Immunodeficiency Diseases

18. Bortin, M., and Rimm, A. Severe combined immunodeficiency disease. *JAMA* 238:591, 1977.
    Characterization of the disease and results of transplantation (N = 69).

19. Mitchell, B., and Kelley, W. Purinogenic immunodeficiency diseases: Clinical features and molecular mechanisms. *Ann. Intern. Med.* 92:826, 1980.
    ADA deficiency is expressed as severe combined immunodeficiency; PNP deficiency results in isolated T-cell defect.

20. Rubinstein, A., Acquired immunodeficiency syndrome in infants. *Am. J. Dis. Child.* 137:825, 1983.
    A brief editorial with references to reported cases and a table of findings in AIDS prodrome and AIDS. (Findings in infants and children compared with those in adults: Pediatrics *72:430, 1983.)*

21. Hill, H. The syndrome of hyperimmunoglobulinemia E and recurrent infections. *Am. J. Dis. Child.* 136:767, 1982.
    Job's syndrome: recurrent abscesses; related to abnormal PMN chemotactic function and allergic mediator release?

Disorders with Associated Immune Defects

22. Saulsbury, F., et al. Combined immunodeficiency and vaccine-related poliomyelitis in a child with cartilage-hair hypoplasia. *J. Pediatr.* 86:868, 1975.
    Makes two points: syndrome recognition can alert you to an immune defect that is not yet clinically apparent; live-virus vaccine can be devastating to an immune-deficient child.

23. Perry, G., et al. The Wiskott-Aldrich syndrome in the United States and Canada (1892–1979). *J. Pediatr.* 97:72, 1980.
    Immunodeficiency with thrombocytopenia and eczema; 301 case histories reviewed.

24. McFarlin, D., Strober, W., and Waldmann, T. Ataxia-telangiectasia. *Medicine* (Baltimore) 51:281, 1972.
    Cerebellar ataxia, ocular and cutaneous telangiectasia, and frequent sinopulmonary infections.

25. Giacoia, G., et al. Picture of the month: Chédiak-Steinbrinck-Higashi syndrome. *Am. J. Dis. Child.* 135:949, 1981.
    Frequent pyogenic infections associated with partial albinism and large granules in white blood cells. (Pictured are a patient, stained bone marrow specimen, and granule-containing white blood cells.)

26. Katz, M., and Stiehm, E. Host defenses in malnutrition. *Pediatrics* 59:490, 1977.
    An editorial review of B cell, T cell, phagocytic, and complement function. (Clinical relevance: Am. J. Dis. Child. *134:824, 1980.)*

100. IMMUNIZATIONS AND VACCINE-PREVENTABLE DISEASES
Kenneth B. Roberts

The administration of immunizing agents exemplifies pediatricians' commitment to preventive medicine. The success of the immunizing agents is reflected in the present rarity of such diseases as paralytic poliomyelitis; yet within the past decade, basic tenets of the immunization program have come under reevaluation. Routine vaccination to protect against smallpox has been discontinued because the risk of contracting the disease in the

United States is now less than the risks attributed to the vaccine. Concern has been expressed about live poliovirus vaccine being more dangerous at present than the equally effective killed virus vaccine; questions still remain about the appropriate use of rubella vaccine and, particularly in Great Britain, of pertussis vaccine. To be used in an entire population, an immunizing agent should be effective and long lasting, safe (or at least much less harmful than the natural disease), and practical to administer in terms of cost, route, and number of doses required.

Diphtheria is now an uncommon disease in the United States. The disease is caused by a toxin elaborated by *Corynebacterium diphtheriae*. The case fatality rate in unimmunized persons is 10 percent (15% under age 5), despite the availability of antibiotics to which the organism is susceptible. Once symptoms have appeared, penicillin or erythromycin are adjuncts only, the primary therapy being antitoxin administration and support. The usual site of disease is the upper respiratory tract and the characteristic sign is the thick, tenacious membrane caused by the necrosing action of the diphtheria toxin. Toxin also reaches distant sites, such as the myocardium and the central nervous system.

The toxoid used for immunization is effective in preventing disease but does not affect carriage of the organisms; thus, fully immunized persons may, if exposed, become infected with the agent and infect others. Because the reactions to diphtheria toxoid appear to increase with the age of the host, the dose of toxoid is decreased after age 6; immunity can be maintained throughout life by the administration of booster doses every 10 years.

Tetanus, like diphtheria, is a disease that results from the effect of a bacterial toxin. The bacterium, *Clostridium tetani*, is a spore-forming, anaerobic, gram-positive bacillus found in soil and feces. Only about 100 cases of tetanus are reported each year in the United States. The toxin causes sustained muscular contraction, leading to such clinical signs as rigidity, spasm, opisthotonos, laryngospasm, and trismus (thus the common name "lockjaw"). Once signs develop, the disease progresses to a fatal outcome in 60 to 70 percent of cases. Neonatal disease may occur if maternal immunity is lacking and infection is introduced at the time of delivery. The organism is sensitive to penicillin, but tetanus immune globulin (or tetanus antitoxin if the globulin is not available) is required once the disease is established.

Tetanus toxoid has an exceptional record as an immunizing agent for both effectiveness and safety. After a primary series, boosters are required only every 10 years, although many clinicians choose to administered toxoid 5 years or more following the last booster if a deep and dirty wound is sustained, particularly a puncture wound contaminated with soil.

Pertussis (whooping cough) is caused by *Bordetella pertussis*; it is not clear at present whether an indistinguishable clinical syndrome is also caused by adenoviruses. The disease is highly contagious. Prior to the use of pertussis vaccine in the United States, whooping cough was a major cause of death in infants; 7 times as many babies died from pertussis as from meningitis, for example. At present, only 1000 to 2000 cases are reported annually. The earliest clinical stage of pertussis is a 1- to 2-week period of coryza, indistinguishable from the common cold. The paroxysmal stage follows, during which the child has the characteristic series of coughs, commonly leading to suffusion of the face, conjunctival hemorrhages, cyanosis, and petechiae; convulsions, presumably from anoxia, but perhaps in part due to small intracranial hemorrhages or encephalitis, are not rare. During the series of coughs, the child is unable to draw air in; as the paroxysm abates, there is an inspiratory gasp, the classic "whoop." The paroxysmal stage lasts 1 to 2 weeks and is followed by a several-week convalescence, during which time a milder cough is present.

Of persons who die from pertussis, 35 percent are less than 3 months of age and 75 percent are under 1 year, underscoring the seriousness of the infection in infancy. The diagnosis is suggested by the clinical course and by a marked increase in total circulating white cells, 70 to 80 percent of which may be small mature lymphocytes. The sedimentation rate is normal or decreased, and the chest roentgenogram may show a pattern of central involvement known as the "shaggy heart sign." The organism is cultured on a special medium (Bordet-Gengou with antibiotic added), but may be recovered only during the catarrhal stage and early in the paroxysmal stage. The fluorescent antibody technique is more rapid than culture but is associated with an unacceptable rate of false-positives in many laboratories.

Neither antibiotics nor pertussis hyperimmune globulin is effective in ameliorating the clinical course once the paroxysmal stage is reached; erythromycin appears to be effective in shortening the period of contagiousness, however. The vaccine is crude, requires multiple inoculations, and is only temporarily effective, with 95% of those vaccinated being susceptible 12 years after vaccination. In addition, the vaccine is associated with a high incidence of complications, particularly fever and local reactions. The incidence of encephalitis associated with the use of this vaccine is not precisely known but is estimated to be approximately 1 in 100,000 doses, with residua apparent 1 year later in one-third of those affected.

Diphtheria toxoid, pertussis vaccine, and tetanus toxoid, or DPT, are usually combined in the primary series of three doses given 8 weeks apart beginning at 2 months of age. Reactions to DPT immunization usually occur within the first 24 hours and frequently include fever, local swelling, redness, and tenderness. Evolving neurologic disease is a contraindication to giving pertussis vaccine; a neurologic or other severe reaction (collapse, shocklike state, screaming for 3 or more hours, temperature of 40.5°C or greater) after a dose of vaccine contraindicates future doses. The immunization schedule presently recommended has been selected on the basis of optimal response to the antigens and practical considerations about the timing of visits for health supervision in the first year of life. Booster doses are required at 18 months and prior to school entry.

Whereas 25 years ago, thousands of infants and children contracted *poliomyelitis* annually, there have been less than 35 cases reported each year in the past 10 years. Poliovirus is a neurotropic enterovirus that, once ingested, multiplies in the gastrointestinal tract. Its particular affinity for anterior horn cells in the spinal cord leads to weakness and paralysis, although the majority of infected persons do not have a clinically detectable neurologic deficit.

Killed virus vaccine administered by intramuscular injection was introduced in the 1950s, but was replaced early in the next decade by trivalent live attenuated oral vaccine. The vaccine currently used has the theoretical advantage of inducing local secretory IgA, and the route of administration mimics the natural disease. Proponents of the killed virus vaccine point out that children with immunodeficiency are endangered by the attenuated but still live vaccine and refer to the success in eradication of poliomyelitis accomplished by countries in which the killed agent has been used exclusively. Vaccine-associated poliomyelitis does occur, at a rate of approximately 1 case per 1 million doses. The oral live attenuated trivalent vaccine remains the immunizing agent chosen by the American Academy of Pediatrics and the United States Public Health Service and is administered along with diphtheria toxoid, pertussis vaccine, and tetanus toxoid to infants and preschool children. Although breast milk may contain antibodies against poliovirus, the live vaccine can be given to breast-fed babies without alteration in their feeding schedule. Other live viral vaccines can be given with the third or fourth dose of poliomyelitis vaccine.

The diagnosis of *measles* is commonly misapplied to any maculopapular eruption when, in fact, the clinical syndrome of measles is distinctive and should not be confused with such disparate conditions as miliaria (prickly heat), enteroviral exanthem, or rubella. The disease is ushered in by low-grade fever, followed by conjunctivitis, coryza, cough, and then the characteristic enanthem of bluish-white dots on an erythematous base located primarily on the buccal mucosa (Koplik spots). The rash appears initially on the face and upper trunk; at this time the face is swollen and the child is miserable. Fever and cough become more prominent, and the rash progresses caudad, becoming confluent over the face and upper trunk during the second and third days. In all, the rash lasts 5 to 7 days and the illness 7 to 10 days. Encephalitis complicates recovery in 1 in 1000 children with measles, and death may occur from the encephalitis or from pneumonia. Subacute sclerosing panencephalitis (SSPE), the prototype of a slow virus infection, is a debilitating late complication of infection with measles virus.

The vaccine currently used is an attenuated live virus vaccine; virus multiplication occurs after subcutaneous administration. Fever appears in 5 to 15 percent of children 5 to 6 days after inoculation but is rarely present on the first day after vaccination. Encephalitis as a complication appears to be a thousand times less common after the vaccine than after natural disease; subacute sclerosing panencephalitis is also less frequent after vaccine than after natural disease. Transplacentally acquired maternal antibody interferes with the immunogenicity of the vaccine. The recommended age for immunization currently is 15 months.

Mumps is common in children, but only two-thirds of those infected have clinical disease. Parotitis is by far the most familiar manifestation, but encephalitis complicates 3 cases in 1000, more commonly in males than females and with a slightly higher incidence after adolescence. A complete, usually unilateral hearing loss may result from the neurologic involvement. The incidence of orchitis may be as high as 20 percent in postpubertal males but is rarely bilateral; thus, the risk of sterility is overstated. Pancreatitis is rare in children. The mumps vaccine in current use is live attenuated virus and is usually combined with measles and rubella vaccines.

Rubella, or German measles, was considered a mild disease of relatively little importance until the epidemic of 1964–1965, when the previously recognized capacity of rubella virus to act as a teratogen was strikingly demonstrated: an estimated 20,000 to 50,000 infants were born with congenital rubella syndrome. The manifestations—mild in some newborns but devastating in others—include the following: growth retardation; eye defects (cataracts, glaucoma, retinopathy, and microphthalmia); cardiac defects (patent ductus arteriosus, septal defects, pulmonary stenosis, especially of the peripheral pulmonary arteries); deafness; thrombocytopenic purpura; hepatitis; bone lesions; cerebral defects (retardation, microcephaly); organomegaly; and others. Rubella acquired later in life is usually a mild illness, characterized by a maculopapular eruption and posterior auricular adenopathy.

The main clinical feature that distinguishes rubella from enteroviral infections is the former's occurrence in winter and spring rather than in late summer and early autumn. A clinical diagnosis of rubella is unreliable; serologic documentation is mandatory. In adults, a mild prodrome may be recognized, and arthralgias may be associated with the clinical illness, particularly in adult women; nevertheless, the diagnosis is still usually difficult and serum specimens (acute and convalescent) should be tested if rubella infection is suspected.

Rubella vaccine is a live attenuated virus. The main side effects, arthralgias and peripheral neuritis, appear to increase in frequency with age from less than 10 percent in young children to nearly 33 percent in adult women. In the United States, current recommendations are to vaccinate preschool children over the age of 12 months and susceptible adult women in the immediate postpartum period; because of the theoretical risk to the fetus, pregnancy is a contraindication to the administration of vaccine. In other countries it is considered preferable to allow natural infection to occur during childhood and to vaccinate during early puberty. The concept of "herd immunity" on which the American system is based has been challenged, but there does seem to have been a decrease in the number of cases of both rubella and congenital rubella syndrome since the introduction of vaccine.

In 1976, the threat of a "swine flu" pandemic focused attention on *influenza* as vaccine preventable. Clinically, influenza is characterized by fever, myalgia, and cough; pneumonia is usually a serious complication only in children with underlying chronic disease. Influenza is also a cause of severe croup in infants, and Reye syndrome (see Chap. 10) has been related to outbreaks of influenza B.

In children, influenza vaccine is recommended routinely only for those with heart, lung, or renal disease. Doses of whole influenza A virus vaccine sufficiently immunogenic to protect against disease may also be toxic; two fractional doses of purified ("split-product") vaccine are utilized in children under age 12 years. Unlike the viral vaccines that have been discussed, influenza vaccine does not contain live virus.

All the immunizing agents that have been mentioned are effective, but a large number of children in this country remain unimmunized. Work continues on vaccines against *Haemophilus influenzae,* the meningococcus, and the pneumococcus, the three most frequent causes of meningitis in infants and children (see Chap. 3); currently available agents are poorly immunogenic in infants under 2 years of age.

General

1. *Report of the Committee on Infectious Diseases* (19th ed.). Evanston, Ill.: American Academy of Pediatrics, 1982.
   The "Red Book"; a concise cookbook of immunization and diseases.

2. Centers for Disease Control. General recommendations on immunization. *Ann Intern. Med.* 98:615, 1983.

The Public Health Service view of issues such as timing, adverse reactions, etc. (? pages). CDC recommendations for prevention of specific diseases published in Ann Intern. Med. *include: diphtheria, tetanus, and pertussis 95:723, 1981; polio 96:630 1982; mumps 98:192, 1983; rubella 101:505, 1984; influenza 101:218, 1984 (updated annually); hepatitis B 97:379, 1982; and pneumococcal infections 101:348, 1984 These and reference 1 are the places to start.*

3. Fulginiti, V. Controversies in current immunization policy and practices. *Curr Probl. Pediatr.* 6(6), 1976.

An excellent, concise discussion of eight controversial issues, emphasizing technolog: and the basic knowledge gap (35 pages, 107 references); the author discusse. additional current controversies: J. Pediatr. 101:487, 1982.

4. Hirtz, D., Nelson, K., and Ellenberg, J. Seizures following childhood immunizations *J. Pediatr.* 102:14, 1983.

Forty immunization-related seizures were noted in the Collaborative Perinata Project; 10 were associated with pertussis, 10 with measles, and the other 20 witt various agents.

Timing

5. Phillips, C. Children out of step with immunization. *Pediatrics* 55:877, 1975.

A review emphasizing that there is no need to "restart" a primary series in a chil already "partially immunized."

6. Brickman, H., et al. The timing of tuberculin test in relation to immunization witt live viral vaccines. *Pediatrics* 55:392, 1975.

Screening for tuberculosis is not invalidated by simultaneous administration o vaccines.

Diphtheria

7. Hodes, H. Diphtheria. *Pediatr. Clin. North Am.* 26:445, 1979.

From history to prevention, including everything in between.

8. Miller, L., et al. Diphtheria immunization. *Am. J. Dis. Child.* 123:197, 1972.

Diphtheria immunization (toxoid) does not affect rate of infection, just disease: full: immune persons had one-thirtieth as much disease as nonimmune persons ani one-twelfth as much as partially immune persons.

Tetanus

9. Weinstein, L. Tetanus. *N. Engl. J. Med.* 289:1293, 1973.

A concise review. For a longer review, see Pediatr. Clin. North Am. 26:415, 1979.

10. Bass, J. Optimal antibiotic and antitoxin treatment of tetanus? *J. Pediatr.* 85:583 1974.

Problems with hyperimmune globulin are discussed; the author suggests tha oxytetracycline, rather than penicillin, should be the drug of choice in treatment.

11. Ipsen, J. Tetanus: Still here? *N. Engl. J. Med.* 280:614, 1969.

An editorial perspective on use and abuse (overuse) of toxoid and the epidemiology o tetanus.

12. Jacobs, R., Lowe, R., and Lanier, B. Adverse reactions to tetanus toxoid. *JAMA* 247:40, 1982.

A review of 740 charts of patients with a history of "adverse reaction": nature o reaction responses to skin tests, and, in some cases, results of challenge recorded (Reactivity seems correlated with high titer of antibody: J. Infect. Dis. 144:376, 1981.

Pertussis

13. Olson, L. Pertussis. *Medicine* (Baltimore) 54:427, 1975.

A lengthy (42 pages, 410 references) review of all aspects as of 1975. (Even better—ani more current—is C. Manclark, and J. Hill, (eds.), International Symposium o1 Pertussis. *Bethesda: DHEW/NIH, 1979. (DHEW publication number [NIH 79–1830.) This is essentially a 400-page textbook on pertussis. For a brief up-to-dat review, see* Pediatr. Infect. Dis. 3:182, 1984.)

14. Brooksaler, F., and Nelson, J. Pertussis. *Am. J. Dis. Child.* 114:389, 1967.
    A review of 190 confirmed cases.
15. Nelson, J. The changing epidemiology of pertussis in young infants. *Am. J. Dis. Child.* 132:371, 1978.
    The role of adults as reservoirs of infection is emphasized (including hospital staff: JAMA 221:264, 1972). (The degree of contagiousness in families is high: J. Pediatr. 103:359, 1983. For a provocative review of the many "epidemiologic anomalies" of pertussis, see Am. J. Med. Sci. 222:333, 1951.)
16. Pittman, M. Pertussis toxin: The cause of the harmful effects and prolonged immunity of whooping cough. A hypothesis. *Rev. Infect. Dis.* 1:401, 1979.
    Proposes that many of the active "factors" produced by B. pertussis are actually a single toxin and that disease involves two distinct steps, attachment and toxin production, each amenable to host defense. Also see Pediatr. Rev. 3:467, 1984.
17. Baraff, L., Wilkins, J., and Wehrle, P. The role of antibiotics, immunizations, and adenoviruses in pertussis. *Pediatrics* 61:224, 1978.
    A compact review of all three issues.
18. Cody, C., et al. Nature and rates of adverse reactions associated with DTP and DT immunizations in infants and children. *Pediatrics* 68:650, 1981.
    Results of 15,752, DTP injections. (Also see Pediatrics 63:256, 1979; for more on contraindications, see JAMA 251:2070, 1984, and Pediatrics 74:303, 1984.)
19. Miller, D., et al. Pertussis immunisation and serious acute neurological illness in children. *Br. Med. J.* 282:1595, 1981.
    The National Childhood Encephalopathy Study estimates rate of encephalopathy from pertussis vaccine to be 1 : 110,000 previously normal children, with 1 : 310,000 abnormal 1 year later.
20. Hinman, A., and Koplan, J. Pertussis and pertussis vaccine: Reanalysis of benefits, risks, and costs. *JAMA* 251:3019, 1984.
    An update of an earlier analysis by the Centers for Disease Control (N. Engl. J. Med. 301:906, 1979) based on more current data; vaccine still appears cost-effective. (For more on "the risks and benefits debate," see Epidemiol. Rev. 4:1, 1982, for a 24-page review with 83 references or Rev. Infect. Dis. 1:927, 1979, for a shorter, readable review.)

Polio

21. Moore, M., et al. Poliomyelitis in the United States, 1969–1981. *J. Infect. Dis.* 146:558, 1982.
    A review of the 203 reported cases.
22. Nightengale, E. Recommendations for a national policy on poliomyelitis vaccination. *N. Engl. J. Med.* 297:249, 1977.
    With an editorial (p. 275); evaluates the use of live vaccine, vaccine-related disease, liability, and consent. (IPV vs. OPV: Rev. Infect. Dis. 2:228, 243, 258, 277, 1980; worldwide control: Rev. Infect. Dis. 6[Suppl. 2], 1984.)

Measles

23. Witte, J., and Axnick, N. The benefits from 10 years of measles immunization in the United States. *Public Health Rep.* 90:205, 1975.
    Estimated savings of $1.3 billion in the United States in the first 20 years of measles vaccine availability.
24. Landrigan, P., and Witte, J. Neurologic disorders following live measles-virus vaccination. *JAMA* 223:1459, 1973.
    No greater than in controls (~ 1 in 1 million) and on the order of a thousand times less frequent than after natural measles.
25. Modlin, J., et al. Epidemiologic studies of measles, measles vaccine, and subacute sclerosing panencephalitis. *Pediatrics* 59:505, 1977.
    The risk of subacute sclerosing panencephalitis following measles and measles vaccination is discussed. (More on the epidemiology of SSPE: J. Pediatr. 94:231, 1979.)
26. Brodsky, A. Atypical measles. *JAMA* 222:1415, 1972.
    Refers to a syndrome in the recipients of vaccine on exposure to wild virus.

27. Brunell, P. Measles immunization: 12 or 15 months? *Pediatrics* 62:1038, 1978.
   An editorial review of the issues and the evidence (accompanies two articles, pp. 955 and 961).
28. Herman, J., Radin, R., and Schneiderman, R. Allergic reactions to measles (rubeola) vaccine in patients hypersensitive to egg protein. *J. Pediatr.* 102:196, 1983.
   It appears safe to immunize a child who has no clinical reaction to egg white regardless of the ovalbumin skin test response; management of the child who has clinical allergic reaction to egg white is discussed.
29. Hinman, A., et al. Progress in measles elimination. *JAMA* 247:1592, 1982.
   Overview of the project and status report. (Also see Rev. Infect. Dis. 5(3), 1983.)

Mumps

30. Lerner, A. Guide to immunization against mumps. *J. Infect. Dis.* 122:116, 1970.
   A good review of the disease as well as an orientation to vaccination.
31. Hayden, G., et al. Current status of mumps and mumps vaccine in the United States. *Pediatrics* 62:965, 1978.
   Documents a drop in mumps-caused morbidity associated with the introduction of a safe and effective vaccine. (Mumps vaccine is cost-effective: Am. J. Dis. Child. 136:362, 1982.)
32. Brickman, A., and Brunell, P. Susceptibility of medical students to mumps: a comparison of serum neutralizing antibody and skin test. *Pediatrics* 48:447, 1971.
   Confirms the worthlessness of the skin test—and of the history; only 1 percent of medical students who claimed to have no history of mumps were susceptible serologically.
33. Brunell, P., et al. Parotitis in children who had previously received mumps vaccine. *Pediatrics* 50:441, 1972.
   Vaccine failures may relate to the fact that not all parotitis is mumps (especially consider parainfluenza virus).
34. Levitt, L., et al. Central nervous system mumps. *Neurology* 20:829, 1970.
   Distinguishes the syndromes of aseptic meningitis and meningoencephalitis. (CNS mumps with low CSF glucose, prolonged pleocytosis, and high protein mimicking bacterial meningitis: N. Engl. J. Med. 280:855, 1969.)

Rubella

35. Heggie, A., and Robbins, F. Natural rubella acquired after birth. *Am. J. Dis. Child.* 118:12, 1969.
   The clinical features and complications of natural rubella; part of an excellent symposium (pp. 5–410) summarizing knowledge as of 1969 (including congenital rubella).
36. Tartakow, J. The teratogenicity of maternal rubella. *J. Pediatr.* 66:380, 1965.
   First trimester: 16.7 percent major defects, 8.3 percent minor defects, 48.6 percent abortuses, 12.6 percent prematures; second trimester: 3.3 percent major defects, 13.4 percent minor defects; third trimester: 0 major defects, 14.3 percent minor defects. (Also see J. Pediatr. 87:1078, 1975, 94:763, 1979, and Lancet 2:781, 1982.)
37. Preblud, S., et al. Current status of rubella in the United States, 1969–1979. *J. Infect. Dis.* 142:776, 1980.
   The good news is a decline in children young enough to have received vaccine; the bad news is no decline in those old enough to have "escaped" vaccine (such as hospital personnel: N. Engl. J. Med. 303:541, 1980; say, you're not susceptible to rubella, are you?).
38. Preblud, S., et al. Fetal risk associated with rubella vaccine. *JAMA* 246:1413, 1981.
   None observed; 95 percent confidence limits estimate maximal risk of 3 percent.
39. Polk, B., et al. A controlled comparison of joint reactions among women receiving one of two rubella vaccines. *Am. J. Epidemiol.* 115:19, 1982.
   Arthralgia/arthritis occurred as frequently with RA 27/3 (26%) as with the formerly used HPV-77:DE 5 (29%), but the onset of symptoms was earlier and the duration briefer.
40. Hinman, A., et al. Rational strategy for rubella vaccination. *Lancet* 1:39, 1983.
   A review of presumptions on which the American and the United Kingdom plans were based and a proposal for a new plan based on current knowledge.

Influenza

41. Aach, R., and Kissane, J. (eds.). CPC: The medical complications of influenza. *Am. J. Med.* 50:105, 1971.
    A review in dialogue form between a teacher and medical students.
42. Hall, C., and Douglas, R. Respiratory syncytial virus and influenza. *Am. J. Dis. Child.* 130:615, 1976.
    Influenza activity in the community is associated with an increased hospitalization rate for respiratory disease in adults but not in children; an increase is noted for croup, however. (Also see J. Pediatr. 81:1148, 1972, and N. Engl. J. Med. 296:829, 1977.)
43. Sanford, J., et al. Amantadine: Does it have a role in the prevention and treatment of influenza? *Clin. Pediatr.* (Phila.) 19:416, 1980.
    Report of the National Institutes of Health Consensus Development Conference. (Use in children: Pediatr. Infect. Dis. 1:44, 1982.)
44. Kilbourne, E. Influenza pandemics in perspective, *JAMA* 237:1225, 1977.
    The difficulties in predicting what "flu" will do.

Bacterial Vaccines

45. Harrison, H., and Fulginiti, V. Bacterial immunizations. *Am. J. Dis. Child.* 134:184, 1980.
    A nine-page review of agents to prevent cholera, plague, anthrax, tuberculosis, and tularemia, as well as pneumococcal and meningococcal infections, diphtheria, tetanus, and pertussis.

101. INFECTIONS OF BONES AND JOINTS

Kenneth B. Roberts

In the preantibiotic era, skeletal infections usually resulted in crippling or death. Today, despite improved techniques for early diagnosis and the availability of effective therapeutic regimens, many children still endure lasting sequelae because of failure to recognize and treat skeletal infections promptly.

Bones and joints can become infected by either of two mechanisms: by direct inoculation (as by a penetrating wound or an adjacent focus of infection) or, more commonly, by hematogenous "seeding" of organisms during bacteremia.

Osteomyelitis results when organisms circulating in the bloodstream enter the bone and lodge in the distal end of the metaphysis where the circulation is sluggish. A self-perpetuating cycle is initiated, as inflammation further compromises blood supply, and an abscess is formed within the confines of the rigid bone. Pus, under pressure, spreads through the haversian and Volkmann canals, extending disease within the bone and outward between the bone and periosteum. At this stage there is "point tenderness," an important diagnostic sign reflecting disease that is well localized to the small area of deep soft-tissue swelling and underlying inflammation of the metaphysis (metaphysitis). By the third day of disease, pus has collected beneath the periosteum, and bone destruction is present; deep swelling has extended to the muscles.

It is not until the tenth to twelfth day of illness that bone destruction and periosteal new bone formation are evident on x-ray examination. Radionucleotide scanning may give evidence of inflammation from the first day of illness and may be useful when the disease is suspected and clinical signs are equivocal.

The child with osteomyelitis is usually febrile, with an elevated white blood cell count and increased sedimentation rate. History of skeletal pain or—particularly in infants—unwillingness to move a limb or bear weight obligates the clinician to make a particularly thorough examination for bone tenderness. Once bone infection is established, it may serve as a continuing source of organisms and perpetuate the initial bacteremia; systemic signs of sepsis may dominate the clinical presentation. Under such circumstances it is imperative to begin therapy for septicemia while considering possible foci of infection, including the bones.

Blood culture yields the organism in more than 50 percent of patients with osteomyelitis. *Staphylococcus aureus* is the most common organism in all age groups, and initial therapy therefore includes the intravenous administration of a penicillinase-resistant penicillin. *Salmonella* osteomyelitis is unusually common in patients with sickle cell disease, but is rare in the general population. Antibiotic therapy for osteomyelitis is prolonged (3 weeks or more) to achieve satisfactory results; treatment of relapses or of chronic osteomyelitis is often unsatisfactory, emphasizing the need for effective management of the acute infection. There is no general agreement as to the role of operative decompression in the early stage of osteomyelitis: some physicians and surgeons are content with a clinical diagnosis, perhaps supplemented by a positive nuclear scan or a roentgenogram that suggests deep soft-tissue swelling; others advocate needle aspiration of the suspected area of involvement, providing a diagnostic specimen for Gram stain and culture; still others argue for formal creation of a "bone window" under general anesthesia, to provide diagnostic specimens and achieve the greatest amount of decompression. There is more general agreement that once the infection has become well established, an operation is needed.

The diagnosis of secondary osteomyelitis, that associated with a contiguous focus of infection, is often difficult to establish and requires frequent reevaluation for signs of bone involvement as the superficial focus responds to antibiotic therapy. Penetrating wounds may cause indolent infections, particularly in the bones of the foot, where *Pseudomonas* is often the culprit.

When organisms from the bloodstream infect a joint and produce septic arthritis, they elicit an exuberant inflammatory response, with upward of 50,000 white cells/cu mm of synovial fluid; the majority of these cells are polymorphonuclear leukocytes. The concentration of sugar is decreased, and there is a poor mucin clot. There are two adverse consequences of this septic inflammation: enzymes that destroy articular cartilage are released, and intraarticular pressure increases, sufficient in the hip to compromise blood flow to the femoral head and cause an avascular necrosis. The clinical presentation may be similar to that described for osteomyelitis except that the site of infection is more obviously involved. Erythema, swelling, and local warmth are characteristic, as is the posture assumed by the child to decrease motion and provide a maximal opportunity for distention of the affected joint. Thus, flexion and limitation are the rule, and the child with arthritis of the hip will have abduction and external rotation as well. Diagnostic aspiration of the joint is mandatory, both to provide a diagnostic specimen and to relieve pressure. If septic arthritis of the hip (or the shoulder, although this is much less common) is present, arthrotomy and lavage is an indicated operative procedure. If the joint is more readily accessible (e.g., a knee or an elbow), repeated needle arthrocenteses may be adequate.

As in osteomyelitis, *S. aureus* is the most common organism, but other bacteria must also be considered in patients in certain age groups: coliforms in neonates; *Haemophilus influenzae* in infants; and *Neisseria gonorrheae* in adolescents. Antibiotic coverage for the more common organisms is generally effective against other pathogens, such as streptococci (both groups A and B) and pneumococci. Direct instillation of antibiotics into the synovial fluid is unnecessary, since the agents commonly used pass from the bloodstream into the synovial fluid in therapeutic concentrations. The duration of therapy is usually 2 to 3 weeks.

Septic arthritis can also be caused by a penetrating injury with inoculation of the joint or by spread from an adjacent focus of osteomyelitis. The latter rarely occurs, however, unless the hip or shoulder is involved or the patient is less than 18 months of age; this is because the site of infection, the metaphyseal portion of the bone, is extraarticular in all but the hip and shoulder joints, and vessels in the involved area do not penetrate the epiphyseal plate except in early infancy.

In one series, sequelae were discovered in one-fourth of the patients. *S. aureus* and *H. influenzae* were associated with equal proportions of residua, and no particular age groups seemed to fare worse than others. The outcome was affected by a delay in treatment, and children whose hip or ankle was infected were more impaired than those with septic arthritis of the knee.

The outlook for normal skeletal development and function in children with untreated osteomyelitis or septic arthritis is dismal. At best, current antibiotic therapy is prolonged, and delays in initiating appropriate treatment can seriously compromise the outcome. The clinician must therefore be alert to the possibility of these diseases, recognize skeletal infection prior to signs of bone or joint destruction, and initiate appropriate therapy promptly.

Traditionally, antibiotic therapy has been administered parenterally, but in the past several years, the efficacy of high-dose oral therapy has been demonstrated. Because of the problems resulting from inadequate treatment, present recommendations for oral therapy include ensured patient compliance and the ability to monitor serum bactericidal activity and adjust dosage as needed.

General
1. Aronoff, S., and Scoles, P. Treatment of childhood skeletal infections. *Pediatr. Clin. North Am.* 30:271, 1983.
   A general review of osteomyelitis and septic arthritis.
2. Prober, C. Oral antibiotic therapy for bone and joint infections. *Pediatr. Infect. Dis.* 1:8, 1982.
   A review of the published experience with oral treatment, leading to recommendations and caveats.

Osteomyelitis
3. Waldvogel, F., Medoff, G., and Swartz, M. Osteomyelitis: A review of clinical features, therapeutic considerations and unusual aspects. *N. Engl. J. Med.* 282:198, 260, 316, 1970.
   A thorough, extensive review, brought up to date by the first author in N. Engl. J. Med. 303:360, 1980.
4. Dich, V., Nelson, J., and Haltalin, K. Osteomyelitis in infants and children. *Am. J. Dis. Child.* 129:1273, 1975.
   A review of the cases of 163 infants and children, concluding that treatment for less than 3 weeks is inadequate.
5. Capitanio, M., and Kirkpatrick, J. Early roentgen observations in acute osteomyelitis. *AJR* 108:488, 1970.
   The x-ray findings in three stages of osteomyelitis: days 1 to 3, 3 to 10, and 10 or more.
6. Treves, S., et al. Osteomyelitis: Early scintigraphic detection in children. *Pediatrics* 57:173, 1976.
   The role of bone scans in establishing the diagnosis is discussed. (Problems in scanning and gallium versus phosphate: J. Bone Joint Surg. 65-A:431, 1983.)
7. Ogden, J., and Lister, G. The pathology of neonatal osteomyelitis. *Pediatrics* 55:474, 1975.
   Infection can spread across the growth plate in this age group.
8. Edwards, M., et al. An etiologic shift in infantile osteomyelitis: The emergence of the group B streptococcus. *J. Pediatr.* 93:578, 1978.
   Group B streptococcal osteomyelitis contrasted with non-GBS osteomyelitis. (Also see: Pediatrics 62:535, 1978, and Pediatrics 53:505, 1974.)
9. Edwards, M., et al. Pelvic osteomyelitis in children. *Pediatrics* 61:62, 1978.
   A diagnosis to consider in a child with fever and a limp. (Signs and symptoms depend on direction inflammation takes: J. Bone Joint Surg. 61-A:1087, 1979.)
10. Bolivar, R., Kohl, S., and Pickering, L. Vertebral osteomyelitis in children: Report of four cases. *Pediatrics* 62:549, 1978.
    Back pain was an uncommon symptom.
11. Fischer, G., et al. Diskitis: A prospective diagnostic analysis. *Pediatrics* 62:543, 1978.
    A confusing entity; clinical signs are vague, etiology is uncertain, and treatment plans are debated.
12. Jacobs, R., et al. Management of *Pseudomonas* osteochondritis complicating puncture wounds of the foot. *Pediatrics* 69:432, 1982.
    Emphasizes value of surgical debridement. (Pseudomonas may also cause arthritis in MTP joints of foot following puncture: J. Pediatr. 94:429, 1979. Where does the Pseudomonas come from? Negative results from culturing children's feet, their shoes, and nails found on the ground: J. Pediatr. 91:161, 1977.)
13. Givner, L., Luddy, R., and Schwartz, A. Etiology of osteomyelitis in patients with major sickle hemoglobinopathies. *J. Pediatr.* 99:411, 1981.
    Salmonella!

Septic Arthritis

14. Nelson, J. The bacteriology and antibiotic management of septic arthritis in infants and children. *Pediatrics* 50:437, 1972.
    Emphasizes the role of coliforms and gram-positive cocci in neonates, H. influenzae in infants, and S. aureus thereafter; recommendations for treatment are offered (221 patients).
15. Howard, J., Highgenboten, C., and Nelson, J. Residual effects of septic arthritis in infancy and childhood. *JAMA* 236:932, 1976.
    Evaluation at discharge was unreliable; 27 percent had sequelae, as frequently after H. influenzae as after S. aureus.
16. Curtiss, P. The pathophysiology of joint infections. *Clin. Orothop.* 96:129, 1973.
    A basic review.
17. Chung, S., and Pollis, R. Diagnostic pitfalls in septic arthritis of the hip in infants and children. *Clin. Pediatr.* (Phila.) 14:758, 1975.
    The joint of concern.
18. Nelson, J. Antibiotic concentrations in septic joint effusions. *N. Engl. J. Med.* 284:349, 1971.
    Methicillin, ampicillin, penicillin, and cephalothin enter the joint fluid well. Other reports add to the list such antibiotics as kanamycin (Clin. Pharmacol. Ther. 12:858, 1971), gentamicin and carbenicillin (N. Engl. J. Med. 285:178, 1971), and clindamycin (Pediatrics 55:213, 1975), as well as some oral agents (J. Pediatr. 92:131, 1978).
19. Pittard, W., Thullen, J., and Fanaroff, A. Neonatal septic arthritis. *J. Pediatr.* 88:621, 1976.
    Role of umbilical catheterization? Emphasizes Candida as a pathogen. (Also remember the gonococcus in this age group: Pediatrics 53:436, 1974.)
20. Keiser, H., et al. Clinical forms of gonococcal arthritis. *N. Engl. J. Med.* 279:234, 1968.
    The forms are (1) septicemic (positive blood culture; negative joint fluid culture) and (2) septic arthritis (negative blood culture, positive joint fluid culture).

102. INFECTIOUS MONONUCLEOSIS
Kenneth B. Roberts

The diagnosis of infectious mononucleosis traditionally has been based on three characteristic findings: (1) a specific clinical syndrome, (2) atypical lymphocytes, and (3) heterophile antibodies. To this list, some clinicians added the requirement of abnormal liver function test results. It now seems clear that the etiologic agent in infectious mononucleosis is the Epstein-Barr virus (EBV), a herpesvirus; demonstration of EBV infection serves to confirm the diagnosis, but the three original requirements continue to maintain a position of central importance.

The classic clinical syndrome in adolescents and adults consists of fever, lymphadenopathy, exudative pharyngitis, and splenomegaly. The lymphadenopathy is generalized, with notable enlargement of the posterior cervical nodes. The tonsillopharyngitis may be confused with diphtheria or steptococcal infection; an aid in differential diagnosis is the longer prodrome present in infectious mononucleosis and the relatively later appearance of palatal lesions. Serum transaminase levels are almost universally elevated during clinical disease, but jaundice is much less common than transaminase abnormalities. Signs of hepatitis may dominate the clinical presentation in some patients, and the correct diagnosis may be delayed. Rash is an infrequent occurrence unless ampicillin is administered; under ordinary circumstances the antibiotic is associated with rash in 10 percent of patients, but those with infectious mononucleosis have nearly a 10-fold increase in the incidence of this complication. Periorbital edema occurs in one-third of patients, and a multitude of other clinical problems involving virtually every organ system, has been reported.

Infants rarely demonstrate the full-blown syndrome just described; infection with EBV is common, particularly in the lower socioeconomic groups, but is usually asymptomatic. The age-dependent nature of the response to EBV infection is not adequately explained at present.

The atypical lymphocytes in infectious mononucleosis have been classified by Downey as monocytoid, plasmacytoid, and blastoid. All three cell types have abundant cytoplasm that may contain large vacuoles or appear "foamy." The cells are characteristically indented by neighboring erythrocytes. When a child has atypical lymphocytes, splenomegaly, and generalized lymphadenopathy, and particularly when thrombocytopenic purpura is also present (a not infrequent complication), the diagnosis of leukemia may be suspected; careful attention to the morphology of the lymphocytes may help establish the correct diagnosis, but examination of bone marrow aspirate is often required.

Patients with infectious mononucleosis produce antibodies that agglutinate sheep red cells; this peculiar reactivity of human antibody against sheep protein is the basis for the term *heterophile antibody*. The antibody is predominantly of the IgM class and is absorbed by bovine red blood cells but not by guinea pig kidney cells, permitting a distinction from the heterophile antibody produced by patients with serum sickness.

Over the past 10 years, considerable evidence has been accumulated to incriminate EBV as the cause of infectious mononucleosis. Epstein-Barr virus can be recovered from throat washings of patients with infectious mononucleosis, lending scientific support to the designation of this illness as the "kissing disease." The cytomegalovirus, also a member of the herpesvirus group, and the protozoan *Toxoplasma gondii* may induce atypical lymphocytes and produce a clinical syndrome compatible with infectious mononucleosis, but neither agent is associated with heterophile antibodies.

There is no specific therapy for infectious mononucleosis. The two major complications in the acute disease are upper airway obstruction and splenic rupture. Convalescence may be prolonged, particularly in those patients whose disease had an insidious onset. Recurrences are virtually unheard of, and the prognosis for complete recovery is excellent.

Reviews

1. Rapp, C., and Hewetson, J. Infectious mononucleosis and the Epstein-Barr virus. *Am. J. Dis. Child.* 132:78, 1978.
   A readable review with data well presented (90 references).
2. Shurin, S. Infectious mononucleosis. *Pediatr. Clin. North Am.* 26:315, 1979.
   Another general review.
3. Karzon, D. Infectious mononucleosis. *Adv. Pediatr.* 22:231, 1976.
   Exhaustive (34 pages, 105 references).
4. Dirckx, J. Infectious mononucleosis. *JAMA* 226:78, 1973.
   A letter urging that all diagnostic criteria be met before reporting yet another bizarre manifestation of infectious mononucleosis!

Laboratory Diagnosis

5. Paul, J., and Bunnell, W. The presence of heterophile antibodies in infectious mononucleosis. *Rev. Infect. Dis.* 4:1062, 1982.
   The 1932 classic reprinted along with excerpts from the history of infectious mononucleosis (p. 1068) and an editorial (p. 1069).
6. Fleisher, G., et al. Incidence of heterophile antibody responses in children with infectious mononucleosis. *J. Pediatr.* 94:723, 1979.
   Of 68 infants and children with clinical infectious mononucleosis, 38 had evidence of EB virus infection; heterophile antibody responses by age presented.
7. Fleisher, G., Paradise, J., and Lennette, E. Leukocyte response in childhood infectious mononucleosis caused by Epstein-Barr virus. *Am. J. Dis. Child.* 135:699, 1981.
   The number of lymphocytes and atypical lymphocytes does not vary significantly with age of the patient.
8. Rocchi, G., et al. Quantitative evaluation of Epstein-Barr virus-infected mononuclear peripheral blood leukocytes in infectious mononucleosis. *N. Engl. J. Med.* 296:132, 1977.

It takes 3 months for the number of infected cells to decline to control levels. (EBV infects B cells, but the atypical lymphocytes are T cells: N. Engl. J. Med. *291:1145, 1974.)*

9. Radetsky, M. A diagnostic approach to Epstein-Barr virus infections. *Pediatr. Infect. Dis.* 1:425, 1982.
   Discussion of the leukocyte count, heterophile antibody measurement, and EB virus serology with a proposed diagnostic approach. (Recommendations for the diagnosis of infectious mononucleosis in adolescents and young adults: J. Clin. Microbiol. *17:619, 1983.)*

Epstein-Barr

10. Andiman, W. The Epstein-Barr virus and EB virus infections in childhood. *J. Pediatr.* 95:171, 1979.
    Emphasis is on the virus; for more on the biology and chemistry of EB virus, see J. Infect. Dis. *146:506, 1982.*

11. Miller, G., Niederman, J., and Andrews, L. Prolonged oropharyngeal excretion of Epstein-Barr virus after infectious mononucleosis. *N. Engl. J. Med.* 288:229, 1973.
    So it is spread by kissing!

12. Ginsburg, C., Henle, G. and Henle, W. An outbreak of infectious mononucleosis among the personnel of an outpatient clinic. *Am. J. Epidemiol.* 104:571, 1976.
    More infectious than is often appreciated.

13. Fleisher, G., et al. Intrafamilial transmission of Epstein-Barr virus infections. *J. Pediatr.* 98:16, 1981.
    Findings suggest an incubation period of 4 to 6 weeks.

14. Fleisher, G., et al. Primary infection with Epstein-Barr virus in infants in the United States: Clinical and serologic observations. *J. Infect. Dis.* 139:553, 1979.
    Asymptomatic infection and clinical infectious mononucleosis syndrome have different antibody profiles.

15. Goldberg, G., et al. In utero Epstein-Barr virus (infectious mononucleosis) infection. *JAMA* 246:1579, 1981.
    A case report raising the specter of a congenital EB syndrome of multiple congenital anomalies.

16. MacKinney, A., and Cline, W. Infectious mononucleosis. *Br. J. Haematol.* 27:367, 1974.
    A review of the evidence for the concept of infectious mononucleosis as a self-limited neoplasm.

Prognosis

17. Chretien, J., et al. Predictors of the duration of infectious mononucleosis. *South. Med. J.* 70:437, 1977.
    That which is slowest to develop (onset of symptoms to diagnosis) is slowest to resolve.

"Heterophil-Negative" (Clinical) Infectious Mononucleosis

18. Klemola, E., et al. Infectious-mononucleosis-like disease with negative heterophil agglutination test: Clinical features in relation to Epstein-Barr virus and cytomegalovirus antibodies. *J. Infect. Dis.* 121:608, 1970.
    Epstein-Barr virus and cytomegalovirus are both causes of heterophil-negative infectious mononucleosis, but the latter is not associated with the tonsillar form. Also see Am. J. Med. *63:947, 1977.*

19. Jones, T., Kean, B., and Kimball, A. Toxoplasmic lymphadenitis. *JAMA* 192:87, 1965.
    The most common form of acquired toxoplasmosis is lymphadenitis. (Serologic diagnosis of toxoplasmosis: J. Infect. Dis. *142:256, 1980.)*

20. Zuelzer, W., and Kaplan, J. The child with lymphadenopathy. *Semin. Hematol.* 12:323, 1975.
    Miscellaneous causes of lymphadenopathy.

103. TUBERCULOSIS
Kenneth B. Roberts

The incidence of tuberculosis has decreased markedly in the United States as a result of improved social conditions and specific antituberculous chemotherapy. A major triumph has been the virtual elimination of milkborne tuberculosis, transmitted to children from infected cows. In certain subgroups of the population, however, tuberculosis is still all too common, and there is a danger that the correct diagnosis may be overlooked if tuberculosis is considered only as a historical curiosity, a rare disease. Accurate diagnosis and treatment are necessary not only for the individual child but also as an integral part of tuberculosis eradication, since the child, once infected, is at lifelong risk for the development of the disease and for infecting others.

Tuberculosis is acquired by inhaling small droplet nuclei contaminated with *Mycobacterium tuberculosis*. The usual source is an infected adult, coughing with sufficient force to expel and propel 5-μ particles; small children with tuberculosis are unable to propel the particles with much force and so are rarely infectious to others. *M. tuberculosis*, once inhaled into the lung, elicits an inflammatory response, producing a small area of pneumonia that is rarely recognized clinically. After 3 to 8 weeks, the tuberculin reaction becomes positive, signaling a host response to the infection. At this stage it is still unusual for clinical signs of illness to be recognized, except in infants, nearly half of whom may be symptomatic. The area of pulmonary involvement is usually not identified on a chest roentgenogram, but *M. tuberculosis* organisms may be recovered from early morning gastric aspirates in 10 to 25 percent of children; if a lesion is demonstrable on x-ray film, the rate of bacteriologic confirmation is increased to as high as 80 to 90 percent. In some infants and children the primary infection is not well contained, and an area of caseation enlarges, ultimately spilling into the bronchi and leaving a cavity (progressive primary pulmonary tuberculosis). If the bronchus is occluded, either by endobronchial disease or by extrinsic compression from enlarged nodes, the so-called collapse-consolidation lesion is formed.

During the initial phase of infection, prior to the development of hypersensitivity to tuberculin, the bacilli gain access to the circulation and are distributed throughout the body. The majority of infants and children contain their primary infection well, but distant foci persist in a dormant stage.

Miliary tuberculosis is not synonymous with the early bacteremia, but represents a massive hematogenous seeding, usually of a large pulmonary vein by a caseous focus. Despite the extensive characteristic pulmonary involvement seen on the chest roentgenogram, auscultation may give few clues to the degree of involvement. Organomegaly is often present.

The most serious complication of miliary tuberculosis is meningitis, but meningitis more often occurs as an isolated event, from contamination of the subarachnoid space by tubercle bacilli in an adjacent subcortical focus. Classically, three clinical stages of tuberculous meningitis are described. During the first stage, the child has general signs of illness without neurologic signs or sensorial abnormalities; fever is virtually always present, and vomiting and apathy are noted in half the patients. Stage II is marked by neurologic signs and signs of meningeal irritation, but without the sensorial changes that are the hallmarks of stage III disease. Prognosis is related to clinical stage, in that children in whom the diagnosis is made prior to stage II have a better outcome than do the others.

The cerebrospinal fluid (CSF) of patients with tuberculous meningitis contains an increased number of mononuclear cells, a decreased concentration of glucose, and an increased concentration of protein; the fluid is often under increased pressure. Even with successful therapy, the CSF does not return to normal rapidly; in one-half the patients the glucose is still abnormally low at the end of the first week, and it is months before the protein concentration and number of cells return to normal. In addition to specific antituberculous therapy, corticosteroids are administered, particularly to patients with a high concentration of protein in the CSF or markedly increased CSF pressure, in an attempt to prevent early mortality from "coning."

Miliary tuberculosis and tuberculous meningitis occur with maximal frequency in the first months following primary infection, but clinical disease of the pericardium, peritoneum, kidneys, and skeleton are usually delayed a matter of years. Once the diagnosis of tuberculosis is considered clinically, additional support is provided by the demonstration of a positive reaction to 5 Tuberculin Units (TU) of intracutaneously administered tuberculin (PPD-S, Purified Protein Derivative Standard); 10 mm of induration 48 hours after inoculation is considered a positive reaction, but under certain circumstances, such as recent exposure to tuberculosis or severe illness compatible with tuberculosis, 5 mm of induration may be a more appropriate criterion. The significance of a reaction between 5 and 10 mm may be difficult to determine; the response may be caused by mycobacteria other than *M. tuberculosis,* such as the bacillus Calmette-Guérin (BCG) strain or the so-called atypicals; often, the history or the simultaneous administration of different mycobacterial antigens as skin tests along with PPD-S will help resolve confusion.

The treatment is largely determined by the extent of disease. For the child with a positive tuberculin reaction but no evidence of active disease, isoniazid for 1 year as the sole therapy prevents the development of active disease; the protection appears to be long-lasting, and toxicity, including hepatitis, is rare in children. Mild pulmonary disease demonstrable by a chest roentgenogram prompts the addition of a second oral medication. For more advanced disease, a third drug, classically streptomycin, previously was recommended; at present, the combination of isoniazid and rifampin appears to be at least as effective as the older three drug regimens and has the advantage of better entry into the CSF. Data are being accumulated on "short-course" therapy in children. Regimens, such as isoniazid and rifampin daily for 1 month followed by twice weekly for 8 months, appear to be effective. Because the duration of therapy is shorter than the standard course and supervised administration on an ambulatory basis is feasible, short-course therapy offers the potential of maximizing compliance.

Public health investigation of new cases remains an important activity in the control of tuberculosis. Household contacts of a person with newly diagnosed active disease have about a 3 percent risk of the development of active tuberculosis within 1 year if not treated; the rate is twice that high for infants and young children. Since 3 to 8 weeks are required after exposure before hypersensitivity to tuberculin develops, the tuberculin test must be repeated in exposed persons if there is a negative reaction at the time contact with the source of infection is broken. The administration of isoniazid is a logical preventive measure while waiting for the 8 weeks to elapse before determining whether or not infection has occurred.

Reviews

1. Gutman, L. Tuberculosis. In S. Krugman, and S. Katz, (eds.), *Infectious Diseases of Children* (7th ed.). St. Louis: Mosby, 1981.
   A revision of the encyclopedic reviews from previous editions by Edward Sewell and Edith Lincoln (51 pages, 125 references); another extensive review by a renowned pediatric "tuberculologist" (Margaret Smith) in R. Feigin, and J. Cherry, (eds.), Textbook of Pediatric Infectious Diseases (Vol. I). Philadelphia: Saunders, 1981. P. 1016. (44 pages, 253 references).

2. American Thoracic Society. Diagnostic standards and classification of tuberculosis and other mycobacterial diseases (14th edition). *Am. Rev. Resp. Dis.* 123:343, 1981.
   The Bible; discusses transmission, pathogenesis, diagnosis, bacteriology, and classification.

3. Smith, M. Tuberculosis in adolescents. *Clin. Pediatr.* (Phila.) 6:9, 1967.
   An overview of special considerations in teenagers.

Historical Perspective

4. Koch, R. The etiology of tuberculosis. *Rev. Infect. Dis.* 4:1270, 1982.
   The author's observations, his postulates (as they are now called), and his conclusion; first published in 1882.

5. Comroe, J. T.B. or not T.B.? I. The cause of tuberculosis. II. The treatment of tuberculosis. *Am. Rev. Resp. Dis.* 117:137, 379, 1978.
   A history of tuberculosis traced through various "major" textbooks, from Laennec (1819) through Osler to the present.

6. Glassroth, J., Robins, A., and Snider, D. Tuberculosis in the 1980s. *N. Engl. J. Med.* 302:1441, 1980.
   A state of the art review: where we are now.

Skin Test

7. American Thoracic Society. The tuberculin skin test. *Am. Rev. Resp. Dis.* 124:356, 1981.
   This is where to read about the skin test. (Should a tuberculin test be routine in office practice?: Pediatrics *64:965, 1979.)*
8. Edwards, L., Acquaviva, F., and Livesay, V. Identification of tuberculous infected. *Am. Rev. Respir. Dis.* 108:1334, 1973.
   "Doubtful" (5–9 mm) reactions to tuberculin may be clarified by simultaneously testing with PPD-S and a PPD derived from "atypical" mycobacteria.
9. Fine M., et al. Tuberculin skin test reactions. *Am. Rev. Respir. Dis.* 106:752, 1972.
   Using the classification of "positive," "doubtful," or "negative," correlation between tine test and PPD was 96 percent (7.7% false-positive tine, 1.6% false-negative).

Prophylaxis

10. American Thoracic Society. Preventive therapy of tuberculous infection. *Am. Rev. Respir. Dis.* 110:371, 1974.
    Who should take INH and how they should be managed.
11. Hsu, K. Thirty years after isoniazid: Its impact on tuberculosis in children and adolescents. *JAMA* 251:1283, 1984.
    The final report of a 30-year study involving nearly 2500 children for a total of 15,943 person-years; no child who received INH prophylaxis before age 4 developed active disease during follow-up. As therapy for existing disease, INH was effective and protective.
12. Comstock, G. New data on preventive treatment with isoniazid. *Ann. Intern. Med.* 98:663, 1983.
    Editorial report of study relating benefit of INH in reducing the rate of active TB to duration of therapy: 12 weeks resulted in "slight reduction," 24 weeks in 65 percent reduction, 52 weeks in 75 percent reduction, and 52 weeks with good compliance in 93 percent reduction.
13. O'Brien, R., et al. Hepatotoxicity from isoniazid and rifampin among children treated for tuberculosis. *Pediatrics* 72:491, 1983.
    An article to read before prescribing INH and rifampin; INH by itself infrequently causes hepatotoxicity, but the addition of rifampin to INH, particularly in children with more serious forms of TB, results in an incidence of hepatotoxicity (3.3%) approximating the rate in adults. Recommendations given.

Treatment

14. Lorin, M., Hsu, K., and Jacob, S. Treatment of tuberculosis in children. *Pediatr. Clin. North Am.* 30:333, 1983.
    An overview of prophylaxis, treatment of various forms of TB, and management of an infant born to a mother with TB. (Brief summary statements regarding antitubercular drugs: Med. Lett. Drugs. Ther. *24:17, 1982.)*
15. Abernathy, R., et al. Short-course chemotherapy for tuberculosis in children. *Pediatrics* 72:801, 1983.
    A series of 50 children treated with INH and rifampin daily for 1 month followed by twice weekly for 8 months. (Although 9 months is effective, 6 months is not: Am. Rev. Resp. Dis. *129:573, 1984.)*
16. Snider, D., et al. Treatment of tuberculosis during pregnancy. *Am. Rev. Resp. Dis.* 122:65, 1980.
    A review of the relative safety of antituberculous drugs.

Meningitis/Miliary

17. Sumaya, C., et al. Tuberculosis meningitis in children during the isoniazid era. *J. Pediatr.* 87:43, 1975.
    Quantitates the sequelae. (For other series, see Pediatrics *56:1050, 1975, and* Am. J. Dis. Child. *130:364, 1976; INH plus rifampin:* J. Pediatr. *87:983, 1975.)*
18. Schuit, K. Miliary tuberculosis in children. *Am. J. Dis. Child.* 133:583, 1979.
    The clinical and laboratory manifestations in 19 patients.

Newborns; BCG

19. Kendig, E. The place of BCG vaccine in the management of infants born of tuberculous mothers. *N. Engl. J. Med.* 281:520, 1969.
   Strongly advocates the use of BCG.
20. Avery, M., and Wolfsdorf, J. Approaches to newborn infants of tuberculous mothers. *Pediatrics* 42:519, 1968.
   This balanced view of choices also leans toward BCG.

Epidemiology

21. Hinman, A., et al. Changing risks in tuberculosis. *Am. J. Epidemiol.* 103:486, 1976.
   The greatest risk (in New York State) for the development of pulmonary or miliary tuberculosis is between ages 20 and 24, but the greatest risk for dying from tuberculosis is before age 5.

104. ROCKY MOUNTAIN SPOTTED FEVER
Kenneth B. Roberts

Before 1900, Idaho physicians recognized a distinct febrile exanthem that was referred to as "Snake River measles." The present name, Rocky Mountain spotted fever (RMSF), stems from the work of Howard Taylor Ricketts in the Bitter Root Valley of Montana and the subsequent establishment in that state of the Viral and Rickettsial Disease Center. The incidence of RMSF in the Rocky Mountain states 40 to 50 years ago was 100 times what it is there now, while the incidence in the Mid-Atlantic region remains essentially unchanged; thus, the incidence of the disease now is 10 to 20 times higher in the East than in the Rocky Mountain states.

The infecting organism, *Rickettsia rickettsii,* is roughly 1 μ in length and 0.2 to 0.3 μ in width. It is capable of growing in both the nucleus and the cytoplasm of infected cells of ticks and mammals. Ticks can become infected by either of two mechanisms: transovarially or by feeding on an infected host. Once infected, the tick carries the organism for several years and serves not only as a vector but also as a reservoir of the disease. In certain areas of the Mid-Atlantic seaboard, as many as 5 percent of ticks are infected.

Ticks require three different hosts in their life cycle. After the tick eggs hatch, the larvae migrate to vegetation and await the first host. If the larvae are successful in negotiating a host, they engorge themselves on its blood, fall off, and molt to a new stage. The nymphs engorge themselves on a second host, fall off, and molt again. The adults then find a final host for feeding (tick control is complicated by the adult tick's ability to survive up to 4 years without feeding). When the adults feed, attachment may last for 3 to 12 hours, but at least $1\frac{1}{2}$ to 2 hours are required before the tick injects any infected material from its stomach contents into the host. A rational, effective means of protection against RMSF is for people living in areas where ticks are present to inspect themselves (and their children) every few hours.

Rocky Mountain spotted fever is a true infectious vasculitis. The organism invades and multiplies in endothelial cells, resulting in damage that is clinically manifested by edema and petechiae; in severely ill patients, fluid balance and maintenance of adequate intravascular volume is a difficult problem in management. Vascular lesions are most readily appreciated in the skin, but also occur in other tissues, notably the myocardium and central nervous system.

The classic presentation is an ill patient with headache and fever. The headache is described as excruciating in severity and is generalized, although frequently more intense frontally. Fever is low grade in the morning but high (40–40.6° C, 104–105° F) during the day; the course of fever may be as short as 2 days in very mild disease or as long as 3 weeks in severe untreated disease. Myalgia may be prominent, with the abdominal muscles commonly affected; arthralgias may also be present. In addition to headache, about 50 percent of the patients have neurologic signs, such as lethargy, restlessness, and insomnia.

The rash of RMSF characteristically appears 2 to 6 days after the onset of fever. The initial lesions are pink macules (which may become papular) on the extremities, especially on the wrists, ankles, palms and soles. After 6 to 12 hours, the rash extends centripetally to the trunk; only later do petechiae appear. If the rash progresses, hemorrhagic lesions coalesce and may lead to gangrene and slough (purpura fulminans).

The diagnosis becomes clear as the disease progresses but may be difficult in the early stages, when treatment is most effective. The character and distribution of the rash may suggest atypical measles, but this disorder may be distinguished by its pulmonary manifestations and occurrence in the winter-spring months. Skin lesions caused by meningococcemia are often painful when stroked, and the organism may be seen if the lesion is aspirated and the specimen Gram stained. The rash of enteroviral infection is usually generalized, and fever is not as prominent as in RMSF. The RMSF complement fixation test and Weil-Felix reaction are not helpful early, since they are not positive until the second week; if therapy is begun early and is effective, there may be further delay in antibody rise. Recently, a technique has been described for demonstrating rickettsiae in skin biopsy specimens by immunofluorescence; the technique takes only a few hours, but is not yet generally available.

Treatment with chloramphenicol or tetracycline shortens the duration of fever and improves the survival rate. Patients who survive the first 24 hours after the initiation of antibiotic therapy rarely die later.

A vaccine is available, but its efficacy is questionable. Prevention, as noted, is usually based on removal of ticks before they introduce infected material into the host. Crushing the tick in the process of removing it is to be avoided, since infected material may be squeezed from the tick into the "wound." An abrasion is sufficient for inoculation; a penetrating bite is not required.

RMSF is the most common of the rickettsioses in the United States. It is preventable and treatable, yet the case fatality rate remains 5 to 10 percent. It appears clear that earlier recognition is required, so that appropriate therapy may be administered.

Reviews
1. Kelsey, D. Rocky Mountain spotted fever. *Pediatr. Clin. North Am.* 26:367, 1979.
   Start with this excellent review.
2. Riley, H. Rickettsial diseases and Rocky Mountain spotted fever. *Curr. Prob. Pediatr.* 11(5, 6), 1981.
   Encyclopedic two-issue review, with more than 30 pages on RMSF.

Epidemiology, Clinical Features, and Diagnosis
3. Helmick, C., Bernard, K., and D'Angelo, L. Rocky Mountain spotted fever: Clinical, laboratory, and epidemiological features of 262 cases. *J. Infect. Dis.* 150: 480, 1984.
   Centers for Disease Control review, 1977-1980. (Overview of 1981-1983: p. 609.)
4. Hattwick, M., et al. Fatal Rocky Mountain spotted fever. *JAMA* 240:1499, 1978.
   Associated with delay in diagnosis and treatment; causes for delay discussed and need for presumptive treatment stressed.
5. Wilfert, C., et al. Epidemiology of Rocky Mountain spotted fever as determined by active surveillance. *J. Infect. Dis.* 150:469, 1984.
   Active surveillance in an endemic area: Seek and ye shall find.
6. Bradford, W., and Hawkins, H. Rocky Mountain spotted fever in childhood. *Am. J. Dis. Child.* 131:1228, 1977.
   A report on 138 children; low serum sodium concentration and thrombocytopenia are stressed as helpful clues to diagnosis.
7. Woodward, T., et al. Prompt confirmation of Rocky Mountain spotted fever: Identification of rickettsiae in skin tissues. *J. Infect. Dis.* 134:297, 1976.
   Prompt, but not widely available.
8. Philip, R., et al. A comparison of serologic methods for diagnosis of Rocky Mountain spotted fever. *Am. J. Epidemiol.* 105:56, 1977.
   The complement fixation test appears definitely less sensitive than newer (less widely available!) tests.

9. Marx, R., et al. Rocky Mountain spotted fever: Serologic evidence of previous subclinical infection in children. *Am. J. Dis. Child.* 136:16, 1982.
   Mild or asymptomatic subclinical cases apparently occur.
10. Westerman, E. Rocky Mountain spotless fever: A dilemma for the clinician. *Arch. Intern. Med.* 142:1106, 1982.
   Headache, myalgias, and fever—but no rash!

Organ Involvement
11. Marin-Garcia, J., Gooch, W., and Coury, D. Cardiac manifestations of Rocky Mountain spotted fever. *Pediatrics* 67:358, 1981.
   Cardiac involvement is frequent and warrants attention.
12. Gorman, R., Saxon, S., and Snead, O. Neurologic sequelae of Rocky Mountain spotted fever. *Pediatrics* 67:354, 1981.
   Behavioral disturbances and learning disabilities but no seizures.

Prevention
13. Lennette, E. Rocky Mountain spotted fever. *N. Engl. J. Med.* 297:884, 1977.
   Editorial review of an article on laboratory acquisition from aerosols (p. 859) and summary of the status of vaccine against RMSF.

105. STREPTOCOCCAL INFECTIONS
Kenneth B. Roberts

The streptococcus is a pyogenic gram-positive organism capable of elaborating extracellular products that are pathogenic, such as erythrogenic toxin (the cause of scarlet fever), and immunogenic, such as streptolysin O (to which antistreptolysin O [ASO] antibodies are formed). Streptococci are classified into groups on the basis of differences in the carbohydrate constituents in the cell wall. Group A streptococci cause tonsillopharyngitis, impetigo, sepsis, erysipelas, pneumonia, and scarlet fever and lead to acute glomerulonephritis and rheumatic fever. Group B organisms have emerged as a major cause of neonatal sepsis in the past decade. Group D streptococci are a cause of subacute bacterial endocarditis and urinary tract infection. The other groups are infrequently incriminated in human infection.

Group A streptococci are classified further on the basis of the ability of colonies to hemolyze red blood cells: alpha hemolysis is characterized by the persistence of "ghost" cells microscopically and a greenish tinge macroscopically; beta hemolysis is complete; gamma is the designation given to nonhemolytic organisms. In the discussion to follow, the organisms considered are beta-hemolytic, group A streptococci.

Streptococcal pharyngitis is spread by close contact with an individual shedding the organism. The bacteria multiply in the nasopharynx of the susceptible host, and after 24 to 48 hours the typical clinical syndrome develops in 60 percent; the illness is so mild in 20 percent that the symptoms are overlooked, and 20 percent are completely asymptomatic. In infants the disease is usually a nasopharyngitis with a profuse nasal discharge. In somewhat older children, signs and symptoms become referable to the tonsils and pharynx, but abdominal complaints are frequent as well. School-age children manifest the classic syndrome of fever, headache, and sore throat, described more as pain on swallowing than a feeling of pharyngeal irritation. Hoarseness and cough are not features; their presence argues strongly for a nonstreptococcal cause of the illness. Examination of the pharynx usually reveals an intensely red throat with moderate or marked exudate, although the exudate may not be present on the first day. Petechiae on the palate early in the course strongly suggest a streptococcal origin, and the presence of the rash of scarlet fever is virtually diagnostic. Tender anterior cervical lymph nodes at the angle of the jaw are particularly noteworthy, since they imply a more invasive infection and correlate with ASO antibody rises. The definitive diagnosis of streptococcal infection is established by throat culture.

The ability of antibiotics to modify the clinical course once disease is established is still debated, but there is no controversy about treatment for the prevention of acute rheumatic fever: the incidence of this nonsuppurative complication can be reduced 10-fold, although not eliminated, if treatment successfully eradicates the streptococci from the pharynx. The short delay inherent in processing a culture does not negate the benefit of treatment. Penicillin is the drug of choice; for patients truly allergic to penicillin, erythromycin is the preferred alternative. The recommended treatment is a single injection of long-acting benzathine penicillin or oral penicillin on a 2- or 4-times-a-day schedule for 10 days. There are fewer failures with benzathine than with oral penicillin (even when compliance with the oral regimen is ensured), but the pain associated with the injection has limited its general use. Combinations of benzathine and procaine penicillin are now available that in appropriate doses are as effective as benzathine alone and are less painful.

After the acute infection, some children continue to carry streptococci in their throat, regardless of the regimen of initial treatment or retreatment. The organisms carried differ biologically from those that caused the initial infection by virtue of the loss of M protein (the cell-wall constituent by which group A streptococci are typed); this information is reassuring, since M protein appears to be a "virulence factor." However, M-typing is not a readily available laboratory procedure, so in practice, carriers are identified by the demonstration of repeated positive cultures. At the time of clinical illness, it is often impossible to determine whether the child is a carrier or has acquired a new, virulent streptococcal strain.

The exact mechanism by which acute rheumatic fever is produced remains unknown, and the significance of a few streptococci in the throat is controversial. Antistreptolysin O (ASO) antibodies only corroborate (retrospectively) the occurrence of a streptococcal infection and do not appear to play a direct etiologic role in rheumatic fever. There is no way at present to estimate the individual child's risk for the development of acute rheumatic fever, but children who have a family history of rheumatic heart disease or who have had a previous bout of rheumatic fever deserve particular attention.

The growth of streptococci on normal skin is limited by the effect of sebum. Once the skin is traumatized, however, streptococci may multiply and produce the nonbullous lesions of impetigo. The earliest stage of the lesion is a vesicle that is rarely noticed; pustules form rapidly and are covered by characteristic thick, amber-colored crusts. Lymphadenopathy is common, but systemic signs of illness are infrequent. Antistreptolysin O (ASO) titer rises are unusual after impetigo; retrospective serologic evidence of the infection can be obtained by measuring anti-DNAse B antibodies.

Staphylococci commonly are present in the lesions along with the streptococci but are not of clinical significance. Lesions that require specific antistaphylococcal measures are bullous and are seldom accompanied by regional lymphadenopathy. Once group A streptococci have established infection in the skin, spread to the upper respiratory tract occurs; staphylococci more often colonize the upper respiratory tract first and then spread to the skin.

The therapy of impetigo has traditionally included vigorous scrubbing and the use of antibacterial soap, but neither has been proved effective, and scrubbing may even delay healing. Topical therapy with bacitracin ointment effects a less rapid response than systemic penicillin or erythromycin.

Acute rheumatic fever does not follow streptococcal infection of the skin, but acute glomerulonephritis can. As noted in Chapter 69, not all strains of streptococci are nephritogenic; those that are cause glomerulonephritis with equal frequency after pharyngitis or impetigo. It is questionable whether antibiotic treatment can prevent glomerulonephritis.

The development of a streptococcal vaccine has been hampered by the large number of antigenically distinct strains and the concern that a vaccine might inadvertently produce rheumatic fever or glomerulonephritis.

General

1. Wannamaker, L. Differences between streptococcal infections of the throat and of the skin. *N. Engl. J. Med.* 282:23, 78, 1970.
   A classic two-part review (G. Peter, and A. Smith, N. Engl. J. Med. 297:311, 365, 1977, a more recent two-part review, is good but does not replace this as number 1).

2. Wannamaker, L. Changes and changing concepts in the biology of group A streptococci and in the epidemiology of streptococcal infections. *Rev. Infect. Dis* 1:967, 1979.
   An overview of many issues by one of the premier "strep-ologists," followed by two pages of discussion (pp. 974–975).
3. Powers, G., and Boisvert, P. Age as a factor in streptococcosis. *J. Pediatr.* 25:481 1944.
   Nasopharyngitis in early childhood; "scarlet fever" and systemic disease later.

Scarlet Fever
4. Trousseau, A. Scarlatina, *Rev. Infect. Dis.* 1:1016, 1979.
   The master clinician's 1873 lecture; please refrain from using his recommendations for treatment!

Pharyngitis: General
5. Peebles, T. Identification and treatment of group A-hemolytic streptococcal infections. *Pediatr. Clin. North Am.* 18:145, 1971.
   A discussion of unresolved issues.
6. Pantell, R. Pharyngitis: Diagnosis and management. *Pediatr. Rev.* 3:35, 1981.
   A thoughtful consideration of the various options: Culture or not, treat or not.
7. Glezen, W., et al. Group A streptococci, mycoplasmas, and viruses associated with acute pharyngitis. *JAMA* 202:455, 1967.
   What causes pharyngitis at what age.

Pharyngitis: Diagnosis
8. Taranta, A., and Moody, M. Diagnosis of streptococcal pharyngitis and rheumatic fever. *Pediatr. Clin. North Am.* 18:125, 1971.
   Excellent review, plus 78 references.
9. Breese, B., and Disney, F. The accuracy of diagnosis of beta streptococcal infections on clinical grounds. *J. Pediatr.* 44:670, 1954.
   A classic: 75 percent accuracy in predicting positive cultures; 77 percent accuracy in predicting negative cultures.
10. Stillerman, M., and Bernstein, S. Streptococcal pharyngitis. *Am. J. Dis. Child* 101:476, 1961.
    An analysis of various clinical syndromes.
11. Ross, P. Throat swabs and swabbing technique. *Practitioner* 207:791, 1971.
    Quantitates the "sampling" error in swabbing throats infected with streptococci.
12. Kaplan, E. The group A streptococcal upper respiratory tract carrier state: An enigma. *J. Pediatr.* 97:337, 1980.
    Definition, epidemiology, and clinical implications.

Pharyngitis: Treatment
13. Nelson, J. The effect of penicillin therapy on the symptoms and signs of streptococcal pharyngitis. *Pediatr. Infect. Dis.* 3:10, 1984.
    Clinical improvement was faster with penicillin than with placebo.
14. Catanzaro, F., et al. The role of the streptococcus in the pathogenesis of rheumatic fever. *Am. J. Med.* 17:749, 1954.
    Persistence of streptococci is the key factor; rheumatic fever can still be prevented even if the onset of penicillin therapy is delayed 9 days.
15. Breese, B., Disney, F., and Tapley, W. Penicillin in streptococcal infections. *Am. J Dis. Child.* 110:125, 1965.
    If the total daily dose is kept constant, administration twice a day is as effective as administration 4 times a day; neither oral regimen is as effective as an injection of benzathine penicillin.
16. Mohler, D., et al. Studies in the home treatment of streptococcal disease. *N. Engl. J. Med.* 254:45, 1956.
    Of patients receiving oral therapy for less than 4 days, 75 percent had positive throat cultures; of those who received 7 days, 11 percent had positive cultures. (And 10 days of antibiotic appears better than 7: JAMA 246:1790, 1981.) Again, an injection of benzathine penicillin was more effective than penicillin by mouth.

17. Charney, E., et al. How well do patients take oral penicillin? *Pediatrics* 40:188, 1967.
    Not as well as we would like.
18. Rosenstein, B., et al. Factors involved in treatment failures following oral penicillin therapy of streptococcal pharyngitis. *J. Pediatr.* 73:513, 1968.
    Multiple possible causes are considered, tested, and rejected.
19. Kaplan, E. Rationality in reculturing after antibiotic treatment for streptococcal pharyngitis: Can we throw away the culture plates? *Pediatr. Infect. Dis.* 1:75, 1982.
    By all means.

Impetigo
20. Dillon, H. Impetigo contagiosa: Suppurative and non-suppurative complications. *Am. J. Dis. Child.* 115:530, 1968.
    The clinical, bacteriologic, and epidemiologic characteristics are reviewed.
21. Dillon, H. The treatment of streptococcal skin infections. *J. Pediatr.* 76:676, 1970.
    Systemic treatment is more effective than local treatment.
22. Ferrieri, P., Dojani, A., and Wannamaker, L. Benzathine penicillin in the prophylaxis of streptococcal skin infections: A pilot study. *J. Pediatr.* 83:572, 1973.
    There was a reduction of 38 percent in the incidence of impetigo during the 6 weeks after injection.

Nonsuppurative Sequelae
23. Stollerman, G. Nephritogenic and rheumatogenic group A streptococci. *J. Infect. Dis.* 120:258, 1969.
    Focuses on the streptococcal strains; also see J. Pediatr. 92:325, 1978.
24. Krause, R. Prevention of streptococcal sequelae by penicillin prophylaxis: A reassessment. *J. Infect. Dis.* 131:592, 1975.
    A review of the relationship between the streptococcus and rheumatic fever.
25. Weinstein, L., and LeFrock, J. Does antimicrobial therapy of streptococcal pharyngitis or pyoderma alter the risk of glomerulonephritis? *J. Infect. Dis.* 124:229, 1971.
    A review of the data leaves the question unanswered.
    Also see Rheumatic Fever, Chapter 54, and Acute Poststreptococcal Glomerulonephritis, Chapter 69.

106. ENTERIC INFECTIONS
Kenneth B. Roberts

Acute diarrhea is a common problem in infants and chidren and is frequently associated with infection, either intestinal or extraintestinal (so-called parenteral diarrhea). Other etiologies include overfeeding, medications, inflammatory bowel disease, cystic fibrosis, and other cases of malabsorption (see Chap. 64).

Organisms in the intestine generally produce diarrhea by one of two mechanisms: Some, like cholera, remain in the lumen and produce an enterotoxin that acts on the mucosa of the small bowel to cause a profuse secretory watery diarrhea; others, like *Shigella*, penetrate the epithelial cell and cause inflammation, and mucus and inflammatory cells can be found in the stool. The clinical syndrome suggests the mechanism by which diarrhea is produced and gives clues to the causative organism.

Shigella is most frequently a pathogen in children between 1 and 5 years of age; it rarely causes disease in the first days of life. The organism proliferates in the small bowel 8 to 40 hours after ingestion and causes fever and watery diarrhea. Shortly thereafter the colon is invaded, stool cultures become positive, the temperature begins to return toward normal, and the characteristic bloody, mucoid stools appear. Tenesmus may be prominent, reflecting mucosal destruction. One-fourth of the patients will have only watery diarrhea; another fourth will have high fever but few gastrointestinal complaints. Between 10 and 45 percent of children have a convulsion. Bacteremia is rare, and mortality is less than 1 percent. The diagnosis of shigellosis is suggested by the presence of polymorphonuclear leukocytes in a stained stool specimen and an increased number of band forms in the peripheral blood, irrespective of the total white blood cell count; a positive stool culture confirms the diagnosis. Ampicillin therapy reduces the duration of fever, diarrhea, positive cultures, and days in the hospital. Within the past several years, however, strains have been identified that are resistant to ampicillin, so the clinician must rely on susceptibility testing.

Salmonellae are said to infect more living creatures than any other organism because of their ubiquitous distribution and ability to infect animals as well as humans. Roughly one-third of the contacts of a known *Salmonella* excreter (half the contacts under the age of 5 years) become culture positive. Of human clinical infections, 70 percent or more are acute uncomplicated gastroenteritis; the remainder are "enteric fever," bacteremia, or a prolonged carrier state.

The incubation period prior to enteritis is 6 to 48 hours. The diagnosis of *Salmonella* as the responsible organism is suggested by the passage of green stools that are particularly malodorous; polymorphonuclear leukocytes may be observed in the stool, but blood or mucus is rarely present. Vomiting is more prominent than in other bacterial gastroenteritides. Although the enteritis is generally self-limited (2–5 days), shedding of the organism in the stool occurs for weeks and often much longer, particularly in infants. Antibiotics are not indicated for the treatment of uncomplicated gastroenteritis and may serve to prolong the period of shedding and increase the relapse rate. Unlike *Shigella*, *Salmonella* causes disease in the neonatal period and is a particular problem in nurseries and institutions. Newborns, older compromised hosts, and infants whose infection is associated with failure to thrive may warrant antibiotic therapy.

The classic enteric fever is typhoid, a disease only of humans. The organism multiplies rapidly in the gastrointestinal tract and penetrates the epithelium, assuming an intracellular location within 24 hours. Mesenteric lymph nodes halt the progress of the organism but permit continued multiplication. The organisms reach the bloodstream by the end of the first week and infect the biliary tract. Two days after the bacteremia, fever occurs, accompanied shortly thereafter by headache and abdominal pain; chills and sweats are uncommon, but myalgias, malaise, and anorexia are pronounced. The course is usually more abrupt in infants than in adults, "rose spots" are less common, and there is greater prominence of both gastrointestinal and central nervous system signs. Despite in vitro sensitivity to gentamicin, this agent is ineffective in treating disease or even sterilizing the bloodstream. Chloramphenicol appears to be the drug of choice when the organism is sensitive, but it is associated with a 10 to 20 percent relapse rate and a 2 to 3 percent carrier rate; clinical response may not be evident until the third to fifth day of illness. At present, there is no satisfactory treatment of the carrier state.

Bacteremia occurs with salmonellae other than *S. typhosa*, particularly *S. choleraesuis*. The association between sickle cell disease and *Salmonella* osteomyelitis should be remembered when *Salmonella* is isolated from the blood of a child.

Escherichia coli can cause diarrhea by either of the two mechanisms: elaborating an enterotoxin or invading the mucosa. *E. coli* can also cause diarrhea by a third mechanism, involving attachment with neither toxin production nor invasion. Of these three mechanisms, the most frequent is the production of toxin; this appears to be the major cause of traveler's diarrhea. Both heat-labile and heat-stable enterotoxins have been identified. The organism attaches to the epithelial surface of the small intestine mucosa but does not damage it; after only approximately 30 minutes, toxin has stimulated adenyl cyclase to decrease the absorption of sodium, increase the secretion of chloride, and induce a profuse loss of water. The capacity to produce toxin is conferred by an episome (R factor), which is transferred from organism to organism. The identification of enterotoxigenic or enteroinvasive *E. coli* requires tests not commonly performed in clinical laboratories. Doxycycline, trimethoprim-sulfamethoxazole, or bismuth subsalicylate can be used to prevent traveler's diarrhea; once clinical disease is apparent, it is not clear that any specific treatment is more effective than supportive therapy alone.

"New" bacterial pathogens, recognized in the past several years, include *Campylobacter* and *Yersinia*; *Clostridium difficile*, the organism incriminated in antibiotic-associated pseudomembranous colitis, has been isolated from the stools of infants, but it is not clear whether it is a pathogen in such circumstances. *Campylobacter* causes a dysentery syndrome similar to that caused by *Shigella*; the differential white blood cell count may show a shift to the left as in *Shigella* infection, although usually to a less marked degree. Treatment with erythromycin does not appear to affect the clinical course but does decrease the duration of shedding of the organism. *Yersinia* is notable since it may produce a clinical picture indistinguishable from appendicitis. Disease confined to the gastrointestinal tract is usually self-limited and does not require treatment.

Viral agents have recently been implicated as the major causes of diarrhea in children, particularly the rotavirus. This infection is most common in infants during the winter and is associated with significant vomiting and dehydration. Other viruses, such as the Norwalk agent, are capable of causing outbreaks of diarrheal disease as well. No specific therapy is available.

Supportive management of the patients with diarrhea requires replacement of fluid and electrolyte losses. Glucose and electrolyte solutions taken orally usually maintain fluid balance and isotonicity, but occasionally intravenous treatment is required. Potent pharmacologic agents designed to slow or halt intestinal motility are dangerous in infants, since they permit fluid to pool in the intestine unnoticed; the diarrhea ceases, but dehydration may progress. In addition, animal studies suggest that diarrhea is a physiologic protective mechanism, at least against bacterial infection.

Reviews; Traditional Enteric Pathogens

1. Grady, G., and Keusch, G. Pathogenesis of bacterial diarrheas. *N. Engl. J. Med.* 285:831, 891, 1971.
   An easy-to-read, straightforward review (254 references).
2. DuPont, H., and Hornick, R. Clinical approach to infectious diarrhea. *Medicine* (Baltimore) 52:265, 1973.
   A concise presentation of practical clinical, pathologic, laboratory, and epidemiologic aspects; advocates fecal leukocyte examinations (see Ann. Intern. Med. 76:697, 1972.)
3. Nelson, J., and Haltalin, K. Accuracy of diagnosis of bacterial diarrheal disease by clinical features. *J. Pediatr.* 78:519, 1971.
   Dallas housestaff accurately differentiated bacterial from nonbacterial diarrheas 72 percent of the time on clinical grounds and "guessed" the organism two-thirds of the time; should be read in conjunction with references 1 and 2 for interpretation.
4. Ashkenazi, S., et al. Differential leukocyte count in acute gastroenteritis: An aid to early diagnosis. *Clin. Pediatr.* (Phila.) 22:356, 1983.
   The absolute band count and the ratio of bands to total neutrophils are highest with Shigella, *then* Campylobacter *and* Salmonella; *infections with these three organisms can be distinguished from* E. coli *or nonbacterial gastroenteritis.*

Shigella

5. Wilson, R., et al. Family illness associated with *Shigella* infection: The interrelationship of age of the index patient and the age of household members in acquisition of illness. *J. Infect. Dis.* 143:130, 1981.
   There was at least one secondary culture-positive case in two-thirds of the families; beware the young child with Shigella!
6. Weissman, J., et al. Shigellosis: To treat or not to treat? *JAMA* 229:1215, 1973.
   Discussion and recommendations from the Centers for Disease Control and the Dallas group.
7. Barrett-Connor, E., and Connor, J. Extraintestinal manifestations of shigellosis. *Am. J. Gastroenterol.* 53:234, 1970.
   A catalogue of findings in 330 patients. (More on the CNS manifestations: Clin. Pediatr. [Phila.] 21:645, 1982.)

Salmonella

8. Rosenstein, B. Salmonellosis in infants and children. *J. Pediatr.* 70:1, 1967.
   Emphasis is on the spread among household contacts and the problems of oral treatment. (For more on the duration of positive cultures after infection, see Rev. Infect. Dis. 6:345, 1984.)
9. Nelson, J., et al. Treatment of *Salmonella* gastroenteritis with ampicillin, amoxicillin or placebo. *Pediatrics* 65:1125, 1980.
   The antibiotics were of no benefit and apparently some harm; the authors'

recommendations for antibiotic therapy in Salmonella syndromes are expressed in an editorial: Am. J. Dis. Child. 135:1093, 1981.

10. Hornick, R., et al. Typhoid fever: Pathogenesis and immunologic control. N. Engl. J. Med. 283:686, 739, 1970.
The paper on this subject, noting the authors' careful observations in experimental typhoid, including treatment with chloramphenicol. (Typhoid in children: Pediatrics 56:606, 1975; clinical manifestations often more severe in infants than in older children: Clin. Pediatr. [Phila.] 20:448, 1981.)

11. Baine, W., et al. Institutional salmonellosis. J. Infect. Dis. 128:357, 1973.
Centers for Disease Control update of an earlier study (N. Engl. J. Med. 279:674, 1968) that implicated person-to-person spread to children; the case fatality rate for nurseries was 7 percent; for pediatric wards, 3 percent.

12. Black, P., Kunz, L., and Swartz, M. Salmonellosis: A review of some unusual aspects. N. Engl. J. Med. 262:811, 864, 921. 1960.
Catalogue of foci of Salmonella infections, with brief discussions. (More on Salmonella bacteremia in infants: Am. J. Dis. Child. 135:1096, 1981, and J. Pediatr. 96:57, 1980.)

E. Coli

13. Neter, E. Enteropathogenicity of Escherichia coli. Am. J. Dis. Child. 129:666, 1975.
A two-page editorial status report on enterotoxins and invasive strains, accompanying a study of the incidence of different forms in children, page 668.

14. Guerrant, R. Yet another pathogenic mechanism for Escherichia coli diarrhea? N. Engl. J. Med. 302:113, 1980.
Attachment without invasion or toxin production! (For the summary of a workshop on these organisms, see J. Infect. Dis. 147:1108, 1983.)

15. Nelson, J. Duration of neomycin therapy for enteropathogenic Escherichia coli diarrheal disease: A comparative study of 113 cases. Pediatrics 48:248, 1971.
Treatment for 3 to 5 days is as good as treatment for 7 to 10 days but a question about the need for any antibiotics at all is raised.
Also see reference 26.

Viruses

16. Blacklow, N., and Cukor, G. Viral gastroenteritis. N. Engl. J. Med. 304:397, 1981.
Norwalk agent, rotavirus, and miscellaneous others; the role of each in one hospital quantitated: Am. J. Dis. Child. 131:733, 1977 (companion editorial on p. 729).

17. Steinhoff, M. Rotavirus: The first five years. J. Pediatr. 96:611, 1980.
Eleven pages, three half-page electron micrographs, and 100 references. (Rotavirus is the major cause of gastroenteritis requiring hospitalization: Am. J. Dis. Child. 134:777, 1980.)

18. Kaplan, J., et al. Epidemiology of Norwalk gastroenteritis and the role of Norwalk virus in outbreaks of acute nonbacterial gastroenteritis. Ann. Intern. Med. 96:756, 1982.
Of 74 outbreaks of acute nonbacterial gastroenteritis investigated, 42 percent were due to Norwalk virus; clinical epidemiologic characteristics are summarized.

"New Agents"

19. San Joaquin, V., and Marks, M. New agents in diarrhea. Pediatr. Infect. Dis. 1:53, 1982.
The long course (13 pages, 237 references); for the short course, see Pediatr. Infect. Dis. 1:S57, 1982. Another review of "new" bacterial agents: Rev. Infect. Dis. 5:246, 1983.

20. Rettig, P. Campylobacter infections in human beings. J. Pediatr. 94:855, 1979.
One of many recent reviews; also see Pediatrics 64:898, 1979, and N. Engl. J. Med. 305:1444, 1981.

21. Blaser, M., et al. Campylobacter enteritis in the United States. Ann. Intern. Med. 98:360, 1983.
Clinically similar to Salmonella and Shigella yet epidemiologically different. (Signs and symptoms are age-related: abdominal distention without fever in young infants, abdominal pain and fever in children: Clin. Pediatr. [Phila.]22:98, 1983.)

22. Robins-Browne, R., et al. Treatment of *Campylobacter*-associated enteritis with erythromycin. *Am. J. Dis. Child.* 137:282, 1983.
    This article and the one after it (p. 286) agree: erythromycin decreases the period of shedding but does not affect the clinical course. (Clue to diagnosis is appearance as "gull wings" in Gram-stained stool specimen: Ann. Intern. Med. 96:62, 1982.)
23. Kohl, S. *Yersinia enterocolitica* infections in children. *Pediatr. Clin. North Am.* 26:433, 1979.
    A thorough review of the epidemiology, clinical syndromes, bacteriology, serology, host response, treatment, and control (90 references).
24. Feigin, R. Antimicrobial agent-induced pseudomembranous colitis. *Pediatr. Rev.* 3:147, 1981.
    A recent review; also see Pediatr. Clin. North Am. 26:261, 1979. (Is Clostridium difficile pathogenic in infants? J. Pediatr. 100:393, 1982.)

Special Situations

25. Pickering, L., and Woodward, W. Diarrhea in day care centers. *Pediatr. Infect. Dis.* 1:47, 1982.
    A practical review of the problem in day care centers and beyond.
26. Steffen, R., et al. Epidemiology of diarrhea in travelers. *JAMA* 249:1176, 1983.
    Get two copies of this and the companion editorial (p. 1193), one for you and one for your travel agent. (For a summary of approaches to prevention and treatment, see Ann. Intern. Med. 102:260, 1985.)

Treatment

27. Pickering, L. Antimicrobial therapy of gastrointestinal infections. *Pediatr. Clin. North Am.* 30:373, 1983.
    Considers non-specific therapy as well as specific treatment of antimicrobial-associated colitis, traveler's diarrhea, and infections caused by various bacteria and protozoa (105 references).
28. Finberg, L. Treatment of dehydration in infancy. *Pediatr. Rev.* 3:113, 1981.
    The emphasis is on parenteral therapy. (The author comments on oral rehydration for diarrhea: J. Pediatr. 101:497, 1982, and 105:939, 1984; also see N. Engl. J. Med. 306:1103, 1982, and Pediatrics 75:358, 1985.)
29. Wendland, B., and Arbus, G. Oral fluid therapy: Sodium and potassium content and osmolality of some commercial "clear" soups, juices and beverages. *Can. Med. Assoc. J.* 121:564, 1979.
    Includes fruit juices, fruit drinks, and commercially prepared chicken soup (but not my mother's). (For electrolyte concentration of various flavors of Kool-Aid and gelatin products, see Clin. Pediatr. [Phila.] 9:508, 1970.)
30. Ginsberg, C. Lomotil (diphenoxylate and atropine) intoxication. *Am. J. Dis. Child.* 125;241, 1973.
    Signs of atropinism occur early; CNS and respiratory depression (from diphenoxylate) occur later. (Also see Pediatrics 53:495, 1974; by decreasing motility, diphenoxylate may interfere with host defenses against offending agent? JAMA 226:1525, 1973.) Not a drug for infants!

---

107. GONORRHEA

Kenneth B. Roberts

Gonorrhea is the most frequently reported infectious disease in this country, with cases numbering in the millions each year. The causative organism, *Neisseria gonorrhoeae*, appears as a gram-negative diplococcus; on smears of clinical specimens, it is often located within polymorphonuclear leukocytes. Special media and techniques are used to foster the growth of this fastidious organism; an important practical advance has been the introduction of Transgrow, which permits inoculation of specific agar in a carbon dioxide-enriched environment for transportation to a reference laboratory.

Until recently, all gonococci were considered sensitive to penicillin, although increasing amounts of the drug have been required with each passing decade to effect a cure. Some gonococci now have been isolated with documented penicillin resistance; the full epidemiologic potential of these organisms has not yet been realized. Ampicillin and amoxicillin are also effective against gonococci but have the same limitations as penicillin. Alternative drugs include tetracycline and spectinomycin. Doses and routes of administration vary with the clinical manifestation of disease.

Widespread prophylaxis against gonorrheal ophthalmia neonatorum is practiced in delivery rooms. The most popular form of prevention is the instillation of silver nitrate solution in the manner described nearly 100 years ago by Credé. Because of the rising incidence of gonorrhea, particularly in teenagers and young adults, there has been renewed concern about contamination of the newborn's eyes with gonococci from the maternal genital tract. Prophylaxis is not 100 percent effective, so it is to be expected that gonococcal ophthalmia may be on the increase. Without prophylaxis, ophthalmia occurs on the second postpartum day, but nowadays it is most frequently appreciated at the end of the first week of life, perhaps delayed by the silver nitrate instillation. The hallmark of the disease is rapid progression, with thick, purulent exudate, early corneal ulceration and, ultimately, blindness; mild cases also occur, however. Treatment includes systemic antibiotics. Ophthalmia may also occur later in life, from direct inoculation, and requires aggressive treatment.

Infection of prepubescent children by the gonococcus is infrequent. It seems that gonorrhea can be spread by other than sexual means, but it is not clear whether or not this is common; sexual abuse must be considered. The clinical manifestation of gonorrhea in prepubertal girls is vulvovaginitis; puberty is associated with changes in the vaginal mucosa and secretions that protect against this form of clinical illness thereafter. The converse is also true: disease of the cervix and fallopian tubes, common in postpubertal women, is not seen before puberty.

Most gonococcal infections of the genital tract in women are asymptomatic. With menstruation, a transient endometritis can be established, with progression to bilateral endosalpingitis and pelvic peritonitis, abscess, pyosalpinx or hydrosalpinx, and, infrequently, perihepatitis (the Fitz-Hugh-Curtis syndrome). The clinical syndrome of pelvic inflammatory disease may be easy to diagnose in an acutely ill patient with fever, abdominal tenderness, tenderness on manipulation of the cervix, and many gram-negative intracellular diplococci on smear of the purulent cervical discharge. Often, however, the differentiation from other causes of severe abdominal pain is difficult (see Acute Abdomen, Chap. 8). Particularly when the right tube is involved more than the left, laparotomy may be required to differentiate pelvic inflammatory disease (PID) from appendicitis; recently, laparoscopy has been suggested as a more benign procedure for definitive diagnosis. Antibiotic therapy usually effects a dramatic improvement within 3 to 4 days, but it is impossible to determine the extent of damage to the tubes by the clinical response. Recurrent or chronic pelvic inflammatory disease is a cause of infertility, and chronic pain may prove so incapacitating as to require salpingectomy.

In the male, genital gonococcal infection is manifested by urethritis with a purulent discharge. Epididymitis and prostatitis are the common complications.

In both sexes, other mucosal sites may be primarily infected, notably the pharynx and rectum. Most infections are asymptomatic, but exudative pharyngitis and proctitis are known complications; it is likely that only a small proportion of gonococcal infections in these sites are properly diagnosed.

Disseminated disease is said to occur more commonly with asymptomatic than with symptomatic gonorrhea. The two most common manifestations are dermatitis and arthritis. The skin lesions are characteristically maculopapular on an erythematous base with a central purplish coloration. They are uncommon in the scalp and oral mucosa, but may be present on the palms and soles. Two forms of gonococcal arthritis are recognized clinically, although some believe them to be different stages of a single pathologic process: in the hematogenous form, many joints are affected but synovial fluid is characteristically sterile despite gonococcemia and clinical signs of sepsis. In contrast, in patients with the septic arthritis form, a single large joint is usually affected, with an abundant effusion that is positive on culture; the patient is not systemically ill, and the blood is sterile. In either form, intravenously administered penicillin produces a rapid clinical response—so rapid in fact as to be virtually diagnostic. Tenosynovitis is also characteristic of gonococcal infection and responds as predictably to appropriate anti-biotic therapy.

The increasing resistance to penicillin and the specter of gonococci that are totally resistant to penicillin make it imperative that the antibiotic be given in full dosage, with probenecid (to maintain high blood levels of penicillin by blocking renal excretion), and that "proof of cure" be obtained by repeated cultures at multiple sites 2 weeks after treatment. At present, there is no gonococcal vaccine, and only personal measures are available to help protect a person against gonorrhea. The high incidence of gonococcal infection, with the majority of cases escaping medical attention because of a lack of symptomatic disease, the usual mode of transmission, and the lack of unlimited resources combine to make the prospect for control of gonorrhea gloomy indeed.

Sexually Transmitted Diseases: General

1. Washington, A., Mandell, G., and Wiesner, P. Treatment of sexually transmitted diseases. *Rev. Infect. Dis.* 4(6), 1982.
   The entire issue is on treatment guidelines and various related topics. (For a quick summary of the treatment of sexually transmitted diseases, see Med. Lett. Drugs Ther. *26:5, 1984.*
2. Bell, T. Major sexually transmitted diseases of children and adolescents. *Pediatr. Infect. Dis.* 2:153, 1983.
   An extensive review, preceded (p. 146) by an article on office and laboratory diagnosis of sexually transmitted diseases.

Gonorrhea

3. Hook, E., and Holmes, K. Gonococcal infections. *Ann. Intern. Med.* 102:229 1985.
   Thorough review (14 pages, 157 references).
4. Litt, I., Edberg, S., and Finberg, L. Gonorrhea in children and adolescents: A current review. *J. Pediatr.* 85:595, 1974.
   Useful, but add reference 6 or 1. (Same with Am. J. Dis. Child. *125:233, 1973.)*

Diagnosis

5. Wald, E. Gonorrhea: Diagnosis by gram stain in the female adolescent. *Am. J. Dis. Child.* 131:1094, 1977.
   The use of Gram stain for presumptive diagnosis is discussed.

Treatment

6. Centers for Disease Control. Sexually transmitted diseases: Treatment guidelines, 1982. *Rev. Infect. Dis.* 4:729, 1982.
   The official "recommended treatment schedules" for various forms of GC: p. 731.
7. McCormack, W. Penicillinase-producing *Neisseria gonorrhoeae*: A retrospective. *N. Engl. J. Med.* 307:438, 1982.
   Less than 0.5 percent of the reported cases are due to PPNG; spectinomycin is the drug of choice. (Spectinomycin in prepubertal children: Am. J. Dis. Child. *134:359, 1980.)*

Neonates

8. Bernstein, G., Davis, J., and Katcher, M. Prophylaxis of neonatal conjunctivitis. *Clin. Pediatr.* (Phila.) 21:545, 1982.
   Compares silver nitrate, erythromycin, and tetracyline; gives erythromycin the edge.

Children

9. Deitch, S., et al. Gonorrhea in prepubertal children. *Pediatrics* 71:553, 1983.
   A brief statement by the American Academy of Pediatrics Committee on Early Childhood, Adoption, and Dependent Care recommending that abuse be presumed.
10. Emans, S. Vulvovaginitis in children and adolescents. *Pediatr. Rev.* 2:319, 1981.
    The evaluation of vaginal discharge in prepubertal children and adolescents. (Also see Clin. Pediatr. *[Phila.] 19:799, 1980.)*

Adolescents

11. Klein, J. Update: Adolescent gynecology. *Pediatr. Clin. North Am.* 27:141, 1980.
    Gonorrhea in perspective with other infections and other gynecologic problems of

adolescence. (Also see Pediatr. Clin. North Am. *28 [2], 1981 and* Curr. Prob. Pediatr. *8 [12], 1978.)*

12. Shafer, M., Irwin, C., and Sweet, R. Acute salpingitis in the adolescent female. *J. Pediatr.* 100:339, 1982.
    A thorough review of risk factors, organisms, pathogenesis, diagnosis and treatment. (Also see Clin. Pediatr. *[Phila.] 19:791, 1980.)*

13. Bowie, W., and Jones, H. Acute pelvic inflammatory disease in outpatients: Association with *Chlamydia trachomatis* and *Neisseria gonorrhoeae*. *Ann. Intern. Med.* 95:685, 1981.
    Among patients with mild PID, Chlamydia *was incriminated more frequently than GC. (More on* Chlamydia: Pediatr. Rev. *3:77, 1981, and* Pediatr. Clin. North Am. *26:269, 1979.)*

14. Litt, I., and Cohen, M. Perihepatitis associated with salpingitis in adolescents. *JAMA* 240:1253, 1978.
    The Fitz-Hugh-Curtis syndrome.

15. Wiesner, P., et al. Clinical spectrum of pharyngeal gonococcal infection. *N. Engl. J. Med.* 288:181, 1973.
    From asymptomatic to exudative. (A higher dose is required to treat pharyngeal GC than to treat genital GC: JAMA *239:1631, 1978.)*

16. Hein, K., Marks, A., and Cohen, M. Asymptomatic gonorrhea: Prevalence in a population of urban adolescents. *J. Pediatr.* 90:634, 1977.
    A reminder.

Disseminated Disease

17. Holmes, K., Counts, G., and Beaty, H. Disseminated gonococcal infection. *Ann. Intern. Med.* 74:979, 1971.
    An encyclopedic review.

18. Keiser, H., et al. Clinical forms of gonococcal arthritis. *N. Engl. J. Med.* 279:234, 1968.
    They include the septicemic form (positive culture of blood, joint fluid negative) and septic arthritis form (negative culture of blood, joint fluid positive). (Or are these sequential stages: J. Rheumatol. *2:83, 1975?)*

19. Handsfield, H., Wiesner, P., and Holmes, K. Treatment of the gonococcal arthritis-dermatitis syndrome. *Ann. Intern. Med.* 84:661, 1976.
    The response is usually dramatic even with less than "mega" doses.

20. Wilkens, R., et al. Reiter's syndrome. *Arthritis Rheum.* 24:844, 1981.
    Something to think about in your differential diagnosis.

Males

21. Holmes, K., Johnson, D., and Trostle, H. An estimate of the risk of men acquiring gonorrhea by sexual contact with infected females. *Am. J. Epidemiol.* 91:170, 1970.
    The fun is not in knowing the answer (22%) but in trying to figure out, as you walk to the library, how to design a study to find out!

22. Rosenfeld, W., and Litman, N. Urogenital tract infections in male adolescents. *Pediatr. Rev.* 4:257, 1983.
    A discussion by bug and by clinical syndrome.

INDEX

Abdomen, acute, 24–27. *See also specific disorder*

Abdominal mass, 338, 339, 342

Abdominal pain
acute, 24–27. *See also specific disorder*
recurrent, 92–94, 95–96

Abducens palsy, and increased intracranial pressure, 32
and brain tumor, 351
in meningitis, 10

Abetalipoproteinemia, 220, 223

ABO incompatibility, 128

Abscess
brain
versus brain tumor, 351
and cyanotic heart disease, 173, 174, 176
and increased intracranial pressure, 32
intraabdominal, 26
lung, 199, 206
pelvic, and gonorrhea, 388
peritonsillar, 190
thyroid, 266

Absence spells, 285–286, 288

Abuse, child. *See* Child abuse

Abuse, sexual. *See* Sexual, abuse

Acanthocytosis, 220

Accidents, 39–42. *See also* Burns; Ingestion(s); *specific cause*

Acetaminophen, 43, 44, 45

Acetazolamide, in increased intracranial pressure, 32

N-Acetylcysteine, in acetaminophen overdose, 44, 45

Acetylsalicylic acid. *See* Salicylate

Achilles tendon, in cerebral palsy, 295

Acquired immune deficiency syndrome (AIDS), 325, 362

Acrodermatitis enteropathica, 221, 223

ACTH (adrenocorticotropic hormone)
in adrenal hyperplasia, 259, 260, 261
in infantile spasms, 286, 288

Actinomycin D
in Ewing sarcoma, 354
in Wilms tumor, 339, 340, 341

Activated prothrombin complex, in hemophilia, 324, 325

Acute abdomen, 24–27. *See also specific disorder*

Acute tubular necrosis (ATN), 27, 28, 234

Acyclovir, in neonatal herpes, 143, 145

Addiction, maternal, and withdrawal in neonate, 119–120, 121, 122, 123

Adductor tenotomy, in cerebral palsy, 295

Adenine arabinoside, in neonatal herpes infection, 143, 145

Adenoidectomy, 189, 190, 193

Adenoids, 189

Adenotonsillectomy, 190, 193

Adenovirus
and pertussis, 363, 367
and pneumonia, 199

Adenyl cyclase
and asthma, 202
and diarrhea, 384

ADH. *See* Antidiuretic hormone (ADH)

Adrenal hemorrhage, and septicemia, 7

Adrenal hyperplasia, congenital, 259–262
and hypertension, 185, 260
and precocious pseudopuberty, 99, 259
and pseudohermaphroditism, 98, 259

Adrenal tumor
versus hyperplasia, 259–260
and precocious pseudopuberty, 99
and short stature, 63

Adrenarche, 99, 101

Adrenocorticotropic hormone. *See* ACTH (adrenocorticotropic hormone)

Adrenogenital syndrome. *See* Adrenal hyperplasia, congenital

Adriamycin
in Ewing sarcoma, 354
in neuroblastoma, 344
in osteogenic sarcoma, 354
in Wilms tumor, 339, 340

Agammaglobulinemia, 361
Swiss type. *See* Immune deficiency, severe combined

Aganglionic megacolon. *See* Hirschsprung disease

AIDS. *See* Acquired immune deficiency syndrome (AIDS)

Airway
and resuscitation, 3
and status epilepticus, 34
upper, obstruction of. *See* Upper airway obstruction

Alae nasi, flaring of, in pneumonia, 199

Albinism, in Chédiak-Steinbrinck-Higashi syndrome, 362

Albuterol, 204

Alcohol
and fetus, 121, 277, 280
and hypoglycemia, 267
intoxication, versus diabetic ketoacidosis, 21

Alcohol—*Continued*
  and motor vehicle fatalities, 41
  withdrawal, in neonate, 119, 121
Aldosterone, in hypertension, 185. *See
    also* Mineralocorticoids, in adrenal
    hyperplasia
Alkalosis
  in cystic fibrosis, 207
  "rebound" after alkali treatment for
    respiratory failure, 17
  in Reye Syndrome, 29
  in salicylate intoxication, 43
Allopurinol, in uric acid nephropathy,
    337
Alopecia, in leukemia, 338
Alpha-fetoprotein
  in biliary atresia, 213, 214
  in congenital nephrotic syndrome, 246,
    248
  in neonatal hepatitis, 213, 214
  in spinal dysraphism, 290
Alpha-keto acids
  in renal failure, 253
  in Reye syndrome, 29
Alpha-1-antitrypsin deficiency, 201, 202,
    213, 214
Alport syndrome, 236, 238, 240, 252
Alternative pathway. *See* Properdin,
    pathway, in immune system
Amantadine, in influenza, 369
Amebiasis, versus ulcerative colitis, 224
Amino acids
  disorders of, 273–274, 276. *See also
    specific disorder*
    hypoglycemia in, 267
    seizures in, 122
  in nutrition, 65, 133
  in renal failure, 253
  in Reye syndrome, 29, 30
Aminoglycoside antibiotics, 150. *See also
    specific indication*
Aminophylline. *See* Theophylline
Aminopterin, as teratogen, 277
Aminotransferase
  in hepatitis, 216
  in infectious mononucleosis, 372
  and salicylate, 304
Ammonia
  and high protein feedings, 131
  in renal failure, 253
  in Reye syndrome, 29, 30, 31
  in urea cycle disorders, 273, 274, 276
Amniocentesis, 108, 129. *See also* Pre-
    natal diagnosis
Amphetamines, in attention deficit disor-
    der, 80
Amyloidosis, 305
ANA. *See* Antinuclear antibodies
Anabolic steroids. *See* Androgens
Anaerobic bacteria

  and intraabdominal abscess, 25, 26
  and neonatal septicemia, 148–149
Anal atresia, 137
Anal fissures, and encopresis, 86
Analgesics. *See specific drug; specific
    indication*
Anaphylactoid purpura. *See* Henoch-
    Schönlein syndrome
Anaphylaxis, and cow milk intolerance
    67, 220
Androgens, 101
  in adrenal hyperplasia, 259
  and growth, 62, 63, 65
  and sexual differentiation, 97–98
Androstenedione, 260, 262
Anemia, 317–318. *See also specific
    disorder*
Anergy. *See* Delayed hypersensitivity
Anesthesia, and cardiopulmonary arres
    3, 4, 190
Angioedema, and cow milk intolerance,
    67
Angioneurotic edema, 67
Aniridia, and Wilms tumor, 338
Ankylosing spondylitis. *See* Spondylitis
    ankylosing
Annular pancreas, 137
Anomalies, congenital, 153–156. *See al*
    Malformation syndromes; *specific
    anomaly*
Anorectic drugs, and obesity, 72, 74
Anthrax vaccine, 369
Antibiotic-associated pseudomembrano
    colitis, 384, 387
Antibiotics, 9, 12. *See also specific
    indication*
  in neonate, 150
Antibody-coated bacteria, in urinary
    tract infection, 249, 251
Anticonvulsants, 123, 288. *See also
    specific drug*
Antidepressants, withdrawal from, in
    neonate, 119
Antidiuretic hormone (ADH)
  in cystic fibrosis, 207
  in meningitis, 10, 12
Antihistamines
  in Henoch-Schönlein syndrome, 330
  in otitis media, 192, 193, 194
  in upper respiratory tract infection,
    189, 191
Antihypertensive drugs, in hypertensio
    183–184, 186
Anti-inflammatory drugs, 304
Antimalarial drugs, in systemic lupus
    erythematosus, 306, 308
Antinuclear antibodies, 301, 306, 307
Antipyretics, 43–45. *See also specific
    drug*
Antistreptolysin O (ASO), 180, 380, 38

ntitussive drugs, in upper respiratory
    tract infection, 189, 191
ntiviral drugs
  in bronchiolitis, 196, 198
  in neonatal herpes, 143, 145
  in upper respiratory infection, 189, 191
nuria. *See* Renal failure
nus. *See also* Perianal disease, in
    Crohn disease
  atresia of, 137
  fissures, 86
  imperforate, 136, 137
orta
  coarctation of, 116, 117, 118
    and gonadal dysgenesis, 98
    and heart failure, 19, 116
    and hypertension, 183
    and necrotizing enterocolitis, 134
    and patent ductus arteriosus, 178
    and transposition of the great arte-
      ries, 175
  supravalvar stenosis, in Williams syn-
    drome, 280
ortic arch
  interrupted, 118
  right, in tetralogy of Fallot, 173
ortic valve
  atresia, 116, 117, 118
  stenosis, 19, 116, 117, 118, 178
    and endocarditis, 169
pgar score, 105, 106
phthous ulcers, in Crohn disease, 227
pley's law, in recurrent abdominal
    pain, 93
pnea. *See also* Cardiopulmonary arrest;
    associated disorder
  infantile, 57
  of prematurity, 108
ppendicitis, 24–26
  versus Crohn disease, 227
  versus diabetic ketoacidosis, 21
  versus myocarditis, 163
  versus pelvic inflammatory disease,
    388
  versus sickle cell disease, 319
pt test, 151
queduct of Sylvius, 291
queductal stenosis, 292
ra-A, in neonatal herpes infection, 143,
    145
rnold-Chiari malformation, and hydro-
    cephalus, 289, 292
rrhythmias, cardiac. *See* Cardiac
    dysrhythmias
rteriovenous fistula, and heart failure
    in neonate, 116
rthritis, 303
  in Crohn disease, 227, 229
  gonococcal, 388, 390
  juvenile rheumatoid (JRA), 301–305

myocarditis in, 163, 165
  pericarditis in, 164, 166
  versus rheumatic fever, 179
  and psoriasis, 301–302, 303
  in rheumatic fever, 179, 180, 182
  after rubella vaccine, 368
  septic, 370, 371, 372
    versus juvenile rheumatoid arthritis,
      302
    in neonate, 149
  of spine. *See* Spondylitis, ankylosing
  in systemic lupus erythematosus, 305,
    306
  in ulcerative colitis, 224, 225, 227
Articulation, and otitis media, 194
Ascorbic acid. *See* Vitamin(s), C
Aseptic meningitis, 10, 11, 12, 368
Aseptic necrosis. *See* Avascular necrosis,
    of femoral head
ASO. *See* Antistreptolysin O (ASO)
Aspergillus
  and asthma, 203
  in chronic renal failure, 254
  in cystic fibrosis, 206
Aspiration pneumonia. *See* Pneumonia,
    aspiration
Aspirin. *See* Salicylate
Asthma, 201–205
  versus bronchiolitis, 196, 197, 202
  and cow milk intolerance, 67, 220
  and recurrent pneumonia, 201
  status asthmaticus, 16–19
Astrocytoma, 351, 352
Asymmetric septal hypertrophy, 21
Asymmetric tonic neck reflex, in cerebral
    palsy, 294
Ataxia
  in lead poisoning, 46
  in meningitis, 10
  and neuroblastoma, 342, 343
Ataxia-telangiectasia, 362
Atenolol, in supraventricular tachy-
    cardia, 163
Athetosis, in cerebral palsy, 295
ATN. *See* Acute tubular necrosis (ATN)
Atrial
  contraction, premature, 160
  fibrillation, 160, 162
  flutter, 160, 162
  septal defect
    in congenital rubella syndrome, 365
    rarely cause of endocarditis, 167
    and tetralogy of Fallot, 172
  septostomy, in transposition of great
    arteries, 114, 176, 177
  tachycardia, 159–160, 160–163
Atrioventricular node, 159, 160
Atropine
  in cardiopulmonary resuscitation, 5
  poisoning, 387

Attention deficit disorder, 78–82
  and cerebral palsy, 295
  and congenital cytomegalovirus, 142
Atypical lymphocytes
  in hepatitis, 216
  in infectious mononucleosis, 372, 373, 374
Atypical measles, 367
  versus Rocky Mountain spotted fever, 379
Automobile accidents, 39, 40, 41
AV node, 159, 160
Avascular necrosis, of femoral head, 154, 302, 319, 370
Azathioprine
  in renal transplantation, 254
  in systemic lupus erythematosus, 306, 308
Azulfidine. See Sulfasalazine

Babinski sign, in cerebral palsy, 295
Bacilli, gram-negative. See Gram-negative bacilli
Bacillus Calmette-Guérin (BCG), 376, 378. See also Tuberculosis, vaccine
Baclofen, in cerebral palsy, 295
Bacteremia, 6–9. See also specific disorder; specific organism
Bacterial endocarditis. See Endocarditis
Bacterial tracheitis, 15
BAL (British anti-lewisite), in lead poisoning, 47
Barbiturates. See also Phenobarbital
  coma, therapeutic, 31, 33, 34, 37
  and neonatal withdrawal, 119, 122
Basilar skull fraction, 36, 37
Basophilic stippling, in lead poisoning, 46
Bassen-Kornzweig disease. See Abetalipoproteinemia
Battered child. See Child abuse
Bayley scales, 75, 318
BCG. See Bacillus Calmette-Guérin (BCG)
Beclomethasone, in asthma, 202, 204
Bedwetting. See Enuresis
Behavior modification, and obesity, 72, 74
Behavior problems, in preschool children, 85. See also specific problem
Berger disease, 236, 238, 254, 331
Beta cell. See Islet (of Langerhans) cell
Beta-adrenergic
  agonists, in asthma, 17, 202, 204
  blockers, 186. See also specific drug; specific indication
Bicarbonate, sodium
  in cardiopulmonary arrest, 4, 5
  in diabetic ketoacidosis, 22, 23
  in respiratory failure, 67

Bile acids, in neonatal hepatitis/biliary atresia, 213
Biliary atresia, 213–215
Bilirubinuria, in hepatitis, 216
Biofeedback
  and fecal soiling, 88, 291
  and headaches, 95
Birth control pills
  and hypertension, 183
  and precocious pseudopuberty, 99
Birthmarks, 107
Bladder
  control, 85, 87, 89, 91
  exstrophy of, 139, 141
  neurogenic, and urinary tract infection, 249, 250
  tumor of, 236
Blalock-Taussig shunt, in tetralogy of Fallot, 173
Bleeding. See also specific disorder
  emergencies, 324
  intracranial. See Epidural hematoma; Subdural hematoma
  in neonate, 151, 152, 153
  in neonate, 150–153
Blindness. See also Vision
  after cardiac arrest, 5
  from congenital toxoplasmosis, 141–142
  from gonococcal ophthalmia, 388
  from iridocyclitis, in juvenile rheumatoid arthritis, 301
  in Tay-Sachs disease, 275
Blood culture, 7, 169. See also Bacteremia
Blood pressure, 182, 184–185. See also Hypertension
Blueberry muffin lesions, in congenital rubella syndrome, 142
Bonding, 78, 106–107
Bone marrow. See also specific disorder
  dysfunction, in Shwachman syndrome, 222
  suppression, and hepatitis, 216
  transplantation
    in immune deficiency, 360
    in leukemia, 337
Bone pain
  and bone tumors, 354
  in leukemia, 355
  in neuroblastoma, 342
  in osteomyelitis, 369
  and recurrent pains (abdominal, head), 96, 97
  in sickle cell disease, 319
Bone tumors, 354–355
Bordetella pertussis, 363. See also Pertussis
Bordet-Gengou medium, in pertussis, 36
Bowel training, 85–86, 87

ᴮD. *See* Bronchopulmonary dysplasia (BPD)

aces
in cerebral palsy, 295, 297
in spinal dysraphism, 289, 290
ᴬachial palsy, in neuroblastoma, 342
adycardia, 160
ain
abscess. *See* Abscess, brain
death, 5
stem glioma, 352–353
tumors, 351–353
  and increased intracranial pressure, 32
  and seizures, 34
ᴬanched-chain ketoaciduria. *See* Maple syrup urine disease
ᴮeast-feeding, 66, 67–68. *See also* Milk, human
and hypernatremic dehydration, 234
and obesity, 73
stools, 86, 218
ᴮeast milk. *See* Breast-feeding; Milk, human
ᴮeath hydrogen, 220, 222
ᴬitish anti-lewisite (BAL), in lead poisoning, 47
ᴿonchiectasis, 201
in asthma, 203
in cystic fibrosis, 205
ᴿonchiolitis, 195–198
versus asthma, 196, 197, 202
ᴿonchitis, chronic, versus asthma, 203
ᴿonchopulmonary dysplasia (BPD), 108, 111, 112
ᴿonchoscopy, and foreign bodies, 14, 15
ᴿudzinksi sign, in meningitis, 10
ᴿushfield spots, in Down syndrome, 278
ᴬffy coat, Gram stain of, in septicemia, 6, 7–8, 147, 150
ᴬllous impetigo, 381
ᴬllous myringitis, 194
ᴬndle of His, 159, 160
ᴬndle of Kent, and Wolff-Parkinson-White syndrome, 159–160
ᴬrkitt lymphoma, 349, 350
ᴬrns, 39, 40, 42. *See also* Smoke inhalation
and child abuse, 49, 50
and septicemia, 6
ᴬrsa of Fabricius, 359

admium
as cause of interstitial nephritis, 250
as uremic toxin, 253
alcifications
intracranial, in congenital infection, 141, 142
intraperitoneal, in meconium ileus, 138

subcutaneous, in dermatomyositis/polymyositis, 310, 311
Calcium. *See also* Hypercalcemia; Hypercalciuria, and hematuria; Hypocalcemia
and lead poisoning, 46
metabolism
  in neonate, 120
  in renal failure, 253
salts, in resuscitation, 4
Calories, required
by infants failing to thrive, 70
by normal infants, 65
by premature or ill infants, 131
Campylobacter, 384–385, 386–387
Cancer, 335–355. *See also specific disease; specific site*
as cause of fever of unknown origin (FUO), 43
second, after treatment, 338, 341
Candida
in chronic renal failure, 254
in immune deficiency, 360, 362
in septic arthritis, 372
skin test, 362
Captopril, 20, 184, 186
Carbamazepine, 285. *See also* Anticonvulsants
Carbohydrates. *See also specific carbohydrate*
in infant nutrition, 65, 131
malabsorption of, 219–220, 222
metabolism
  disorders of, 274–275, 276–277. *See also specific disorder*
  in renal failure, 255
Carbon tetrachloride, and renal failure, 27
Cardiac arrest. *See* Cardiopulmonary arrest
Cardiac dysrhythmias, 159–163
and cardiopulmonary arrest, 3, 4
and heart failure, 19, 20
  in neonate, 116
and isoproterenol use in asthma, 17, 18
and myocarditis, 163
and sudden infant death syndrome, 56, 57
after surgery
  for tetralogy of Fallot, 174
  for transposition of great arteries, 176
and theophylline overdose, 203
Cardiac failure. *See* Heart, failure
Cardiac surgery. *See* Heart, surgery
Cardiac tamponade
in pericarditis, 164, 165
in status asthmaticus, 17

Cardiomyopathy. *See* Myocardiopathy
Cardiopulmonary arrest, 3–5
    after tonsillectomy and adenoidectomy,
        190
Carotene, in malabsorption, 220
Carotid massage, and supraventricular
        tachycardia, 159
Cartilage hair hypoplasia, and immune
        deficiency, 362
CAT scan. *See* Computerized axial to-
        mography (CAT scan)
Cataplexy, 83
Cataracts
    in congenital rubella syndrome, 142,
        365
    in galactosemia, 274
Catecholamines, and neuroblastoma,
        341–342, 344
Cattell scales, 75
Cavernous sinus thrombosis, in men-
        ingitis, 10
Celiac disease, 220, 221, 222
Cephalhematoma, and hyper-
        bilirubinemia, 125
Cerebellar ataxia. *See* Ataxia
Cerebral edema. *See also* Increased in-
        tracranial pressure
    in diabetic ketoacidosis, 22, 24
    and head trauma, 38
    in hypernatremic dehydration, 233
    in Reye syndrome, 30
    and seizures, 122
    in status epilepticus, 34
Cerebral palsy, 75, 294–297
    and congenital infections, 140, 141
    and encopresis, 87
    and hyperbilirubinemia, 124
    and phenylketonuria, 274
Cerebrospinal fluid, 11, 291. *See also*
        specific disorder
Cerebrovascular accident (CVA)
    in cyanotic heart disease, 173, 174
    and hypertension, 184
    in sickle cell disease, 319–320, 322
Chédiak-Steinbrinck-Higashi syndrome,
        362
Chelating agents, in lead poisoning, 47,
        48
Chest
    pain, 92, 95, 97
        and cardiac dysrhythmia, 160
        and pericarditis, 164
    shieldlike, in gonadal dysgenesis, 98
Chickenpox. *See* Varicella
Chicken soup, 191, 387
Child abuse, 48–51
    and failure to thrive, 69, 70
    and head trauma, 37
    and maternal narcotic addiction, 120
Child neglect, 50, 69

Chlamydia trachomatis, 144, 146, 390
    and myocarditis, 163, 165
    and pelvic inflammatory disease, 390
    and pneumonia, 146, 199, 201
Chlorambucil
    in nephrotic syndrome, 245, 247–248
    in systemic lupus erythematosus, 300
Chloride
    in cystic fibrosis, 207
    in diarrhea, familial disorder of, 221
Chlorothiazide, in heart failure, 117. *See
        also* Diuretics
Choanal atresia, 139, 140
Cholangiography, 213, 214
Cholangitis, 214
Choledochal cyst, 214
Cholelithiasis. *See* Gallstones
Cholera, 369, 383
Cholesterol
    in acute poststreptococcal glomeru-
        lonephritis, 239
    in nephrotic syndrome, 244
    as precursor of steroid compounds, 251
Cholestyramine, 213, 215
Chondrodysplasia, 62
Chondrosarcoma, 354
Chordee, and hypospadias, 154
Chorea
    versus attention deficit disorder, 79
    in cerebral palsy, 295
    in rheumatic fever, 179, 180, 181
Chorioretinitis, and congenital infection,
        141, 143, 145
Choroid plexus
    and production of cerebrospinal fluid,
        291
    tumor of, 292
Christmas disease. *See* Hemophilia B
Chromosome(s)
    disorders, 98, 100, 280. *See also specific
        disorder*
    and sex differentiation, 97–98
Chronic active hepatitis, 216, 217, 218
Chronic nonspecific diarrhea, 219,
        221–222
Chronic persistent hepatitis, 216
Circumcision, 106, 107
    and bleeding, in hemophilia, 151, 323
Cirrhosis
    in biliary atresia, 214
    in cystic fibrosis, 207
    and hepatitis, 217
    in ulcerative colitis, 225, 227
Cis-platinum, and acute renal failure, 237
Cleft lip, 154, 155
Cleft palate, 154, 155
    and otitis media, 193
Clinitest
    and galactosemia, 274
    and malabsorption, 219, 222

Clitoris
  in adrenal hyperplasia, 259
  bifid, and exstrophy of bladder, 139
Clonazepam, 286. *See also*
      Anticonvulsants
Clostridium, and necrotizing entero-
      colitis, 135
Clostridium difficile, 384, 387
Clostridium tetani, 363. *See also* Tetanus
Clotting factors. *See also* Disseminated
      intravascular coagulation;
      Hemophilia
  in hemolytic-uremic syndrome, 243
  in neonate, 150
  in Reye syndrome, 30
Clubbing
  in Crohn disease, 227
  in cystic fibrosis, 206
Cluster headache, 95
Coarctation of the aorta. *See* Aorta, co-
      arctation of
Cognitive development, 74, 75, 77. *See
      also* Mental retardation
Cognitive stimulation, 78
Cold agglutinins, in *Mycoplasma pneu-
      moniae,* 199
Cold, common. *See* Upper respiratory
      tract infection (URI)
Colectomy
  in Crohn disease, 228
  in ulcerative colitis, 224, 225, 226
Colic, 66, 68
  and attention deficit disorder, 79
  in cow milk allergy, 67
  versus normal crying, 68
  and urinary tract infection, 249
Coliforms. *See* Gram-negative bacilli
Colon, irritable. *See* Irritable bowel
      syndrome
Complement 359, 360, 361, 362. *See also*
      specific disorder
Computerized axial tomography (CAT
      scan), 33, 293. *See also specific
      disorder*
Concussion, 36
Conditioning techniques, and enuresis,
      90, 92
Congenital anomalies. *See* Anomalies,
      congenital
Congenital dislocation of hip, 105, 106,
      154, 155–156
Congenital infections, 141–146. *See also
      specific infection*
  and heart disease, 165
  and neonatal hepatitis, 213, 215
Congenital stridor, 13
Congestive heart failure. *See* Heart,
      failure
Conjunctivitis, and *Chlamydia,* 146
Constipation, 66, 86–87, 88

Constitutional delay of growth and ado-
      lescence, 62, 64, 99
Constrictive pericarditis, 164–165, 167,
      220
Continuous positive airway pressure
      (CPAP), 108, 109, 178
Contraception
  and breast-feeding, 68
  counseling, 100
Contraceptives, oral
  and hypertension, 183
  and precocious pseudopuberty, 99
Contusion, cerebral, 36
Convulsions. *See* Seizures
Coombs test
  in erythroblastosis, 129
  in hemolytic-uremic syndrome, 242
  and hyperbilirubinemia, in neonate,
      125
Copper deficiency, in neonates, 131, 133
Cor pulmonale. *See also* Pulmonary
      hypertension
  in bronchopulmonary dysplasia, 111
  in cystic fibrosis, 206, 209
  as form of progressive heart failure, 20
  and tonsillar hypertrophy, 189
Cornelia de Lange syndrome, 280
Coronary arteries
  and heart failure in neonate, 117
  and tetralogy of Fallot, 173, 174
  and transposition of great arteries, 176
Corrected transposition of great arteries,
      175
  and congenital heart block, 160
Cortical blindness, after cardiac arrest, 5
Corticosteroids. *See* Glucocorticoids
Cortisol, 21, 259
Corynebacterium diphtheriae, 363. *See
      also* Diphtheria
Costochondritis, 95, 97
Cot death. *See* Sudden infant death
      syndrome
Cough suppressants. *See* Antitussive
      drugs, in upper respiratory tract
      infection
Countercurrent immunoelectrophoresis
      antigen detection tests, 6, 10, 11
Cow milk. *See* Milk, cow
Coxsackie virus. *See also* Enterovirus
      infection
  and congenital infection, 144
  and diabetes mellitus, 269
  and hemolytic-uremic syndrome, 243
  and hepatitis, in neonate, 215
  and myopericarditis, 163, 164, 165
CPAP. *See* Continuous positive airway
      pressure (CPAP)
Cranial nerve VI palsy. *See* Abducens
      palsy, and increased intracranial
      pressure

Craniopharyngioma, 99, 351, 352, 353
Creatinine clearance, clinical cor-
    relations, 252
Cretinism. See Hypothyroidism
Cri du chat syndrome, 280
Crib death. See Sudden infant death
    syndrome
Crohn disease, 227–230
    versus Henoch-Schönlein syndrome,
        330
    versus ulcerative colitis, 224
Cromoglycate, sodium, in asthma, 202,
    204
Cromolyn, in asthma, 202, 204
Croup, 13, 14–15
    and influenza, 365, 369
Cry, hoarse, in hypothyroidism, 262
Crying, in infancy, 68
Cryptorchidism. See Testes, undescended
    (cryptorchidism)
Cushing syndrome
    and hypertension, 183
    and obesity, 72
    and short stature, 63
Cushing triad, in increased intracranial
    pressure, 32
CVA. See Cerebrovascular accident
    (CVA)
Cyanide poisoning, from nitroprusside,
    184
Cyanosis, 113, 114. See also specific
    cause
Cyanotic heart disease, 112–116. See also
    specific disorder
Cyclic AMP (adenosine monophosphate),
    and asthma, 202
Cyclic vomiting, 95, 97
Cyclophosphamide, 247
    in Ewing sarcoma, 354
    in nephrotic syndrome, 245, 247
    in neuroblastoma, 342, 344
    in non-Hodgkin lymphoma, 349
    in systemic lupus erythematosus, 306
Cyclosporine, 256
Cystic fibrosis, 205–210. See also Me-
    conium ileus
    and malabsorption, 220, 222
    and pneumonia, 199, 200, 201
Cystinosis, as cause of renal failure, 252
Cytomegalovirus
    congenital infection, 142, 145
        and heart disease, 165
        and neonatal hepatitis, 213, 215
    and hepatitis, 215
    in immunosuppressed host, 199
        in leukemia, 336
        after renal transplantation, 254
    and infectious mononucleosis, 373, 374

Dactylitis, in sickle cell disease, 319, 321

Dandy-Walker syndrome, 292, 293
Dantrolene, in cerebral palsy, 295
Deafness. See Hearing loss
Death. See also Mortality; specific
    disorder
    brain, 5
    dying and mourning, 51–55
    perinatal, 54
    sudden, and cardiac dysrhythmias,
        160, 162, 174. See also Sudden in-
        fant death syndrome
Decadron. See Dexamethasone
Decongestants
    in otitis media, 192, 193, 194
    in upper respiratory tract infection,
        189, 191
Defibrillation, 4
Delayed hypersensitivity, 360, 361–362
    to tuberculin. See Tuberculin test
        (PPD)
Delinquency, and attention deficit disor-
    der, 80, 81
Dental
    bleeding, in hemophilia, 324
    manipulation, and endocarditis, 167,
        168, 170
Denver Developmental Screening Test,
    75, 76–77
Depakene. See Valproic acid
Dermatomyositis, 309–310, 311
Dexamethasone
    and head injury, 38
    in increased intracranial pressure, 32
Diabetes insipidus
    and enuresis, 89
    as cause of hypernatremic dehydration,
        233
    and hypothalamic tumor, 351
Diabetes mellitus, 269–273
    and congenital rubella, 142
    in cystic fibrosis, 206–207
    and enuresis, 89
    ketoacidosis in. See Diabetic
        ketoacidosis
    and interstitial nephritis, 250
    maternal. See Infant of diabetic
        mother
    and urinary tract infection, 250
Diabetic ketoacidosis, 21–24
    and acute abdominal pain, 21, 23, 25
    versus hypernatremic dehydration, 233
Dialysis, 256
    in acute renal failure, 28
    in chronic renal failure, 252–256
    hemodialysis, 253–254, 255, 256
        and ammonia, 31
        and hepatitis B, 217
    and hypernatremic dehydration, 233
    peritoneal
        and amino acid disorders, 274

and ammonia, 31
and hemolytic-uremic syndrome, 242, 244
and salt poisoning, 234, 235
and uric acid neuropathy, 335
Diamox. *See* Acetazolamide, in increased intracranial pressure
Diaphragmatic hernia, 138–139, 140
Diarrhea
  acute infectious, 383–387. *See also specific agent*
  chronic, 218–223. *See also specific disorder*
  in hemolytic-uremic syndrome, 242
  and hypernatremia, 233
  traveler's, 384, 387
Diazepam
  administered through E-T tube, 5
  in cerebral palsy, 295
  in narcotic withdrawal, in neonate, 119, 121, 123
  in seizures, 286. *See also* Anticonvulsants
  in neonate, 124
  in status epilepticus, 34, 36
Diazoxide
  in hypertension, 184, 186
  in hypoglycemia, 267, 268
Diencephalic syndrome, 351, 353
Di George syndrome, 361
Digitalis, 20, 21, 161. *See also specific disorder*
Digoxin. *See* Digitalis
Diiodohydroxyquin. *See* Antimalarial drugs, in systemic lupus erythematosus
Dilantin. *See* Phenytoin
Dimercaprol (BAL), in lead poisoning, 47
Dimethyltriazenoimidazole-carboxamide (DTIC), in neuroblastoma, 342, 344
Diphenoxylate, in diarrhea, 387
Diphenylhydantoin. *See* Phenytoin
Diphtheria, 363, 366
  versus infectious mononucleosis, 372
  and myocarditis, 163, 164, 165
Diphtheria toxoid, 363, 364, 366, 369
  as skin test for delayed hypersensitivity, 361, 362
Dipyridamole, in hemolytic-uremic syndrome, 242, 244
Disaccharides. *See* Carbohydrates; *specific disaccharide*
Diskitis, 371
Disseminated intravascular coagulation
  in erythroblastosis, 130
  and hemolytic-uremic syndrome, 243
  in herpes infection, in neonate, 143
  in necrotizing enterocolitis, 134–135, 151, 152

in neonate, 151, 152, 153
in respiratory distress syndrome, 108
and Reye syndrome, 29
in septicemia, 7, 9
  in neonate, 148, 151
Diuretics, 186. *See also specific indication*
Diving reflex, and supraventricular tachycardia, 159, 163
Divorce, 51, 53, 93
Dobutamine, 5, 20
DOCA (desoxycorticosterone acetate), in adrenal hyperplasia, 260
Done nomogram, in salicylate intoxication, 44
Dopamine
  in cardiopulmonary resuscitation, 4, 5
  in neuroblastoma, 241, 244
  in septic shock, 7
"Double bubble" sign, in duodenal atresia, 137
Down syndrome, 278–279, 280
  and duodenal atresia, 137
  and endocardial cushion defect, 171
  mourning behavior in parents, 51
  and ventricular septal defect, 170
Driver education, 41
Drowning, 16, 18, 39, 40, 41, 42
Drugs. *See also specific class of drug; specific drug*
  in breast milk, 68
  dosages, and renal failure, 255
  withdrawal reaction, in neonate, 119–120, 121, 122, 123
DTIC. *See* Dimethyltriazenoimidazole-carboxamide (DTIC), in neuroblastoma
Dubowitz score, 106
Ductus arteriosus, 177. *See also* Patent ductus arteriosus (PDA)
  and tetralogy of Fallot, 173
  and transposition of great arteries, 175
Duhamel procedure, in Hirschsprung disease, 138
Duodenal
  atresia, 137, 140
  hematoma, and child abuse, 49
  stenosis, 137
  web, 137
Dwarfism
  deprivation, 50, 63, 64, 69
  primordial, 62, 64
  psychosocial, 50, 63, 64, 69
D-xylose test, in malabsorption, 220, 223
Dysdiadochokinesis, 79
Dyslexia, 82
Dysmorphic syndromes. *See* Malformation syndromes
Dysrhythmias, cardiac. *See* Cardiac dysrhythmias

EACA. *See* Epsilon-aminocaproic acid (EACA), in hemophilia
Ebstein anomaly, 114, 115, 159, 175
ECHO virus, and congenital infection, 215. *See also* Enterovirus infection
Eczema
  and cow milk intolerance, 67, 220
  in phenylketonuria, 274
  in Wiskott-Aldrich syndrome, 360, 362
EDTA (ethylenediaminetetraacetate), in lead poisoning, 47
Edwards syndrome, 280
EEG. *See* Electroencephalogram (EEG)
Electroencephalogram (EEG), 287. *See also specific disorder*
Emboli
  in cardiac dysrhythmias, 162
  in endocarditis, 167, 169
  in nephrotic syndrome, 247
Empyema, 198, 199, 200
Encephalitis
  versus brain tumor, 351
  and congenital rubella, 142
  and measles, 364, 367
  and measles vaccine, 364, 366, 367
  and mumps, 365, 368
  and pertussis, 363
  and pertussis vaccine, 364, 367
  versus Reye syndrome, 29
  and status epilepticus, 35
Encephalopathy
  hypertensive, 184
    in acute poststreptococcal glomerulonephritis, 239
    in membranoproliferative glomerulonephritis, 245
  and increased intracranial pressure, 32, 33
  in lead poisoning, 46, 47, 48
  in Reye syndrome, 29, 30, 31
  and status epilepticus, 34
  toxic, 32, 33
Encopresis, 86–87, 88
Endocardial cushion defect, 117, 171, 172
Endocardial fibroelastosis, 116, 164, 165
Endocarditis, 167–170. *See also specific aspect; specific disorder*
End-stage renal disease. *See* Renal failure, chronic
Enemas, 86, 87
Enteric fever, 384
Enterococcus, in endocarditis, 168, 169
Enterohepatic recirculation, of bilirubin, 125
Enterokinase deficiency, as cause of malabsorption, 220
Enteropathogenic *Escherichia coli,* 384, 386
Enterotoxin, 383, 384, 386
Enterovirus infection. *See also* Coxsackie virus; ECHO virus, and congenital infection; *specific enterovirus*
  and heart disease, 165
  and hemolytic-uremic syndrome, 243
  and hepatitis, in neonate, 215
  versus measles, 364
  meningitis (aseptic), 10, 12
  in neonate, 144
  versus Rocky Mountain spotted fever, 379
  versus rubella, 365
Enuresis, 88–92
  and sleep, 83, 84, 85
  and urinary tract infection, 249
Ependymoma, 352, 353
Epicanthic folds, in Down syndrome, 278
Epididymis
  in cystic fibrosis, 207
  and gonorrhea, 388, 390
Epidural hematoma, 32, 36–37
Epiglottitis, 13–14, 15
Epilepsy. *See* Seizures
Epinephrine
  in asthma, 202
    status asthmaticus, 16, 17
  in cardiopulmonary resuscitation, 3, 5
  in diabetes, 21
  and hypoglycemia, 266
  and neuroblastoma, 341, 344
Episcleritis, in Crohn disease, 227
Epispadias, 139, 156
Epsilon-aminocaproic acid (EACA), in hemophilia, 324
Epstein-Barr virus, 374
  and Burkitt lymphoma, 349
  and hepatitis, 215
  and infectious mononucleosis, 372, 373, 374
Ergotamine, in migraine, 95
Erysipelas, 380
Erythema marginatum, 180, 181
Erythema nodosum, in inflammatory bowel disease, 225
Erythroblastosis fetalis, 128–130
Erythrocyte protoporphyrin, 46, 47, 315, 316, 317
Escherichia coli (E. coli). See also Gramnegative bacilli
  and diarrhea, 384, 386
  and leukemia, 335
  and nephrotic syndrome, 245
  and septicemia, 6
    in neonate, 149
  in urinary tract infection, 249
Esophageal
  atresia, 136–137, 140
  varices, in cystic fibrosis, 207
Estrogen
  and gonadal dysgenesis, 98
  treatment for tall girls, 63, 64–65

Ethamsylate, and intraventricular hemorrhage, 153
Ethosuximide, in seizures, 286
Eustachian tube, 190, 192, 193, 194
Evans syndrome, 327
Ewing sarcoma, 354, 355
Exchange transfusion. *See* Transfusion, exchange
Exercise
  and asthma, 204
  and cardiac dysrhythmias, 160, 174
  and diabetes mellitus, 269, 270
  and heart failure, 19
  and hypertension, 186
  and myocarditis, 164
  urine abnormalities following, 235, 237
Expectorants, 191
  in asthma, 202
  in pneumonia, 199
Exstrophy of bladder, 139, 141
Extramembranous glomerulonephritis, 246, 248

Factors, clotting. *See* Clotting factors; *specific disorder*
Failure to thrive, 69–91. *See also* Growth; *specific cause*
Fanconi syndrome, and lead poisoning, 46
Fat
  in infant nutrition, 65
  malabsorption of, 220, 222–223
Fatty acids, and hyperbilirubinemia in neonate, 125
Fears, of preschoolers, 83
Febrile seizures, 43, 285, 287
Fecolith, and appendicitis, 25
Feingold diet, 80, 81, 82
Ferritin, 315, 316, 317
Fertility
  and cryptorchidism, 155, 156
  and cystic fibrosis, 207
  after death of infant, 57
  and immunosuppressives, 245
  and mumps, 365
  and pelvic inflammatory disease, 388
  and sickle cell disease, 321, 322
Fetal alcohol syndrome, 121, 280
  and ventricular septal defect, 170
Fetal hydantoin syndrome, 280
Fetal monitoring, 106
Fever, 42–45. *See also specific disorder*
  and seizures, 43, 285, 287
  of unknown origin, 43, 45
Fibrin split products, 243. *See also* Disseminated intravascular coagulation
Fibrosarcoma, 354
Firearms, 39
Fisting, persistent, in cerebral palsy, 294

Fitz-Hugh-Curtis syndrome, 388, 390
Fluoride, 68. *See also* Minerals, in infant nutrition
Focal segmental glomerular sclerosis, 245, 248, 254
Folate deficiency
  and heart disease, 20
  in prematures, 131, 133
Folic acid. *See* Folate deficiency
Fontanelle
  in hydrocephalus, 292
  in hypothyroidism, 262
  and increased intracranial pressure, 32
  in meningitis, 10
Food poisoning, and acute abdomen, 25
Foramen ovale, 175
Foreign body, 14, 15, 202
Formula, in infant nutrition, 66, 68, 133. *See also* Milk, cow
Fragile-X syndrome, 78, 281
Free erythrocyte protoporphyrin (FEP), 46, 47, 315, 316, 317
Fresh-frozen plasma
  in bleeding neonate, 151, 152
  in neonatal sepsis, 150
Friction rub, in pericarditis, 164
Friedreich ataxia, as cause of myocardiopathy, 164
Fructose intolerance, 174, 175
Funerals, 54
Fungus. *See also specific fungus*
  and cell-mediated immunity, 359
  in immunosuppressive host, 254
  and leukemia, 335
  and meningitis, 10
Furosemide. *See also* Diuretics
  in acute poststreptococcal glomerulonephritis, 241
  in acute renal failure, 28
  in heart failure, in neonate, 117
  in increased intracranial pressure, 22
  and patent ductus arteriosus, 178–179

Galactosemia, 118, 274–275, 276–277
Gall bladder, 215
Gallop rhythm, 19
Gallstones
  in Crohn disease, 227, 229
  and recurrent abdominal pain, 92
  in sickle cell disease, 321
Gamma globulin. *See* Human immune serume globulin (HISG); Immunoglobulin(s)
Ganglion cells
  in Hirschsprung disease, 128
  in neuroblastoma, 341, 344
Ganglioneuroblastoma, 341
Ganglioneuroma, 341
Gangliosidosis, 275
Gastric bypass, for obesity, 72, 74

Gastroesophageal reflux. *See* Reflux, gastroesophageal
Gastroschisis, 137–138, 140
Gender identity, 98, 99, 100
Genetic counseling, 280. *See also specific disorder*
Genetics, 279. *See also specific disorder*
Genital organs, external
   in adrenal hyperplasia, 98, 259, 260, 261, 262
   and sexual differentiation, 97–98
German measles. *See* Rubella
Gestational age
   assessment of, 105, 106
   and bilirubin-binding capacity, 126
   and incidence of hypoglycemia, 120
   and outcome, 110
   small for. *See* Intrauterine growth, retardation
Gianotti-Crosti syndrome, 217
Giardia lamblia, 219, 221, 223
Glaucoma, in congenital rubella syndrome, 365
Glioblastoma multiforme, 352
Glioma, brainstem, 352, 353
Glomerulonephritis, 239–241
   acute poststreptococcal, 239–241
   chronic, 248. *See also specific disorder*
   and chronic renal failure, 252
   in endocarditis, 167, 169, 240
   in Henoch-Schönlein syndrome, 329, 330
   and hepatitis B, 216, 217
   hereditary. *See* Alport syndrome
   membranoproliferative, 240, 245, 248, 252, 254, 308
   membranous, 246, 248, 308
   mesangial proliferative, 246, 248
   mesangiocapillary. *See* membranoproliferative
   postinfectious, 240
   rapidly progressive, 27
   in systemic lupus erythematosus, 305, 306, 308
   and Wilms tumor, 338
Glomerulopathy, membranous, 246, 248, 308
Glomerulosclerosis, focal, segmental, 245, 248, 254
Glucagon, 21
Glucocorticoids, 308. *See also* Adrenal hyperplasia, congenital; *specific therapeutic indication*
Glucose 6-phosphate dehydrogenase (G-6-PD) deficiency, as cause of neonatal hyperbilirubinemia, 125
Glucuronyl transferase, 124, 125, 126
Gluten enteropathy. *See* Celiac disease
Glycerol, in increased intracranial pressure, 32, 34

Glycogen storage diseases, 274, 276
   and hypoglycemia, 118, 267, 276
   as cause of myocardiopathy, 164
Glycosylated hemoglobin, 270, 271
Goiter, 263, 264, 265
Gold salts
   as a cause of acute renal failure, 27
   in juvenile rheumatoid arthritis, 302, 305
Gonadal
   agenesis, 98
   dysgenesis, 62, 98, 100, 280
Gonadotropins, 99
Gonococcus. See *Neisseria gonorrhoeae*
Gonorrhea, 387–390. *See also* Pelvic inflammatory disease (PID); *specific agent*
G-6-PD deficiency, and neonatal hyperbilirubinemia, 125
Gram stain, 11. *See also specific infection; specific organism*
Gram-negative bacilli. *See also specific organism*
   and leukemia, 335
   and pericarditis, 164
   and septic arthritis, 370, 372
   and septicemia, 6
   in neonate, 6, 147, 148
Granulocytopenia. *See* Neutropenia
Granulomas, in Crohn disease, 228
Granulosa cell tumor, and precocious pseudopuberty, 99
Graves disease, 263, 265
Grief, parental, 52–53, 54
   and Down syndrome, 51, 279, 280
   and leukemia, 336
   and mental retardation, 55
   and sudden infant death syndrome, 52, 54, 56, 57
Group A beta-hemolytic *Streptococcus.* See *Streptococcus,* group A beta-hemolytic
Group B *Streptococcus.* See *Streptococcus,* group B
Growth, 61–65. *See also* Failure to thrive; *specific disorder*
Growth hormone
   in adrenal hyperplasia, 262
   deficiency
      and hypoglycemia, 267
      and pituitary tumor, 63, 351
   in diabetes, 21
   in disorders of growth, 62–63, 64, 65
   in obesity, 71
Guanidines, as uremic toxins, 253
Guillain-Barré syndrome, versus polymyositis, 310
Gynecomastia
   and chest pain, 95
   in Klinefelter syndrome, 98

Habilitation
  in cerebral palsy, 296
  of handicapped child, 76
Haemophilus influenzae, 8
  antibiotics against, 8
  bacteremia/septicemia, 6, 7, 8
  in cystic fibrosis, 205
  in epiglottitis, 14
  in meningitis, 9, 10, 11, 12
  in otitis media, 192
  in pericarditis, 164, 166
  in pneumonia, 198, 200
  in septic arthritis, 370, 372
  in sickle cell disease, 320
Haemophilus influenzae vaccine, 7,
    10–11, 365
Hamartoma, and gonadotropin prod-
    uction, 99
Hand-foot syndrome, in sickle cell dis-
    ease, 319, 321
Hashimoto thyroiditis, 263, 265
Haversian canal, and osteomyelitis,
    369
HCG. *See* Human chorionic gonadotropin
    (HCG), and cryptorchidism
Head trauma, 36–38
  and increased intracranial pressure,
    32, 33–34, 37
  and seizures, 34, 37, 38
Headache, 92, 94–95, 96–97. *See also re-
    lated disorder; specific cause*
Hearing, 75, 77
Hearing loss, 77
  versus attention deficit disorder, 79
  in cerebral palsy, 295
  in congenital rubella syndrome, 142,
    365
  and cytomegalovirus, 142, 145
  and hereditary nephritis. *See* Alport
    syndrome
  in kernicterus, 126, 295
  and meningitis, 10, 12
  and mumps, 365
  and otitis media, 192, 193, 194
  and toxoplasmosis, 141, 142
Heart
  attack. *See* Myocardial infarction, in
    systemic lupus erythematosus
  block, 159, 160, 161, 162, 307, 309
  dysrhythmias. *See* Cardiac
    dysrhythmias
  failure, 19–21. *See also related disor-
    der; specific cause*
    in neonate, 116–118. *See also related
      disorder; specific cause*
  surgery. *See also specific disorder;
    specific procedure*
    cardiac dysrhythmias following, 159,
      160, 161, 162. *See also specific
      disorder*

  and endocarditis, 167, 168, 169
  postpericardiotomy syndrome, 164,
    166
  and renal failure, 28
  transplantation, 19, 21
Heimlich maneuver, 15
Hemarthrosis, in hemophilia, 323–324,
    325
Hematuria, 235–238. *See also specific
    disorder*
Hemihypertrophy, and Wilms tumor,
    338, 340
Hemiplegia
  in cerebral palsy, 294
  in sickle cell disease, 321
Hemolytic-uremic syndrome, 241–244
  as cause of acute renal failure, 27
  as cause of chronic renal failure, 252
Hemophilia, 150–151, 153, 323–325
  and hepatitis B, 219
Hemophilia B, 150–151, 323
Hemoptysis, 198, 206, 209
Hemorrhage. *See* Bleeding; *specific bleed-
    ing disorder*
Hemorrhages, splinter, in endocarditis,
    167
Hemorrhagic disease of newborn, 151,
    153
Hemotympanum, and basilar skull frac-
    ture, 36
Henoch-Schönlein syndrome, 328–331
  and acute abdominal pain, 25
  versus acute poststreptococcal glomer-
    ulonephritis, 240, 329
  and chronic renal failure, 252, 330
  versus rheumatic fever, 179, 329
Heparin
  in disseminated intravascular coagu-
    lation, 7, 9, 152
  in hemolytic-uremic syndrome, 242,
    244
Hepatic failure. *See* Liver, failure
Hepatitis, 215–218
  and glomerulonephritis, 248
  and hemophilia, 325
  and infectious mononucleosis, 215, 216,
    372
  and isoniazid/rifampin, 376, 377
  neonatal, 213–215
    and bleeding, 151
    and congenital infections, 365
    and hyperbilirubinemia, 125
  versus Reye syndrome, 29, 215
  and thrombocytopenic purpura, 326
Hepatitis B immune globulin (HBIG),
    217, 218
Hepatitis B vaccine, 146, 217, 218, 366
Hepatoblastoma, and gonadotropin pro-
    duction, 99
Hepatocellular carcinoma, 216

Heredity. *See* Genetics

Hermaphroditism, 98, 100

Hernia
diaphragmatic, 138–139, 140
inguinal, 24, 156
umbilical, 156
in hypothyroidism, 262

Heroin, maternal addiction to
and incidence of respiratory distress
syndrome, 107, 109
and withdrawal, in neonate, 119–123

Herpes simplex
and chronic renal failure, 254
in neonate, 142–143, 145, 215

Herpes zoster. *See also* Varicella
and abdominal pain, 25
and chronic renal failure, 254
and Hodgkin disease, 346, 348
and leukemia, 336
in neonate, 145

Herpesvirus(es). *See* Cytomegalovirus;
Epstein-Barr virus; Herpes simplex; Herpes zoster

Heterophile antibodies, 372, 373, 374

Hexosaminidase A, 275

Hip click. *See* Ortolani procedure

Hirschsprung disease, 24, 87, 88, 138, 140

Histiocytoses, 346, 350

Histocompatibility antigens (HLA), 307
in diabetes mellitus, 269
in juvenile rheumatoid arthritis, 301
and renal transplantation, 254
in systemic lupus erythematosus, 307
in ulcerative colitis, 225

HLA. *See* Histocompatibility antigens
(HLA)

Hodgkin disease, 345–348

Holter monitor, 161

Holt-Oram syndrome, 170

Homosexuality, and hepatitis B, 217

Homovanillic acid (HVA), in neuroblastoma, 342

Horner syndrome, in neuroblastoma, 342

Hospital-acquired infection
hepatitis, 218
and isolation, 338
respiratory syncytial virus, 197
Salmonella, 386

Human chorionic gonadotropin (HCG),
and cryptorchidism, 155, 156

Human immune serum globulin (HISG),
218, 360, 361
in hepatitis, 217
in idiopathic thrombocytopenic purpura, 326, 328

Human milk. *See* Milk, human

Hurler syndrome, as a cause of myocardiopathy, 164

Hutchinson teeth, in congenital syphilis,
143

HVA. *See* Homovanillic acid (HVA), in
neuroblastoma

Hyaline membrane disease. *See* Respiratory distress syndrome

Hydantoin. *See* Phenytoin

Hydralazine
in heart failure, 20
in hypertension, 183, 184
and systemic lupus erythematosus, 307

Hydrocarbon pneumonia, 201

Hydrocephalus, 291–294
and brain tumors, 352
and congenital toxoplasmosis, 141
and increased intracranial pressure, 32
and intraventricular hemorrhage, 152
and meningitis, 10
and precocious puberty, 99
and seizures, 122
in spinal dysraphism, 289, 291

Hydronephrosis. *See also* Urinary tract,
obstruction of
in Crohn disease, 227, 229
and hematuria, 235
and recurrent abdominal pain, 92
versus Wilms tumor, 339

Hydrops fetalis, 128, 129

Hydroxychloroquine. *See* Antimalarial
drugs, in systemic lupus
erythematosus

Hydroxylase deficiency. *See* Adrenal hyperplasia, congenital

17-Hydroxyprogesterone, 259, 260, 261

3-Hydroxysteroid dehydrogenase, 260

Hyperactivity. *See also* Attention deficit
disorder
and cow milk intolerance, 67
and lead poisoning, 46

Hyperalimentation. *See* Nutrition,
parenteral

Hyperbilirubinemia, in neonate,
124–128. *See also related disorder*

Hypercalcemia
in non-Hodgkin lymphoma, 349
in Williams syndrome, 280

Hypercalciuria, and hematuria, 238

Hyperglycemia. *See also* Diabetes
mellitus
from diazoxide, 184
in hypernatremic dehydration, 233
and methylprednisolone, 34
post-hypoglycemia. *See* Somogyi effect

Hyperkalemia
in acute renal failure, 27
in adrenal hyperplasia, 259
in cardiopulmonary arrest, 3, 4
in chronic renal failure, 253
in non-Hodgkin lymphoma, 349

Hyperlipidemia
and abdominal pain, 25
and diabetic ketoacidosis, 21

and obesity, 71
and renal failure, 255
Hypernatremia, 234
    and dehydration, 233–235
    and seizures, in neonate, 122
Hyperoxia test, 113, 115
Hypersensitivity, delayed. See Delayed
        hypersensitivity
Hypersensitivity pneumonitis, 201
Hypertension, 182–186. See also specific
        disorder
Hyperthyroidism, 263–264, 265–266
    versus attention deficit disorder, 79
    as cause of heart failure in neonate,
        116
    as cause of myocardiopathy, 163
Hyperventilation, in increased intra-
        cranial pressure, 32, 34
Hypnagogic hallucinations, 83
Hypnosis, and enuresis, 90, 92
Hypoalbuminemia. See Hypoproteinemia
Hypocalcemia. See also Calcium
    in chronic renal failure, 253
    in hypernatremic dehydration, 233,
        235
    in neonate, 119, 120–121
        with disseminated intravascular co-
            agulation, 152
        and hypoglycemia, 118, 267
        with respiratory distress syndrome,
            108
Hypogammaglobulinemia, 361
    and congenital rubella, 142
Hypoglycemia, 266–269. See also specific
        disorder
    in neonate, 118–119, 120, 123,
        266–267, 268. See also related dis-
        order; specific cause
Hypokalemia
    in cystic fibrosis, 207
    in diabetic ketoacidosis, 22
    in hypernatremic dehydration, 233,
        235
    in ulcerative colitis, 226
Hypomagnesemia. See Magnesium
Hyponatremia
    and adrenal hyperplasia, 259
    in diabetic ketoacidosis, 23
    and feedings, 131
    in meningitis, 10
    in Rocky Mountain spotted fever, 379
    and seizures, in neonate, 122
Hypoparathyroidism. See Parathyroid
        gland
Hypopituitarism. See Pituitary gland
Hypoplastic left heart syndrome, 20, 114,
        116, 118, 178
Hypoproteinemia
    in cystic fibrosis, 207
    in malabsorption, 220

    in neonate
        with biliary atresia/neonatal hepa-
            titis, 214
        with erythroblastosis, 128
    and nephrotic syndrome, 244
    in ulcerative colitis, 226
Hypospadias, 98, 154, 156
Hypothermia, therapeutic, in increased
        intracranial pressure, 31, 32, 34
Hypothyroidism, 262–263, 264–265
    and cardiac dysrhythmia, 159
    and encopresis, 87
    and growth retardation, 62
    and hyperbilirubinemia, in neonate,
        125
    as cause of myocardiopathy, 163, 165
    and obesity, 72
    after treatment of Hodgkin disease,
        346
Hypsarrhythmia, 286, 288

Ibuprofen, in juvenile rheumatoid ar-
        thritis, 302, 304
Icterus. See Hyperbilirubinemia, in
        neonate
Idiopathic thrombocytopenic purpura.
        See Thrombocytopenic purpura, id-
        iopathic (ITP)
Ileal atresia, 24, 137, 140
Illness, child's concept of, 77
Imipramine
    in enuresis, 89, 91
    in narcolepsy, 83
Immotile cilia syndrome, 201
Immune deficiency, 359–362
    acquired. See Acquired immune
        deficiency syndrome (AIDS)
    and malabsorption, 221, 223
    and polio vaccine, 360, 362, 364
    and recurrent pneumonia, 200, 201
    and septicemia, 6
    severe combined, 221, 362
Immunoglobulin(s), 359, 360, 361. See
        also Human immune serum glob-
        ulin (HISG)
    hyperimmune
        hepatitis B, 217, 218
        pertusis, 364
        RhoGAM, 128, 130
        tetanus, 363, 366
        varicella-zoster, 245
    IgA
        deficiency, and malabsorption, 221,
            223
        and Henoch-Schönlein syndrome,
            329, 331
        nephropathy (Berger disease), 236,
            238, 254, 331
        and polio vaccine, 364
        and tonsils, 189

Immunoglobulin(s)—*Continued*
  IgE
    in asthma versus bronchiolitis, 196,
      197, 202
    and recurrent infections, 362
  IgG, and cystic fibrosis, 208
  IgM, in congenital infections, 141, 144
Immunization, 362–369. *See also specific*
    disease; specific organism
Immunosuppressive drugs. *See also*
    specific drug
  and cancer, 245, 345
  in chronic thrombocytopenic purpura,
    326, 328
  in Crohn disease, 229
  in nephrotic syndrome, 245, 247–248
  and renal transplantation, 254, 256
  in systemic lupus erythematosus, 306,
    308, 309
  in ulcerative colitis, 225
Immunotherapy, in asthma, 205
Imperforate anus, 136, 137
Impetigo, 381, 383
  bullous, 381
Imuran. *See* Azathioprine
Inborn errors of metabolism, 273–277
Incontinence
  of feces
    in anal atresia, 137
    in spinal dysraphism, 289, 291
  of urine
    versus enuresis, 88, 89
    in exstrophy of bladder, 141
    in spinal dysraphism, 289
Increased intracranial pressure, 31–34.
    See also Cerebral edema; *specific*
    disorder
Indomethacin. *See also* Anti-
    inflammatory drugs
  and acute renal failure, 27
  and arthritis, 302, 304
  and ductus arteriosus, 178, 179
Infant of diabetic mother
  and hypoglycemia, 266
  and respiratory distress syndrome, 107
Infantile spasms, 286, 288
Infection(s). *See also specific infection*
  congenital, 141–146
    and heart disease, 165
    and neonatal hepatitis, 213
  recurrent, 359, 360, 362
Infectious mononucleosis, 372–374
  and hepatitis, 215
  versus Hodgkin disease, 345
  and myocarditis, 163
  and thrombocytopenic purpura, 326,
    327, 373
Infertility. *See* Fertility
Inflammatory bowel disease, 224–230.
    See also specific disorder

and growth retardation, 62–64
  and malabsorption, 221, 223
Influenza, 365, 366, 369
  as cause of myocarditis, 163
  and pneumonia, 199, 200
Influenza B, and Reye syndrome, 29, 30,
    365
Influenza vaccine, 365, 366
Ingestion(s), 39, 40, 42. *See also specific*
    toxic agent
  versus child abuse, 49
INH. *See* Isoniazid (INH)
Injury control, 39, 40
Insulin
  in chronic renal failure, 253
  in cystic fibrosis, 206–207
  in diabetes mellitus, 269, 270, 271,
    272, 273
  in diabetic ketoacidosis, 21, 22, 23
  in erythroblastosis, 130
  and hypoglycemia, 267, 268
    in neonate, 118, 119, 120, 266, 267
  and obesity, 71, 74
Intercourse, and urinary tract infection,
    249
Interferon, and upper respiratory tract
    infection, 191
Interstitial nephritis, 27, 250
Intestinal. *See also specific disorder*
  atresia, 24, 137, 140
  disease, and parenteral nutrition, 132,
    135, 137, 138, 228
  lymphangiectasia, 165, 220
  malrotation, 24, 138, 139
  strictures
    in Crohn disease, 228
    in necrotizing enterocolitis, 134
Intracranial
  calcifications, 141, 142
  hemorrhage. *See* Bleeding, intracranial
  pressure, increased. *See* Increased in-
    tracranial pressure
Intrauterine growth, 61
  retardation, 107
    and congenital infections, 141, 143
    and hypoglycemia, 120, 267
    and maternal addiction, 120
    and persistence of fetal circulation,
      113
    and postnatal growth (primordial
      dwarfism), 62, 64
Intrauterine transfusion, 129
Intravenous alimentation, *See* Nutrition,
    parenteral
Intussusception, 24, 26
  in cystic fibrosis, 206, 209
  in Henoch-Schönlein syndrome, 329,
    330
Ipecac, and supraventricular tachycardia,
    159

Iridocyclitis, 227, 301, 303, 304
Iron
    deficiency of, 315–319
        and celiac disease, 222
        and gastrointestinal effects, 221, 223
        and heart disease, 20
        and lead poisoning, 46
    in nutrition
        in neonates and infants, 65–66, 68
        in prematures, 131, 133
Irradiation. *See also specific indication*
    mediastinal, and constrictive peri-
        carditis, 167
    as teratogen, 277, 278, 279
Irritable bowel syndrome, 92, 219, 221,
    224
Islet (of Langerhans) cell. *See also*
        Insulin
    adenoma of, 120, 267
    transplantation, in diabetes mellitus,
        270, 272
Isolation, 338
Isoniazid (INH)
    and lupuslike syndrome, 307
    in tuberculosis, 376, 377
Isoproterenol
    in asthma, 202
        in status asthmaticus, 17, 18
    in cardiopulmonary resuscitation, 4
    in septic shock, 7
ITP. *See* Thrombocytopenic purpura, id-
        iopathic (ITP)

Janeway lesions, in endocarditis, 167
Jatene procedure, for transposition of
        great arteries, 176
Jaundice. *See* Hyperbilirubinemia, in
        neonate
Jejunal atresia, 24, 137, 140
Jejunoileal bypass, in obesity, 72, 74
Job syndrome, 362
Jones criteria, in rheumatic fever, 180,
        181
JRA. *See* Arthritis, juvenile rheumatoid
        (JRA)

Kasai procedure, in biliary atresia, 213,
        214
Kawasaki disease, 310, 312
Kell antigen, and erythroblastosis, 128
Keratitis, interstitial, in congenital syph-
        ilis, 143
Keratoconjunctivitis, herpetic, in neo-
        nate, 143
Keratopathy, band, in chronic renal fail-
        ure, 252
Kernicterus, 108, 124, 126–127
    and cerebral palsy, 124, 295
    and erythroblastosis, 129
Kernig sign, in meningitis, 10

Ketoacidosis, diabetic. *See* Diabetic
        ketoacidosis
Ketogenic diet, and seizures, 288
17-Ketosteroids, in adrenal hyperplasia,
        259
Ketotic hyperglycinemia, and neonatal
        seizures, 122
Ketotic hypoglycemia, 267, 268–269
Kidney(s). *See also* Urinary tract; *specific
        disorder; specific renal entry*
    hypoplastic-dysplastic, 237, 252
    polycystic, 235, 237
    transplantation of, 248, 252, 253, 254,
        255, 256. *See also specific disorder;
        specific indication*
    tumors of, 338–341
Klebsiella. See also Gram-negative bacilli
    in septicemia, 6
    in urinary tract infection, 249
Klinefelter syndrome, 98, 100, 280
Kool-Aid, composition of, 387
Koplik spots, in measles, 364

Lactase deficiency, 69
    after diarrhea, 66
    and malabsorption, 219, 220
    and phototherapy, 127
    in premature infant, 131
    and recurrent abdominal pain, 92–93,
        96
Lactic dehydrogenase, urinary, in uri-
        nary tract infection, 249
Lactobacillus, in bowel flora, breast- ver-
        sus bottle feeding, 66
Lactose
    and calcium absorption, 131
    intolerance of. *See* Lactase deficiency
    in milk, 65
Language, 74, 75, 77
    and chronic otitis, 193, 194
Laryngomalacia, 13, 15
Lasix. *See* Furosemide
Latex agglutination antigen detection
        tests, 6, 10, 11
Laxatives, 86, 87
Lazarus syndrome, 53
Lead poisoning, 45–48
    and attention deficit disorder, 46, 48,
        79
    versus brain tumor, 351
    and increased intracranial pressure, 32
    versus iron deficiency, 315
    as cause of nephritis, 250
Learning problems, 79–82. *See also asso-
        ciated disorder*
Leg
    pain. *See* Bone pain
    ulcers, in sickle cell disease, 320
Legionella pneumophila, 199, 201
Lens. *See* Cataracts

Leukemia, 335–338
  in Down syndrome, 278
  as cause of fever of unknown origin
    (FUO), 43
  versus idiopathic thrombocytopenic
    purpura, 326, 327
  versus infectious mononucleosis, 373
  in non-Hodgkin lymphoma, 348, 349,
    350
  versus rheumatic fever, 179
  in Wilms tumor, 341
Leukopenia, in systemic lupus eryth-
    ematosus, 305, 308
Levamisole, in upper respiratory tract
    infection, 191
Levodopa
  in cerebral palsy, 295
  and growth hormone, 64
Leydig cell tumor, and precocious pseu-
    dopuberty, 99
Lidocaine, in cardiac dysrhythmias, 160
Limb pain. See Bone pain
Limulus lysate test, for endotoxin, 6, 10
Lipoid nephrosis. See Nephrotic
    syndrome
Lipoma, and spina bifida occulta, 289
Lipoprotein-X, 213, 214
Listeria, in neonate, 148
Liver. See also specific disorder
  failure
    and acetaminophen, 44
    in biliary atresia, 214
    in hepatitis, 215
    and myoclonic seizures, 286
    and Reye syndrome, 30
  and parenteral nutrition, 132, 133, 213
  and salicylate, 304
  transplantation of, 213, 215
  tumor
    and gonadotropin production, 99
    and hepatitis B, 216
Lockjaw. See Tetanus
Lomotil. See Diphenoxylate, in diarrhea
Ludwig angina, 15
Lumbar puncture, 11. See also Cere-
    brospinal fluid
  contraindicated, with increased intra-
    cranial pressure, 32
  meningitis after, in child with bacte-
    remia, 8
  in neonate, 150
Lung(s), hypoplasia in, and diaphrag-
    matic hernia, 140. See also specific
    disorder; specific pulmonary entry
Luteinizing hormone-releasing hormone,
    and cryptorchidism, 155, 156
Lymphadenopathy, causes of, 346, 350,
    374. See also specific disorder
Lymphangiectasia, intestinal, 165, 220
Lymphangiography, in Hodgkin disease,
    346, 347

Lymphocyte(s)
  atypical
    in hepatitis, 216
    in infectious mononucleosis, 372,
      373, 374
  in immune system, 359, 360
  in pertussis, 363
  reduced number in intestinal lymph-
    angiectasia, 220
Lymphoid hyperplasia, obstruction of Eu-
    stachian tube, 192
Lymphoma
  Burkitt, 349, 350
  Hodgkin, 345–348
  non-Hodgkin, 348–350
    and bone, 354
    and renal failure, 28
Lysosomal storage diseases, 275, 277

Magnesium
  in neonate, 119, 120, 121
  as toxin in chronic renal failure, 253
Malabsorption, 218–223. See also specific
    disorder; specific nutrient
Malformation syndromes, 277–281
Malrotation, 24, 138, 139
Maltsupex, 86
Mannitol
  in acute renal failure, 28
  and increased intracranial pressure, 32
    in Reye syndrome, 31
Manometrics, and constipation, 87, 88
Maple syrup urine disease, 121, 273, 276
Mastoiditis, 192, 194
Mathematical skills, 77
Maturation, sexual. See Puberty
MCV. See Mean corpuscular volume
    (MCV)
Mean corpuscular volume (MCV), 315,
    316, 317
Measles, 364, 367, 368
  versus Hodgkin disease, 345
  as cause of myocarditis, 163
  and pneumonia, 199
  and thrombocytopenic purpura, 326
Measles vaccine, 364–365, 367–368
Meckel diverticulum, 24, 92
Meconium ileus
  in neonate, 24, 138, 140, 206
    and hyperbilirubinemia, 125
  in older child, 209
Meconium plug, 206
Mediastinum
  air in. See Pneumomediastinum
  in Hodgkin disease, 346
  irradiation, and pericarditis, 167
  mass in
    in neuroblastoma, 342
    in non-Hodgkin lymphoma, 348, 349,
      350
    in T cell leukemia, 336, 348

Medical students, and spelling ability, 82
Medium-chain triglycerides, 131, 132, 133
Medullary cystic disease, 252
Medulloblastoma, 351–352, 353
Megacolon, 86
  aganglionic. See Hirschsprung disease
  congenital. See Hirschsprung disease
  toxic, 224–225, 226, 228, 229
Membranoproliferative glomeru-
      lonephritis. See Glomeru-
      lonephritis, membranoproliferative
Membranous glomerulopathy, 246, 248, 308
Menarche, 99. See also Puberty
Meningioma, 352, 353
Meningitis, 9–12
  and head trauma, 36–37
  and hydrocephalus, 292
  and increased intracranial pressure, 32
  due to mumps, 368
  in neonate, 123, 147, 148, 149
    and seizures, 122
  and pericarditis, 164
  and septicemia, 8
  in sickle cell disease, 320, 321–322
  in spinal dysraphism, 289, 290
  and status epilepticus, 35
  tuberculous, 375, 377
Meningocele. See Spinal dysraphism
Meningococcal vaccine, 365, 369
Meningococcus. See Neisseria
      meningitidis
Meningoencephalitis
  in congenital herpes, 143
  in mumps, 368
Meningomyelocele. See Spinal
      dysraphism
Mental retardation, 75–76, 77–78. See
      also specific cause
Mercury, as nephrotoxin, 27, 250
Mesangial proliferative glomeru-
      lonephritis, 246, 248
Mesangiocapillary glomerulonephritis.
      See Glomerulonephritis,
      membranoproliferative
Mesenteric lymphadenitis, 25, 26
Metabolic disorders, 273–277. See also
      specific disorder
Metanephrines, in neuroblastoma, 342
Metaproterenol, and asthma, 17. See also
      Beta-adrenergic, agonists, in
      asthma
Methadone, maternal addiction, and
      withdrawal of neonate, 119, 121,
      122, 123
Methemoglobinemia, as cause of cy-
      anosis, 113
Methimazole, in thyroid disease, 263
Methotrexate
  in leukemia, 335, 338

  in non-Hodgkin lymphoma, 349
  in osteogenic sarcoma, 354
Methoxamine, in tetralogy of Fallot, 173
Methyldopa, in hypertension, 183
Methylphenidate
  in attention deficit disorder, 79, 80, 81
  in narcolepsy, 83
Methylxanthines, in asthma, 202
Metrizamide, 136, 289
Microcephaly, and congenital infections,
      141, 365
Microphthalmia, in congenital rubella
      syndrome, 365
MIF. See Müllerian inhibiting factor (MIF)
Migraine, 94–95, 96–97
Miliaria, versus measles, 364
Miliary tuberculosis, 375, 377, 378
Milk
  breast. See human
  cow
    versus human, 131, 133
    intolerance, 66, 67, 68–69, 220, 222
    and iron, 66, 69, 316, 318
    stools, 86
  human
    versus cow, 131, 133
    drug transfer in, 68
    and hyperbilirubinemia, 125, 126
    and hypoproteinemia, in cystic
        fibrosis, 207
    and iron absorption, 66, 68, 316, 318
    and necrotizing enterocolitis, 134,
        135
    and septicemia in neonate, 66
  soy-based, 68
Mineral oil, 87, 88
Mineralocorticoids, in adrenal hyper-
      plasia, 259, 260
Minerals, in infant nutrition, 65, 67, 68,
      131, 133. See also specific mineral
Minimal brain dysfunction. See Atten-
      tion deficit disorder
Minimal cerebral dysfunction. See Atten-
      tion deficit disorder
Minimal change nephrotic syndrome,
      237, 244–245, 246, 247–248
Minoxidil, in hypertension, 184, 186
Mist therapy, 196, 197, 199
Mitral valve
  atresia, 116
  cleft, 171
  prolapse
    and chest pain, 95
    and endocarditis, 169
    and heart failure, 19
Mixed connective tissue disease,
      310–311, 312
Mom, my, 191, 387
Mongolism. See Down Syndrome
MOPP therapy, in Hodgkin disease, 346,
      347

Moro reflex, 105, 294
Morphea, 310
Morphine, for spells, in tetralogy of
    Fallot, 173
Mortality. *See also specific disorder*
    accidents, as most common cause in
        children beyond neonatal period,
        39
    malformations, as most common cause
        in full-term neonates during neo-
        natal period, 277
    respiratory distress syndrome, as most
        common cause in premature in-
        fants, 107
    sudden infant death syndrome, as most
        common cause between age 1
        month and 1 year, 55
Mother-infant bonding. *See* Bonding
Motor vehicle accidents, 39, 40, 41
Mottling, in hypothyroidism, 262
Mourning, 52–53, 54. *See also* Grief,
    parental
Mouth. *See* Oral
Mucocutaneous candidiasis, 360, 362
Mucocutaneous lymph node syndrome.
    See Kawasaki disease
Mucolipidoses, 275, 277
Mucopolysaccharidoses, 275, 277
    as cause of myocardiopathy, 164
Mucus
    in cystic fibrosis, 205
    plugging by, in asthma, 203
Mulberry molars, in congenital syphilis,
    143
Mulibrey nanism, 165, 167
Müllerian inhibiting factor (MIF), 97
Mumps, 365, 366, 368
    and diabetes mellitus, 269, 271
    meningitis, 10, 368
    as cause of myocarditis, 163
    skin test, 362, 368
    and thrombocytopenic purpura, 326
Mumps vaccine, 366, 368
Muscle
    pain
        in influenza, 365
        in Rocky Mountain spotted fever,
            378, 380
        in typhoid fever, 384
    relaxants, 4
Muscular dystrophy
    versus dermatomyositis/polymyositis,
        310
    as cause of myocardiopathy, 163–164
Mustard procedure, in transposition of
    great arteries, 176, 177
Mycobacteria, atypical, 376, 377
Mycobacterium tuberculosis, 375. *See also*
    Tuberculosis
Mycoplasma pneumoniae, 200

as cause of otitis media, 192, 194
    as cause of pharyngitis, 382
    as cause of pneumonia, 198, 199, 200
Myectomy, in Hirschsprung disease, 138
Myelodysplasia. *See* Spinal dysraphism
Myelomeningocele. *See* Spinal
    dysraphism
Myocardial infarction, in systemic lupus
    erythematosus, 307
Myocardiopathy, 21, 165
    and dysrhythmias, 160
    and heart failure, 19
    versus myocarditis, 163–164, 165
Myocarditis, 163–164, 165
    in congenital rubella, 142
    and dysrhythmias, 159, 160, 161
    and heart failure, 19, 20
    in rheumatic fever, 179, 180, 182
    in rheumatoid arthritis, 301, 304, 305
    in Rocky Mountain spotted fever, 378,
        380
Myoclonic seizures, 286
Myoglobin, and iron, 315
Myringotomy, in otitis media, 192
Mysoline. *See* Primidone, in seizure
    disorders

Naloxone, 5, 9
Narcolepsy, 83, 84
Narcotic addiction, and withdrawal in
    neonate, 119, 121, 122, 123
Nasopharyngeal ulcers, in systemic lu-
    pus erythematosus, 305
Nasopharyngitis, streptococcal, 380, 382
NEC. *See* Necrotizing enterocolitis
    (NEC)
Neck
    stiff. *See* Nuchal rigidity
    webbed, in gonadal dysgenesis, 98
Necrotizing enterocolitis (NEC), 134–136
    as cause of acute abdomen, 24
    and disseminated intravascular coagu-
        lation, 134–135, 151, 152
    and feeding, 132
Neisseria gonorrhoeae, 387. *See also*
    Gonorrhea
    in septic arthritis, 370, 372
    in septicemia, 6
Neisseria meningitidis, 8
    in meningitis, 9, 10
    in pericarditis, 164
    in septicemia, 6, 7, 8–9
        versus Rocky Mountain spotted fe-
            ver, 379
Neisseria meningitidis vaccine, 7, 10–11,
    365, 369
Neonatal hepatitis. *See* Hepatitis,
    neonatal
Nephritis, interstitial, 250. *See also*
    Glomerulonephritis

Nephroblastoma. *See* Wilms tumor
Nephrocalcinosis, as cause of interstitial nephritis, 250
Nephrosis. *See* Nephrotic syndrome
Nephrotic syndrome, 237, 244–248
  and Henoch-Schönlein syndrome, 329
  in systemic lupus erythematosus, 305
Nesidioblastosis, and hypoglycemia, 268
Neural tube. *See* Spinal dysraphism
Neuroblastoma, 341–345
  versus Ewing sarcoma, 354
  versus Wilms tumor, 339
Neurocutaneous syndromes, and brain tumors, 352
Neurofibromatosis, 353
  and brain tumors, 352, 353
  and infantile spasms, 286
Neurogenic bladder, and urinary tract infection, 249, 250
Neurologic signs, soft, 79, 81
Neutropenia, 361
  in leukemia, 335, 337
  in necrotizing enterocolitis, 136
  and septicemia, 6, 335, 337
    in neonate, 147, 150
  in Shwachman syndrome, 220
Neutrophil
  dysfunction of, 361
  normal number, 361
    in neonate, 149
  reduced. *See* Neutropenia
  transfusions, in neonatal sepsis, 148, 150
Night terrors, 83, 84
Night waking, 82–83, 84
Nightmares, 83, 84, 85
Nitrogen mustard. *See* Chlorambucil; Cyclophosphamide; MOPP therapy, in Hodgkin disease
Nitroprusside, 20, 184, 186
Nocardia, and renal transplantation, 254
Nodules
  subcutaneous
    in neuroblastoma, 342
    in polyarteritis nodosa, 310
    in rheumatic fever, 180
  thyroid, 264, 266
Non-Hodgkin lymphoma. *See* Lymphoma
Noonan syndrome, 280
Norepinephrine, in neuroblastoma, 341, 344
Norwalk agent, and diarrhea, 385, 386
Nose, polyps of, in cystic fibrosis, 206, 209
Nosocomial infection. *See* Hospital-acquired infection
Nuchal rigidity, 11
  and brain tumor, 351
  in hypernatremic dehydration, 233
  in meningitis, 10

5-Nucleotidase, 213
Nutrition. *See also* Failure to thrive; Obesity
  in children with heart disease, 21, 132, 134
  maternal, 68
  for normal infant, 65–69
  parenteral, 133
    in cystic fibrosis, 209
    in intestinal disease, 132, 135, 137, 138, 228
    liver toxicity versus neonatal hepatitis, 132, 133, 213
    in neonate, 132, 133–134
  for premature and ill infant, 130–134
Nystagmus
  and brain tumor, 351
  in chronic renal failure, 252

Obesity, 71–74
  in adult versus juvenile diabetes mellitus, 269
  and hypertension, 183, 185
Occupational therapy, and cerebral palsy, 295, 296
Odor(s), in metabolic diseases, 275
Omphalitis, and neonatal septicemia, 147
Omphalocele, 137–138, 140
Oncovin. *See* Vincristine
Ophthalmia neonatorum, gonorrheal, 388, 389
Opisthotonos
  in cerebral palsy, 294
  in increased intracranial pressure, 32
  in tetanus, 363
Opsoclonus, and neuroblastoma, 342, 343
Opsonins, 360
  in neonate, 146
  in nephrotic syndrome, 245
Optic glioma, 353
Optometric exercises, 80, 82
Oral
  anomalies, 107
  ulcers
    in Crohn disease, 227
    in systemic lupus erythematosus, 305
    in ulcerative colitis, 225
Orchiopexy, 155
Orchitis, in mumps, 365
Orthostatic proteinuria, 237, 238
Orthotics. *See* Braces
Ortolani procedure, 105, 106, 154
Osler nodes, in endocarditis, 167, 169
Osmolarity, increased
  of feedings, and necrotizing enterocolitis, 132, 135
  in hypernatremic dehydration, 223, 234
  and sodium bicarbonate, 5

Osmols, idiogenic, in hypernatremic dehydration, 233, 234
Osteitis, in congenital syphilis, 144
Osteodystrophy, in renal failure, 253, 255
Osteogenic sarcoma, 354, 355
Osteomyelitis, 369–370, 371
    versus Ewing sarcoma, 354
    in neonate, 149
    in sickle cell disease, 319, 321, 384
Otitis media, 192–195
    and cleft palate, 154, 155
    in neonate, 149, 194
Otoscopy, pneumatic, 192
Ovarian tumor, and precocious pseudopuberty, 99
Ovaries, and sexual differentiation, 97
Ovary, torsion of, 25
Oxalosis, as cause of chronic renal failure, 252, 254
Oxytocin, and hyperbilirubinemia, 126

Pacemaker, cardiac, 19, 159, 160, 163
Palpitations, in cardiac dysrhythmias, 159
Pancreas, 222. See also Islet (of Langerhans) cell; Pancreatitis
    annular, 137
    in cystic fibrosis, 205, 206, 209, 220, 222
    in Shwachman syndrome, 220, 222
    transplantation of, and diabetes mellitus, 273
Pancreatitis, 26
    in chronic renal failure, 252
    and corticosteroids, 254
    in mumps, 365
Papillary necrosis, in sickle cell disease, 320, 321
Papilledema
    in hydrocephalus, 292
    in increased intracranial pressure, 32
    and Reye syndrome, 30
Papular acrodermatitis, 216, 217
Parainfluenza virus
    and bronchiolitis, 196
    and croup, 13, 14
    and parotitis, 368
    and pneumonia, 199
Paraldehyde, in status epilepticus, 35, 36
Parasite(s), in stool, in malabsorption, 219. See also specific parasite
Parathyroid gland
    and Di George syndrome, 361
    function, and hypocalcemia in neonate, 119
    hormone (PTH)
        in neonate, 120
        in renal failure, 253
Paregoric, in neonatal narcotic withdrawal, 119, 121, 123

Parenteral nutrition. See Nutrition, parenteral
Parotitis, 365, 368
Paroxysmal supraventricular tachycardia, 159–163
Paroxysms, of coughing, in pertussis, 363
Partial thromboplastin time
    in hemophilia, 323
    in neonate, 150
Patau syndrome, 280
Patent ductus arteriosus (PDA), 116, 117, 177–179
    and bronchopulmonary dysplasia, 111
    in congenital rubella syndrome, 142, 365
    and heart failure, 116
    and necrotizing enterocolitis, 134
    and respiratory distress syndrome, 108, 109, 110
    and transposition of great arteries, 177
Patterning, 78, 80, 82
Pavor nocturnus. See Night terrors
PDA. See Patent ductus arteriosus (PDA)
PE tube. See Tympanostomy tube
Pel-Ebstein fever, in Hodgkin disease, 346
Pelvic inflammatory disease (PID), 25, 26, 388, 390
Penicillamine
    in juvenile rheumatoid arthritis, 302
    in lead poisoning, 47
Penis, normal size in fetus and newborn, 100. See also Circumcision; specific disorder
Peptic ulcer. See Ulcer(s), peptic
Perceptual deficits, 79
Perchlorate, and thyroid disease, 266
Perianal disease, in Crohn disease, 228
Pericarditis, 163, 164–167
    as cause of acute abdomen, 25
    in chronic renal failure, 253
    and intestinal lymphangiectasia, 165, 220
    in juvenile rheumatoid arthritis, 301, 304
    in rheumatic fever, 179, 180
    in systemic lupus erythematosus, 305, 308
    tuberculous, 375
Pericardium, 165, 166
Perihepatitis, gonococcal, 388, 390
Periostitis, in congenital syphilis, 144
Peripheral pulmonary artery stenosis
    in congenital rubella syndrome, 142, 365
    and tetralogy of Fallot, 173
Peritoneal dialysis. See Dialysis, peritoneal
Peritonitis
    and appendicitis, 24
    in nephrotic syndrome, 245, 247

pelvic, in gonorrhea, 388
and peritoneal dialysis, 254
tuberculous, 375–376
Peritonsillar abscess, and tonsillectomy, 190
Persistence of fetal circulation (PFC), 113, 115, 140
Pertussis, 363, 366, 367
and thrombocytopenic purpura, 326
Pertussis immune globulin, 364
Pertussis vaccine, 363, 364, 366, 367, 369
Petit mal. See Absence spells
Peyer patches, and immunoglobulin production, 359
PFC. See Persistence of fetal circulation (PFC)
Phagocytes (phagocytosis), in immune system, 6, 359, 360, 361, 362
in neonate, 146
Phakomatoses. See Neurocutaneous syndromes, and brain tumors
Pharyngitis, 382
gonococcal, 388, 390
in infectious mononucleosis, 372, 374
due to Mycoplasma, 382
streptococcal, 380–381, 382–383
viral, 382
Phenobarbital. See also Anticonvulsants; Barbiturates
in biliary atresia/neonatal hepatitis, 213
in hyperbilirubinemia, 126
and intraventricular hemorrhage, 153
in seizure disorders, 285, 286, 287
in neonate, 124
in status epilepticus, 34
toxicity, 288
in withdrawal syndrome, 119
Phenolphthalein, in urine, versus hematuria, 235
Phenylalanine, 274. See also Phenylketonuria
Phenylalanine hydroxylase, 274. See also Phenylketonuria
Phenylephrine
and supraventricular tachycardia, 159
and tetralogy of Fallot, 173
Phenylketonuria, 273, 274, 276
and infantile spasms, 286
Phenytoin. See also Anticonvulsants
in digitalis toxicity, 162
and fetus, 277, 280
versus Hodgkin disease, 345
metabolism, 44
in seizures, 285, 286
in neonate, 124
in status epilepticus, 34–35
and systemic lupus erythematosus, 307
toxicity, 286
Pheochromocytoma, 185
Phosphorus

in acute renal failure, 28
in chronic renal failure, 253
in diabetic ketoacidosis, 23
in nutrition, 131
in perinatal period, 120
and seizure, in neonate, 121
Photosensitivity, in systemic lupus erythematosus, 305
Phototherapy, in neonatal hyperbilirubinemia, 125–126, 127–128, 129, 130
Physical therapy
in cerebral palsy, 295, 296
in dermatomyositis/polymyositis, 310
in hemophilic arthropathy, 324
in juvenile rheumatoid arthritis, 302, 304
in spinal dysraphism, 289
Phytohemagglutinin, 360
Piaget, 77
Pica, and lead poisoning, 46, 47
Pickwickian syndrome, 72, 74
PID. See Pelvic inflammatory disease (PID)
Pinealoma, 352
Pituitary gland
and emotional deprivation, 50, 63, 64
gigantism, 63
and hypoglycemia, 267
and sexual maturation, 99
and short stature, 62, 63, 64
and thyroid disease, 262, 263
tumor, 63, 351
PKU. See Phenylketonuria
Placebo, in upper respiratory tract infection, 189
Plague vaccine, 369
Plasma cells, in immune system, 359
Plasma, fresh-frozen
in bleeding neonate, 151, 152
in neonatal sepsis, 150
Plasmapheresis, 130, 309
Plasminogen, in respiratory distress syndrome, 110
Platelet(s). See also Thrombocytopenia; Thrombocytopenic purpura
in chronic renal failure, 252
in hemolytic-uremic syndrome, 242, 243
and hemophilia, 323, 324
in neonate, 150, 152
and phototherapy, 127
and salicylate, 44
in von Willebrand disease, 323, 325
Pleuritis, in systemic lupus erythematosus, 305
Pneumatic otoscopy, and otitis media, 192
Pneumatocele, in staphylococcal pneumonia, 199
Pneumatosis intestinalis, in necrotizing enterocolitis, 134

Pneumococcal vaccine, 7, 8, 365, 366, 369
    and meningitis, 10–11
    and nephrotic syndrome, 245
    and otitis media, 193
    and sickle cell disease, 321, 322
Pneumococcus. See *Streptococcus pneumoniae*
Pneumocystis carinii
    in leukemia, 336
    pneumonia, 199, 210
    in systemic lupus erythematosus, 307
Pneumomediastinum
    in asthma, 18, 203
    diagnosis by transillumination, 110
Pneumonia, 198–201
    aspiration, 201
        in dermatomyositis/polymyositis, 309
    infectious, 198–201
        versus appendicitis, 25
        in asthma, 203
        in bronchiolitis, 195
        in leukemia, 336, 337
        in measles, 364
        in sickle cell disease, 320, 321
        in tuberculosis, 375
    in neonate
        in congenital rubella syndrome, 142
        as cause of death in bronchopulmonary dysplasia, 111
        and esophageal atresia, 136
        in group B streptococcal sepsis, 147
        versus respiratory distress syndrome, 108, 147
    as cause of respiratory failure in infants, 16
Pneumothorax
    in asthma, 17, 18, 203
    in bronchiolitis, 196
    in cystic fibrosis, 209
    diagnosis by transillumination, 110
    and lung aspirate, 198
    in respiratory distress syndrome, 108
Poisoning. See Ingestion(s)
Poliomyelitis, 364, 366, 367
Poliomyelitis vaccine, 363, 364, 366, 367
    and immunodeficiency, 360, 362, 364
Polyarteritis nodosa, 310, 311, 312
    as cause of glomerulonephritis, 240
    and hepatitis B, 216, 217
Polycystic disease of kidneys, 235, 237
Polycythemia
    as cause of cyanosis in neonate, 113
    and hyperbilirubinemia in neonate, 125
    and necrotizing enterocolitis, 134
    in persistence of fetal circulation, 113
    and seizure in neonate, 122
    and tetralogy of Fallot, 174
    and Wilms tumor, 338

Polyhydramnios, and esophageal atresia, 136
Polymyositis, 309, 310, 311
Polyps, nasal, in cystic fibrosis, 206, 209
Pompe disease, as cause of myocardiopathy, 164
Ponderal index, in obesity, 72
Porphyria, as cause of abdominal pain, 25
Portal systemic shunt, in cystic fibrosis, 209
Portal vein, air in, in necrotizing enterocolitis, 134
Posterior fossa tumors, 351, 352, 353
Postpericardiotomy syndrome, 164, 166
Postural drainage
    and asthma, 202
    and cystic fibrosis, 207, 209
Potassium, 23. See also Hyperkalemia; Hypokalemia
PPD (purified protein derivative). See Tuberculin test (PPD)
P–R interval
    in rheumatic fever, 180
    in Wolff-Parkinson-White syndrome, 160, 161
Prader-Willi syndrome, 281
Prazocin, in heart failure, 20
Precocious puberty. See Puberty, precocious
Prednisone. See Glucocorticoids; *specific indication*
Pregnancy
    and anticonvulsants, 288
    and asthma, 204
    and hepatitis B, 217
    nutrition in, 68
    and sickle cell disease, 322
    and tuberculosis, 377
    and urinary tract infection, 249
Pregnanetriol, in adrenal hyperplasia, 259, 260
Premature atrial contraction, 160
Premature ventricular contraction, 160
Prenatal diagnosis, 276. See also *specific disorder*
Prenatal visit, 105
Priapism, in sickle cell disease, 320, 321
Primidone, in seizure disorders, 285. See also Anticonvulsants
Primitive reflexes, in cerebral palsy, 294, 296
Primordial dwarfism, 62, 64
Probenecid, in gonorrhea, 389
Procainamide, and lupuslike syndrome, 307
Procarbazine, in Hodgkin disease, 346, 347
Proctitis, gonococcal, 388
Prolapse of rectum, in cystic fibrosis, 207, 209

Prolonged rupture of membranes. *See* Rupture of membranes, prolonged

Properdin
  loss of urine, in nephrotic syndrome, 245
  pathway, in immune system, 361

Propranolol. *See also* Beta-adrenergic, blockers
  in cardiac dysrhythmias, 159, 160, 162
  and growth hormone, 64
  in hypertension, 183, 186
  in hyperthyroidism, 263
  in migraine, 95
  in tetralogy of Fallot, 173, 174

Proptosis
  in hyperthyroidism, 263
  in neuroblastoma, 342

Propylthiouracil, in hyperthyroidism, 263

Prostaglandins
  and action of antipyretics, 43
  and ductus arteriosus, 114, 116, 117, 173, 177, 178, 179

Prostatitis, in gonorrhea, 388, 390

Protein. *See also* Amino acids
  malabsorption of, 220, 223
  in nutrition, 65, 131, 133

Proteinuria, 235–238, 244, 247. *See also* Nephrotic syndrome; *specific disorder*

Proteus, in urinary tract infection, 249

Prothrombin time
  in hemophilia, 323
  in hepatitis, 216
  in malabsorption, 220
  in neonate, 150
  in Reye syndrome, 29

Pruritus
  in chronic renal failure, 253
  in Hodgkin disease, 346

Pseudohermaphroditism, 98, 100
  and hypospadias, 154
  and Wilms tumor, 338, 340

Pseudomembranous colitis, 384, 387

Pseudomonas. See also Gram-negative bacilli
  in cystic fibrosis, 199, 205, 209
  in leukemia, 335
  in osteomyelitis, 370, 371
  in septicemia, 6, 7
    in neonate, 148
  in urinary tract infection, 249

Pseudopuberty, 99, 101

Pseudotumor cerebri (benign intracranial hypertension), 32, 33

Pseudotumor, hemophilic, 325

Psoriasis, and arthritis, 301–302, 303

Psychometric testing, 77, 79, 81

Pubarche, 99, 101

Puberty, 98, 100–101
  delayed, 99

  in chronic renal failure, 252
  in sickle cell disease, 322
  and manifestations of gonorrhea, 388, 389
  precocious, 99
    in adrenal hyperplasia, 260, 262
    and hypothalamic tumor, 351
    and short stature, 63
  and short stature, 62

Pulmonary artery stenosis, peripheral
  in congenital rubella syndrome, 142, 365
  in tetralogy of Fallot, 173

Pulmonary function tests, 203. *See also specific disorder*

Pulmonary hypertension. *See also* Cor pulmonale
  in diaphragmatic hernia, 139
  in patent ductus arteriosus, 177
  in persistence of fetal circulation, 113, 115
  in transposition of great arteries, 176
  in ventricular septal defect, 171

Pulmonary insufficiency of prematurity, 111, 112

Pulmonary valve
  atresia, 113, 115, 172, 178
  stenosis, 19, 113, 114, 115
    and endocarditis, 169
    and tetralogy of Fallot, 172
    and transposition of great arteries, 175, 176

Pulmonary vascular disease. *See* Pulmonary hypertension

Pulmonary venous return, total anomalous, 114, 115

Pulsus paradoxus, 166
  in pericarditis, 164, 166
  in status asthmaticus, 17, 18

Purified protein derivative (PPD). *See* Tuberculin test (PPD)

Purpura
  anaphylactoid. *See* Henoch-Schönlein syndrome
  chronic thrombocytopenic, 328
  fulminans
    in Rocky Mountain spotted fever, 379
    in septic shock, 7
  in hemolytic-uremic syndrome, 242
  in Henoch-Schönlein syndrome, 328
  idiopathic thrombocytopenic (ITP). *See* Thrombocytopenic purpura, idiopathic (ITP)
  in meningococcemia, 6, 9
  thrombocytopenic. *See* Thrombocytopenic purpura

Pyelonephritis. *See* Urinary tract, infection of

Pyloric stenosis, versus adrenal hyperplasia, 259

Pyoderma gangrenosum, in ulcerative colitis, 225
Pyridoxine, and seizures in neonate, 122, 123
Pyrimethamine, in toxoplasmosis, 141
Pyruvate kinase deficiency, as cause of neonate hyperbilirubinemia, 125

Q-oTc interval, and neonatal hypocalcemia, 121
Quetelets' index, in obesity, 72
Quinidine, in cardiac dysrhythmias, 159
Quinsy, 190
Q–T interval, prolongation of, 57, 160, 161, 162

Racemic epinephrine, 13, 14, 15
Radiotherapy. See Irradiation
Rashkind procedure, in transposition of great arteries, 176
Rastelli operation, in transposition of great arteries, 176
Red-eye syndrome, in chronic renal failure, 252
Reed-Sternberg cell, 345
Reflexes
  deep tendon
    in cerebral palsy, 295
    in hypothyroidism, 263
    loss of, and vincristine, 339
  primitive, in cerebral palsy, 294, 296
Reflux
  gastroesophageal
    and asthma, 201
    and recurrent pneumonia, 201
    and sudden infant death syndrome, 56, 57
  vesicoureteral
    and chronic renal failure, 252
    and urinary tract infection, 249, 250, 251
Regional enteritis or ileitis. See Crohn disease
Reiter syndrome, 390
Rejection, of transplanted kidney, 254
Relactation, 67, 133
Relaxation therapy, 95, 205
Renal artery stenosis, and hypertension, 183
Renal disease, and hypertension, 183, 185
Renal failure. See also Dialysis; Kidney(s); Urinary tract
  acute, 27–29. See also specific disorder
  chronic, 252–256. See also specific disorder
  drug doses in, 255
  and hypertension, 184
Renal stones
  in Crohn disease, 227, 229

as cause of hematuria, 235
  and interstitial nephritis, 250
  and renal failure, 27
Renal transplantation. See Kidney(s), transplantation of
Renal tubular acidosis, 62, 64
Renin
  in acute poststreptococcal glomerulonephritis, 241
  in acute renal failure, 28
  in chronic renal failure, 252
  in hemolytic-uremic syndrome, 241
  in hypertension, 183
  and Wilms tumor, 338
Reserpine, in hypertension, 184
Respiratory arrest. See Cardiopulmonary arrest; Respiratory failure
Respiratory distress syndrome, 107–110
Respiratory failure, 16–19. See also specific cause
Respiratory rate, related to blood gases
  in bronchiolitis, 195
  in croup, 13, 14
Respiratory syncytial virus, 196–197
  and asthma, 202
  in bronchiolitis, 196, 197
  versus influenza, 369
  as cause of otitis media, 194
  as cause of pneumonia, 199, 200
Resuscitation, 3–5
  in neonate, 3, 4, 106
Retardation, mental. See Mental retardation
Reticulum cell sarcoma, 354
Retina
  and abetalipoproteinemia, 220
  in child abuse, 49, 50
  in congenital rubella syndrome, 142, 365
  in congenital syphilis, 143
  in congenital toxoplasmosis, 141, 145
  in hypertension, 184
Retrolental fibroplasia, 108, 109–110
Retropharyngeal masses, 15
Reye syndrome, 29–31
  versus diabetic ketoacidosis, 21, 269
  versus hepatitis, 215
  and increased intracranial pressure, 30, 31, 32
  and influenza B, 29, 30, 365
Rh disease, 128, 129, 130
Rhagades, in congenital syphilis, 143
Rheumatic fever, 179–182
  as cause of acute abdomen, 25
  and group A beta-hemolytic Streptococcus, 380, 381, 382, 383
  versus Henoch-Schönlein syndrome, 329
  versus infectious myocarditis, 163
  versus rheumatoid arthritis, 302

Rheumatic heart disease
  and atrial fibrillation, 160
  and heart failure, 19
Rheumatoid arthritis. *See* Arthritis
Rheumatoid factor
  in endocarditis, 167
  in rheumatoid arthritis, 301
Rhinitis
  allergic, 191
  in congenital syphilis, 143
Rhinorrhea
  and otitis media, 192
  in upper respiratory tract infection,
    189
Rhinovirus, 189, 190, 191
Rhinovirus vaccine, 191
RhoGAM, 128, 130
Ribavirin, in bronchiolitis, 198
Riboflavin deficiency, and phototherapy,
    127
Rickets
  in biliary atresia, 214, 215
  in chronic renal failure, 253
  and nutrition, 66, 131, 133
  and parenteral nutrition, 133
  as cause of short stature, 62
Rickettsia rickettsii, 378. *See also* Rocky
    Mountain spotted fever
Rifampin
  in prophylaxis, against meningococcus
    and *H. influenzae*, 7
  in tuberculosis, 376, 377
  in urine, versus hematuria, 235
Right middle lobe syndrome, 200
Ritalin. *See* Methylphenidate
Rocky Mountain spotted fever, 378–380
Rocky Mountain spotted fever vaccine,
    379, 380
Rose bengal test, in biliary atresia, ver-
    sus neonatal hepatitis, 213
Rose spots, in typhoid fever, 6, 384
Rotavirus
  and diarrhea, 385, 386
  in neonate, 144
Roth spots, in endocarditis, 167
Rubella, 365, 366, 368
  congenital, 142, 145, 365, 368
    and neonatal hepatitis, 213
    and patent ductus arteriosus, 177
    and ventricular septal defect, 170
  versus measles, 364
  as cause of myocarditis, 163
  and thrombocytopenic purpura, 326
Rubella vaccine, 363, 365, 366, 368
Rubeola. *See* Measles
Rumination, 69
Rupture of membranes
  and herpes infection of neonate, 143
  prolonged
    and incidence of respiratory distress

syndrome, 107, 109
  favors lung disease (versus heart) in
    cyanotic neonate, 113
  and septicemia, 147

SA node. *See* Sinoatrial (SA) node
Saber shins, in congenital syphilis, 144
Sabin-Feldman dye test, for toxoplas-
    mosis, 141
Sacroilitis. *See* Spondylitis, ankylosing
Saddle nose, in congenital syphilis, 143
Salbutamol, in asthma, 17, 202
Salicylate, 44, 45
  as analgesic/anti-inflammatory drug
    in juvenile rheumatoid arthritis,
      302, 304
    in rheumatic fever, 180, 182
    in systemic lupus erythematosus,
      306
    in ulcerative colitis. *See*
      Sulfasalazine
    in upper respiratory tract infection,
      191
  as antipyretic, 43, 44, 45
  and bleeding (effect on platelets)
    in hemolytic-uremic syndrome, 242,
      244
    in hemophilia, 324
    in neonate, 151
  and hyperbilirubinemia, in neonate,
    125
  intoxication by, 40, 42, 43, 44, 45
    versus asthma, 202
    versus diabetic ketoacidosis, 21, 269
    and hypoglycemia, 267
  and Reye syndrome, 29, 31, 45
  as teratogen, 277
Salmonella, 384, 385–386
  bacteremia/septicemia, 7, 9
  in osteomyelitis and sickle cell disease,
    319, 321, 370, 371
Salmonella typhosa, 6. *See also* Typhoid
    fever
Salpingitis. *See* Pelvic inflammatory dis-
    ease (PID)
Salt
  losing, in adrenal hyperplasia, 259,
    260, 261
  poisoning, 233, 234, 235
  restriction
    and glomerulonephritis, 239
    and heart failure, 20
    and hypertension, 183, 185
    and nephrotic syndrome, 244
  wasting, in chronic renal failure, 252
SC disease, 319, 321
  and hematuria, 235
Scarlet fever, 380, 382
School problems, 82. *See also* Attention
    deficit disorder; Learning problems

Scleroderma, 310, 311–312
Scoliosis
    acute, in appendicitis, 24
    in cerebral palsy, 295, 297
    after radiotherapy, in Wilms tumor,
        339
Seizures, 285–288. *See also related
        disorder*
    in neonate, 121–124
    status epilepticus, 34–36
Self-flagellation. *See* Index, self-inflicted
Senning procedure, in transposition of
        great arteries, 176, 177
Separation, 52, 83, 98
    parental. *See* Divorce
Sepsis. *See* Septicemia
Septal defects. *See* Atrial, septal defect;
        Ventricular, septal defect (VSD)
Septicemia, 6–9. *See also related disor-
        der; specific organism*
    in neonate, 146–150
Sequestration crisis, in sickle cell dis-
        ease, 319, 320–321
Serum hepatitis. *See* Hepatitis
Serum sickness
    and hepatitis B, 216, 217
    heterophile antibody in, versus infec-
        tious mononucleosis, 373
    versus rheumatic fever, 179
Setting sun sign, in hydrocephalus, 293
Sex
    in adrenal hyperplasia, 259, 260
    steroids, 259, 260
Sex chromosome disorders, 98, 100, 280.
        See also specific disorder
Sexual
    abuse, 49, 50–51, 389, 390
    differentiation, 97–98, 100
    maturation. *See* Puberty
Sexuality, 97, 99–100, 101
Sexually transmitted diseases, 389. *See
        also specific disease*
SGOT (serum glutamic oxaloacetic trans-
        aminase). *See* Aminotransferase
SGPT (serum glutamic pyruvic trans-
        aminase). *See* Aminotransferase
Shaggy heart sign, in pertussis, 363
Shigella (and shigellosis), 383–384, 385
    and hemolytic-uremic syndrome, 242,
        243
Shock, 5, 9
    septic, 7, 9, 150
        in neonate, 147, 148
Short bowel syndrome, 136
Short stature, 61–65. *See also specific
        cause*
Shunt for hydrocephalus, 292, 293
Shwachman syndrome, 220, 222
Sibling
    and death, 54
    of retarded child, 76

Sick sinus syndrome, 160, 161, 162
Sickle cell disease, 319–322
    as cause of acute abdomen, 25
    and elevated erythrocyte porphyrin,
        versus lead poisoning, 46
    and meningitis, 10, 11
    and osteomyelitis, 370, 371, 384
    versus rheumatic fever, 179
    and septicemia, 6
Sickle trait, 238, 319, 322
    and hematuria, 235, 238
Silver nitrate, in gonorrheal ophthalmia
        prophylaxis, 388, 389
Simian crease, in Down syndrome, 278
Sinoatrial (SA) node, 159
    and cardic dysrhythmias, 159–162
Sinus bradycardia, 160
Sinusitis, 189, 191
    in cystic fibrosis, 206, 209
    and headaches, 94, 95
Skin test. *See* Delayed hypersensitivity
Skin turgor, in hypernatremic dehy-
        dration, 233
Skull fracture, 36
    basilar, 36, 37
    depressed, 36
    growing, 38
SLE. *See* Systemic lupus erythematosus
        (SLE)
Sleep, 82–85
    apnea, and sudden infant death, 56, 84
    disturbed, after head trauma, 37
    and enuresis, 89, 91
    hypoxemia, in cystic fibrosis, 210
    and stimulants, in attention deficit dis-
        order, 80
    and upper airway obstruction, 16,
        83–84, 85
Small for gestational age. *See* Intra-
        uterine growth, retardation
Smallpox vaccination, discontinued,
        362–363
Smoke inhalation, 16, 39, 201. *See also*
        Burns
Smoking, parental, and childhood
        asthma, 205
Snake River measles, 378
Snuffles, in congenital syphilis, 143
Soave procedure, in Hirschsprung dis-
        ease, 138
Sodium, 234. *See also* Hypernatremia;
        Hyponatremia; Salt
Soft neurologic signs, 79, 81
Somatomedin, 63, 64
Somatostatin, 63
Somnambulism, 83, 85
Somogyi effect, 272
Soup, chicken
    composition of, 387
    in upper respiratory tract infection,
        191

Soy-based formula. *See* Milk, soy-based
Spasmodic croup, 13, 14
Spectinomycin, 389
Speech. *See* Language
Spelling, and medical students, 82
Spells, in tetralogy of Fallot, 172, 173, 174
S-persistence of fetal hemoglobin, 319
Spherocytosis, as cause of neonatal hyperbilirubinemia, 125
Sphingolipidoses, 275
Spina bifida. *See* Spinal dysraphism
Spinal cord tumors, 352
Spinal dysraphism, 288–291
 and nutrition, 134
 and urinary tract infection, 250
Spinal tap. *See* Lumbar puncture
Spirometry, 203
Spironolactone, and hyperkalemia, in chronic renal failure, 253. *See also* Diuretics
Spleen
 in cystic fibrosis, 207
 in Hodgkin disease, 346
 in idiopathic thrombocytopenic purpura, 326, 327
 in infectious mononucleosis, 372, 373
 rupture of
  in erythroblastosis, 130
  in infectious mononucleosis, 373
 and septicemia, 6
 in sickle cell disease, 320, 321
Splinter hemorrhages, in endocarditis, 167
Spondylitis, ankylosing, 303
 in inflammatory bowel disease, 225, 227
 in juvenile rheumatoid arthritis, 301, 303
Sponging, to reduce fever, 43, 44
Squatting, in tetralogy of Fallot, 174
SS disease. *See* Sickle cell disease
SSPE. *See* Subacute sclerosing panencephalitis (SSPE)
Staphylococcus, and urinary tract infection, 249
Staphylococcus aureus
 in bacterial tracheitis, 15
 in cystic fibrosis, 199, 205
 in endocarditis, 167, 168
 and leukemia, 335
 in osteomyelitis, 370
 in pericarditis, 164, 166
 in pneumonia, 198–199, 200
 in septic arthritis, 370, 372
 in septicemia, 6, 7
  in neonate, 6, 148
 in skin infection, 381
Staphylococcus epidermidis
 in neonatal sepsis, 149
 in shunt infection, 292
Status asthmaticus, 16–19

Status epilepticus, 34–36
Steatorrhea. *See* Fat, malabsorption of
Sterility. *See* Fertility
Sternocleidomastoid retraction, in asthma, 16, 18, 203
Steroids. *See* Glucocorticoids; Mineralocorticoids, in adrenal hyperplasia; Sex steroids
Sβ-thalassemia, 319, 321
Still disease, 301, 303
Stimulants, in attention deficit disorder, 79–80, 81
Stones. *See* Gallstones; Renal stones
Stools, time of first passage, 107
Streptococcus
 in endocarditis
  nutritionally deficient, 168
  satelliting, 169
  viridans group, 167, 168, 169
 and mesenteric lymphadenitis, 25
Streptococcus fecalis, in urinary tract infection, 249
Streptococcus, group A beta-hemolytic, 380–383
 and acute poststreptococcal glomerulonephritis, 239, 240, 241
 antibodies against extracellular products of, 180
 and Henoch-Schönlein syndrome, 329, 331
 infection of skin (impetigo), 180, 381, 383
 in otitis media, 192
 pharyngitis, 180, 380–381, 382–383
  versus infectious mononucleosis, 372
 in pneumonia, 199, 200
 in rheumatic fever, 179, 180, 181, 182
 in septic arthritis, 370
 and tonsillectomy, 189
Streptococcus, group B
 in osteomyelitis, in neonate, 371
 versus respiratory distress syndrome, 108, 147, 148
 in septic arthritis, in neonate, 370, 372
 in septicemia, in neonate, 6, 147, 148
Streptococcus, group D, 149, 380
Streptococcus pneumoniae, 8
 bacteremia/septicemia, 6, 7, 8
 in meningitis, 9, 10, 11, 12
 in nephrotic syndrome, 245
 in otitis media, 192, 193
 in pericarditis, infrequency of, 164
 in pneumonia, 198, 200
 in septic arthritis, 370
 in sickle cell disease, 320, 321, 322
Streptococcus pneumoniae vaccine. *See* Pneumococcal vaccine
Streptokinase, in hemolytic-uremic syndrome, 242
Streptokinase-streptodornase skin test, 362

Stridor, 13, 14, 15
Stroke. *See* Cerebrovascular accident
   (CVA)
Subacute bacterial endocarditis, 167, 170
Subacute sclerosing panencephalitis
   (SSPE)
  epidemiology of, 367
  and measles, 364, 367
  and measles vaccine, 364, 367
  as cause of myoclonic seizures, 286
Subarachnoid hemorrhage. *See* Bleeding
Subcutaneous
  emphysema in asthma, 17, 203
  nodules. *See* Nodules, subcutaneous
Subdural effusion
  and head trauma, 38
  and meningitis, 10, 12
Subdural hematoma
  versus brain tumor, 351
  and child abuse, 49
  and head trauma, 36, 38
  and hypernatremic dehydration, 233
  and increased intracranial pressure, 32
Subglottic stenosis, 15
Sucrase-isomaltase deficiency, 219, 222
Sudden death. *See* Death, sudden, and
   cardiac dysrhythmias
Sudden infant death syndrome, 55–57
  and mourning, 53, 54, 57
  and neonatal drug withdrawal, 120
Suicide, 39
Sulfasalazine, 227
  in Crohn disease, 228
  in ulcerative colitis, 225
Supraventricular tachycardia, 159–160,
   161–163
Surfactant, 107, 108, 109, 110
Sweat, in cystic fibrosis, 207, 208
Swenson procedure, for Hirschsprung disease, 138
Swine flu, 365
Swiss-type agammaglobulinemia. *See*
   Immune deficiency, severe
   combined
Sydenham chorea, 181
Syncope, and cardiac dysrhythmia, 159,
   160, 162
Syndromes. *See* Malformation syndromes; *specific syndrome*
Syphilis
  congenital, 143–144, 146
   and neonatal hepatitis, 213
  secondary, as cause of nephritis, 248
  serologic test for, in systemic lupus
   erythematosus, 305
Systemic lupus erythematosus (SLE),
   305–309
  and autoimmune thrombocytopenia, in
   neonate, 151
  as cause

  of chronic renal failure, 252
  of glomerulonephritis, 240
  versus dermatomyositis/polymyositis,
   310
  versus idiopathic thrombocytopenic
   purpura, 326, 327
  and membranous glomerulopathy, 248
  and myocarditis, 163
  versus rheumatic fever, 179
  versus rheumatoid arthritis, 302
Systemic sclerosis, 310, 311, 312

T and A, 190, 193
Tamponade, cardiac, 164, 165
Tanner stages, 99, 101
Tay-Sachs disease, 275, 277
TE (tracheoesophageal) fistula, 136–137,
   140
Teeth. *See* Dental
Tegretol. *See* Carbamazepine
Temper tantrums, and attention deficient
   disorder, 79
Temperament
  and night waking, 84
  and toilet training, 86
Tenosynovitis, in gonorrhea, 388
Tensilon, and supraventricular tachycardia, 159
Teratogens, 277, 279. *See also specific*
   teratogen
Testes
  in adrenal hyperplasia, 259
  ectopic, 155
  in Klinefelter syndrome, 98
  in leukemia, 335, 338
  retractile, 155
  and sexual differentiation, 97
  torsion of
   and abdominal pain, 25, 26–27
   and cryptorchidism, 155
   in Henoch-Schönlein syndrome, 331
  tumor in
   and cryptorchidism, 155
   and precocious pseudopuberty, 99
  undescended (cryptorchidism), 154,
   155, 156
  versus adrenal hyperplasia, 259
Testicular feminization syndrome, 98
Testosterone, 259, 338. *See also*
   Androgens
Tetanus, 363, 366
Tetanus immune globulin, 363, 366
Tetanus toxoid, 363, 364, 366, 369
Tetralogy of Fallot, 114, 172–174
  development of, from ventricular septal defect, 172
  as cause of endocarditis, 167
Thalassemia
  and hepatitis B, 217

versus iron deficiency, 315
versus lead poisoning, 46
'helarche, 99, 101
'heophylline, 204
  in asthma, 17, 18, 202, 204
  in bronchiolitis, 197
'hrombocytopenia. *See also* Platelet(s);
    Thrombocytopenic purpura
  and actinomycin D, 339
  in hemolytic-uremic syndrome, 242
  in leukemia, 335, 337
  in neonate, 151
    in congenital infection, 141, 142
    in necrotizing enterocolitis, 134, 136
    in septicemia, 147
  in Rocky Mountain spotted fever, 379
  in systemic lupus erythematosus, 305,
    308
  in Wiskott-Aldrich syndrome, 360, 362
'hrombocytopenic purpura, 326, 327
  chronic, 328
  in congenital rubella syndrome, 365
  idiopathic (ITP), 325–328
  in infectious mononucleosis, 326, 327,
    373
  in leukemia, 326, 335
  in neonate, 151, 153, 326
  in systemic lupus erythematosus, 305,
    326
  thrombotic, versus hemolytic-uremic
    syndrome, 242
'hromboplastin time, partial. *See* Partial
    thromboplastin time
'hrombosis
  and disseminated intravascular coagu-
    lation, in neonate, 152, 153
  in nephrotic syndrome, 245, 247
'hrombotic thrombocytopenic purpura,
    242
'hymoma, versus Hodgkin disease, 345
'hymus, in immune system, 359, 360,
    361
'hyroid disorders, 262–266. *See also* Hy-
    perthyroidism; Hypothyroidism
'icks, in Rocky Mountain spotted fever,
    378
'odd paralysis, after seizure, 286
'oe walking, in cerebral palsy, 294
'ofranil. *See* Imipramine
'oilet training, 85–86, 87, 89, 91
  in retarded children, 76
'olazoline, in persistence of fetal circu-
    lation, 115
'onsillectomy, 190, 191–192
  and Hodgkin disease, 347
'onsils
  and frequent upper respiratory infec-
    tions, 189
  in immune system, 189, 360
  obstructive, and sleep apnea, 84

TORCHES syndrome, 141. *See also* Cyto-
    megalovirus; Herpes simplex; In-
    fection(s), congenital; Rubella;
    Syphilis; Toxoplasmosis
Total anomalous pulmonary venous re-
    turn, 114, 115
Toxemia of pregnancy, and hypo-
    glycemia, in neonate, 267
Toxic granulation of neutrophils, in sep-
    sis, 6, 147
Toxic megacolon. *See* Megacolon, toxic
Toxoplasma gondii, 141, 373
Toxoplasmosis
  acquired, versus infectious mono-
    nucleosis, 373, 374
  congenital, 141–142, 144–145
    and neonatal hepatitis, 213
Tracheitis, bacterial, 15
Tracheoesophageal fistula, 136–137, 140
Tracheostomy, in upper airway obstruc-
    tion, 13, 14, 15
Tranquilizers, in attention deficit disor-
    der, 80
Transaminase. *See* Aminotransferase
Transfusion
  of blood components. *See specific indi-
    cation; specific disorder*
  and cytomegalovirus, 142
  exchange, 128
    in amino acid disorders, 274
    and ammonia, 31
    and disseminated intravascular co-
      agulation, 152
    and erythroblastosis, 129, 130
    and hyperbilirubinemia, 125, 128
    and hypocalcemia, 119
    in necrotizing enterocolitis, 134, 135
    and neonatal sepsis, 150
    and respiratory distress syndrome,
      110
    in Reye syndrome, 29
  and hepatitis, 216, 217, 218
  intrauterine, 129
Transgrow, 387
Transillumination, 110, 292
Transplantation. *See specific organ*
Transposition of great arteries, 113,
    175–177
  corrected, 175
  and congenital heart block, 160
Treponema pallidum, 143. *See also*
    Syphilis
Tricuspid atresia, 114, 115
Triglycerides, medium-chain, 131, 132,
    133
Trismus, in tetanus, 363
Trisomy 13, 280
Trisomy 18, 280
  and biliary atresia/neonatal hepatitis,
    213

Trisomy 21. *See* Down syndrome
Truncus arteriosus, 114, 116, 117, 118
TSH (thyroid-stimulating hormone). *See* Thyroid disorders
Tuberculin test (PPD), 376, 377, 378
  and live viral vaccines, 366
  and pneumonia, 199
Tuberculosis, 375–378
  as cause
    of fever of unknown origin, 43
    of meningitis, 10
    of pericarditis, 164
  vaccine, 369. *See also* Bacillus Calmette-Guérin (BCG)
Tuberous sclerosis, 353
  and brain tumors, 352, 353
  and infantile spasms, 286
  and precocious puberty, 99
Turner syndrome. *See* Gonadal, dysgenesis
Tylenol. *See* Acetaminophen
Tympanic membranes, in otitis media, 192, 193, 194
Tympanometry, 192, 193
Tympanostomy tube, 190, 193, 195
Typhoid fever, 384, 386
Tyrosine in phenylketonuria, 274

Ulcerative colitis, 224–227
  versus Crohn disease, 224, 227
  versus hemolytic-uremic syndrome, 242
Ulcer(s)
  gastric, 26
  leg, in sickle cell disease, 320
  nasopharyngeal, in systemic lupus erythematosus, 305
  oral. *See* Oral, ulcers
  peptic, 26
  and recurrent abdominal pain, 92
Ulrich-Noonan syndrome, 280
Upper airway obstruction, 13–16, 42
  in infectious mononucleosis, 373
  and obesity, 74
  as cause of respiratory failure, 16
  and sudden infant death syndrome, 55–56
  by tonsils, 189
Upper respiratory tract infection (URI), 189–191
  and thrombocytopenic purpura, 326
Urea
  in increased intracranial pressure, 32
  in sickle cell disease, 320
  as uremic toxin, 253
Urea cycle defects, 273, 274, 276. *See also* Ammonia
Ureaplasma urealyticum, 199, 201
Uremia. *See* Renal failure, chronic

Urethra
  and gonorrhea, 388, 390
  valves, posterior, 249
URI. *See* Upper respiratory tract infection (URI)
Uric acid
  and interstitial nephritis, 250
  nephropathy
    and acute renal failure, 27
    in leukemia, 335, 337
    in non-Hodgkin lymphoma, 349
Urinary tract. *See also* Kidney(s); *specific disorder; specific renal entry*
  infection of, 248–252
    as cause of acute abdomen, 25
    and constipation, 87, 88
    and diarrhea in infant, 219, 249
    and enuresis, 89
    and hematuria, 235
    in neonate, 149, 249
    and recurrent abdominal pain, 92
    and spinal dysraphism, 289
  obstruction of. *See also* Hydronephrosis
    and acute renal failure, 27
    and chronic renal failure, 252
    and non-Hodgkin lymphoma, 349
Urobilinogen, in hepatitis, 216
Urticaria
  in Henoch-Schönlein syndrome, 328
  in hepatitis B, 216
Uveitis, in Crohn disease, 227

Vagus, stimulation, and supraventricular tachycardia, 159
Valium. *See* Diazepam
Valproic acid, 35, 285, 286. *See also* Anticonvulsants
Vanillylmandelic acid (VMA), in neuroblastoma, 342, 344
Varicella. *See also* Herpes zoster
  and leukemia, 336
  as cause of myocarditis, 163
  and nephrotic syndrome, 245
  and pneumonia, 199
  and Reye syndrome, 29, 30
  and thrombocytopenic purpura, 326
Varicella-zoster. *See* Herpes zoster
Varicella-zoster immune globulin, 245
Varices, esophageal, in cystic fibrosis, 207
Vas deferens, in cystic fibrosis, 207
Vasculitis, 310, 311, 312
  and renal failure, 27, 252
Vasoactive intestinal peptide, 342
Vasodilators
  in heart failure, 20
  in hypertension, 183–184
VATER syndrome, 136, 137, 140
Vegetarian diet, 67

entricular
  contraction, premature, 160
  fibrillation, 160
  septal defect (VSD), 116, 117, 170–172
    in congenital rubella syndrome, 365
    and endocarditis, 167, 168, 169
    and patent ductus arteriosus, 178
    in tetralogy of Fallot, 172
    and transposition of great arteries,
      175, 176
  tachycardia, 160
erapamil, and cardiac dysrhythmia,
    159, 162
ertigo, 95
idarabine. See Adenine arabinoside, in
    neonatal herpes infection
incristine
  in Ewing sarcoma, 354
  in Hodgkin disease, 346, 347
  in leukemia, 335
  in neuroblastoma, 342, 344
  in non-Hodgkin lymphoma, 349
  in Wilms tumor, 339, 340
isceral larva migrans versus asthma,
    202
ision, 77. See also Blindness
  decreased acuity versus attention
    deficit disorder, 79
itamin(s), 66, 67, 68, 131, 133
  B₁₂, 131
  C
    and false-negative test for blood, 235
    and upper respiratory tract infection,
      189, 191
  D. See also Rickets
    and lead poisoning, 46
    and milk, 66, 68, 131
    and renal failure, 253, 255, 256
  E, and iron, 131, 133
  fat-soluble, and malabsorption, 207,
    220
  K, and neonate, 150, 151, 153
  pyridoxine, and seizures, 122, 123
  riboflavin, and phototherapy, 127
MA. See Vanillylmandelic acid (VMA),
    in neuroblastoma
ocal cord paralysis, 15
olkmann canals, and osteomyelitis, 369

Volvulus, and malrotation, 138
  as cause of acute abdomen in neonate,
    24, 138
von Gierke disease, 267
von Recklinghausen disease. See
    Neurofibromatosis
von Willebrand disease, 323, 325
VSD. See Ventricular, septal defect
    (VSD)
Vulnerable child syndrome, 53, 54
Vulvovaginitis, 388, 389

Waldeyer ring, 189
Walking, age of, 77
Warfarin
  and bleeding in neonate, 151
  as teratogen, 277
Water intoxication, in meningitis, 10
Waterhouse-Friderichsen syndrome, 7
Wechsler scales, 75
Wegener granulomatosis, 310
Weil-Felix reaction, in Rocky Mountain
    spotted fever, 379
Wheezing, differential diagnosis of, 202,
    203
Whooping cough. See Pertussis
Williams syndrome, 280
Williams-Campbell syndrome, 201
Wilms tumor, 338–341
Wilson-Mikity syndrome, 110, 111, 112
Wiskott-Aldrich syndrome, 360, 362
Withdrawal reaction, from drugs, in neo-
    nate, 119–120, 121, 122, 123
Wolffian duct, 97
Wolff-Parkinson-White syndrome, 114,
    159–163

Xylocaine, 4

Yersinia
  and diarrhea, 384, 385, 387
  and mesenteric lymphadenitis, 25

Zarontin. See Ethosuximide, in seizures
Zinc. See also Minerals, in infant
    nutrition
  in acrodermatitis enteropathica, 223
  and neonate, 123, 133